AF443338

TRENDS IN VASCULAR SURGERY

Edited by

William H. Pearce, MD
Violet R. and Charles A. Baldwin Professor of Vascular Surgery
Northwestern University, Feinberg School of Medicine
Chief, Division of Vascular Surgery
Northwestern Memorial Hospital
Chicago, IL

Jon S. Matsumura, MD
Assistant Professor of Surgery
Northwestern University, Feinberg School of Medicine, Northwestern University
Northwestern Memorial Hospital
Chicago, IL

James S. T. Yao, MD, PhD
Magerstadt Professor of Surgery
Northwestern University, Feinberg School of Medicine, Northwestern University
Northwestern Memorial Hospital
Chicago, IL

PRECEPT PRESS
Chicago, Illinois

07 06 05 04 03 1 2 3 4 5
ISBN: 0-944496-70-9

Library of Congress Cataloging-in-Publication Data

Trends in vascular surgery / edited by William H. Pearce, Jon S. Matsumura, James S.T. Yao.
    p. ; cm.
Includes bibliographical references and index.
   ISBN 0-944496-70-9
   1. Blood-vessels-Surgery.
   [DNLM: 1. Vascular Diseases—surgery. 2. Vascular Surgical Procedures. WG 170 T794 2003] I. Pearce, William H. II. Matsumura, Jon. III. Yao, James S. T.

RD598.5 .T745 2003
617.4'13—dc21

2002015935

Printed in the United States of America

Editor: Susan Parmentier
Compositor: Type Shoppe II Productions, Ltd.
Indexer: Rita Tatum
Printer: Data Reproductions

Contents

Contributors

Francisco Alcocer, MD
Instructor
University of Alabama School of
  Medicine
University of Alabama Hospital
Birmingham, AL

Karen L. Andrews. MD
Mayo Medical School
Mayo Clinic and Foundation
Rochester, MN

George Andros, MD
Section Vascular Surgery
Providence Saint Joseph Medical Center
Burbank, CA

J. Fritz Angle, MD
Associate Professor of Radiology
University of Virginia Medical School
Department of Radiology
University of Virginia Health Systems
Charlottesville, VA

William H. Baker, MD
Professor of Surgery
Loyola University Stritch School of
  Medicine
Loyola University Medical School
Maywood, IL

Dennis F. Bandyk, MD
Vascular Surgery Fellow
Division of Vascular and Endovascular
  Surgery
University of South Florida College of
  Medicine
Tampa, FL

Jeffrey V. Behar, MD
University of Virginia Medical School
University of Virginia Health Systems
Charlottesville, VA

Peter Bell, MD
Professor of Surgery
Department of Vascular and
  Endovascular Surgery
Leicester Royal Infirmery
Leicester, United Kingdom

Peter A. Blume, MD
Yale University School of Medicine
New Haven, CT

Amman Bolia, MD
Consultant Vascular Radiologist
Department of Vascular and
  Endovascular Surgery
Leicester Royal Infirmery
Leicester, United Kingdom

Andrew N. Bowser, MD
Professor of Surgery
Division of Vascular and Endovascular
  Surgery
University of South Florida College of
  Medicine
Tampa, FL

David C. Brewster, MD
Clinical Professor of Surgery
Harvard Medical School
Massachusetts General Hospital
Boston, MA

Dorothy L. Cage, MSN, ACNP
Nurse Practitioner
University of Virginia Medical School
Department of Radiology
University of Virginia Health Systems
Charlottesville, VA

Jeffrey P. Carpenter, MD
Associate Professor of Surgery and
  Radiology, Division of Vascular
  Surgery, Department of Surgery
Hospital of the University of
  Pennsylvania
Philadelphia, PA

Elliot L. Chaikof, MD, PhD
Division of General Vascular Surgery,
  Department of Surgery
Emory University School of Medicine
Atlanta, GA

Kenneth J. Cherry, Jr., MD
Professor of Surgery
Mayo Medical School
Division of Vascluar Surgery
Mayo Clinic and Foundation
Rochester, MN

Mitchell J. Cohen, MD
Resident, Department of General Surgery
Rush Presbyterian St. Lukes Medical
  Center
Chicago, IL

M.P. Colgan, MD
Department of Vascular and
  Endovascular Surgery
St.James Hospital
Dublin, Ireland

Michael S. Conners III, MD
Section of Vascular Surgery
Oschner Clinic and Foundation
New Orleans, LA

Michael S. Conte, MD
Assistant Professor
Harvard Medical School
Brigham and Women's Hospital
Boston, MA

Mark K. Eskandari, MD
Assistant Professor
Northwestern University, Feinberg
  School of Medicine
Northwestern Memorial Hospital
Chicago, IL

Guy Fishwick, MD
Consultant Vascular Radiologist
Department of Vascular and
  Endovascular Surgery
Leicester Royal Infirmery
Leicester, United Kingdom

Gail L. Gamble, MD
Mayo Medical School
Mayo Clinic and Foundation
Rochester, MN

Peter Gloviczki, MD
Chair, Division of Vascular Surgery,
  Professor of Surgery
Mayo Medical School
Director, Gonda Vascular Center
Mayo Clinic and Foundation
Rochester, MN

Richard M. Green, MD
Professor & Chair
Division of Vascular Surgery, University
  of Rochester Medical Center
Rochester, NY

Roy K. Greenberg, MD
Director, Endovascular Research,
  Department of Vascular Surgery
The Cleveland Clinic Foundation
Cleveland, OH

Lazar J. Greenfield, MD
Professor of Surgery
Interin Vice President for Medical Affairs
  and
Chief Executive Officer
University of Michigan
Ann Arbor, MI

M. Grouden, MSc, MP
Department of Vascular and
  Endovascular Surgery
St.James Hospital
Dublin, Ireland

Klaus D. Hagspiel, MD
Associate Professor
University of Virginia Medical School
Department of Radiology
University of Virginia Health Systems
Charlottesville, VA

Norman R. Hertzer, MD
Department of Vascular Surgery
The Cleveland Clinic Foundation
Cleveland, OH

Larry H. Hollier, MD
Julius H. Jacobson II Professor & Chair,
  Department of Surgery
Mt. Sinai School of Medicine
New York, NY

Glenn R. Jacobowitz, MD
Assistant Professor of Surgery
New York University School of Medicine
New York Uninversity Medical Center
New York, NY

William D. Jordan, Jr., MD
Associate Professor and Chief
University of Alabama School of
  Medicine
University of Alabama Hospital
Birmingham, AL

Riyad Karmy-Jones, MD
Associate Professor
University of Washington School of
  Medicine
Harborview Medical Center
Seattle, WA

Richard R. Keen, MD
Chief Division of Vascular Surgery
Cook County Hospital
Chicago, IL

John D. Keen, MD
Radiologist
Aurora BayCare Medical Center
Green Bay, WI

Timothy F. Kresowik, MD
Professor of Surgery
University of Iowa College of Medicine
Principal Care Coordinator
Iowa Foundation for Medical Care
Iowa City, IA

Rebecca A. Kresowik, BLS
Vice President, Government Quality
  Improvement Programs
Iowa Foundation for Medical Care
West Des Moines, IA

William C. Krupski, MD
Professor of Surgery
University of Colorado Health Sciences
  Center
Chief, Vascular Surgery
University of Colorado Hospital
Denver, CO

Gregory J. Landry, MD
Assistant Professor of Surgery
Division of Vascular Surgery, Oregon
  Health Sciences University
Portland, OR

John C. Lantis II, MD
Assistant Professor of Surgery
Columbia University College of
  Physicians and Surgeons
New York Presbyterian Hospital
New York, NY

Frank A. Lederle, MD
Professor of Medicine
Veterans Affairs Medical Center
Minneapolis, MN

Daniel A. Leung, MD
Assistant Professor
University of Virginia Medical School
Department of Radiology
University of Virginia Health Systems
Charlottesville, VA

Evan C. Lipsitz, MD
Albert Einstein School of Medicine
Division of Vascular Surgery,
  Department of Surgery, Montefiore
  Medical Center
New York, NY

P. Madhavan, FRCS (Edin)
Department of Vascular and
  Endovascular Surgery
St.James Hospital
Dublin, Ireland

B. Mahendran, FRCS (Edin)
Department of Vascular and
  Endovascular Surgery
St.James Hospital
Dublin, Ireland

Alan H. Matsumoto, MD
Professor and Executive Chair
University of Virginia Medical School
Director, Division of Angiography,
  Interventional Radiology and Special
  Procedures
University of Virginia Health Systems
Charlottesville, VA

Jon S. Matsumura, MD
Assistant Professor of Surgery
Northwestern University, Feinberg
  School of Medicine, Northwestern
  University
Northwestern Memorial Hospital
Chicago, IL

John H. Matsuura, MD
Director of Vascular Fellowship
Atlanta Medical Center
Atlanta, GA

Mary McGrae McDermott, MD
Assistant Professor of Medicine
Northwestern University, Feinberg
  School of Medicine
Northwesterm Memorial Hospital
Chicago, IL

Mark Meissner, MD
Associate Professor
University of Washington School of
  Medicine
Harborview Medical Center
Seattle, WA

Kevin Molloy, MD
Clinical Research Fellow
Department of Vascular and
  Endovascular Surgery
Leicester Royal Infirmery
Leicester, United Kingdom

Gregory L. Moneta, MD
Professor of Surgery
Division of Vascular Surgery, Oregon
  Health Sciences University
Portland, OR

Samuel R. Money, MD, FACS, MBA
Head, Section of Vascular Surgery
Oschner Clinic and Foundation
New Orleans, LA

D. J. Moore, MD, FRCSI
Department of Vascular and
  Endovascular Surgery
St.James Hospital
Dublin, Ireland

Mark D. Morasch, MD
Assistant Professor
Northwestern University, Feinberg
  School of Medicine
Northwestern Memorial Hospital
Chicago, IL

Nicholas J. Morrissey, MD
Assistant Professor of Surgery, Division
  of Vascular Surgery
Mt. Sinai School of Medicine
New York, NY

Leila Mureebe, MD
Assistant Professor
University of Missouri
University of Missouri Health Care
Columbia, MO

Sasan Najibi, MD
Section Vascular Surgery
Providence Saint Joseph Medical Center
Burbank, CA

Thomas C. Naslund, MD
Associate Professor of Surgery
Chief, Division of Vascular Surgery
Vanderbuilt University Medical Center
Nashville, TN

Mark R. Nehler, MD
Assistant Professor of Surgery
University of Colorado Health Sciences
  Center
Vascular Surgery Section
University of Colorado Hospital
Denver, CO

Audra A. Noel, MD
Mayo Medical School
Mayo Clinic and Foundation
Rochester, MN

Robert W. Oblath, MD
Section Vascular Surgery
Providence Saint Joseph Medical Center
Burbank, CA

Takao Ohki, MD, PhD
Albert Einstein School of Medicine
Division of Vascular Surgery,
  Department of Surgery, Montefiore
  Medical Center
New York, NY

Kenneth Ouriel, MD
Professor of Surgery
Ohio State University
Chairman, Department of Vascular
  Surgery
The Cleveland Clinic Foundation
Cleveland, OH

William H. Pearce, MD
Violet R. and Charles A. Baldwin
  Professor of Vascular Surgery
Northwestern University, Feinberg
  School of Medicine
Chief, Division of Vascular Surgery
Northwestern Memorial Hospital
Chicago, IL

Malcolm O. Perry, MD
Professor Emeritus
University of Texas Southwestern
  Medial School
Dallas, TX

Mary C. Proctor, MD
Senior Research Associate
Department of Surgery
University of Michigan
Ann Arbor, MI

John J. Ricotta, MD
Professor & Chairman of Surgery, Chief
  of Surgery
Department of Medicine, School of
  Medicine, SUNY Stoney Brook
Chief of Surgery
Stoney Brook Hospital
Stony Brook, NY

Thomas S. Riles, MD
George David Stewart Professor and
  Chair, Department of Surgery
New York University School of Medicine
New York Uninversity Medical Center
New York, NY

Heron E. Rodriguez, MD
Assistant Professor of Surgery and
  Radiology
Loyola University Stritch School of
  Medicine
Loyola University Medical School
Chicago, IL

Thom W. Rooke, MD
John and Krehbiel Professor of Vascular
  Medicine
Mayo Medical School
Head, Section of Vascular Medicine
Mayo Clinic and Foundation
Rochester, MN

David Rosenthal, MD
Chief of Vascular Surgery
Medical College of Georgia
Clinical Professor of Surgery
Atlanta Medical Center
Atlanta, GA

Albert D. Sam II, MD
Division of Vascular Surgery
Northwestern University, Feinberg School
  of Medicine, Northwestern University
Northwestern Memorial Hospital
Chicago, IL

Joseph R. Schneider, MD, PhD
Associate Professor, Vascular Surgery
Northwestern University, Feinberg
  School of Medicine
ENH Medical Group
Skokie, IL

Gregor D. Shanick, MD, FRACS
Department of Vascular and
  Endovascular Surgery
St.James Hospital
Dublin, Ireland

Maureen K. Sheehan, MD
Loyola University Stritch School of
  Medicine
Loyola University Medical School
Maywood, IL

Thomas A. Shuster, MD
Vascular Fellow
University of Missouri
Columbia, MO

Donald Silver, MD
Professor Emeritus
University of Missouri
Medical Director Surgical Services
University of Missouri Health Care
Columbia, MO

David J. Spinosa, MD
Associate Professor
University of Virginia Medical School
Department of Radiology
University of Virginia Health Systems
Charlottesville, VA

James C. Stanley, MD
Professor of Surgery
Head, Section of Vascular Surgery
University of Michigan Medical School
Ann Arbor, MI

S. William Stavropoulos, MD
Assistant Professor of Radiology and
  Surgery, Division of Interventional
  Radiology, Department of Radiology
Hospital of the University of
  Pennsylvania
Philadelphia, PA

Timothy M. Sullivan, MD
Director of Endovascular Practice
Mayo Clinic and Foundation
Rochester, NY

Vita Sullivan, MD
Department of Surgery, Section of
  Vascular Surgery
University of Michigan Medical Center
Ann Arbor, MI

Bauer E. Sumpio, MD, PhD
Professor & Chief of Vascular Surgery
Yale University School of Medicine
New Haven, CT

Lloyd M. Taylor, Jr., MD
Professor of Surgery
Division of Vascular Surgery, Oregon
  Health Sciences University
Portland, OR

Thomas T. Terramani, MD
Division of General Vascular Surgery,
  Department of Surgery
Emory University School of Medicine
Atlanta, GA

Matthew M. Thompson, MD, FRCS
Consultant Vascular and Endovascular
  Surgeon
Department of Vascular and
  Endovascular Surgery
Leicester Royal Infirmery
Leicester, United Kingdom

Britt H. Tonnessen, MD
Section of Vascular Surgery
Oschner Clinic and Foundation
New Orleans, LA

Gustavo Torres, MD
Section Vascular Surgery
Providence Saint Joseph Medical Center
Burbank, CA

Jonathan B. Towne, MD
Professor of Surgery
Medical College of Wisconsin
Milwaukee. WI

William D. Turnipseed, MD
Professor
University of Wisconsin Medical School
University of Wisconsin Hospital and
  Clinics
Madison, WI

R. James Valentine, MD
Frank H. Kidd, Jr., MD distiunguished
  Professor in Surgery & Vice Chair,
  Department of Surgery
The University of Texas Southwestern
  Medical Center
Zale Lipsky University Hospital and
  Packland Memorial Hospital
Dallas, TX

Paul S van Bemmelen, MD, PhD
Associate Professor of Surgery
School of Medicine SUNY Stony Brook,
  Stony Brook, NY
Chief of Vascular Surgery
VA Medical Center, Northport, NY

Frank J. Veith, MD
Professor of Surgery
Albert Einstein School of Medicine
Division of Vascular Surgery,
  Department of Surgery, Montefiore
  Medical Center
New York, NY

Thomas W. Wakefield, MD
S. Martin Lindenauer Collegiate
  Professor of Vascular Surgery
University of Michigan Medical Center
Ann Arbor, MI

Eric D. Wellons, MD
Department of Vascular Surgery
Atlanta Medical Center
Atlanta, GA

Michael A. West, MD, PhD
Professor of Surgery
Northwestern University, Feinberg
  School of Medicine, Northwestern
  University
Chief, Division of Trauma and Critical
  Care
Northwestern Medical Faculty
  Foundation
Chicago, IL

James S. T. Yao, MD, PhD
Magerstadt Professor of Surgery
Northwestern University, Feinberg
  School of Medicine, Northwestern
  University
Northwestern Memorial Hospital
Chicago, IL

Preface

Dedication-James A. DeWeese, MD

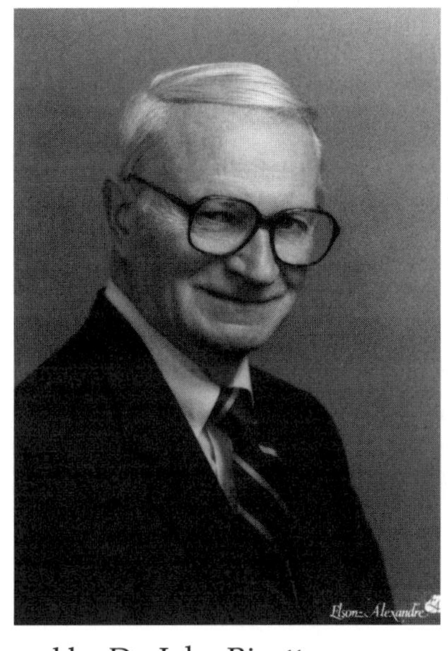

Advances in surgery rest on new technology. Hence, treatment modalities for vascular problems continue to evolve. It is hoped that this symposium will provide practicing vascular surgeons up-to-date and relevant information regarding newer approaches in the treatment of patients with vascular disease. All invited contributors are experts in their own field.

Like us, all of the contributors to this symposium are admirers of Dr. James DeWeese, who has touched almost all the topics discussed here. We thank the participants as well as the invited contributors for joining us for the celebration of this truly remarkable surgeon.

We dedicate this volume to Dr. James A. DeWeese in honor of his many contributions in vascular surgery. In ensuing chapters, his accomplishments as a leader in vascular surgery and as an educator will be described by Dr. Malcolm Perry and by Dr. John Ricotta.

James Arville DeWeese was born and educated in Kent, Ohio. After completing Kent State High School, he attended Harvard College and Kent State University. He graduated from University of Rochester Medical School in 1949 and remained there for his entire surgical career. Together with Dr. Charles Rob, who came to Rochester in 1961, Dr. DeWeese established Rochester University Medical School as the premiere learning center for vascular surgery.

Contributions by James DeWeese are multiple and include advances in the treatment of arterial and venous disorders. In the venous field, he wrote about the use of ascending phlebography, patterns of venous thrombosis, ilio-femoral venous thrombosis, and the Adams-DeWeese vena cava clip for prevention of pulmonary embolism. He also described intermittent compression of the subclavian vein, thus establishing the concept of thoracic outlet compression. Later, he reviewed his experience in subclavian venous thrombectomy. As arterial surgery developed, he again became a pioneer in the treatment of arterial problems. His report on autogenous vein graft and, later, on the meticulous ten-year follow-up remains a classic. He and Charles Rob were among the first to describe an arterialized in-situ saphenous vein graft prepared by disrupting the valves. His use of a canine model to compare various prosthetic with biological grafts firmly established the superior patency of venous bypass graft. His description of pulse-disappearing phenomenon shed light on the basic physiological basis for intermittent claudication. As surgical treatment of cerebrovascular disease evolved, he contributed to the expansion of the role of surgery in the treatment of carotid stenosis and subclavian steal syndrome. His clear insights into the pathophysiology of intimal hyperplasia have been invaluable. He is perhaps best remembered for his analysis of sexual dysfunction following aortic surgery. He maintains a keen interest in aortic aneurysm, up to the current development of endovascular graft.

In addition to contributions in the scientific literature, Dr. DeWeese has published several important articles on training and certification in vascular surgery. These documents provided a blueprint for vascular surgery to emerge as a distinct specialty. The Optimal Resources for Vascular Surgery Report defined the training for vascular surgery and also the standard for medical instrumentation leading to the development of the vascular laboratory. In subsequent years, he and others wrote extensively about training and certification in vascular surgery. The path to an independent vascular surgery board is tortuous at best; these documents and Dr. DeWeese's statesmanship have paved the way to making this undertaking a reality.

In summary, James DeWeese has touched every aspect of vascular surgery. The Division of Vascular Surgery is honored to have the opportunity to recognize this outstanding surgeon, leader, and educator.

William H. Pearce
Jon S. Matsumura
James S.T. Yao

I

James A. DeWeese, MD: A Tribute

1

The Educator

John J. Ricotta, MD

Dr. James DeWeese is a man of many accomplishments. He is a superb clinician, an accomplished technical surgeon, a prolific writer, and one of the founding leaders of vascular surgery. However, when asked to select the most important of his many accomplishments, he chose the training of the many residents and fellows who have had the privilege to work with him at the University of Rochester in general, vascular, and cardiothoracic surgery. In doing so, Jim defined himself as first and foremost an educator, and I believe his residents, fellows, and professional colleagues would agree. The word "educator" derives from two Latin words, which together mean, "to lead out." In Webster's dictionary the word "educate" is defined as "to develop the knowledge, skill, mind, or character of . . . to form or develop." As someone who has devoted his professional life to developing surgeons, forming their knowledge and character, Dr. James DeWeese embodies the spirit of an educator.

An educator must by definition be a master in the chosen field. Equally important, this person must have an historical perspective, an understanding of the cumulative experience that has led to current knowledge. The educator is an historical figure that serves as a conduit in the transmission of knowledge and values between generations. The educator must have a love of learning and be able to engage his or her trainees in an interactive process where both master and student participate and benefit. Finally, the complete educator must be a "mentor," a word that is much used currently. Mentor was a personage of Greek mythology, described as a "loyal friend and advisor" of Odysseus and the teacher of his son Telemachus. The ability to develop a personal relationship with one's trainees that is based on mutual respect, loyalty, and friendship represents the ultimate educational relationship. Jim DeWeese embodies all of these characteristics.

That Dr. DeWeese is a master of his field is widely recognized. He is a prolific contributor to the literature on topics in both vascular and cardiac surgery, has been on the editorial board of the major journals in both cardiac and vascular surgery, and has edited a textbook on operative surgery. His professional colleagues have recognized him by election to the American Board of Surgery, the American Board of Thoracic

Surgery, and the Presidency of 5 professional societies (including the Society for Vascular Surgery and International Society for Cardiovascular Surgery). In addition, he has served as visiting professor at numerous institutions around the world. He is recognized as an excellent clinician, and a skilled technical surgeon. One of the anecdotes told by the residents at the University of Rochester involved Dr. DeWeese standing at the foot of the table while the operation was progressed, closely observing the chief resident or fellow, ready to intervene when necessary. The entire team was comfortable in the knowledge that Dr. DeWeese would be able to fix anything that went awry. His knowledge of the published literature is encyclopedic. Discussion of virtually any vascular topic would end with a suggestion to read one or more articles previously written on the subject along with a suggestion of where to find them. Typically, these references were often to the work of others, and when they did include work done by Dr. DeWeese, he always recognized the contributions of the coauthors.

Dr. DeWeese has a keen historical perspective in which he acknowledges both those who have gone before him and those who will be future leaders in our profession. He was stimulated to enter medicine by his father and brothers, who were physicians. His brother Bill, who was a surgeon at the University of Michigan, played a particularly important role in his decision. Accepted at the University of Rochester School of Medicine after 2 years of college, Dr. DeWeese was heavily influenced by his exposure to faculty there, particularly Dr. George Hoyt Whipple, Dean of the School, and Drs. John Morton, Sr., Merle Scott, and Earle Mahoney in the Department of Surgery. Although he had numerous opportunities to join other academic institutions, Dr. DeWeese has spent his entire professional career at Rochester, where he first benefited from the legacy of his teachers and subsequently embellished that legacy through his own contributions. In so doing, he has worked constructively with the many faculty members at the University of Rochester for the betterment of the Institution. The most obvious example of this was his professional collaboration with Dr. Charles Rob, which began in 1961 and continued for more than 15 years. These efforts established the Department of Surgery at the University of Rochester as one of the premier vascular centers in North America. A lesser, but more personally important collaboration was the one Jim developed between himself and two young faculty members in the 1980s. His ability to organize and coordinate my efforts and those of Dr. Richard Green played an important role is our professional development and continued the strength of vascular surgery at the University of Rochester.

Dr. DeWeese has been equally mindful of the important role that trainees play in the perpetuation of new knowledge. At Rochester he established a series of superb interactive clinical conferences in vascular surgery. These conferences were characterized by a free exchange of ideas, and were devoid of "pronouncements" by the professor that often characterize such events. Jim would always ask the residents their opinion on management and require that they fortify such opinions with references from the literature. As a learning experience it was without peer and many clinical papers were born from those discussions. Dr. DeWeese took his concerns with the education of future vascular surgeons to a national level. In 1969 he was chosen to head a task force on "Optimal Resources for Vascular Surgery," along with Drs. Blaisdell and Foster. The results of this report, which were presented to the Society for Vascular Surgery in 1972, called for defined training and experience in vascular surgery that would ultimately be recognized through a separate certification process. This work eventually led to the establishment of a certificate in Vascular Surgery by the American Board of Surgery and forms the basis of a process that is still in evolution. In discussing this with Jim, it is apparent that in his mind the important issues were not turf but education, that is, how are new trainees best educated in the field.

Dr. DeWeese has served as a mentor to almost 100 residents in cardiothoracic and vascular surgery, as well as many general surgery residents who have chosen to make the treatment of vascular disease a major part of their professional life. Each of these persons regards Jim with the most profound respect, and I am sure none has ever considered himself Jim's equal. However, the relationship Jim has established with his trainees is a very personal one. It is based on shared standards, mutual respect, and recognition of each other's essential humanity. Jim has been able to do this by making it clear to each of his trainees, and junior faculty, that he took them and their concern seriously, that he valued their opinions and recognized their efforts. Perhaps the most consistent professional characteristic displayed by Dr. DeWeese is his willingness to acknowledge the efforts of others. This is done in both public and private fora, locally and on a national level. In so doing he has provided immense opportunities for those who have been privileged to work with him.

During the course of his professional career Dr. James DeWeese has contributed enormously to the development of the field of vascular surgery at multiple levels. As an accomplished surgeon, he has helped many patients lead fuller lives. As a prolific author, he has created new knowledge in both clinical and basic research. As an administrative leader, he has helped shape the direction that vascular surgery will take in the new millennium. However, I must agree with his assessment that his greatest achievement has been the education of young surgeons who will carry on the tradition of excellence he inherited from his own mentors.

2

Leader in Vascular Societies

Malcolm Perry, MD

Leaders have two important characteristics: first, they are going somewhere, and second, they are able to persuade others to go with them. James A. DeWeese was introduced to the Society for Vascular Surgery and the North American Chapter of the International Society for Cardiovascular Surgery by Dr. Merle Scott and his associates Dr. Pearse and Dr. Morton; all were charter members. Dr. DeWeese found an enduring interest in societies, and quickly became involved in the scientific and administrative efforts. The vascular societies and the American Board of Surgery were searching for guidelines to assist in the education of vascular surgeons. A committee composed of DeWeese as chairman, Bill Blaisdell, and John Foster, was charged to define Optimal Resources for Vascular Surgery. Funds were supplied partly by NIH grant 69–29. After an extensive review of the practices and results obtained in a large number of leading institutions where the full range of vascular surgery was being done the report was presented to the sponsoring groups. It was then published in the *Archives of Surgery* in 1972, and became an important reference for establishing and evaluating training programs in vascular surgery.

Dr. DeWeese's thoughtful and dependable work on behalf of vascular surgery led to his election as secretary of the Society for Vascular Surgery in 1972. He served a 4-year term and in 1976 became president-elect of the SVS. As president he presided over the 1978 meeting in Los Angeles. His presidential address "Vascular Surgery-Is It Different?" supported the concept that this discipline requires special, well-designed training programs. He encouraged the members to help develop and preside over programs which would become accredited for the training of vascular surgeons. He then continued to serve on the council for 3 more years. There were a number of important and difficult problems to be solved during this time, and under his direction and help most were solved. As Harry Shumaker wrote in his *History of the Society for Vascular Surgery*, "How extraordinarily well congenial friends with a common objective can get along without fixed rules and regulations."[1] Dr. DeWeese helped others understand the need for cooperation in reaching acceptable solutions to these issues.

Jim had only a short respite without official duties before he became president-elect of the North American Chapter of the International Society for Cardiovascular Surgery. In 1985 he served as president of the ISCVS during the meeting in Baltimore, and then remained on the council until 1989. As many members will recall, during these years vascular surgery was in the midst of important changes, and not all of them were free of pain or controversy. Dr. DeWeese's leadership was critical; he perhaps knew what Coach John Wooden told his championship basketball team at UCLA, "Do not let what you cannot do interfere with what you can do."

Dr. DeWeese was also quite active on the international stage. He was Assistant Secretary-General of the International Society for Cardiovascular Surgery from 1977 through 1987, responsible for the organization and operation of the large biannual congress, 5 days of lectures, symposia, and hundreds of free paper presentations. For his good work he was "rewarded by being elected Secretary-General in 1987, serving until 1995. He became President for the 2-year term of 1995 to 1997. Under his stewardship the Society flourished; the scientific programs were improved by the standards he developed to assist in the selection of papers and the organization of the congress itself. In his presidential address at the World Congress he reviewed the work of some of his predecessors, emphasizing their contributions to the ISCVS. He remains an important member of the Council, offering advice and help gleaned from years of leadership in vascular surgery. His work ethic reminds one of what Irvine Page, M.D. said about surgeons, "I am sure one must be born a surgeon to have all the necessary personality traits; no one could acquire them."[2]

James DeWeese had been a role model for many of us. His hard work, dedication, and attention to detail are unsurpassed. He has always understood that it is wise to keep in mind that no success or failure is necessarily final.

REFERENCES

1. Shumacker, HB. *The Society for Vascular Surgery: A History* 1945–1983. Manchester, MA: The Society for Vascular Surgery.
2. Page, IH. Surgeons through a physician's eye. *Modern Medicine.* June 30, 1969:59–61.

3

Reflections from a Resident and Colleague

Richard Green, MD

The achievements of Jim DeWeese are forever etched in the annals of vascular surgery. His selfless dedication to teaching will live on in the testimony of his trainees and has been eloquently summarized by John Ricotta. His service to our national and international societies has been detailed by Malcolm Perry. What is not generally known or chronicled is the simple fact that Jim DeWeese was first and foremost a surgeon and everything he has accomplished was based on that experience.

I first came in contact with Jim in the late '60s when I was a second year medical student rotating on pathology. I was participating in an autopsy of a man who died in the operating room during an unsuccessful attempt to repair a ruptured abdominal aortic aneurysm. It was about 2 A.M. and Jim entered the room with surgical scrubs on, chewing gum in an aggressive manner, looked around and left without saying anything. Sometime later, a younger surgeon entered and gave us the history. The resident surgeon told us his name was Jock and he worked with Dr. DeWeese. This patient died early in the afternoon and they had been operating all day but wanted to see what happened. It was my first contact with Jim and the impression he made has never left me. He could have been home sleeping.

Jim's entire surgical career was spent at Strong Memorial Hospital where he was chief of both cardiac (1975) and vascular surgery (1987). His practice was a mixture of adult cardiac (Tuesday and Thursday) and peripheral vascular (Wednesday and Saturday) cases. I think that he had difficulty separating these two specialties and that his academic hat was slanted towards vascular surgery but that his clinical preference was for cardiac cases. Nonetheless, he performed an equal number of both reaching 150 cases per year of each specialty during his clinical prime. He was a bone fide cardiovascular surgeon who understood that the diaphragm was an artificial boundary for surgeons who operated on the aorta. Whether the two specialties will once again combine or each will deal with the impact of catheter-based procedures in its own way is a matter that Jim and I have discussed many times over the years.

I often think back to my training in Rochester and the roles that Jim and Charles Rob played. Our major exposure to Jim came in our fourth clinical year although many of us spent a year in the research lab with him learning the basics of arterial suturing, data gathering, and abstract writing. Jim had a tremendous knowledge of anatomy and understood the mechanics of performing a procedure. Jim and his generation were self-taught inventing many of these procedures that we now consider routine. Their genius was in recognizing the need to amalgamate their trial and error experience into the principles of a new specialty and to expand it beyond the walls of the original few centers of excellence. I remember him watching me from afar sew an anastomosis to an external iliac artery in a very obese patient with an aortic aneurysm and telling me that my needle angles were all wrong. He was right. He knew how to do things properly and always had the patience to watch and teach. He could have been home sleeping.

Jim's dedication to his patients, residents (both cardiac and vascular), and to his national responsibilities took its toll. I cannot remember his leaving the hospital before 9 P.M. and having his usual dinner of a candy bar and coffee. I began my fourth year rotation on Jim's service on New Year's Eve. I remember an awful snow storm and a phone call around 11 P.M. Jim was one the phone. He told me we were doing a mitral valve the next morning, that the patient needed to be prepared, that the junior resident could not be trusted, and that I should plan on living in the hospital for the next 4 months. All of these things came to pass. I wasn't alone, though, because he was with me most of the time. A few weeks later we were operating in the middle of the night after a full day and at 2 in the morning it was time to close a femoral arteriotomy. I thought, "Great—I'll get this done and sleep for a couple of hours." No way—he told me to wake up an intern and show him how to close an artery. I did—Jim stayed to watch—we both could have been home sleeping.

Jim was an outstanding diagnostician carefully examining each patient and documenting his findings. He tried to be as objective as possible and carried an oscillometer around with him as well as a stopwatch. What was the capillary filling time? How many flickers were there on the oscillometer? He kept a notebook dedicated for each type of procedure and constantly updated his results. Data were always available for review and they were always accurate. Jim and I had many disagreements about the usefulness of the vascular lab. He always thought that a good bedside evaluation by a competent physician was superior. Sometimes I get the opportunity to review his old office records and still marvel at their completeness and accuracy. Often office days were on weekends and evenings.

It is fitting that this symposium is dedicated in Jim's honor at this time. Vascular surgery is once again struggling with its identity. Jim, because of his unique position as a busy clinical surgeon and national leader, recognized the need to certify a new specialty and to see that its trainees could function in the community as true specialists. We are once again at a crossroads and one hopes that thoughtful leaders will emerge à la Jim Deweese to chart the right course. Hopefully they are not sleeping.

II

Nonoperative Management

4

Leg Symptoms in Peripheral Arterial Disease: Clinical Characteristics and Functional Impairment

Mary McGrae McDermott, MD

Intermittent claudication has been typically considered the most classical manifestation of lower extremity peripheral arterial disease (PAD).[1] However, when non-invasive testing is used to diagnose PAD with the ankle brachial index (ABI), many patients with PAD have exertional leg symptoms other than intermittent claudication while other patients with PAD are asymptomatic.[2-4] Comorbid diseases, such as disc disease, spinal stenosis, and neuropathy are common in patients with PAD and may contribute to the character of leg symptoms reported by patients with PAD. This article reviews the types of leg symptoms commonly associated with PAD and describes the clinical characteristics and functional limitations associated with each category of leg symptoms in PAD. It also describes questionnaires commonly used to classify leg symptoms in patients with PAD.

THE ROSE INTERMITTENT CLAUDICATION QUESTIONNAIRE

In 1962 Dr. Geoffrey Rose developed the Rose intermittent claudication questionnaire for use as an epidemiologic tool, in order to measure the prevalence and significance of intermittent claudication in defined populations.[1] Dr. Rose developed his questionnaire based on observations of 37 patients with physician-diagnosed intermittent claudication and 18 patients without intermittent claudication identified from a hospital practice setting. Features of intermittent claudication according to the Rose questionnaire are exertional calf pain that does not occur at rest, does not subside with walking, and resolves within ten minutes of rest (Table 4–1). In Rose's validation study, the sensitivity and specificity of the Rose claudication questionnaire for a physician diagnosis of intermittent claudication were 92% and 100% respectively.[1] Using the Rose claudication questionnaire, the prevalence of intermittent claudication is 1.3 to 5.0% among community-dwelling men and women age 50 and older.[5-8]

TABLE 4–1. INTERMITTENT CLAUDICATION QUESTIONNAIRES

Original questions in the Rose intermittent claudication questionnaire	Edinburgh claudication questionnaire	San Diego claudication questionnaire
• Do you get pain in either leg on walking?	X	X
• Does this pain ever begin when you are standing still or sitting?	X	X
• Do you get this pain in your calf (or calves?)	X	X
• Do you get it when you walk uphill or hurry?	X	X
• Do you get it when you walk at an ordinary pace on the level?	X	X
• Does the pain ever disappear while you are still walking?		
• What do you do if you get it when you are walking?		
• What happens to it when you stand still?	X	X
• How soon does it resolve with rest? (ten minutes or less vs. more than ten minutes)	X	X

lIntermittent claudication as defined by the Rose claudication questionnaire consists of exertional leg pain that does not begin when standing or sitting still, involves the calves, does not disappear while walking, causes the patient to stop walking, and resolves within 10 minutes of rest. The questions about whether the pain occurs with walking uphill or hurrying and whether the pain occurs while walking at an ordinary pace on the level relate to severity of claudication symptoms. Participants with more severe disease report symptoms when walking at an ordinary pace on the level.

MODIFIED VERSIONS OF THE ROSE CLAUDICATION QUESTIONNAIRE

Recognizing that Rose claudication symptoms may not be particularly sensitive for PAD, Smith et al. studied relationships between "probable" and "possible" intermittent claudication with mortality among 18,388 men age 40–64 participating in the Whitehall study of London Civil Servants.[9] Participants were examined between 1967 and 1969 and were followed prospectively for mortality through January 3, 1985. Baseline measures included the Rose claudication questionnaire and cardiovascular risk factors. At baseline subjects were categorized according to a) no intermittent claudication; b) probable intermittent claudication; c) possible intermittent claudication. Participants with probable intermittent met all criteria for intermittent claudication from the Rose claudication questionnaire. Participants with "possible" claudication met all criteria from the Rose claudication questionnaire except they reported that exertional leg pain subsided while they were walking. The prevalence of "probable" claudication was 0.8% and the prevalence of "possible" claudication was 1.0%. As compared to participants with no intermittent claudication, those with "probable" intermittent claudication had a relative risk for all-cause mortality of 1.72 (95% Confidence-Interval = 1.3–2.3) and those with "possible" intermittent claudication had a relative for all cause mortality of 1.86 (95% Confidence-Interval = 1.5–2.40), adjusting for age, systolic blood pressure, cholesterol, smoking, employment level, and degree of glucose intolerance. As compared to participants with no intermittent claudication, those with "probable" intermittent claudication had a relative risk for cardiovascular disease mortality of 2.69 (95% Confidence-Interval = 2.0–3.7) and those with "possible" intermittent claudication had a relative for all cause mortality of 2.05 (95% Confidence-Interval = 1.5–2.8), adjusting for age, systolic blood pressure, cholesterol, smoking, employment level, and degree of glucose intolerance. Smith et al. concluded that these findings indicated that the category of "possible" intermittent claudication has acceptable validity for a diagnosis of PAD.

In a follow-up study to the Whitehall intermittent claudication report, Criqui et al. assessed the prevalence of intermittent claudication and "possible" intermittent claudication in 567 older community-dwelling men and women from the Lipid Research Clinics cohort.[10] Most participants were age 60 and older. All participants were followed prospectively over 4 years for mortality. Criqui et al. defined "possible" intermittent claudication as exertional leg pain that does not begin at rest but is otherwise not consistent with Rose criteria for intermittent claudication. The relative risk of mortality in participants with Rose intermittent claudication was 1.9 as compared to participants without intermittent claudication. The relative risk of mortality in participants with either Rose or "possible" Rose claudication was 3.7 as compared to participants without intermittent claudication. The relative risk of mortality in participants with large vessel PAD, as measured by non-invasive testing, was 7.5 as compared to participants without large vessel disease. These data by Criqui et al., like those of Smith et al.,[9] are consistent with a low sensitivity of the Rose claudication questionnaire for PAD.

EDINBURGH CLAUDICATION QUESTIONNAIRE

In 1992 Leng et al. devised a modified claudication questionnaire, the Edinburgh Claudication Questionnaire, in effort to develop a claudication questionnaire that was more sensitive than the Rose claudication questionnaire for the diagnosis of intermittent claudication and PAD.[11] To develop their questionnaire, Leng et al. mailed the Rose claudication questionnaire to 586 patients with clinically-diagnosed intermittent claudication identified from a vascular clinic at the Royal Infirmary of Edinburgh in addition to 61 patients with exertional leg pain due to causes other than PAD. The sensitivity of the Rose claudication questionnaire in the combined population of patients with and without PAD was 60%. The specificity was 91%. When the definition of claudication was expanded to include "possible claudication" as defined by Criqui et al. (exertional calf pain that does not begin at rest but which is not otherwise fully consistent with Rose criteria), the sensitivity of the questionnaire increased to 91% but specificity fell to 72%.

Leng et al. analyzed individual responses to the questions in the Rose claudication questionnaire to identify which questions caused a drop in questionnaire sensitivity and which were important to maintain high specificity. Eliminating the question, "does the pain disappear with continued walking" (See Table 4–1) increased the sensitivity of the questionnaire from 60% to 79% without loss of specificity. Based on his findings, Leng et al. eliminated the following questions from the original Rose claudication questionnaire: "Does the pain ever disappear while you are walking?" and "What do you do if you get the pain while walking?" The latter question was eliminated to simplify the questionnaire. Furthermore, this question has relatively low specificity for diagnosing intermittent claudication.

SAN DIEGO CLAUDICATION QUESTIONNAIRE

Criqui et al. revised the original Rose claudication questionnaire by including leg specific (i.e. right vs. left) questions for each leg and by inquiring about exertional thigh and buttock pain. This revised questionnaire, the San Diego claudication questionnaire, has been used in epidemiologic studies to classify the types of leg symptoms reported by patients with PAD.[2–4, 14]

Prevalences of leg symptom categories in several epidemiologic studies are shown in Table 4–2, based on data collected with the claudication questionnaires described above.

PREVALENCE OF ASYMPTOMATIC PERIPHERAL ARTERIAL DISEASE

While most community-dwelling men and women with PAD as measured by ABI <0.90 do not have symptoms of Rose intermittent claudication,[6–8,11,12] it is unclear whether these PAD participants without claudication are asymptomatic or whether they have exertional leg symptoms other than intermittent claudication.[13] McDermott et al. studied the prevalence of asymptomatic PAD in the Women's Health and Aging Study (WHAS), a study of 1,002 disabled women age 65 and older living in and around Baltimore. All participants had functional difficulty in at least two of the following four areas: upper extremity, mobility, higher functioning, and basic self-care. Of 933 women with valid ABI measurements in the WHAS, 327 (35%) had ABI <0.90, consistent with PAD. Of the 327 women with PAD, 198 (61%) reported no exertional leg symptoms (i.e. were asymptomatic). The absence of exertional leg symptoms was similar between women with and women without PAD. As compared to women with

TABLE 4–2: PREVALENCE OF PERIPHERAL ARTERIAL DISEASE AND INTERMITTENT CLAUDICATION IN DEFINED STUDY POPULATIONS.

Study	Screened Population	Prevalence of peripheral arterial disease	Prevalence of leg symptom categories among individuals with peripheral arterial disease
Community dwelling men and women			
Cardiovascular Health Study (15)	5,572 men and women age 65 and older identified randomly from the community	13%	Intermittent claudication—8.6% Asymptomatic—59.1% Atypical exertional leg pain—32.3%
Men and women identified from general medicine practice			
PARTNERS (14)	6,979 men and women in primary care practices across the United States. Participants were either a) aged 50–69 with a history of diabetes mellitus or a 10-year pack year cigarette smoking history or b) age 70 and older.	29%	Newly diagnosed PAD: Intermittent claudication—5.5% Asymptomatic—48.3% Atypical exertional leg pain—46.3% Previously diagnosed PAD: Intermittent claudication—12.6% Asymptomatic—25.8% Atypical exertional leg pain—61.7%
Men and women identified from non-invasive vascular laboratories			
Walking and Leg Circulation Study (WALCS) (2)	Men and women age 55 and older identified from non-invasive vascular laboratories at 3 Chicago-area hospitals	100% by definition	Intermittent claudication—32.6% Asymptomatic—20% Leg pain on exertion and rest—19.1% Atypical exertional leg pain/carry-on—8.9% Atypical exertional leg pain/stop—19.6%

asymptomatic PAD, WHAS participants with exertional leg pain had higher prevalences of comorbidities associated with leg pain, such as knee arthritis, hip arthritis, disk disease, and spinal stenosis.

Thus, WHAS data showed that asymptomatic PAD is common among older disabled women and that the presence vs. absence of leg symptoms in PAD may be influenced by the presence of comorbid diseases affecting the lower extremities. However, data from older disabled women in the WHAS may not be generalizable to patients with PAD who are typically encountered by clinicians. Subsequent studies have shown that the prevalence of asymptomatic PAD ranges from 15% to 30% among patients identified from non-invasive vascular laboratories.[2-4]

PREVALENCE OF INTERMITTENT CLAUDICATION AMONG PATIENTS WITH PAD IDENTIFIED FROM GENERAL MEDICAL PRACTICES

Studies performed in general medicine practices show that most men and women with PAD in these settings do not have classical symptoms of intermittent claudication. McDermott et al. reported that among 26 men and women age 55 and older found to have PAD based on a screening ABI, 3.8% had symptoms consistent with intermittent claudication, 53.8% were asymptomatic, and 42.3% had exertional leg symptoms other than intermittent claudication.[4]

In the PAD Awareness, Risk, and Treatment: New Resources for Survival (PARTNERS) program, 6,979 men and women in 25 cities and 320 primary care practices across the United States were screened with the ABI. Inclusion criteria were: a) age 70 or older or b) age 50–69 with a history of diabetes mellitus or cigarette smoking. Twenty-nine percent of participants screened had an ABI <0.90, consistent with PAD. Participants with PAD were further classified into a) prior diagnosis of PAD or b) new diagnosis of PAD. A prior diagnosis of PAD was determined based on medical record review and primary care physician report. The overall prevalence of intermittent claudication among participants with PAD was 8.7%. Intermittent claudication was more common among PAD participants with a prior diagnosis of PAD vs. a new diagnosis of PAD (12.6% vs. 5.5%, p <0.01). Among participants with PAD, 53% had exertional leg symptoms other than intermittent claudication and 38% had no exertional leg symptoms.[14]

COMORBID DISEASE AND LEG SYMPTOMS IN PERIPHERAL ARTERIAL DISEASE

Newman et al. studied the relation between leg symptoms, ABI, and comorbid disease among men and women participating in the Cardiovascular Health Study (CHS).

The CHS included 5,572 men and women aged 65 and older identified randomly from the community.[15] Measurements included the ABI and the Rose claudication questionnaire. All participants were categorized according to whether they had no exertional leg pain (asymptomatic), intermittent claudication, or exertional leg pain other than intermittent claudication (exertional leg symptoms that were not consistent with Rose claudication). Overall, 78.2% of CHS participants had no exertional leg pain, 20.2% had exertional leg pain other than intermittent claudication, and 1.6% had intermittent claudication.[15] Thirteen percent of CHS participants had PAD (ABI <0.90). The prevalence of ABI <0.90 was 9.8% in participants with no exertional leg pain, 20.8% in participants with exertional leg pain other than intermittent claudication, and 68.9% among those with intermittent claudication. Among all participants, those with exertional leg pain other than intermittent claudication had a higher prevalence of comorbid diseases than participants with no exertional leg pain. In particular, diabetes, heart disease, stroke, depression, and chronic obstructive pulmonary disease were more common among participants with exertional leg pain other than intermittent claudication as compared to the asymptomatic group. Prevalences of comorbid disease were comparable between the intermittent claudication and exertional leg pain other than claudication groups. However, arthritis was more common in the exertional leg pain other than claudication group as compared to the intermittent claudication and asymptomatic groups.[15]

Among CHS participants with PAD, 59% reported no exertional leg symptoms, 32% had exertional leg symptoms other than intermittent claudication, and 9% had intermittent claudication. At lower ABI levels, indicating more severe PAD, the proportion of participants with exertional leg pain and intermittent claudication increased. For example, among participants with ABI <0.70, 43.5% had no exertional leg pain, 43.5% had exertional leg pain other than intermittent claudication, and 13% had intermittent claudication. The authors noted that PAD participants with arthritis did not discriminate between leg pain from arthritis and leg pain from PAD when responding to the Rose claudication questionnaire. Newman et al. concluded that lower extremity arthritis may contribute to leg symptoms reported by patients with PAD.[15]

LEG SYMPTOMS IN PERIPHERAL ARTERIAL DISEASE PATIENTS PARTICIPATING IN THE WALKING AND LEG CIRCULATION STUDY

McDermott et al. studied the prevalence of leg pain categories in patients with PAD identified from three medical centers in the Chicago area.[2] Participants were 460 men and women with PAD and 130 without PAD enrolled in the Walking and Leg Circulation Study (WALCS). PAD participants were identified from non-invasive vascular laboratories at the 3 Chicago medical centers. All were administered the San Diego claudication questionnaire. Leg symptom categories were based on those previously developed by Criqui et al. and included the following categories (Figure 4–1): a) Intermittent claudication; b) pain on exertion and rest (exertional leg symptoms that sometimes begins at rest); c) atypical exertional leg pain/carry-on (exertional leg symptoms that do not begin at rest and do not stop the individual from walking); d) atypical exertional leg pain/stop (exertional leg symptoms that do not begin at rest, but that do stop the individual from walking and do not involve the calves or do not resolve within 10 minutes of rest); e) asymptomatic (no exertional leg pain). McDermott et al. proposed that patients with PAD might be asymptomatic either because they have milder PAD and are minimally limited by extremity atherosclerosis or because they have restricted their activity enough to avoid precipitating exertional leg symptoms. Therefore, two subcategories of asymptomatic PAD patients were defined. An asymptomatic "active" group was defined consisting of PAD patients without exertional leg pain who walked more than six blocks last week. An asymptomatic "inactive" group consisted of PAD patients without exertional leg pain who walked six or

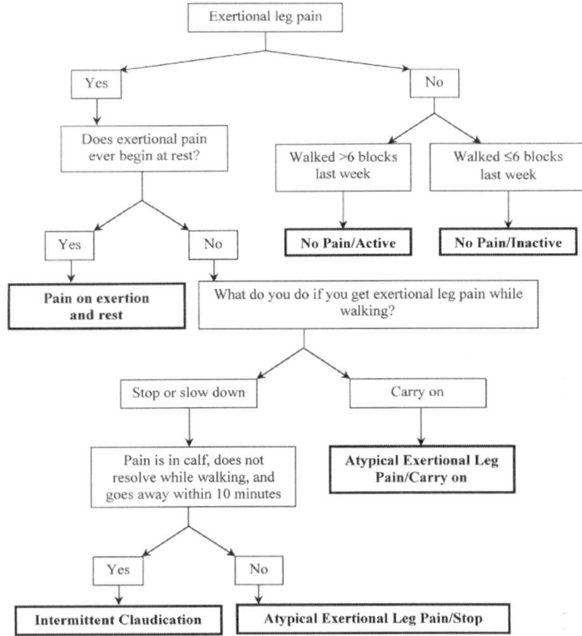

Figure 4–1. Leg symptoms commonly present in peripheral arterial disease

fewer blocks last week. A priori, the asymptomatic "active" group was expected to have better functioning than the asymptomatic "inactive" group. Comorbid diseases were ascertained rigorously using algorithms that combined data from medical record review, patient medications, patient report, a primary care physician questionnaire, and knee x-rays. To learn more about the significance of specific leg pain categories in PAD, characteristics and functional impairment associated with each leg pain category were studied.

CLINICAL CHARACTERISTICS ASSOCIATED WITH LEG PAIN CATEGORIES IN PERIPHERAL ARTERIAL DISEASE

Of the 460 PAD participants in the WALCS, 32% had leg symptoms consistent with intermittent claudication, 19% had pain on exertion and rest, 9% had atypical leg pain/carry on, 20% had exertional leg pain/stop, 14% were in the asymptomatic/active group, and 6% were in the asymptomatic/inactive group. The atypical exertional leg pain/carry on group had a significantly higher ABI than patients with intermittent claudication (0.70 vs. 0.61, p=0.004). There were no other significant differences in average ABI level between leg pain groups. Among the leg pain categories, participants with exertional leg pain/carry-on included a higher proportion of men, were generally healthier, and had better functioning compared to participants with intermittent claudication. Participants with leg pain on exertion and rest included a higher proportion of women, had a greater average number of comorbidities, and had poorer functioning as compared to participants with intermittent claudication (Table 4–3). The leg pain on exertion and rest group also had more neuropathy and a higher prevalence of

TABLE 4–3. CLINICAL CHARACTERISTICS AND FUNCTIONAL IMPAIRMENT ASSOCIATED WITH SPECIFIC LEG SYMPTOM CATEGORIES IN PATIENTS WITH PERIPHERAL ARTERIAL DISEASE.*

Leg symptom group	Clinical characteristics (in reference to intermittent claudication group)	Functional limitations (in reference to intermittent claudication group)	Other
Atypical exertional leg pain/carry on	• Higher ankle brachial index • Lower prevalence of prior lower extremity revascularization • Fewer depressive symptoms	• Greater distance achieved in 6-minute walk test • Low rate of stopping during the 6-minute walk test	
Atypical exertional leg pain/stop	No significant differences as compared to intermittent claudication group during the 6-minute walk test	• Greater distance achieved in 6-minute walk test • Low rate of stopping	
Pain on exertion and rest	• Higher proportion of women • Poorer neuropathy score • Higher prevalence of diabeter • Higher prevalence of spinal stenosis	• Slower walking speed • Shorter 6-minute walk distance • Poorer performance on tandem stand test of balance • Slower time to rise 5 times consecutively from seated position	
No exertional leg pain/active	• Older • Higher ankle brachial index	• Functioning comparable to patients with intermittent claudication	33.3% reported exertional leg symptoms during the 6-minute walk
No exertioal leg pain/inactive	• Older • Higher prevalence of blacks with intermittent claudiation	• Slower walking speed compared to patients	53.6% rep exertional leg symptoms during the 6-minute walk test

*All comparisons are in reference to patients with peripheral arterial disease and intermittent claudication. A monofilament applied to the bottom of the feet was used to determine the neuropathy score. Higher scores indicate a greater number of times the participant was unable to feel the monofilament.

Data are from McDermott et al. JAMA 2001;286:1599–1606.

comorbid diseases influencing leg symptoms such as spinal stenosis and diabetes mellitus (Table 4–3). Thus PAD patients with leg pain on exertion and rest have a higher prevalence of comorbid diseases that also contribute to exertional leg symptoms.

LEG FUNCTIONING IN PERIPHERAL ARTERIAL DISEASE PATIENTS WITHOUT INTERMITTENT CLAUDICATION: THE WALKING AND LEG CIRCULATION STUDY (WALCS)

The entire cohort of patients with PAD who did not have intermittent claudication symptoms had poorer lower extremity functioning than patients without PAD. As compared to PAD patients with intermittent claudication, individuals with atypical leg pain/carry-on had better performance on the 6-minute walk test, adjusting for potential confounders. Just 6.8% of PAD patients with exertional leg pain/carry-on stopped during the 6-minute walk, while 36% of PAD patients with intermittent claudication stopped during the 6-minute walk (p = 0.002). PAD patients with exertional leg pain/carry-on achieved a greater distance in the 6-minute walk compared to the intermittent claudication group (404.3 vs. 328.5 meters, p<0.001). In contrast the pain on exertion and rest group performed consistently more poorly than the intermittent claudication group. As compared to participants with intermittent claudication and adjusting for potential confounders, those with pain on exertion and rest performed more poorly in balance testing, had slower walking velocity, and had poorer performance in the 6-minute walk test. Thus, PAD patients without intermittent claudication have significantly impaired lower extremity functioning compared to individuals without PAD. In addition, PAD patients with leg pain on exertion and rest have poorer functioning than PAD patients with intermittent claudication. These findings are important in part because to date there have been no clinical trials testing the ability of specific interventions to improve lower extremity functioning in PAD patients who do not have classical symptoms of intermittent claudication.

CHARACTERISTICS OF ASYMPTOMATIC PATIENTS WITH PERIPHERAL ARTERIAL DISEASE IN THE WALCS

As compared to PAD patients with intermittent claudication, the two groups of asymptomatic patients with PAD were significantly older (74.7 + 7.8 vs. 70.7 + 8.4, p<0.01 for the active asymptomatic PAD group and 75.5 + 8.7 vs. 70.7 + 8.4, p<0.01 for the inactive asymptomatic PAD group). The inactive asymptomatic PAD group included a significantly higher prevalence of African-Americans as compared to the intermittent claudication group (35.7% vs. 13.3%, p<0.01) and had a significantly poorer neuropathy score.

Adjusting for potential confounders, the asymptomatic inactive group had significantly slower walking speed as compared to the intermittent claudication group (0.78 vs. 0.90 meters/second, p<0.01). However the asymptomatic active group had comparable functioning to the intermittent claudication group.

During the 6-minute walk test, 33.3% of the asymptomatic active group and 53.6% of the asymptomatic inactive group developed exertional leg pain. This finding suggests that many asymptomatic PAD patients do not get exertional leg symptoms because they are too inactive to precipitate exertional leg symptoms. This phenomenon is particularly common among the most inactive asymptomatic PAD patients.

CONCLUSION

While intermittent claudication has been considered the most classical symptom of intermittent claudication, a minority of all PAD patients have classical symptoms of intermittent claudication. Most PAD patients are either asymptomatic or have exertional leg symptoms other than intermittent claudication. Comorbid diseases such as spinal stenosis and neuropathy contribute to the types of leg symptoms reported by patients with PAD. Furthermore, the nature of leg symptoms associated with PAD influences the degree of functional impairment. To date, clinical trials studying interventions to improve functioning in patients with PAD (including exercise and drug treatments) have focused on PAD patients with intermittent claudication. Because PAD patients without intermittent claudication have substantially impaired lower extremity functioning, future work should identify interventions to improve lower extremity functioning in PAD patients who do not have classical symptoms of intermittent claudication.

REFERENCES

1. Rose GA. The diagnosis of ischaemic heart pain and intermittent claudication in field surveys. *Bull Wld Hlth Org*. 1962;27:645–658.
2. McDermott MM, Greenland P, Liu K, et al. Leg symptoms in peripheral arterial disease: associated clinical characteristics and functional impairment. *JAMA*. 2001;286:1599–1606.
3. Criqui MH, Denenberg JO, Bird CE, et al. The correlation between symptoms and non-invasive test results in patients referred for peripheral arterial disease testing. *Vascular Med*. 1996;1:65–71.
4. McDermott MM, Mehta S, Greenland P. Exertional leg symptoms other than intermittent claudication are common in peripheral arterial disease. *Arch Intern Med*. 1999;159:387–392.
5. Schroll M, Munck O. Estimation of peripheral arteriosclerotic disease by ankle blood pressure measurements in a population study of 60-year old men and women. *J Chronic Dis*. 1981;34:261–269.
6. Newman AB, Siscovick DS, Manolio TA, et al. Ankle-arm index as a marker of atherosclerosis in the Cardiovascular Health Study. *Circulation*. 1993;88:837–45.
7. Fowkes FG, Housley E, Cawood EH et al. Edinburgh artery study: Prevalence of asymptomatic and symptomatic peripheral arterial disease in the general population. *Int J Epidemiol*.1991;20(2):384–392.
8. Criqui MH, Fronek A, Barrett-Connor E, et al. The prevalence of peripheral arterial disease in a defined population. *Circulation*. 1985;71(3):510–515.
9. Smith GD, Shipley MJ, Rose GA. Intermittent claudication, heart disease risk factors, and mortality. The Whitehall study. *Circulation*. 1990;82:1925–1931.
10. Criqui MH, Coughlin SS, Fronek A. Noninvasively diagnosed peripheral arterial disease as a predictor of mortality: results from a prospective study. *Circulation*. 1985;72(4):768–773.
11. Leng GC, Fowkes FG. The Edinburgh claudication questionnaire: An improved version of the WHO/Rose questionnaire for use in epidemiological surveys. *J Clin Epidemiol*. 1992; 45(10):1101–1109.
12. Newman AB, Sutton-Tyrrell K, Kuller LH. Lower-extremity arterial disease in older hypertensive adults. *Arteriosclerosis and Thrombosis*. 1993;13:555–562.
13. McDermott MM, Fried L, Simonsick E, et al. Asymptomatic peripheral arterial disease is independently associated with impaired lower extremity functioning. The women's health and aging study. *Circulation*. 2000;101:1007–1012.
14. Hirsch AT, Criqui MH, Treat-Jacobson D, et al. The PARTNERS program: A national survey of peripheral arterial disease detection, awareness, and treatment. *JAMA*. 2001;286: 1317–1324.
15. Newman AB, Naydeck BL, Sutton-Tyrrell K, et al. The role of comorbidity in the assessment of intermittent claudication in older adults. *J Clin Epidemiol*. 2001;54:294–300.

APPENDIX
SAN DIEGO CLAUDICATION QUESTIONNAIRE*

			Right Leg	**Left Leg**
1.	Do you ever get PAIN in either leg or buttock on walking? (If no or uncertain, stop)	No.....	1	1
		Yes.....	2	2
2.	Does this pain ever begin when you are STANDING STILL or SITTING?	No.....	1	1
		Yes.....	2	2
In what part of the leg or buttock do you feel the pain?				
3a.	Pain includes calf	No.....	1	1
		Yes.....	2	2
3b.	Pain includes thigh	No.....	1	1
		Yes.....	2	2
3c.	Pain includes buttock	No.....	1	1
		Yes.....	2	2
4.	Do you get it when you walk UPHILL or HURRY?	No.....	1	1
		Yes.....	2	2
		Never walks uphill or hurries...	3	
5.	Do you get it when you walk at an ORDINARY PACE on the level?	No.....	1	1
		Yes.....	2	2
6.	Does the pain ever DISAPPEAR while you are WALKING?	No.....	1	1
		Yes.....	2	2
7.	What do you do if you get it when you are walking?	Carry on.....	1	
		Stop or slow down.....	2	
8.	What happens if you STAND STILL?	Lessens or relieved.....	1	1
		Unchanged.....	2	2
9	If standing still relieves pain, HOW SOON?	10 minutes or less.....	1	1
		More than 10 minutes.....	2	2

*Coding
No pain: 1 = 1;
Pain on exertion and rest: 1 = 2 and 2 = 2;
Atypical exertional leg pain/carry on: 1 = 2 and 2 = 1 and 7 = 1
Atypical exertional leg pain/stop 1=2 and 2 =1 and 7 = 2 and (3a = 1 or 3a = 3); alternatively 1 = 2 and 2 = 1 and 7 = 2 and 3a = 2 and (6 = 2 or 8 = 2 or 9 = 2);
Intermittent claudication: 1 = 2 and 2 = 1 and 3a = 1 and (4 = 2 or [4 = 3 and 5 = 2]) and 6 = 1 and 7 = 2 and 8 = 1 and 9 = 1.

5

Hypercoagulable States and Arterial Ischemia

Donald Silver, MD, Thomas A. Shuster, DO, and Leila Mureebe, MD

Thrombosis is the most common cause of death in the United States, with there being approximately 2 million deaths each year from arterial or venous thromboses or their consequences.[1] More than 5 million patients were hospitalized in the United States in 1997 with thrombotic disorders. The cost of these disorders has been estimated to be approximately 13 billion dollars.[2] Thrombosis is most often the "final cause" of acute arterial ischemia. It has been estimated that 50% of patients with thromboses have a congenital or acquired coagulation protein or platelet defect that caused the thromboses.

While most of the hypercoagulable disorders contribute to venous thromboembolism, the vascular surgeon should suspect a hypercoagulable disorder in patients with juvenile, idiopathic, recurrent, or multi-located arterial thromboses or unexplained arterial reconstructive failures. Many of these patients have 1 or more acquired or congenital hypercoagulable disorders, which make them likely to experience thrombotic events when exposed to conditions that are tolerated by most individuals.

We will limit this review to the pathophysiology and management of those hypercoagulable disorders which the vascular surgeon is likely to encounter in patients with non-mechanical thrombotic-induced lower extremity, mesenteric, and cerebral ischemia. The concerns of inadequate in-flow or out-flow, technical inadequacies, graft inadequacies, inadequate anti-coagulation, or other cause of early arterial reconstructive failures, while important, are not discussed. If a hypercoagulable disorder is recognized, appropriate management may control the prothrombotic tendency and prevent a thrombosis.

TABLE 5–1: ACQUIRED HYPERCOAGULABLE DISORDERS

Smoking
Antiphospholipid syndrome
Hyperhomocystinemia
Heparin-induced thrombocytopenia
Warfarin
Diabetes mellitus
Hyperlipidemia
Polycythemia vera
Hyperfibrinogenemia
Nephrotic syndrome
Vasculitis

SMOKING

Smoking contributes to arterial thrombosis and atherogenesis through a variety of mechanisms. Nicotine and carbon monoxide are the most harmful constituents. Nicotine results in endothelial damage, leading to platelet deposition and platelet-induced medial and intimal hyperplasia. Carbon monoxide increases the permeability of the endothelium, resulting in increased deposition of lipids in the media and production of atheromas. Smoking reduces the synthesis of prostacyclin and increases blood viscosity, leading to increased tendencies toward coagulation.[3]

ANTIPHOSPHOLIPID SYNDROME

The antiphospholipid syndrome is a common acquired cause of hypercoagulability. It occurs in 1% to 5% of the population and increases with age, with 50% of patients older than 80 years having antiphospholipid antibodies.[4] Patients with these disorders develop antibodies to protein-phospholipid complexes; the patients may have the lupus anticoagulant and/or anticardiolipin antibodies. The antibodies are directed against neoepitopes of plasma proteins, other phospholipid complexes that react with protein C, protein S, or factors XI and XII, and phospholipids on platelets and endothelial cells. The endothelial reaction blocks the antithrombin inactivation of thrombin and the thrombomodulin activation of protein C. The antiphospholipid antibodies may also contribute to the formation of atherosclerotic lesions.[5]

Recurrent venous thrombosis is the usual manifestation of the antiphospholipid syndrome. However, arterial thromboses are known to occur in the brain, eye, heart, and in the periphery. Thrombocytopenia is a common occurrence. The diagnosis of antiphospholipid syndrome includes testing for the lupus anticoagulant, which is manifested with prolongation of the clotting assays, and the anticardiolipin antibodies which are detected with enzyme-linked immunosorbent assays. Patients should undergo both tests.

Management of the antiphospholipid syndrome includes elimination of the risk factors in patients with known antibodies, (e.g., avoid pregnancy, oral contraceptives, major trauma, etc.). Acute thrombotic episodes should be treated with lytic agents and/or heparin. The rate of recurrent thrombosis can be decreased with long-term anti-coagulation. It has been demonstrated that low-dose warfarin therapy is ineffective and that the INR should be 2.5 to 3.5, or higher. Treatment with warfarin should be long-term—certainly until antibodies are no longer present. Recent studies have demonstrated the value of low molecular weight heparin in preventing recurrences of thromboses in patients with the antiphospholipid syndrome.

HEPARIN-INDUCED THROMBOCYTOPENIA

Heparin-induced thrombocytopenia occurs in 2% to 3% of patients who receive heparin therapy. We have recently reported that 21% of patients undergoing vascular reconstruction develop heparin-associated anti-platelet antibodies and 18.2% of these patients have heparin-induced thromboses.[6]

A few patients develop heparin-associated anti-platelet antibodies while receiving heparin. The antibodies of these patients, when exposed to heparin, induce platelet aggregation and thromboses and, rarely, hemorrhage. The antibodies also activate endothelial cells which contribute to the thrombotic tendency. The development of the antibodies is independent of patient age or sex, the route of administration, the type of heparin, or the amount of heparin received. The antibodies usually occur in patients between the fifth and the eighth day during the first exposure and may recur during the first day of a patient's re-exposure to heparin. The clinical manifestations include: a falling platelet count; an increased resistance to anti-coagulation therapy with heparin; or new thrombotic (arterial, rarely venous) or, rarely, hemorrhagic events. The physician must be aware that continued heparin anticoagulation places these patients at risk for a heparin-induced thrombosis. The vascular surgeon should be aware that thrombosis in the operating room or in the recovery room of a technically successful arterial reconstruction may be caused by heparin-induced thrombocytopenia.

The heparin-induced thrombocytopenia syndrome is one of the more common hypercoagulable disorders encountered in patients undergoing vascular surgery. Its management includes the avoidance of all forms of heparin to which the patient is sensitized. Like most drug-induced antibodies, the heparin-associated anti-platelet antibodies usually remit in a few weeks to months; however, we have found that the antibodies may persist for as long as 13 years. Thrombin inhibitors, e.g. lepirudin, have been found to be safe and effective agents for anticoagulating patients with heparin associated antiplatelet antibodies.[7]

WARFARIN-INDUCED THROMBOSIS

Warfarin-induced skin necrosis is the most serious, non-hemorrhagic complication of oral anticoagulation therapy. The necrosis is caused by thromboses and hemorrhages of venules and capillaries within the subcutaneous fat and the overlying skin. The breasts, thighs, buttocks, and legs are most often involved. The administration of warfarin leads to reduction of coagulation factors II, VII, IX, and X and proteins C and S. Protein C and factor VII have short half-lives of approximately 6 hours and are quickly reduced. The other vitamin K dependent factors have significantly longer half-lives, so that therapeutic anti-coagulation requires 3 to 4 days. However, the induced deficiency of protein C induces a hypercoagulable state during the first 2 to 3 days of warfarin therapy. Consequently, it is recommended that patients with risk factors for intravascular thrombosis and especially those patients with protein C and protein S deficiencies, or patients with previous episodes of warfarin-induced skin necrosis, should be protected with heparin for the first 4 days of anti-coagulation with warfarin.

OTHER ACQUIRED HYPERCOAGULABLE DISORDERS

Many clinical disorders predispose patients to thrombosis by activating the coagulation system, inhibiting the fibrinolytic system, or initiating platelet activation. Soft tissue trauma, thermal injuries, and operative dissections predispose one to thrombosis through the release of tissue factor. Sepsis predisposes a patient to thrombosis with the increased production of tissue factor; decrease of antithrombin, protein C and protein S, and thrombomodulin activity; and the increase in production of plasminogen activator inhibitor-1. Patients with hyperlipidemia, myeloproliferative diseases, diabetes, and thrombotic thrombocytopenia are all predisposed to thrombosis through the effects on platelets. Hyperlipidemia activates platelets with an increase of thromboxane A_2, and a decrease of the platelet response to prostacyclin.

CONGENITAL HYPERCOAGULABLE SYNDROMES

Most of the congenital disorders of hypercoagulability contribute to venous thromboembolism. However, a hypercoagulable disorder should also be suspected in patients with juvenile, idiopathic, recurrent, or multi-level arterial thromboses (e.g. 15% to 70% of young patients with arterial occlusive disease may have a hypercoagulable syndrome and unexplained arterial reconstructive failures).[8,9] Some patients who are hypercoagulable have multiple genetic disorders (e.g. the frequent association of factor V Leiden mutation with deficiencies of antithrombin and proteins C and S). The congenital hypercoagulable disorders are listed in Table 5–2. The more prevalent ones are discussed.

TABLE 5–2: CONGENITAL HYPERCOAGULABLE DISORDERS

Anti-thrombin deficiency
Protein C deficiency
Protein S deficiency
Activated protein C resistance
Prothrombin 20210A
Sticky platelet syndrome
Heparin cofactor II deficiency
Hyperhomocystinemia
Dysfibrinogenemia
Increased factors VIII, XI
Abnormal/decreased plasminogen
Decreased plasminogen activator
Increased plasminogen activator inhibitor

ANTITHROMBIN DEFICIENCY

Antithrombin, the major plasma inhibitor of thrombin, also inhibits factors IXa, Xa, Xia, and XIIa. Patients with low levels of antithrombin are not only at risk for venous thromboses, but are also at risk for arterial thromboses. The risk of thrombosis increases as the functional antithrombin level activity decreases to less than 80% of normal, with highest risk occurring when the antithrombin levels are less than 60%. The antithrombin deficiency prevalence is 1:5,000. Heparin is the mainstay of therapy for patients with antithrombin deficiency and acute thrombosis. Increased amounts of heparin are frequently required to achieve a therapeutic aPTT. Antithrombin deficiency management occasionally requires infusions of fresh frozen plasma or antithrombin concentrate. Concentrates are preferred. It is recommended that the antithrombin concentration be adjusted to at least 80% of normal activity during the management of a thromboembolic event with heparin and before surgery in a patient with acquired or congenital antithrombin deficiency.

PROTEIN C AND PROTEIN S DEFICIENCIES

Protein C and protein S are vitamin K-dependent proteins that are synthesized in the liver. Protein C, when activated by thrombin, is a major anticoagulant and significantly enhances fibrolytic activity. Activated protein C degrades activated forms of factor V (Va) and factor VIII (VIIIa). Protein C also decreases plasminogen activator inhibitor activity, thus increasing fibrolytic potential. Protein S has no anticoagulant or fibrolytic potential, but serves as a co-factor for protein C and enhances the expression of the anticoagulant effect of protein C.

Protein C and protein S plasma levels may be decreased in patients with hepatic insufficiency, renal failure, vitamin K deficiency, and disseminated vascular coagulation. Congenital protein C deficiency is transmitted as an autosomal dominant trait, with a prevalence that varies from 1:200 to 1:300. Deficiencies of protein C and protein S usually place the patient at risk for venous thrombosis, with the incidence of thromboembolic events in patients who are heterozygous for protein C varying from 0% to 50%.[10,11] Protein C and protein S deficiencies have been found in 15% to 20% of young patients with peripheral vascular disease.[12] While protein C and protein S deficiencies are predominantly responsible for venous thromboses, they, on rare occasions, contribute to arterial thrombosis. We have had a recent patient with an aortic thrombosis and distal embolization that was caused by a protein S deficiency.

The management of protein C and protein S deficiencies includes prophylaxis with heparin or warfarin during times when the patient is at increased risk for venous thrombosis, and life-long anticoagulation with warfarin for patients who have had recurrent or significant arterial and/or venous thromboses. It should be remembered that cutaneous necrosis is likely to occur when warfarin anticoagulation is offered to patients with protein C deficiency; consequently, those patients should receive heparin therapy during the first 3 to 4 days of warfarin therapy.

ACTIVATED PROTEIN C RESISTANCE

Activated protein resistance (APC-R) is the most common risk factor for venous thrombosis, accounting for 52% to 64% of the inherited causes of thromboses.[13] Many patients previously thought to have functional antithrombin and protein C and protein S deficiencies have been found to also have APC-R.

APC-R is characterized by a poor anticoagulant response to activated protein C. Activated protein C degrades activated clotting factors Va and VIIIa. In most cases of APC-R, the patient has an altered factor V (factor V Leiden) in which the arginine 506 is replaced with a glutamine thus making the Va resistant to degradation of activated protein C and thus favoring thrombosis.

Although, patients with APC-R have a markedly increased risk of venous thrombosis, there is increasing evidence that APC-R is associated with arterial thromboses, especially myocardial infarction. Patients with APC-R and thrombotic risk situations should undergo thrombosis prophylaxis therapy and those patients with recurrent or life-threatening thrombotic episodes should undergo life-long anticoagulation with warfarin.

STICKY PLATELET SYNDROME

The sticky platelet syndrome is a congenital platelet disorder which is inherited as an autosomal dominant and is characterized by platelet hyperaggregability with ADP and/or epinephrine. It is responsible for venous thrombosis and arterial thrombosis, especially coronary artery thrombosis, cerebrovascular thrombosis, retinal vascular thrombosis, and TIAs. It is said to account for 21% of unexplained arterial thrombotic events and 13.2% of unexplained venous thrombotic events.[14] Management of the sticky platelet syndrome consists of aspirin (81 to 321 mg. per day), which normalizes the hyperaggregability and prevents recurrent symptoms.

PROTHROMBIN GENE VARIANT (20210A)

Port et. al., in 1996, demonstrated a nucleotide change (a G to A transition) at position 20210 of the prothrombin gene in 18% of patients with a documented family history of venous thrombophilia.[15] The mutation was found in 4% to 8% of unselected patients with the first episode of deep venous thrombosis.[16] Early reports suggested that the prothrombin 20210G/A genotype was not related to arterial thrombotic disorders. However, subsequent reports have indicated that the allele has a high prevalence rate in selected patients with arterial thrombosis, especially those with coronary and cerebral thromboses.

It has been suggested that the prothrombin 20210A allele and the factor V Leiden mutation will be found in 63% of families with thrombophilia[17] and that ". . . 0.6% to 5% of symptomatic carriers of the Factor V Leiden mutation also carry the prothrombin gene."[18] Management of the prothrombin gene variant has not been defined, but is likely to require long-term anticoagulant therapy with warfarin for those patients with serious and/or recurrent thromboses.

HOMOCYSTINEMIA

Homocystine is formed during the metabolism of methionine. It is metabolized with remethylation to methionine or transsulfuration to cystine. Inherited disorders of either of these metabolic pathways or of metabolic defects related to deficiencies of vitamins folate, B12 or B6 may produce hyperhomocystinemia. Hyperhomocystinemia causes endothelial disruption and dysfunction, platelet activation and thrombus formation. Hyperhomocystinemia-damaged endothelium has reduced nitric oxide production and reduction of antithrombin binding activity of endothelial heparan sulfate. It has been demonstrated that hyperhomocystinemia is associated with arterial thrombosis, accelerated atherosclerosis and recurrent venous thrombosis.

It is estimated that mild hyperhomocystinemia occurs in approximately 5% to 7% of the population.[19] Patients with high homocystine levels should receive folate, 1–5 mg. per day—up to 15 mg per day in patients with renal failure. If the homocystine level does not correct, they should also be offered B12 (1.0 mg per day) and/or B6 (0.5 to 1.0 mg per day).

HEPARIN COFACTOR II DEFICIENCY

Heparin cofactor II, produced in the liver, is a specific inhibitor of thrombin. It inactivates thrombin by binding to it in a one-to-one relationship. Heparin enhances the rate of thrombin inactivation by heparin cofactor II. Patients with heparin cofactor II deficiency are at risk for thrombosis when the cofactor level is 50% or less than normal. Heparin cofactor deficiencies have been reported in a few patients as a risk factor of venous, and, fewer, arterial thromboses.[20]

DEFICIENT PLASMINOGEN AND PLASMINOGEN ACTIVATOR ACTIVITY

Patients with deficiencies of fibrinolytic activity from structural defects in plasminogen or defects in the plasminogen activator system may have arterial and/or venous thromboses. Their management usually requires long-term warfarin therapy.

CLINICAL IMPLICATIONS

Thrombosis is the usual consequence of obstruction (e.g. occluding atherosclerotic plaque, intimal flap, dissection, inadequate anastomosis, external compression, and so forth) to arterial flow. Patients with hypercoagulable disorders occasionally develop arterial thromboses in vessels with adequate lumens and blood flow. The contribution of genetic risk factors to arterial occlusive disease has been inconsistent. The hemostatic risk factors usually act in concert with other environmental/metabolic risk factors. Nevertheless, the more common hypercoagulable conditions are thought to contribute to extremity, mesenteric and cerebral arterial ischemia.

Hypercoagulable-induced extremity ischemia may present as claudication, rest pain, gangrene, and/or tissue loss. Congential and acquired hypercoagulable states contribute to the initial, and perhaps more importantly, recurrent arterial thrombotic events. In a study of hypercoagulable states of lower extremity ischemia, hypercoagulable states were found in 40% of patients who had undergone a prior bypass procedure, 27% of claudicants, and only 11% of control subjects.[21] Donaldson and associates found a high prevalence of hypercoagulable states in patients on the vascular surgical service. They found patients to have antithrombin deficiencies and protein C and protein S deficiencies, abnormal plasminogen, lupus anticoagulants, and HIT.[22] The incidence of bypass graft failure was much more pronounced in the patients with hypercoagulable states (27%) as compared to patients with normal laboratory values (1.6%). Polycythemia vera, the sticky platelet syndrome, heparin-induced thrombocytopenia, APC-R, AT, protein C and protein S deficiencies, antiphospholipid antibodies, and hyperhomocystinemia have all been reported to lead to early bypass graft failures and unexplained arterial thromboses, especially in young patients.[22–25]

Approximately 25% of patients who develop mesenteric ischemia have thrombosis of one or more of their visceral arteries.[26] Mesenteric ischemia usually is caused by progressive occlusive atherosclerotic vascular disease, with reduction in flow beyond the stenosis ultimately resulting in thrombotic occlusion. A recent review of 36 patients with nonoccluded colonic ischemia identified 26 patients to possess one or more prothrombotic abnormalities.[27] Antiphospholipid antibodies,[28] lupus anticoagulant,[29] the prothrombin variant deficiencies in antithrombin, protein C and protein S, as well as the factor V Leiden mutation, have been reported to cause mesenteric ischemia, including splenic and esophageal infarctions.

Stroke is the third most common cause of death and the leading cause of disability. In addition to the usual risk factors, e.g. hypertension, hyperlipidemia, diabetes, smoking, and obesity, coagulation abnormalities are being recognized with increased frequency as contributory, occasionally causative, factors in producing strokes. The patient with an unexplained stroke (including TIA, lacunar infarct, or unexplained dementia), previous episodes of arterial and/or venous thrombosis, and/or a family history for thrombosis is a candidate for coagulation studies.

Cerebral ischemia is a common arterial thrombotic manifestation of the antiphospholipid syndrome, which is present in up to 7% of patients with otherwise unexplained strokes.[30] Hyperhomocystinemia, heparin-induced thrombocytopenia, the prothrombin variant, the sticky platelet syndrome, increased plasminogen activator inhibitor-1, reductions or abnormal plasminogens, and polycythemia vera are known contributing agents for stroke. Deficiencies of antithrombin and protein C and S, as well as the presence of activated protein C resistant have been described in patients with stroke, but their etiologic roles are less clear. If a coagulation abnormality is identified in a patient with an otherwise unexplained stroke, anticoagulant, and/or antiplatelet therapy may be highly beneficial in preventing additional ischemic events.

WHO, WHAT, WHEN TO TEST

A hypercoagulable disorder should be suspected in patients with juvenile, idiopathic, recurrent, or multi-level arterial thromboses and unexplained arterial reconstructive failures. In addition, one should be concerned about patients who develop thromboses in the presence of minimal risk factors, or who develop arterial and venous thrombosis simultaneously, as well as those who develop thrombosis while receiving heparin and/or warfarin.

Some tests can be done during the time of the thrombosis. At that time, one can test for heparin associated antiplatelet antibodies, hyperhomocystinemia, anticardiolipin antibodies, the prothrombin variant, the Leiden mutation, and sticky platelets. Most of the other coagulation and anti-coagulation proteins/factors are consumed during the thrombotic process and testing, at that time, for these substances is unreliable. Most, preferably all, tests should be performed at a time remote in relation to the acute thrombosis and when the patient has not received warfarin therapy for at least a couple of weeks. The authors usually treat the patient with a suspected hypercoagulable disorder with warfarin for 6 months (or longer, until they have been thrombosis free for at least 2 months), at which time the warfarin is discontinued and the patient placed on low molecular weight heparin for 2 weeks. At the end of 2 weeks, heparin is discontinued and 3 to 4 days later blood is obtained for the remaining hypercoagulable disorders, including proteins C and S and antithrombin deficiency, heparin cofactor II, APC-R, factors I, VIII, and XI, plasminogen, plasminogen activators, and plasminogen activator inhibitors.

If the patient is found to have one of the hypercoagulable conditions, he/she should be retested in several months to determine whether the disorder is persistent and, therefore, most likely familial. If it is found to be familial, the family of the patient should also undergo testing and counseling.

The patient and afflicted members of his/her family should receive thrombosis prophylaxis at the times of increased risk. The patient with a major, or 2 or more thromboembolic episodes, should receive long-term anticoagulation. Patients with hyperhomocystinemia should receive vitamin supplementation. Patients with HIT should avoid the sensitizing heparin and patients with protein C deficiency should be protected from warfarin-induced thrombosis.

SUMMARY

Most arterial thromboses have readily defined etiologies and most arterial reconstructive failures are due to technical mishaps. A few patients also have acquired or congenital abnormalities of their coagulation and/or fibrinolytic proteins or platelet function, which increase their risk for arterial thromboses and/or arterial reconstructive failures. These patients should be tested for hypercoagulable disorders and treated appropriately if one is detected.

REFERENCES

1. Bick RL, Kaplan H. Syndromes of thrombosis and hypercoagulability. Congenital and acquired causes of thrombosis. *Med Clin North Am.* 1998;82:409–458.
2. Stassen JM, Nystrom A. A historical review of hemostasis, thrombosis, and antithrombotic therapy. *Ann Plast Surg.* 1997;39:317–329.
3. Roald HE, Lyberg T, Dedichen T, et al. Collagen-induced thrombosis formation in flowing nonanticoagulate human blood from habitual smokers and nonsmoking patients with severe peripheral atherosclerotic disease. *Arterioscler Thromb Vasc Biol.* 1995;15:128–132.
4. Manoussakis MN, Tzioufas AG, Silis MP, et al. High prevalence of anticardiolipin and other autoantibodies in a healthy elderly population. *Clin Exp Immunol.* 1987;69:557–565.
5. Koike T. Antiphospholipid antibodies in arterial thrombosis. *Ann Med.* 2000;32(Suppl 1):27–31.

6. Calaitges JG, Liem TK, Spadone D, et al. The role of heparin-associated antiplatelet antibodies in the outcome of arterial reconstruction. *J Vasc Surg*. 1999;29:785–786.

7. Mudaliar JH, Liem TK, Nichols WK, et al. Lepirudin is a safe and effective anticoagulant for patients with heparin-associated antiplatelet antibodies. *J Vasc Surg*. 2001;34:17–20.

8. Levy PJ, Hornung CA, Haynes JL, et al. Lower extremity ischemia in adults younger than forty years of age: a community-wide survey of premature atherosclerotic arterial disease. *J Vasc Surg*. 1994;19:873–881.

9. Ray SA, Rowley MR, Loh A, et al. Hypercoagulable states in patients with leg ischemia. *Br J Surg*.1994;81:811–814.

10. Allaart CF, Poort SR, Rosendaal FR, et al. Increased risk of venous thrombosis in carriers of hereditary protein C deficiency defect. *Lancet*. 1993;341:134–138.

11. Broekmans AW, Veltkamp JJ, Bertina RM. Congenital protein C deficiency and venous thromboembolism: a study of three Dutch families. *N Engl J Med*. 1983;309:340–344.

12. Eldrup-Jorgensen J, Flanigan DP, Brace L, Sawchuk AP, Mulder SG, Anderson CP, et al. Hypercoagulable states and lower limb ischemia in young adults. *J Vasc Surg*. 1989;9: 334–341.

13. Griffin JH, Evatt B, Wideman C, et al. Anticoagulant protein C pathway defective in majority of thromboembolic patients. *Blood*. 1993;82:1989–1993.

14. Bick RL. Sticky platelet syndrome: A common cause of unexplained arterial and venous thrombosis. *Clin Appl Thrombosis/Hemostasis* 1998;4:77–81.

15. Poort SR, Rosendaal FR, Reitsma PH, Bertina RM. A common genetic variation in the 3'-untranslated region of the prothrombin gene is associated with elevated plasma prothrombin levels and an increase in venous thrombosis. *Blood* 1996;88:3698–3703.

16. Ferraresi P, Marchetti G, Legnani C, et al. The heterozygous 20210 G/A prothrombin genotype is associated with early venous thrombosis in inherited thrombophilias and is not increased in frequency in artery disease. *Arterioscler Thromb Vasc Biol*. 1997;17:2418–2422.

17. Bertina RM. Factor V Leiden and other coagulation factor mutations affecting thrombotic risk. *Clin Chem*. 1997;43:1678–1683.

18. Rosendaal FR, Siscovick DS, Schwartz SM, et al. A common prothrombin variant (20210 G to A) increases the risk of myocardial infarction in young women. *Blood*. 1997;90: 1747–1750.

19. Kang SS, Wong PW, Malinow MR. Hyperhomocyst(e)inemia as a risk factor for occlusive vascular disease. *Annu Rev Nutr*. 1992;12:279–298.

20. Tollefsen DM. Laboratory diagnosis of antithrombin and heparin cofactor II deficiency. *Semin Thromb Hemost*. 1990;16:162–168.

21. Ray SA, Rowley MR, Loh A, et al. Hypercoagulable states in patients with leg ischemia. *Brit J Surg*. 1994;81:811–814.

22. Donaldson MC, Weinberg DS, Belkin M, et al. Screening for hypercoagulable states in vascular surgical practice: a preliminary study. *J Vasc Surg*. 1990;11:825–831.

23. Flinn WR, McDaniel MD, Yao JS, et al. Antithrombin III deficiency as a reflection of dynamic protein metabolism in patients undergoing vascular reconstruction. *J Vasc Surg*. 1984;1:888–895.

24. Levy PJ, Gonzalez MF, Hornung CA, et al. A prospective evaluation of atherosclerotic risk factors and hypercoagulability in young adults with premature lower extremity atherosclerosis. *J Vasc Surg*. 1996;23:36-43, discussion 43–45.

25. de Jong S. Hyperhomocysteinaemia in patients with peripheral arterial occlusive disease. *Clin Chem & Lab Med*. 2001;39:714–716.

26. Lipski DA, Ernst CB. Visceral Ischemic Syndromes. In: Moore WS, ed. *Vascular Surgery: A Comprehensive Review*. 5th edition, Philadelphia: W.B. Saunders Company; 1998:543–553.

27. Koutroubakis IE, Sfiridaki A, Theodoropoulou A. Role of acquired and hereditary thrombotic risk factors in colon ischemia of ambulatory patients. *Gastroenterology*. 2001;121: 561–565.

28. Chamouard P, Grunebaum L, Wiesel ML. Prevalence and significance of anticardiolipin antibodies in Crohn's disease. *Dig Dis Sci*. 1994;39(7):1501–1504.

29. Cappell MS, Seibold JR. Mesenteric thrombosis associated with anticardiolipin antibodies in a patient with systemic lupus erythematosus. *Am J Gastroenterol.* 1992;87(4):520–522.
30. Hughes GRV, Khamashta MA. The antiphospholid syndrome. *J Royal Coll Physicians London.* 1994;28:301–304.

6

Erectile Dysfunction in Atherosclerosis: An Overview

Thom W. Rooke, MD

Erectile dysfunction is a common problem for men at and beyond middle age, especially for those with atherosclerosis.[1] Until recently, therapy for this problem was inefficient, cumbersome, and/or otherwise unacceptable. However, the development of an oral agent (sildenafil, Viagra™) has revolutionized the treatment of this condition. The following will deal with several basic questions regarding erectile dysfunction and its treatment.

WHAT IS ERECTILE DYSFUNCTION?

Erectile dysfunction (ED) is commonly defined as ". . . the inability to obtain and maintain an erection that is satisfactory for sexual activity . . ." It replaces the term "impotence," which was formerly used to describe this condition. Unfortunately, "impotence" is an imprecise word; it has been used in conjunction with erectile failure, premature ejaculation, sterility, and other dissimilar conditions. The new terminology offers a more accurate description of the problem and avoids some of the negative connotations and confusion occasionally associated with the former term.*

---

*The demise of the word "impotent" also stems in no small part from its similarity to the word "important." Sophomoric "humor" involving the substitution of "impotent" for "important" has been horribly overused by bad comics, floundering late-night television hosts, and medical speakers trying desperately to get a cheap laugh from their audience during an out-of-town lecture. The prospect of a person saying—in a slow mock Arkansas drawl—the sentence "President Clinton is a very im-po-tent man . . ." is now thankfully as passé as the word "impotent" itself.

HOW COMMON IS ERECTILE DYSFUNCTION?

The prevalence of erectile dysfunction in men is surprisingly high. The Massachusetts Male Aging Study on Impotence was a community-based, observational survey of men (aged 40–70 years) conducted in the greater Boston area between 1987 and 1989.[2] It revealed that erectile dysfunction is a major health concern among many otherwise healthy men. In this study of 1,290 male patients, 40-year-old men had a roughly 40% incidence of partial or complete erectile dysfunction; this incidence increased by approximately 10% each decade, reaching 70% for men aged 70 years. Complete erectile dysfunction was present in 5% of 40-year-old subjects, and tripled to 15% in those who were 70.

After correction for age, a correlation was noted between the incidence of erectile dysfunction and heart disease, hypertension, diabetes, and cigarette smoking—all of which are classic risk factors for and/or associates of systemic atherosclerosis.

HOW DOES AN ERECTION OCCUR?

A complete discussion of normal erectile physiology is beyond the scope of this work. Briefly, the arterial supply to the penis[3] has both a superficial and deep component; the superficial portion arises from the femoral arteries via the inferior external pudendal artery, and the deep system (which is the major component) arises from the terminal branches of the internal iliac artery via the internal pudendal artery. The superficial and deep systems interconnect. These arteries and their branches supply, among other things, the spongy *corpora cavernosa* within the shaft of the penis. The *cavernosa* are paired structures that consist of extensive interlinking vascular sinuses enclosed within a tough, non-elastic tissue called the *tunica albuginea*.

Erection is accomplished by vasodilation of small penile blood vessels, including the arterioles and sinuses. As these vessels dilate, blood enters and fills the cavernous spaces within the *corpus cavernosum*. The small veins that drain this tissue become compressed as the sinuses/sinusoids expand, creating a situation in which blood enters the *corpus cavernosum* faster than it can exit. The *cavernosum* fills with blood and the penis becomes erect. Contraction of muscular elements within the penis enables intracavernosal blood pressure to reach (or even exceed) systemic blood pressure.

The penis is innervated by autonomic nerves. *Parasympathetic* nerves control vascular tone, arteriolar blood flow, and erection. The *sympathetic* nerves control ejaculation.* The psychological stimuli for triggering autonomic nerve activation are complex, highly variable, and often difficult to understand; conventional examples may be found at the airport newsstand,[4] although some individuals require stimuli that are far more unorthodox.[5]

Parasympathetic stimulation leads to the production of vasodilators in and around the smooth muscle of the penile arterioles and sinuses.[6] The major vasodilator is *nitric oxide* (NO), which acts as the biological endothelium-derived relaxing factor (EDRF). Nitric oxide enters the vascular smooth muscle and stimulates guanylate cyclase; this increases the production of cyclic guanosine monophosphate (cGMP). Increased

---

Medical students are sometimes taught to remember the relationship between **P**arasympathetic nerves (erection control) and **S**ympathetic nerves (ejaculation control) by recalling the mnemonic "**P**oint and **S**hoot."

intracellular levels of cGMP reduce the cytosolic calcium concentration, which triggers vascular smooth muscle relaxation. Cyclic GMP is subsequently degraded by a unique *phosphodiesterase* (PDE type 5), which is relatively specific for the smooth muscle of the *corpus cavernosum* and penile arteries, although small amounts also exist in many other vascular beds.

In summary, penile erection occurs when appropriate stimuli (including parasympathetic nerve activation caused by conscious and unconscious factors) lead to the production of local vasodilators, including nitric oxide. These vasodilators relax the smooth muscle of the penile arterioles and vascular sinuses, causing increased arterial flow into the sinuses. As the blood volume within the *corpus cavernosum* expands, the small venules that drain the sinuses become (relatively) pinched off and obstructed. This leads to gradual engorgement of the sinuses, elevation of intrasinus blood pressure, and erection of the penis. A steady-state is eventually reached within the *corpus cavernosum* between arterial inflow and venous outflow. Erection quits when the stimulus driving vasodilation declines, which allows phosphodiesterase type 5 to degrade cGMP faster than it is produced. As arterial inflow falls and venous outflow increases, a new steady-state is achieved with the penis in a flaccid state.

WHAT CAUSES ERECTILE DYSFUNCTION?

There may be several etiologies for erectile dysfunction.

Psychological

Psychological factors may be the most common and range from minor anxiety states to full-blown psychoses. Fatigue is a frequent issue. Even minor distractions (ie, the kids are still awake in the next room, the baseball game is on, it's been a bad day on Wall Street, etc.) can affect erectile function.

Neurological

Neurological causes include central nervous system abnormalities, spinal cord injuries, peripheral neuropathies (including diabetes), and a host of others.

Endocrine

Endocrine causes, including pituitary and gonadal abnormalities (as well as less common causes such as thyroid, parathyroid, or adrenal disorders) can adversely affect erectile function. These problems are especially important to identify because they are potentially treatable.

Vascular

Vascular abnormalities, especially those attributable to atherosclerosis,[7] are a common and potentially curable cause of erectile dysfunction. Unfortunately, operations to improve potency by revascularizing the pelvis and/or penis may themselves produce erectile dysfunction, presumably by causing nerve damage at the time of surgery.

Other

Other causes, including drug side effects, diabetes, excessive alcohol intake,* heart disease, cigarette smoking,[8] aging, and many other factors can contribute to erectile dysfunction.

WHAT TREATMENTS ARE AVAILABLE FOR ERECTILE DYSFUNCTION?

Folk remedies for erectile dysfunction abound. Oysters, powdered rhinoceros horn, elixirs made from black bear viscera, and countless other foods or nutritional supplements are thought, in certain cultures, to enhance potency. Religious cures are advocated by some, while others seek the cure to erectile dysfunction through the use of enchanted potions,[9] magic, and witchcraft.[10]

When atherosclerosis or other forms of pelvic arterial disease are present, revascularization may improve erectile function. Bypass surgery involving the aortoiliac and/or internal iliac arteries can improve erectile function in certain individuals. More recently, PTA (with or without stents) has enabled revascularization to be performed less invasively and with less risk of damage to pelvic nerves. The potential ability to revascularize distal vessels (such as pudendal and penile arteries) with angioplasty techniques also exists.

In some cases mechanical techniques offer the only methods for achieving (or simulating) erectile function. *External scaffolding* devices that stretch and position the penis in a semi-physiological position have been tried. *Vacuum* devices[11] can be used to draw blood into the penis and cause passive engorgement and rigidity; the blood is "trapped" by positioning a tight-fitting ring around the base of the penis. The ring is removed following ejaculation, allowing the penis to drain and return to its flaccid state. *Silastic rods* can be implanted into the penis to produce a permanent semi-rigid state.[12] These rods can be bent (much like a Gumby™ doll) to approximate the desired shape and angulation necessary for intercourse. Implantable *inflatable prosthetic devices*, including various air bladders and cylinders, can allow the patient to achieve erection by inflating the penis on demand.[13] In many cases, the "pump" used to inflate the bladders can also be implanted beneath the skin.

It is possible to inject vasodilators directly into the *cavernosum* and produce erections. The most popular injectable materials are prostaglandins and/or other similar agents. These drugs are available in prepackaged kits that allow the individual to self-inject a pre-selected dose at an appropriate time. Although this approach is highly effective for many men, it is certainly inconvenient, occasionally painful, and not without side effects; these include the potential for infection, scarring, and other local problems. Adding insult to injury, a rare complication is the production of prolonged (lasting several hours) painful erections that may persist until the injected drug wears off.

---

*This is an especially curious phenomenon because alcohol can paradoxically enhance the desire for an erection while simultaneously inhibiting the physiological ability to obtain one. Some men have been frustrated by alcohol-induced erectile dysfunction; others have been spared from inappropriate and embarrassing (or even perhaps dangerous) sexual activity while "under the influence." Depending upon the circumstances, alcohol's inhibitory response on erectile function may truly be both a blessing and a curse.

WHAT IS SILDENAFIL AND HOW DOES IT WORK?

Sildenafil citrate (Viagra™) was originally developed and evaluated as a potential antianginal agent. According to folklore, investigational testing was discontinued because the drug appeared to be ineffective against angina. But despite the lack of demonstrable efficacy on angina, samples of the study drug continued to disappear (sometimes from locked facilities) after the studies were terminated. The mystery as to why an apparently ineffective drug would have people stealing it was solved when the investigators broadened the scope of their probe and began to inquire about the "unexpected" effects attributable to the study drug. It turned out that male subjects were experiencing a remarkable improvement in erectile function. Needless to say, there was renewed interest in sildenafil.

It was determined that the mechanism of action for sildenafil comes from its ability to selectively inhibit phosphodiesterase type 5.[14] As previously noted, this form of phosphodiesterase is relatively specific to vascular smooth muscle within the penile arteries and *corpus cavernosum*. When nitrous oxide generation stimulates guanylate cyclase to produce increased intracellular levels of cGMP, it is the job of phosphodiesterase type 5 to eventually catalyze the conversion of cGMP (a potent mediator of vasodilation) back to GMP (a non-vasoactive substance). Inhibition of phosphodiesterase type 5 by sildenafil inhibits this breakdown and thus raises intracellular levels of cGMP, which in turn augments smooth muscle relaxation and increases penile blood flow. The result is an enhancement of erectile capability.

The efficacy of sildenafil citrate appears to be dose related.[15] Roughly 25% of men report improved erections when given a placebo; this increases to 63% in men taking 25 mg of sildenafil, 74% in those taking 50 mg, and 82% in those taking 100 mg.[16] The usual dose is 25 to 100 mg, with larger doses used only if inadequate responses occur to lower dosages.

Surprisingly, the effectiveness of sildenafil appears to be relatively independent of the cause of erectile dysfunction. Patients with erectile dysfunction caused by *depression*,[17] *hypertension*,[18] or *spinal cord damage*[19] will respond to oral sildenafil in 70 to 80% of cases. Reduced—but still significant—response rates to sildenafil (40 to 60%) are seen when the etiology is due to *diabetes* or *radical surgical prostatectomy*.[16]

WHAT ARE THE SIDE EFFECTS OF SILDENAFIL?

Nitrate use is an absolute contraindication to sildenafil![20] The purported mechanism of action of sildenafil (i.e., an augmentation of the effects of nitrous oxide) explains why sildenafil might dangerously potentiate the effects of exogenous nitrate administration (which also exerts its effect through elevated nitrous oxide levels). Other generally accepted relative contraindications to sildenafil include: the presence of acute coronary ischemia (even when patients are not on nitrates), congestive heart failure, low blood pressure, low fluid volume status, complicated multidrug antihypertensive regimens, the simultaneous use of other drugs such as erythromycin or diltiazem which may interfere with sildenafil metabolism, or medical conditions such as liver or renal disease which may affect drug metabolism.

Despite the worrisome list of side effects and contraindications, the data suggest that sildenafil may be reasonably safe even for men with significant coronary disease *provided the appropriate warnings and contraindications are followed.*[21]

TABLE 6–1. Sildenafil use in patients with atherosclerosis obliterans/cardiovascular

* Concomitant nitrate use is *absolutely contraindicated*!
* Caution is indicated in patients with:
  —Atherosclerosis obliterans or significant coronary artery disease (even in patients *not* taking nitrates).
  —Congestive heart failure, hypotension, or volume depletion.
  —Complex and/or multidrug antihypertensive programs.
  —Impaired sildenafil metabolism (caused by renal/liver failure, or use of drugs such as cimetidine or diltiazem).
* Stable coronary artery disease is *not* an absolute contraindication to sildenafil use.

Not all side effects from Viagra™ are potentially life threatening.[22] Frequent "nuisance" side effects include headache (17%), flushing (10%), dyspepsia (7%), and nasal decongestion (4%). Another unusual side effect from Viagra is a *bluish tint to the vision*. It appears that cone cells within the retina contain a type of phosphodiesterase that can be inhibited by sildenafil. This inhibition alters retinal blood flow and/or metabolism and contributes to the perception of a blue tint to the visual fields.*

Perhaps the most unanticipated side effects from sildenafil include certain sociological and marital consequences. While restored or enhanced erectile function may improve many marriages and relationships, it also has been shown to introduce (or reintroduce) problems into others. Specifically, some partners do not appreciate the renewed interest in sex triggered by sildenafil use. In some cases, restoration or enhancement of erectile dysfunction has led to imprudent private and public behavior, marital infidelity, and even divorce.

WHAT HAS BEEN THE PUBLIC REACTION TO SILDENAFIL?

The public response to sildenafil has been impressive. FDA approval for the sale of this drug was granted on March 27, 1988. By the end of the following month, almost 600,000 prescriptions had been filled. Total sales are now measured in the billions of dollars. The drug was an immediate media craze, with hundreds of articles appearing in newspapers, magazines, and television. It was featured on the cover of *TIME* magazine,[23] and was a staple of late night television commentary. Media infatuation with sildenafil may have reached a peak when Pfizer hired Bob Dole to act as a spokesman for the drug; a number of well-known advertisements featuring the former presidential candidate were seen on television and in the printed media.

WHAT IS THIS GOING TO COST AND WHO IS GOING TO PAY FOR IT?

Sildenafil is not cheap. Some mail-order sites charge $10 or more for each tablet. Better values can, of course, be found, but the drug poses a potential payment burden for the individuals using it—and a potential payment nightmare for third party payers.

---

*This bizarre side effect seemingly reinforces the myth that "a connection exists between penile stimulation and visual impairment." In reality, there is no evidence that excessive or repeated sexual stimulation (including masturbation) will cause blindness or otherwise adversely affect vision.

Indeed, HMOs, major insurance companies, and Medicare continue to wrestle with the issue of reimbursement for sildenafil. At this time, there is no uniform national payment policy in effect with regard to this drug

DOES VIAGRA™ WORK FOR WOMEN?

It hasn't been proven. The Internet is full of positive anecdotal reports, and investigators are currently assessing whether sildenafil can augment some measurable parameters of female sexual response. Others remain unconvinced that these changes have any important effect on overall female sexual function.[24] Further study is necessary.

WHAT WILL HAPPEN IN THE FUTURE?

To paraphrase Yogi Berra, "The future is hard to predict . . . especially when it hasn't happened yet." It is certainly to be expected that other oral agents will eventually compete with sildenafil for the erectile dysfunction market. *Uprima* is a medication currently available in Europe. Unlike sildenafil, it works centrally by stimulating dopamine receptors in the hypothalamus and midbrain. Although its application to the FDA was withdrawn in 2000, it remains available in many other countries and can be purchased on the Internet.

Phentolamine (Vasomax) has been used in injectable form to treat erectile dysfunction and is currently undergoing U.S. evaluation as an oral agent (the oral form is already marketed in some countries such as Mexico and Brazil). Like Uprima, it acts on central nerves and can thus produce an effect much more quickly than an intracellular enzyme inhibitor such as sildenafil (Uprima and Vasomax can act in 15 to 20 minutes; sildenafil may take up to an hour). At this time, it remains uncertain when, if ever, these or other drugs will appear on the American market.

REFERENCES

1. NIH Consensus Development Panel on Impotence. *JAMA*. 1993; 270:83–90.
2. Feldman HA, Goldstein I, Hatzichristou DG, et al. Impotence and its medical and psychosocial correlates: results of the Massachusetts Male Aging Study. *J Urol*. 1994 Jan;151(1):54–61.
3. Shetty SD, Farah RN. Anatomy of erectile function. *Textbook of Erectile Dysfunction*. 1999;(3):25–29.
4. *Playboy Magazine*. Playboy Enterprises, Inc., 680 North Shore Drive, Chicago, Illinois, 60611.
5. Marilyn Manson. *Antichrist Superstar*. Interscope Records, 2220 Colorado Avenue, Santa Monica, California, 90404;1996.
6. Zusman RM. Cardiovascular data on sildenafil citrate: introduction. *Am J Cardiol*; 1999;83(5A):1C–2C.
7. Jackson G. Erectile dysfunction and cardiovascular disease. *Int J Clin Pract*. 1999 Jul-Aug.;53(5):36–38.
8. McVary KT, Carrier S, Wessells H. Smoking and erectile dysfunction: evidence based analysis. *J Urol*. 2001 Nov;166(5):1624–1632.
9. *Love Potion # 9*; The Searchers Greatest Hits; Written by Lieber/Stoller; Rhino Records;1985.
10. Pagen Educational Network. P.O. Box 586, Portage, Indiana, 46368.
11. Oakley N; Allen P; Moore KTH. Vacuum devices for erectile impotence. *Textbook of Erectile Dysfunction*. 1999;(34):371–381.

12. Mulcahy JJ. Unitary inflatable, mechanical, and malleable penile implants. *Textbook of Erectile Dysfunction*. 1999;(37):413–421.

13. Carson CC. Inflatable penile prostheses. *Textbook of Erectile Dysfunction*. 1999;(38):423–433.

14. Zusman RM. Cardiovascular data on sildenafil citrate: introduction. *Am J Cardiol*. 1999;83(5A):1C–2C.

15. Goldstein I, Lue TF, Padma-Nathan H, et al. Oral sildenafil in the treatment of erectile dysfunction. *N Engl J Med*. 1998 May 14;338(20):1397–1404.

16. Osterloh I, Eardley I, Carson CC, et al. Sildenafil: a selective phosphodiesterase 5 inhibitor for the treatment of erectile dysfunction. *Textbook of Erectile Dysfunction*. 1999;(26):285–308.

17. Price D. Silfenafil (Viagra™): efficacy in the treatment of erectile dysfunction (ED) in patients with common concomitant conditions. *Int J Impot Res*. 1998;1-:53, 254a.

18. Zusman RM, Prisant LM, Brown MJ. Effect of sildenafil citrate on blood pressure and heart rate in men with erectile dysfunction taking concomitant antihypertensive medication. Sildenafil Study Group. *J Hypertens*. 2000 Dec. 18;(12):1865–1869.

19. Holmgren E, Guiliano FG, Hutling C. Sildenafil (Viagra™) in the treatment of erectile dysfunction (ED) caused by spinal cord injury(SCI): a double-binded, placebo-controlled, flexible-dose, two-way crossover study. *Neurology*. 1998;in press.

20. Cheitlin MD, Hutter AM Jr., Brindis RG, et al. Use of sildenafil (Viagra™) in patients with cardiovascular disease. *J Am Coll Cardiol*. 1999 Jan; 33(1):273–282.

21. Arruda-Olson AM, Mahoney DW, Nehra A, et al. Cardiovascular effects of sildenafil during exercise in men with known or probable coronary artery disease. *JAMA*. 2002;287:719–725.

22. Morales A, Gingell C, Collins M, et al. Clinical safety of oral sildenafil citrate (Viagra™) in the treatment of erectile dysfunction. *Int J Impot Res*. 1998; 10:69–74.

23. *TIME Magazine*. May 4, 1998.

24. Kaplan SA, Reis RB, Kohn IJ, et al. Safety and efficacy of sildenafil in postmenopausal women with sexual dysfunction. *Urology*. 1999 Mar.;53(3):481–486.

7

Mechanical Pump in the Treatment of Chronic Limb-Threatening Ischemia

Paul S. van Bemmelen, MD and John J. Ricotta, MD

This chapter is concerned with treatment of chronic limb-threatening ischemia, as opposed to acute, or "acute on chronic" ischemia. Many chronic patients have diabetes and therefore, a significant part of the threat to the limb consists of severe infectious complications: cellulitis, osteomyelitis, and sepsis, which are outside of the scope of this chapter.

HISTORICAL PERSPECTIVE

The "condensation" of air to "command blood flow" with a manual piston device was already mentioned in the first volume of the Lancet[1] in 1835. Certainly, mechanical devices for the treatment of circulatory insufficiency are among the oldest modalities, preceded only by manual massage.

Even today, many patients with severe peripheral vascular disease will volunteer that they rub their leg to make it feel better. Early descriptions[2] of massage—for poor circulation—have one thing in common with early mechanical devices, namely they are both applied with the patient's torso in a completely upright position. As we will see in the following paragraphs on physiology, the upright position is an essential element for the hydrostatic increase in arterio-venous pressure difference. Figure 7–1 shows a late nineteenth century device, similar to the descriptions by Pierce.[3] Initially, these devices did not have a pneumatic bladder placed on the leg: the pumping was accomplished by passive dorso and plantar flexion of the ankle. This emptied the veins of the calf-muscle pump. Early twentieth century designs had soft rubber pads to rub the lower extremity, using electrical power to empty the veins. Devices in the 1930s were rigid (pyrex glass) boots, which allowed alternation between positive and negative pressure,[4] while observing the skin of the leg and foot.

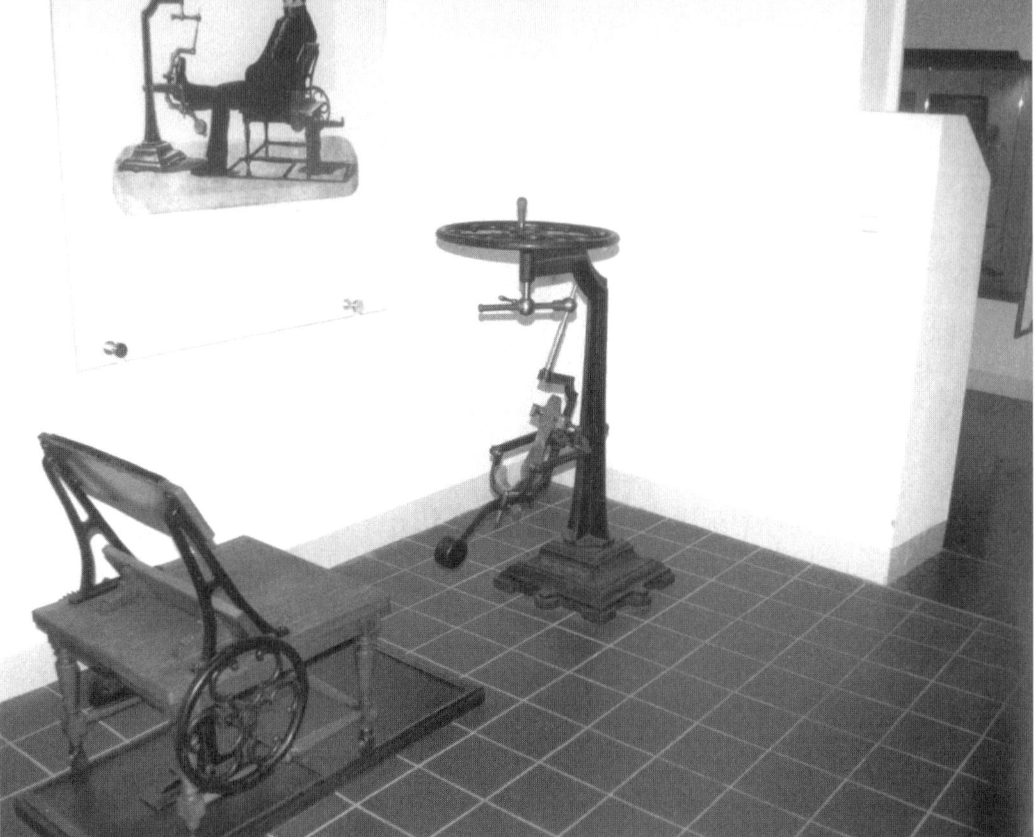

Figure 7–1. Passive ankle-flexion device for improvement of leg circulation; the patient was seated in an upright position. (Photograph by P. van Bemmelen.)

By 1948, a clear description[5] of the physiological principle of increased arterio-venous pressure difference had been published. An unexplained additional flow increase was mentioned in 1959, but the authors[6] blamed their plethysmographic method of flow measurement for this phenomenon, which we now ascribe to endothelial release of vaso-active substances. Indeed, the inherent delays of flow-measuring methods in that era, such as isotope wash-out, plethysmography, calorimetry, and arterio-venous oxygen extraction, prevented the design of compression devices with effective timing.

Flexible pneumatic bladder garments, placed around the lower extremity for the purpose of improving poor circulation were described in 1965. The pump devices at that time[7] consisted of relatively low capacity air pumps, coupled to large inflatable bladders. Therefore a long time was spent on inflating the bladder to a preset pressure. Deflation typically occurred using small and long tubing, which also took up a long amount of time. This is important, because as long as external pressure persists on the skin in excess of 20 mmHg, a decrease in skin perfusion occurs,[8] which negated any positive effects.

These historical efforts preceded the routine use of angiography for patient evaluation, so we can only guess at patient selection with regard to disease level and severity. The advent of "modern" vascular recontructions—femoral endarterectomy, later followed by femoro-popliteal bypass—led to loss of interest in compression therapy. Euphoria about the technical ability to bypass to very distal plantar arteries continued through the 1990s.

At the start of the 21st century, some skeptical minds questioned the hemodynamic impact of bypasses to extremely small unnamed branches at the metatarsal level. In the author's experience, even with patency of these grafts, new ischemic foot lesions can occur.

Other sobering facts are the decreased success rate after multiple repeated bypass surgeries and the absence of reduction in the overall incidence[9] of major amputations, which remain at about 74,000 per year in the US.

PHYSIOLOGICAL MECHANISMS

Post-compression flow increase was directly observed, with capillary microscopy, as early as 1879 in legs of frogs.[10] At that time, however, the distinction between post-occlusion hyperemia and post-compression flow increase was still unclear.

Two separate physiological mechanisms occur in compression treatment and result in acute increase in blood flow: First, due to the increased arterio-venous pressure difference in the (de-)compressed sitting patient and second, an acute vasodilation response. Each mechanism will be discussed in more detail below.

INCREASED ARTERIO-VENOUS PRESSURE DIFFERENCE

Measurement of blood pressure at the ankle or toe level is usually done with the patient in a supine position, therefore little thought is given to the pressure changes that occur due to the more physiological, erect body position.

On the venous side, direct pressure measurement has been commonly practiced, with the patient performing exercise. This resulted in normal values for ambulatory venous pressure, at foot level, in the range of 15–40 mmHg. Neither supine measurement, nor treadmill exercise resembles the most common activity for elderly patients with PVD, which is a passive, sitting position for most waking hours of the day. The effect of added hydrostatic pressure is best illustrated by the following set of diagrams, in which the capillary bed is depicted[11] as a connecting tube between a filled arterial reservoir and a less-filled venous reservoir (Figure 7–2A).

For simplicity, the familiar systolic pressure numbers are used rather than mean arterial pressures. In the supine subject, the venous pressure at the ankle is slightly higher than central venous pressure: about 10 mmHg. The driving force for flow through the connecting tube, that is, perfusion is the difference between arterial and venous pressure: $120 - 10 = 110$ mmHg.

Figure 7–2B illustrates the situation with severe arterial obstruction, in a supine patient. In this example the ankle pressure is reduced to 50 mmHg. Venous pressure remains unchanged, therefore the arterio-venous pressure difference is reduced to $50 - 10 = 40$ mmHg. This decreased perfusion pressure results in decreased flow across the connecting tube.

In the sitting position (Figure 7–3A), the venous pressure is higher than the ambulatory venous pressure during walking. Depending on patient height, the sitting venous pressure is about 60 mmHg when measured at the foot level. Arterial pressure

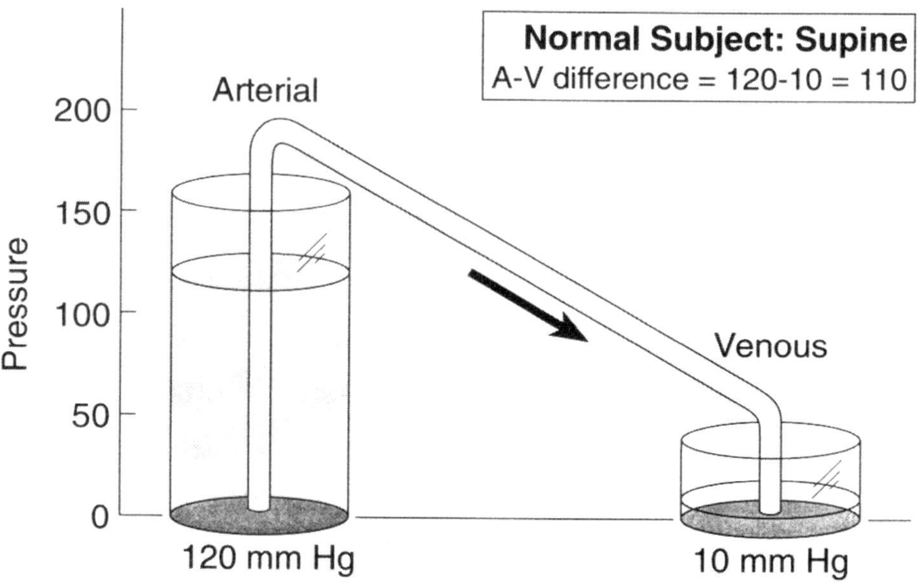

Figure 7–2A. Diagram representing leg perfusion flow in a normal supine subject. The systolic arterial ankle pressure is 120 mmHg; venous pressure is 10 mmHg. The arterio-venous pressure difference is 120 − 10 = 110 mmHg. Flow through the connecting tube, which represents the capillary bed is proportional to the arterio-venous pressure difference. Reproduced from van Bemmelen PS, *VASA* 2000;29:47–52, with permission from Springer Verlag.

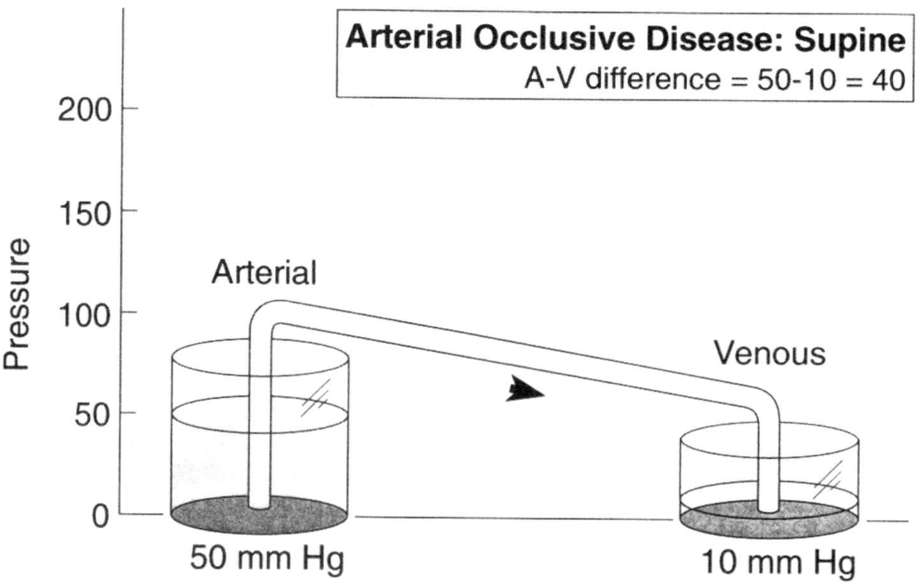

Figure 7–2B. Diagram representing the circulation in a supine patient with severe arterial obstruction and ankle pressure of 50 mmHg. Venous pressure unchanged at 10 mmHg, therefore an arterio-venous pressure difference of 50 − 10 = 40 mmHg and reduced flow through the connecting vascular bed.

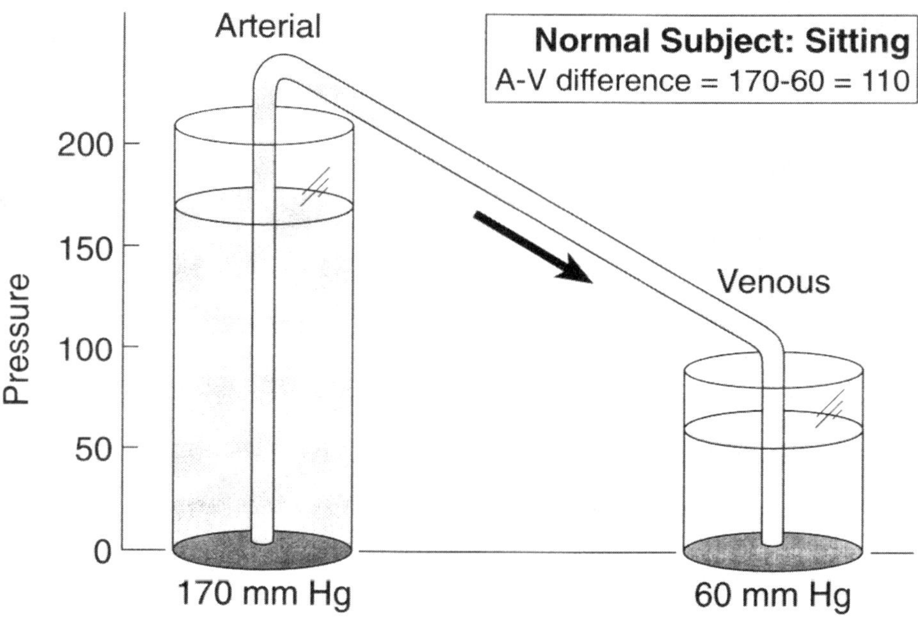

Figure 7–3A. Diagram representing the circulation in a normal subject in a sitting position. A hydrostatic fluid column of 50 mmHg is added to both the arterial and the venous side. The arterio-venous pressure difference equals 170 – 60 = 110 mmHg, which is unchanged from the supine example in Figure 2A. Reproduced from van Bemmelen PS, *VASA* 2000;29:47–52, with permission from Springer Verlag.

at the ankle is increased by the height of the hydrostatic column upon assuming the erect sitting position, that is roughly an addition of 50 mmHg. If we assume a systolic systemic pressure of 120, this adds up to 170 mmHg. The difference between arterial and venous pressure at foot level, or arterio-venous difference (170 – 60) is 110 mmHg, in the normal sitting subject. That is the same perfusion pressure as in the supine example shown in Figure 7–2A.

In the case of arterial obstruction, with the arterial ankle pressure reduced to 50 mmHg in a supine position, we need to add 50 mmHg upon assuming the sitting position (Figure 7–3B), that is 100 mmHg. With the sitting venous pressure unchanged at 60 mm Hg, there is a reduced arterio-venous pressure difference of 100 – 60 = 40 mmHg, with a corresponding reduction in the flow across the capillary network represented by the connecting tube. Note that this is the same reduced perfusion pressure as in the supine patient example shown in Figure 7–2B.

EFFECT OF A SINGLE EXTERNAL COMPRESSION

After a brief compression of the leg and foot with an external pressure that exceeds the venous pressure, the veins will be emptied, and in the presence of intact venous valves, the sitting venous pressure is reduced to about 15 mmHg.[12] For a limited time then, there will be a partial restoration of the arterio-venous pressure difference, in this example: 100 – 15 = 85 mmHg. Increased perfusion will result, due to this "afterload

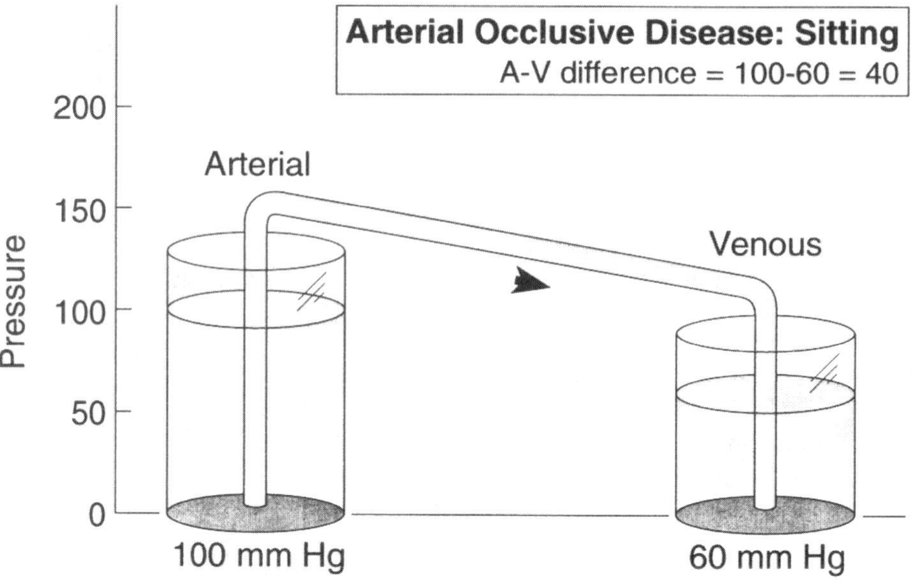

Figure 7–3B. Diagram representing the circulation in the patient with severe arterial occlusive disease (shown in Figure 7–2B) now placed in a sitting position. Again 50 mmHg was added to both the arterial and the venous side, leaving the arterio-venous pressure difference at 100 – 60 = 40 mmHg, which is equal to that in Figure 7–2B.

reduction" as depicted in Figure 3C. This flow augmentation will last until the veins have filled and venous pressure has returned to the initial precompression level. This takes about 14 seconds and at that point another compression is needed to keep the increased perfusion going.

RELEASE OF VASO-ACTIVE SUBSTANCES

This was first postulated based on human studies: Several authors[6, 13] noticed that the flow increase that could be obtained with compression exceeded what would be predicted on the basis of increase in arterio-venous pressure difference alone.

In the absence of vaso-active substance release, one would expect the resistance of the perfused vascular bed to remain constant. Under those conditions, Ohm's law would apply, that is, a doubling in arterio-venous mean pressure difference would result in a doubling of the volume flow. Instead, a 6-fold increase in volume flow has been measured by duplex[13] in normal volunteers. In humans, it is difficult to separate the effect of endothelial dysfunction with regard to nitric oxide release, from the flow restriction due to luminal size reduction, as both of these occur in patients with clinical manifestations of PVD. The short half-life of nitric-oxide and its local effect on neighboring cells makes direct measurements difficult. The conventional wisdom that vasodilation in ischemic legs is already maximal has been refuted by studies on the effect of prostaglandins in critically ischemic legs.[14]

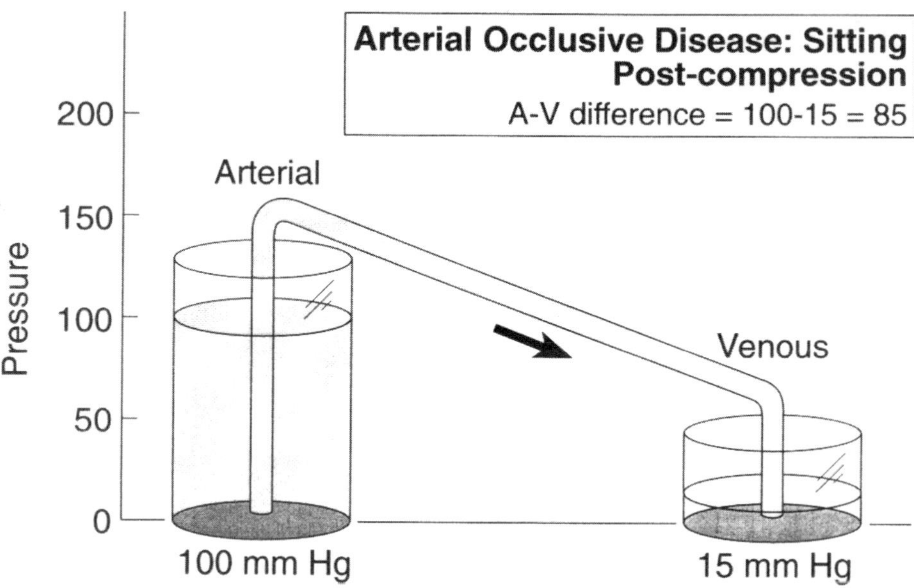

Figure 7–3C. Diagram representing the circulation in the same patient with arterial obstruction as in Figure 7–3B, upon emptying of the venous system with an external compression device, which reduces venous pressure to 15 mmHg. The resulting arterio-venous pressure difference equals 100 – 15 = 85 mmHg, which is more than double compared to Figure 7–3B, and this results in increased flow through the connecting tube, which represents the capillary bed.

ANIMAL STUDIES

Studies in rats with direct observation of the arterioles in the cremaster muscle, have shown a distant systemic vasodilation, in response to intermittent limb compression.[15] The response is shear-stress dependent, rather than related to the pressure level.

This means that the rate of pressure increase is paramount: slow gradual compression has no effect, which explains why older devices, essentially air compressors, were never very successful. A rapid pressure rise (within 0.3 seconds) can be obtained by incorporating a storage tank for compressed air into the device.

Further evidence that the vasodilator response is mediated by nitric oxide was obtained by complete blocking of the vasodilation with mono-methyl-L-Arginine, an inhibitor of nitric oxide synthase.[16]

IN VITRO STUDIES

Rhythmic squeezing of isolated saline-perfused rabbit arterial segments resulted in increased EDRF release as assessed by assay of guanylate cyclase activity.[17] Other basic scientists[18] have been able to elucidate some of the molecular biological mechanisms by subjecting cultured endothelial cells to various forms of mechanical stress. Flowing medium results in a specific orientation of endothelial cells. Repetitive deformation of the cytoskeleton results in mRNA increase for NO synthase. These changes can be observed after relatively short (30 minutes) periods of shear-stress application.

CLINICAL STUDIES

The first duplex time-velocity display, in the popliteal artery of sitting PVD patients,[13] showing increased systolic and diastolic flow velocities, in response to rapid calf compression was published in 1994 (Figure 7–4). This study looked at the optimal pressure levels for compression and whether correlations existed between severity of disease by ankle-brachial pressure index or toe pressure and the post-compression flow augmentation. Based on these findings, an automatically timed cuff inflator with built-in air tank was developed: the arterial assist device (ACI Medical, CA).

After this device became available, several authors[19,20] confirmed the earlier findings in other groups of volunteers. Delis[21] used the device on claudicants and patients with infra-inguinal bypass grafts and found increased volume flow in the grafts.

Increased skin perfusion at the toe level, by Laser Doppler flux-metry, had been described,[22] in response to foot compression alone, in 1993. The same was found by Eze[19] with combined calf and foot compression. A graphic LDF-time display, obtained at the dorsum of the forefoot in ischemic legs, before and during treatment with the arterial assist device was published[11] in the year 2000 (Figure 7–5). Lastly, an increase in capillary red blood cell velocity from 20 to 128 mm/sec (p<0.05) was found at the University of Amsterdam.[23]

The first long-term study in patients[24] for limb salvage was published in 2001. This study consisted of 14 critically ischemic legs, which were not candidates for reconstruction. The limbs included had toe pressure <35 mmHg and 13 of the legs had tissue loss at the forefoot, prior to the start of treatment.

Seven of the limbs had no visible run-off vessels on digital subtraction angiography. In 5 patients, no usable vein conduit could be identified. Nine legs had previous failed ipsilateral bypass (mean number of prior bypasses: 2.0). Three patients were considered to be in too poor general condition to undergo surgery.

The treatment protocol was for a 3-month period; limb salvage occurred in 9 legs (70%) at a maximum follow-up of 2.5 years. Figure 7–6 shows the increase in PVR amplitudes in the 14 legs and Figure 7–7 shows a patient example.

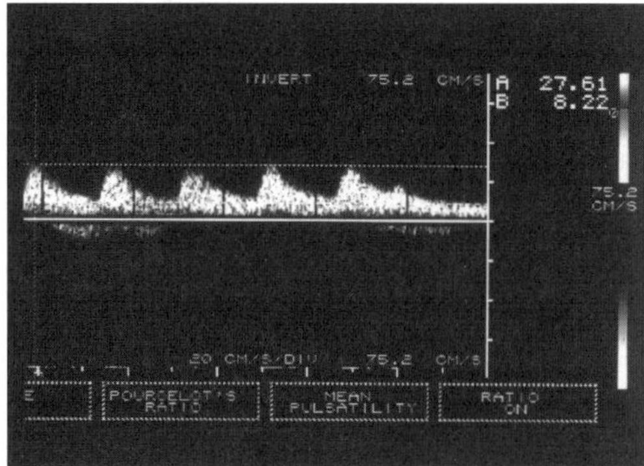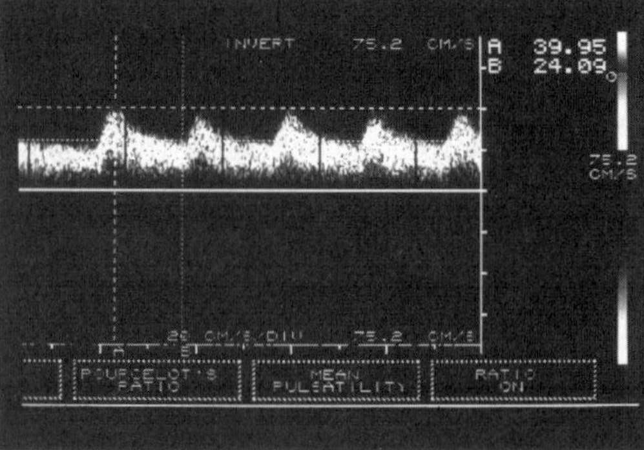

Figure 7–4. Left: Resting flow signal in popliteal artery of seated patient with rest pain and foot ulcer, ABI of 0.3 and toe pressure of 0 mmHg. Signal is mono-phasic with peak systolic velocity of 27.6 cm/sec; end diastolic velocity of 8 cm/sec. Right: Same artery after brief compression of the calf with 120 mmHg external pressure in sitting position. Peak systolic velocity increased to 39.9 cm/sec, and end diastolic velocity increased 3 times to 24 cm/sec. Reproduced from van Bemmelen. *J Vasc Surg.* 1994;19:1052–8, with permission from Mosby.

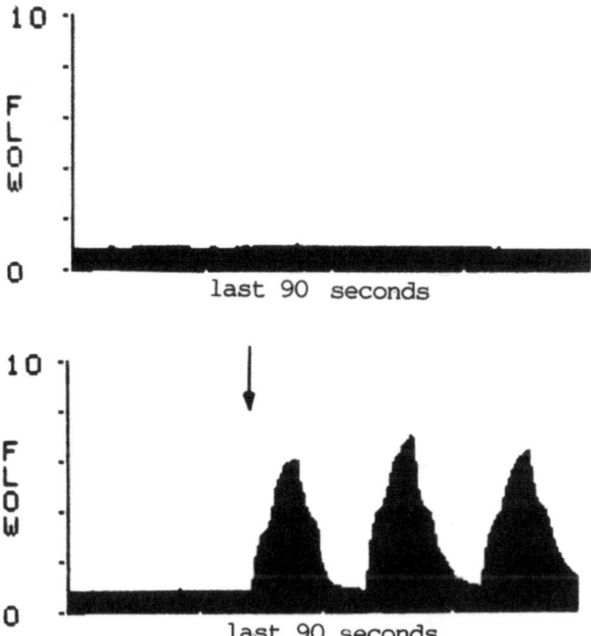

Figure 7–5. Top: Laser-Doppler signal obtained on the dorsum of chronically ischemic foot, shown by angiography to have small vessel disease below the level of the knee (sitting position). Bottom: The arrow indicates activation of the compression device (3 cycles). Reproduced from van Bemmelen. *VASA*. 2000;29:47–52, with permission from Springer Verlag.

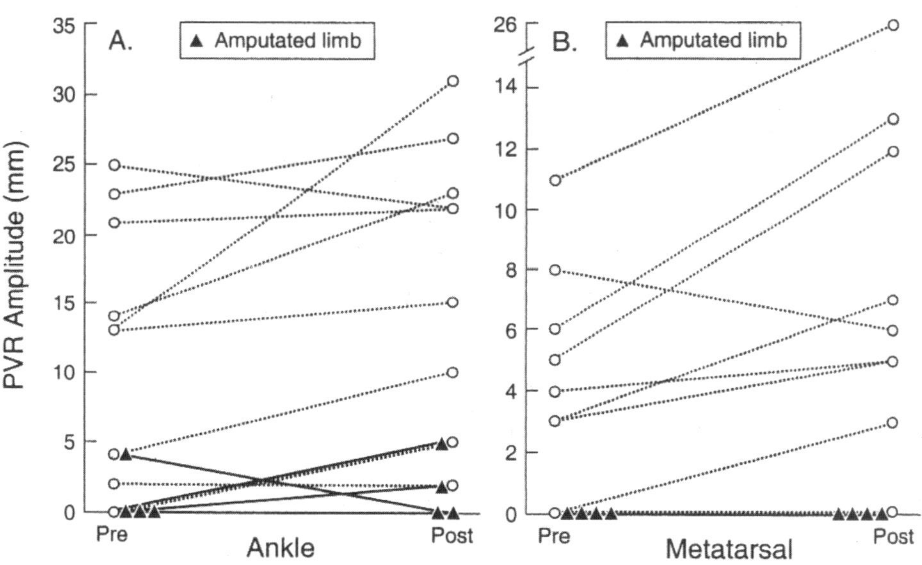

Figure 7–6. Pulse Volume Recording (PVR®, Healthwatch/ Life Sciences Cambridge, Vista, CA) amplitudes at the ankle **(A)** and metatarsal level **(B)** in 14 diseased legs, before and after treatment. Reproduced from van Bemmelen, *Arch Surg*. 2001;136:1280–5, with permission from American Medical Association.

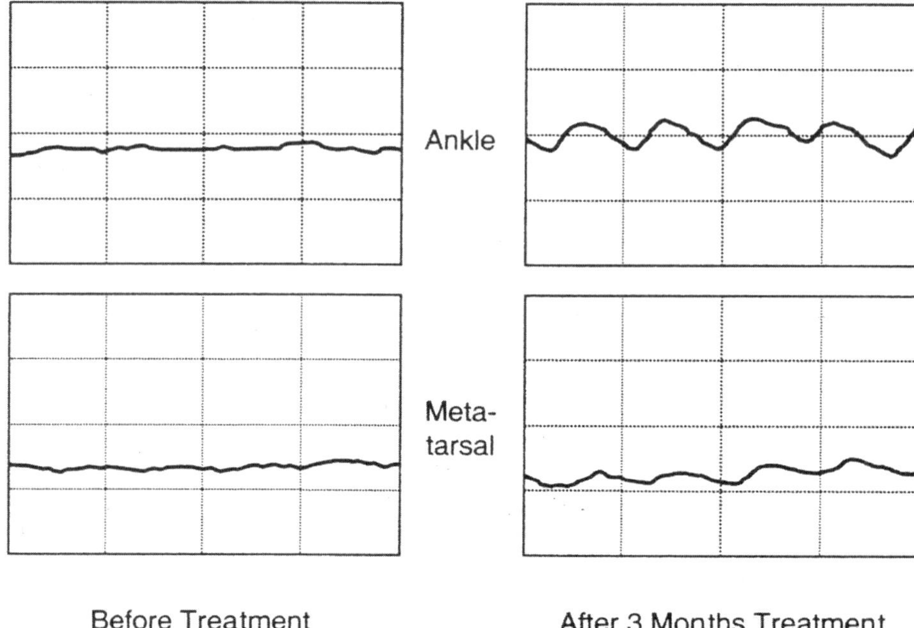

Figure 7–7. Patient example: Pulse volume recording of one of the legs at the ankle **(A)** and metatarsal **(B)** levels before and after 3 months of ArtAssist® treatment. Increase in amplitudes is evident. Reproduced from van Bemmelen, *Arch Surg.* 2001;136:1280–5, with permission from American Medical Association.

Compliance with the compression treatment was associated with lower incidence of below-knee amputation (Figure 7–8). Patients undergoing amputation used the device only for 1.14 hours per day, while patients not undergoing amputation used their device for 2.38 hours a day. Both groups had been instructed to use the device for 4 hours a day; compliance was monitored by an hour counter hidden inside the device. Similar encouraging findings were subsequently reported from Canada on 33 limbs.[25]

Angiographic improvement has been noted in some cases.[26] Repeated arteriography is rarely performed once a patient has been relegated to non-operative treatment. In young patients, it may be worthwhile to repeat arteriography, in order to consider the chances of success of partial foot amputations. TcO_2 measurements were not found to be of much predictive value in these situations as they were noted to change over time in our patients.

PRACTICAL CONSIDERATIONS FOR DAILY USE

Patient Selection

During a 2-year period of clinical application, we found approximately the same number of patients suitable for compression treatment as the number that was suited for primary amputation. Bedridden nursing home patients are not able to sit for the treatment. After severe stroke, the motivation to preserve a non-functioning limb may be absent in the patient. Sometimes, the patient's family is more concerned about limb loss than the patient. When the patient has to rely on others to apply the cuffs to the

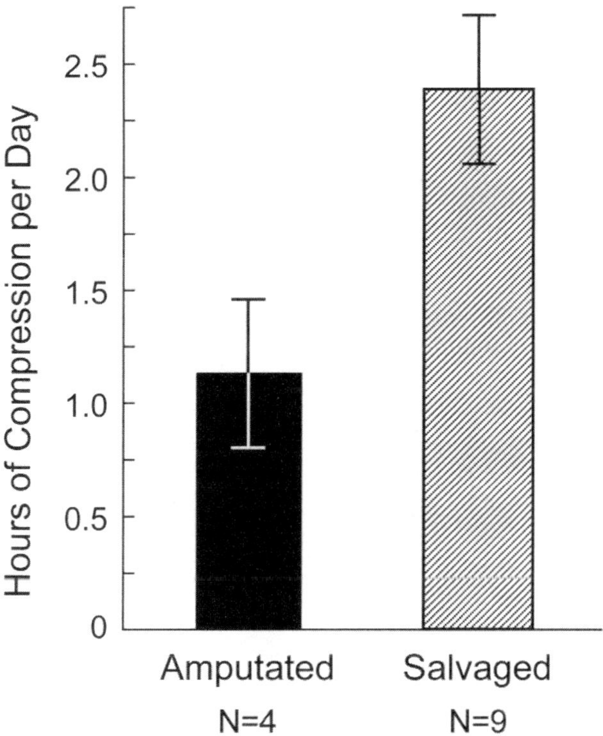

Figure 7–8. Mean (±SE) number of actual hours of compression applied per day in amputated versus salvaged legs, based on hour counter readings. Reproduced from van Bemmelen, *Arch Surg.* 2001;136:1280–5, with permission from American Medical Association.

leg and foot, the compliance is often less than optimal. This was confirmed with the use of an hour counter hidden inside the device. Therefore, the optimal candidate for compression therapy is still independent, but not suitable for revascularization due to poor anatomy, unsuitable conduit or increased operative risk.

The extent of the necrosis at the beginning of the treatment is relevant, as it takes about 2 months to obtain a measurable increase in collateral flow. When dry necrosis is limited to 1 or 2 toes and has progressed slowly, that is over several months prior to presentation, the chances are good that 2 to 3 months of compression treatment can be completed, before wet gangrene involves the entire foot. Unfortunately, sometimes, complete necrosis of the hallux has occurred within 1 week of the first onset of symptoms and the prospects for limb salvage in those cases can be bleak.

Often an area of dry necrosis is surrounded by redness, which can look like active inflammation. A diagnosis of infection-contra-indicating compression-should not be made lightly. If the redness disappears with assumption of a horizontal position, it may just be dependent rubor. Persistent redness, especially when combined with tenderness of the red area, elevated white count, and unstable blood-glucose, point to progressive infection. Usually, dry necrosis that has advanced beyond the MTP joints, does not stay dry for very long (Figure 7–9A). At that point, removal of the dead tissue with an amputation is indicated (Figure 7–9B). With necrosis limited to the toe level only, mild infection of the demarcation area can often be controlled, at least for a while, with antibiotics.

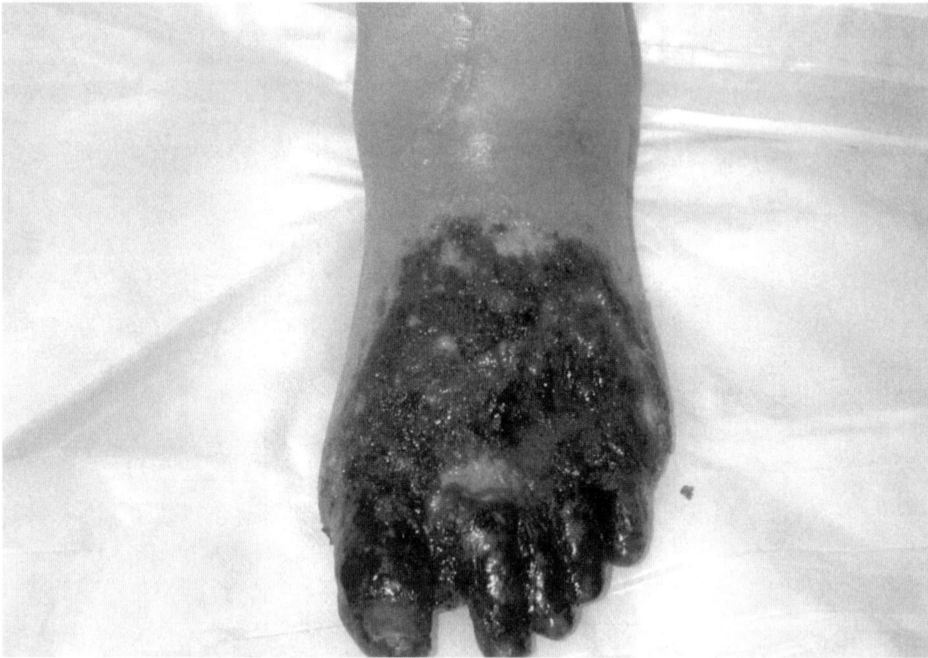

Figure 7–9A. Extensive forefoot necrosis, which has advanced proximal to the MTP joints. Open amputation was performed. Note scar from previously failed dorsalis pedis bypass. This patient received 9 months of compression therapy.

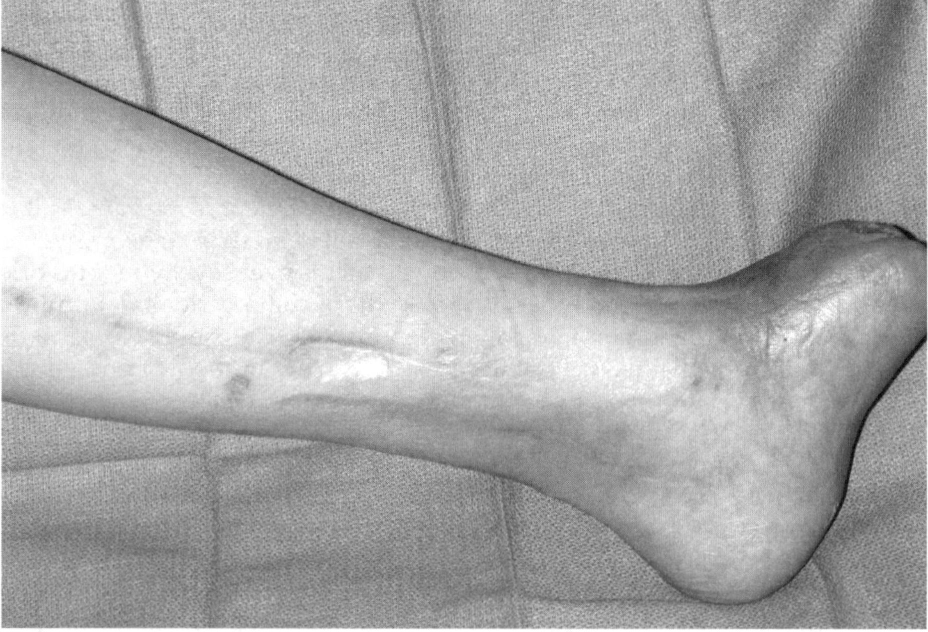

Figure 7–9B. Same patient, medial aspect: After patient developed collaterals and granulation tissue, she had a successful split skin graft. Note the scars of previously failed posterior tibial and peroneal bypasses. After patient resumed ambulation with a forefoot prosthesis, the compression treatment was stopped.

HEMODYNAMIC PARAMETERS

For the selection of critically ischemic legs, the arm blood pressure is a confounding variable, therefore ankle-brachial index should not be used. Perfusion is related to the difference in arterial and venous pressures, therefore the absolute (systolic) ankle pressure is more relevant. Unfortunately, calcification due to diabetes, renal failure, etc. can make this measurement unreliable. Absolute toe pressure is a valuable parameter. However, longitudinal studies with toe pressure are hampered by successive loss of toes, however. In our facility we rely largely on the PVR amplitude at the meta-tarsal level. Originally this recording was obtained with a calibrated air-plethysmograph made by one manufacturer (Life Sciences), which allowed comparison of amplitudes. The mean amplitude at metatarsal level in our patients was 2.9 mm, which was comparable to the 4.0 mm in a large series of patients prior to pedal bypass. Many new different automated systems are currently in use, with electronic calibration and different gain settings, which cannot be compared.

Our experience with trans-cutaneous oxygen measurement has been disappointing, in that large variability occurs within the same patient, depending on probe location. The measurements are time-consuming and can improve with resolution of edema and cellulites.[28]

Angiographical Criteria

It is almost impossible to find a consensus among vascular surgeons, regarding what constitutes an inoperable case of small vessel disease. Zealous surgeons can find unnamed outflow vessels, freeze-dried vein conduits, and other ways to bypass patients who may be in their tenth decade of life. On the other hand, few surgeons look forward to a fifth redo on the same leg. Clearly, the decision to forego further bypass attempts is always tailored to the individual case. Age, functionality, status of the other leg, etc. are all important considerations. Compression treatment at this time is not intended to replace bypass surgery, rather it may prevent, or mitigate some amputations. We do not offer the patient a choice between bypass or compression, instead we inform him/her that (repeat) bypass is not a worthwhile option if this is indeed the case. Only then, is he/she offered the option of compression therapy with the understanding that results of compression are not predictable.

There are no simple angiographic outflow scores that prove absence of operable vessels. Rather we can concentrate on what constitutes a technically satisfactory filling of pedal vasculature. Contrast "bolus-chasing" with delayed exposures is performed. The demonstration of clearly filled small, unnamed, pedal arteries, which are not continuous with an arch, or with the forefoot is more diagnostic than non-visualization (Figure 7–10). In the presence of obstruction proximal to the trifurcation level, it may be prudent to place selective catheters, either pre- or intra-operatively. Color ultrasound imaging of pedal vessels to assess their calcification may be helpful, as well as Magnetic Resonance Angiography (MRA) in selected situations.

Timing of Start of Treatment

Due to the inherent delays in effect of compression therapy when compared to bypass surgery, an early, complete work-up of the patient, presenting with relatively minor

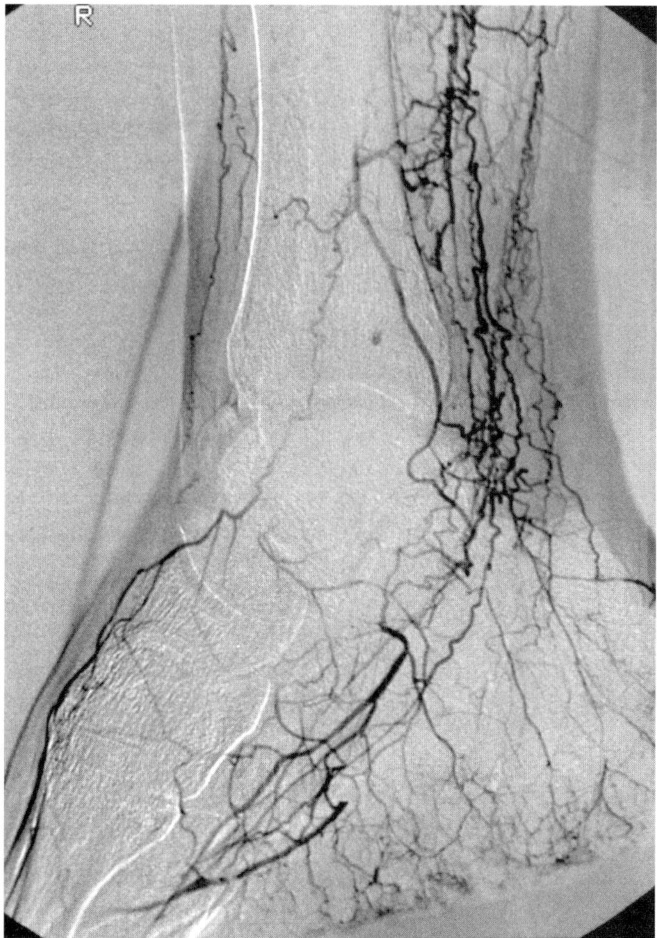

Figure 7–10. Example of technically satisfactory digital-subtraction arteriogram. Lateral view of the ankle and foot, demonstrating well-delineated pedal vessels, with multiple obstructions in a patient, without autogenous vein.

(superficial) looking foot lesions, is of the essence. Worsening of necrosis is common during the first month of compression therapy.

Duration of Treatment/Termination

A minimum of 2 months was required to see measurable increase in PVR amplitude in our patients, which is consistent with other studies. A "standard" treatment of 3 months gives the patient a tangible goal and may benefit compliance. In cases with extensive tissue loss, the threat may not be over after 3 months however, and the treatment was continued in a few cases up to 9 months in order to obtain complete wound closure (see Figure 7–9).

Earlier termination is often associated with poor patient compliance. The treatment typically improves ischemic rest pain, but for the patient with inflammation adjacent to necrotic tissues, the goal of complete pain relief may not be realistic, with compression alone. If the foot is too tender to compress, it is possible to avoid this area and compress the calf only in the initial weeks of treatment.

PRACTICAL APPLICATION FOR NECROSIS OF SPECIFIC AREAS

Forefoot/Toe Necrosis

Somewhat neglected by vascular surgeons, the hallux has a significant role for maintenance of balance and for "push off." Complete removal of the hallux often leads to hammer toe deformity of the second toe, therefore, if it is possible to obtain a viable amputation level in the phalanx itself, this is preferable to complete removal (Figure 7–11). The functional importance of the minor toes is not always clear, but consideration has to be given to inevitable shifts that occur by removing the spacer function of individual toes. As long as the necrosis is limited to the tip and body of the toe, which consist of skin, tendon, bone, and dissecated subcutaneous tissue, the dry necrosis can be treated conservatively for months. Soaking has to be avoided. The toes can be painted daily with Betadine solution (10% povidone-iodine swabsticks) and 2 x 2 gauze pads are placed in between toes to avoid humidity.

Adequate pain medication needs to be provided, especially for patients without neuropathy. Minor episodes of localized infection, manifested by odor or localized redness are treated with prolonged oral antibiotics and frequent visits. Compliance with the compressive regimen is essential and needs to be reinforced at every visit. The hour counter in the device should be inspected during the first couple of weeks to see if patients are indeed approaching the required number of treatment hours. It is not necessary to directly confront the patient about discrepancies, which are common. Rather, gentle pressure has to be exerted to continuously improve compliance.

Non-Healing Toe Amputation Site

Often, a hallux has been amputated as a "litmus test" to see if spontaneous healing can occur. Instead of healing, the wound dehisces, edges break down, and no trace of

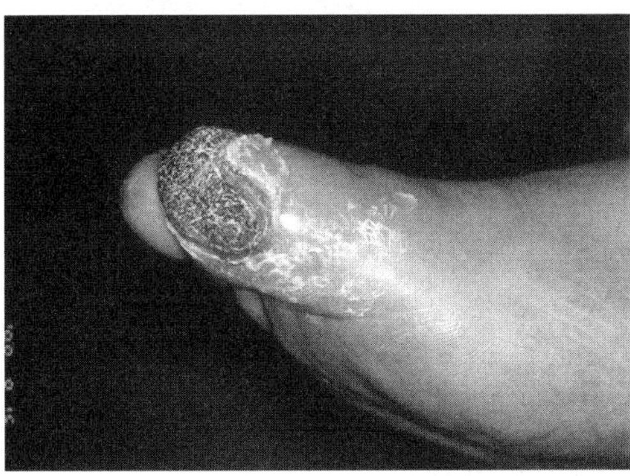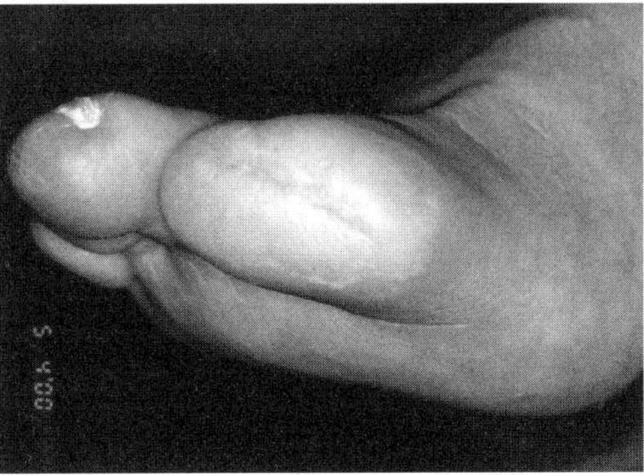

Figure 7–11. Left: Dry necrosis of the hallux tip. Patient started compression at this stage, for a 3-month period. Right: After the PVR® improved, the distal tip of the phalanx was removed, preserving hallux function.

granulation appears for at least a 6-week period. Gradually the metatarsal head becomes exposed amid a fibrous wound base and resection of the metatarsal head with debridement of the wound edges results in a repeat cycle of breakdown and bone exposure. Cultures of these defects usually grow a variety of organisms, which may require systemic antibiotic treatment depending on their virulence and whether the patient has diabetes. With compression treatment, it is important to maintain the status quo in these wounds for a long time, while collaterals develop. This can often be done with topical antibiotics and ointments, such as collagenase. With the improvement of metatarsal PVR amplitude after about 2 months, the base of the defect will begin to form pink granulation tissue. This progresses from the proximal aspect of the wound and ultimate healing occurs by wound contraction, resulting in a cleft-like scar (Figure 7–12).

Necrosis Over Metatarsal Head

This can occur as a separate problem, with an intact toe, for example over the lateral aspect of metatarsal V. This lateral area has minimal soft tissue coverage, which leads to early involvement of the bone. Ideally, the head of MT V should not be resected prior to compression treatment. This is similar to the approach when a bypass is feasible: first revascularize, resect later. A typical case is illustrated in Figure 7–13. Similar areas occur on the medial aspect of MT I.

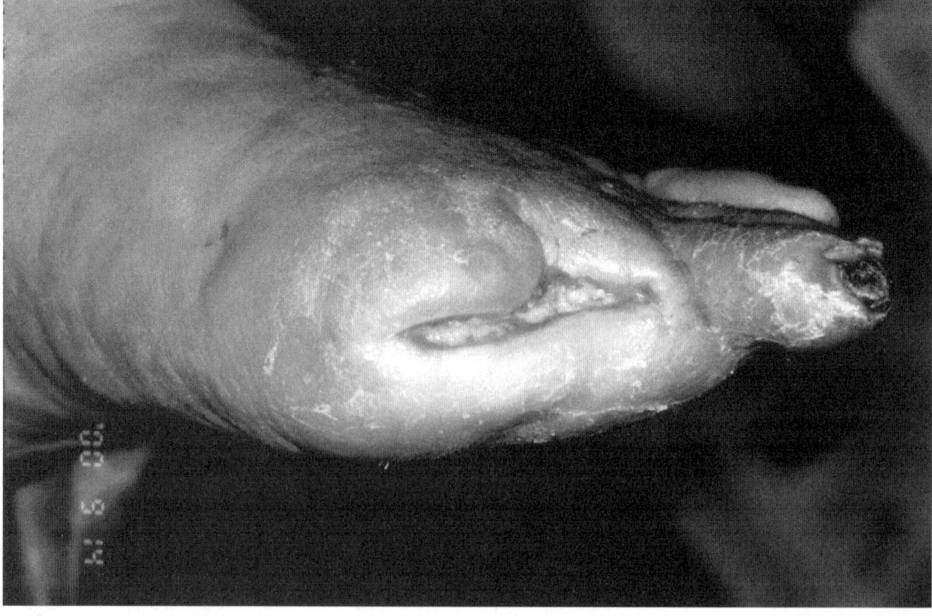

Figure 7–12A. Non-healing hallux amputation site, there is dry necrosis of the tip of the second toe.

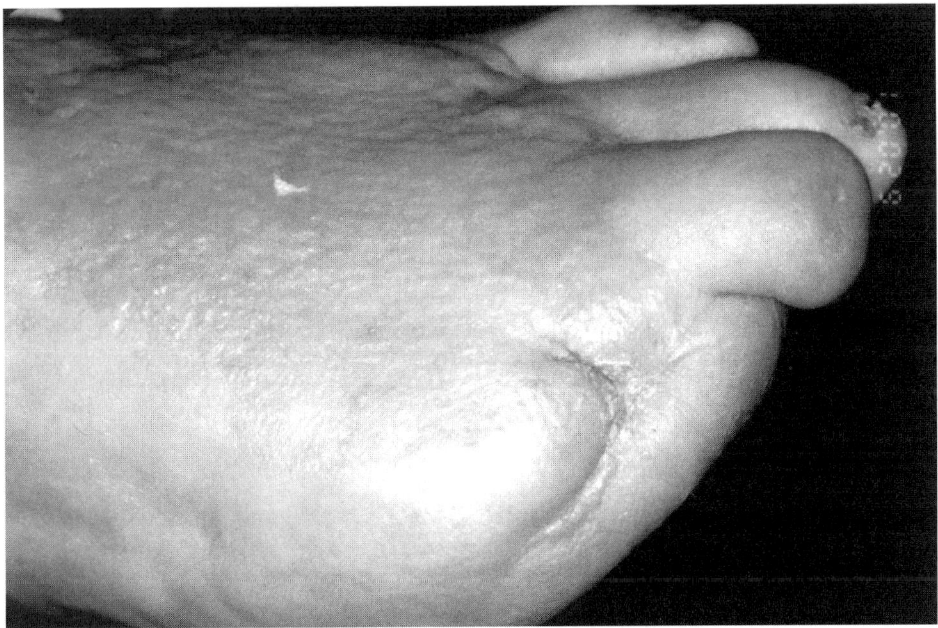

7–12B. After 3 months of treatment both areas were healed.

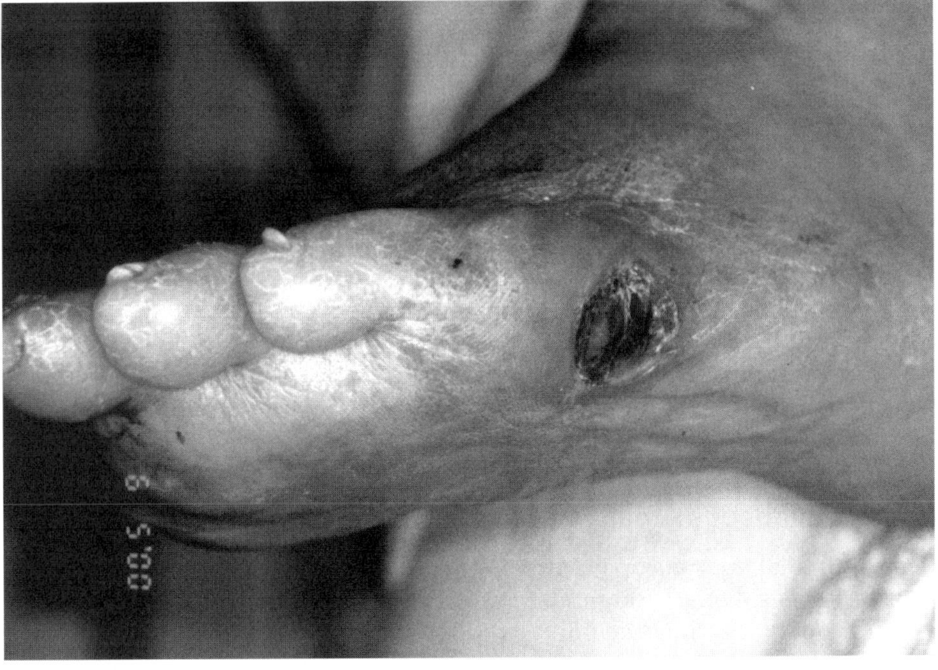

Figure 7–13A. Dry necrosis over the head of the fifth metatarsal bone.

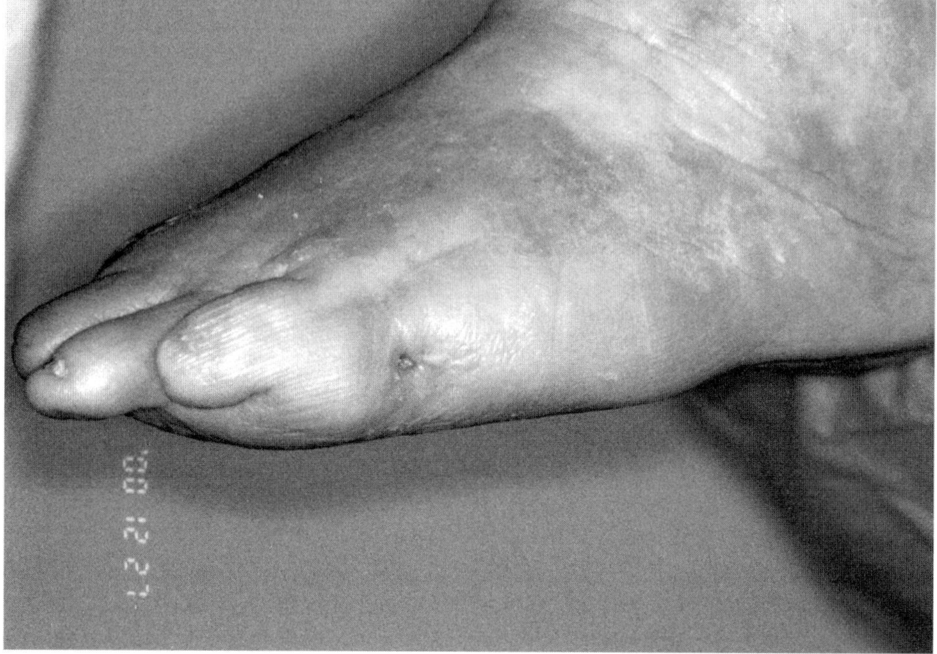

Figure 7–13B. After 3 months compression, the head of MT V was removed via a small dorsal incision.

Heel Ulcers

The ischemic heel ulcer differs from heel decubitus by its location and history: Ischemic lesions start as painful fissures on the very edge of the heel (Figure 7–14) and get progressively larger. They can be located on the medial edge of the heel, which is not weight-bearing in sedentary patients. Decubitus ulcers are located on the postero-lateral surface due to the natural tendency toward external rotation. Often, these occur during or after a recent hospitalization for cardiac or hip surgery. If the patient is able to resume ambulation, dry decubiti tend to be self-limiting and will slowly heal with spontaneous separation of eschar. Therefore, if the heel ulcer is a decubitus, treatment with intermittent compression is not needed, especially if the patient has resumed ambulation.

For the ischemic heel ulcer, treatment with intermittent compression can be useful if the patient is not able to use his natural walking mechanism. The case illustrated in Figure 7–15 is a dialysis patient who previously lost the contra-lateral leg, due to a similar ulcer, which progressed to a gangrenous foot. The arteriographic findings were the same in both legs, namely non-reconstructable disease below the level of the ankle.

Multiple, Simultaneous Areas of Breakdown

In patients with diabetic neuropathy (and in female patients in general), there is a tendency to wear shoes that are too small in size and to wear them too tight, because only then can the patient feel the shoe (with deep sensation). This results in a typical distribution of necrotic areas on the medial side of MT I, the lateral side of MT V, the prominence of the heel, and the dorsum of the (curled up) toes over the inter-phalangeal

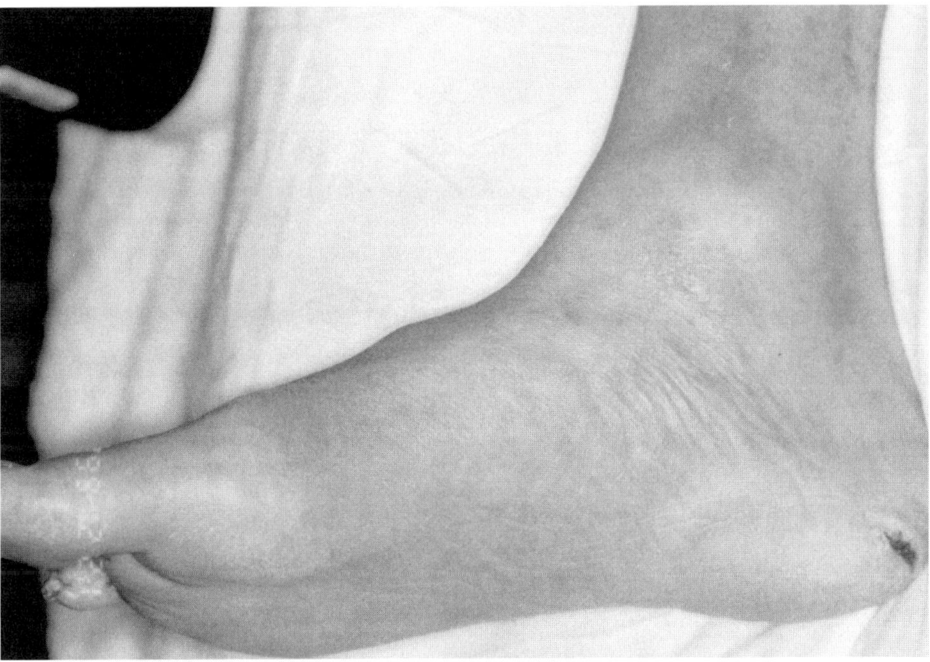

Figure 7–14. Typical ischemic heel fissure at the edge of the heel, after occlusion of 2 distal posterior tibial by-passes. This patient also had severe rest pain and toe necrosis, which resolved with 3 months of compression treatment. At 3-year follow-up, he has not required further treatment.

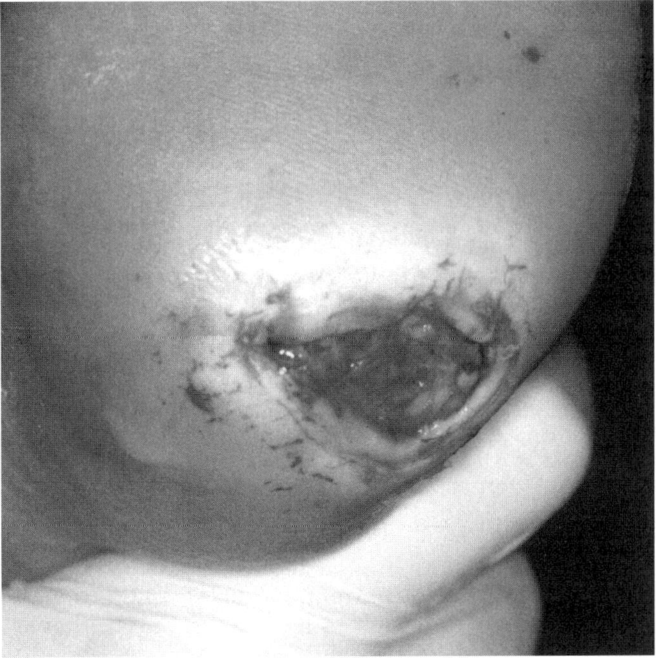

Figure 7–15A. Left: ischemic heel ulcer in diabetic dialysis patient with diffuse below ankle arterial obstruction. A similar, untreated, ulcer on the contra-lateral side resulted in below-knee amputation.

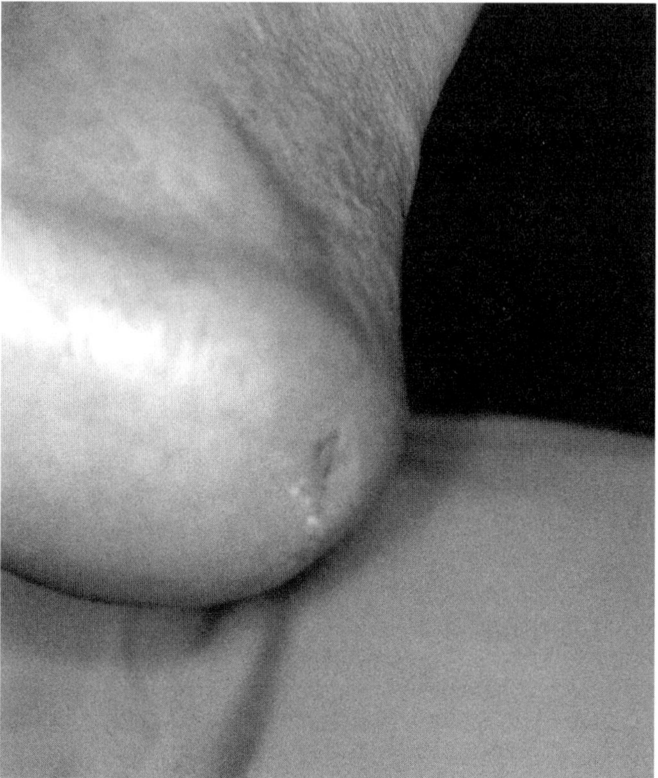

Figure 7–15B. Right: after 3 months of home compression treatment.

joints. Although it is important to recognize this, it is a common misconception to think that elimination of trauma, simply the prevention of recurrent trauma alone, will lead to spontaneous healing of lesions in the chronically ischemic foot. Instead of healing, lesions that have reached the plantar fat pad, take on a life of their own, probably due to low-grade infection or activation of inflammatory adhesion molecules. Therefore, early evaluation and treatment are important. Again, a significant part of the threat to the limb is related to infection, which is outside of the scope of this chapter.

CONCLUSION

Modern mechanical pumps for intermittent compression treatment of chronic arterial insufficiency are the rediscovery of an old tool for non-operative management of this problem. Ongoing developments in the electronic technology, as well as further elucidation of the process of arterio-genesis in response to shear-stress stimuli are likely to lead to further improvements and, hopefully, increased effectiveness of this approach.

REFERENCES

1. Murray J. On the local and general influence on the body of increased and diminished atmospheric pressure. *Lancet.* 1835;1:909–917.
2. Bilz FE. *De nieuwe natuurgeneeswijze.* Amsterdam, Dekam, 1890.
3. Pierce RV: Mechanical aids in the treatment of chronic diseases in: *The people's medical adviser,* 94th edition, Buffalo, World dispensary medical association, 1918:909–912.
4. Herrmann LG, Reed MR. The conservative treatment of arteriosclerotic peripheral vascular diseases. *Ann Surg.* 1934;100:750–760.
5. Scheinberg P, Dennis EW, Robertson, et al. The relation between arterial pressure and blood flow in the foot. *Am Heart J.* 1948;35:409–20.
6. Loane RA. Effect of rhythmically inflating a pneumatic cuff at the ankle on blood flow in the foot. *J Appl Physiol.* 1959;14:411–413.
7. Henry JP, Winsor T. Compensation of arterial insufficiency by augmenting the circulation with intermittent compression of the limbs. *Am Heart J.*1965;70:79–88.
8. Halperin MH, Friedland CK, Wilkins RW. The effect of local compression upon blood flow in the extremities of man. *Am Heart J.* 1948;35:221–237.
9. Feinglass J, Brown JL, LoSasso A, et al. Rates of lower-extremity amputation and arterial reconstruction in the United States, 1979 to 1996. *Am J Public Health.* 1999;89:1222–1227.
10. Roy CS, Brown JG. The blood-pressure and its variations in the arterioles, capillaries and smaller veins. *J of Physiol.* 1879;2:329–359.
11. Van Bemmelen PS, Weiss-Olmanni, Ricotta JJ. Rapid intermittent compression increases the skin circulation in chronically ischemic legs, with infra-popliteal arterial obstruction. *VASA.* 2000;29:47–52.
12. Delis K, Azizi ZA, Nicolaides AN, et al. Determining the optimum intermittent pneumatic compression (IPLC) stimulus for lower limb venous emptying using direct pressure measurements [abstract]. *Br J Surg.* 1996;83(suppl 2):148.
13. Van Bemmelen PS, Mattos MA, Faught, et al. Augmentation of blood flow in limbs with occlusive arterial disease by intermittent calf compression. *J Vasc Surg.* 1994;19:1052–1058.
14. Carlson L, Erikson I. Femoral artery infusion of prostaglandin E1 in severe peripheral vascular disease. *Lancet.*1973:155–156.
15. Liu K, Chen L, Saeber AV, et al. Intermittent pneumatic compression of legs increases microcirculation in distant skeletal muscle. *J Orthop Res.* 1999;17:88–95.
16. Liu K, Chen L, Seaber AV, et al. Influences of inflation rate and duration on vasodilatory effect by intermittent pneumatic compression in distant skeletal muscle. *J Orthop Res.* 1999;17:415–420.
17. Lamontagne D, Pohl U, Busse R. Mechanical deformation of the vessel wall and shear stress determine the basal release of endothelium-derived relaxing factor in the intact rabbit coronary vascular bed. *Circ Res.* 1992;70:123–130.
18. Dai G, Tsukurov O, Orkin RW, et al. An in vitro cell culture system to study the influence of external pneumatic compression on endothelial function. *J Vasc Surg.* 2000;32:977–987.
19. Eze AR, Comerota AJ, Cizek PL, et al. Intermittent calf and foot compression increases lower extremity blood flow. *Am J Surg.* 1996;172:130–135.
20. Labropoulos N, Watson WC, Mansour MA, et al. Acute effects of intermittent pneumatic compression on popliteal artery blood flow. *Arch Surg.* 1998;133:1072–1075.
21. Delis KT, Husmann MJW, Cheshire NJ, et al. Effects of intermittent pneumatic compression of the calf and thigh on arterial calf inflow: a study of normals, claudicants, and grafted arteriopaths. *Surgery.* 2001;129:188–195.
22. Abu Own A, Cheatle T, Scurr JH, et al. Effects of intermttent pneumatic compression of the foot on the microcirculatory function in arterial disease. *Eur J Vasc Surg.* 1993;7:488–492.
23. Ubbink DTh, van Iterson V, Legemate DA. Acute effect of intermittent foot-calf compression on skin microcirculation in patients with severe leg ischemia. Abstract 20th world congress International union of angiology. New York, 2002.

24. van Bemmelen PS, Gitlitz D, Faruqi, et al. Limb salvage using high-pressure intermittent compression-arterial assist device-in cases unsuitable for surgical revascularization. *Arch Surg*. 2001;136:280–285.
25. Louridas G, Saadia R, Spelay J, et al. The ArtAssist® device in chronic lower limb ischemia. A pilot study. *Intern Angiol*. 2002;21:28–35.
26. van Bemmelen PS, Char D, Giron F, et al. Angiographic improvement after rapid intermittent compression treatment [ArtAssist®] for small vessel obstruction. Report of a case. In press.
27. Ballard JL, Eke CC, Bunt TJ, et al. A prospective evaluation of transcutaneous oxygen measurements in the management of diabetic foot problems. *J Vasc Surg*. 1995;22:485–492.

III

Carotid Artery Stenosis

8

Same Day Discharge after Carotid Endarterectomy

Maureen K. Sheehan, MD and William H. Baker, MD

The care of the patient undergoing carotid endarterectomy has undergone significant changes over the past decade. In the late 1980s there was an ebbing of enthusiasm for the operation but in the 1990s NASCET[1] and ACAS[2] proved the efficacy of carotid endarterectomy in treating both symptomatic and asymptomatic patients. Following the publication of these articles, there has been a significant increase in the number of carotid endarterectomies being performed.

During these decades a reduction in Medicare reimbursement and the emergence of HMOs caused a focus on the reduction of hospital costs as well as optimal hospital utilization. In our chronically filled hospital there is always pressure to promptly discharge patients and free up needed beds. The challenge to deliver streamlined and cost efficient medical care was an impetus for numerous institutions to examine the perioperative care for all patients undergoing operations, including patients undergoing carotid endarterectomy. As a result of these institutional examinations, the perioperative care of carotid endarterectomy patients has changed significantly through the last decade.

Currently, carotid endarterectomy is being challenged as the gold standard for the treatment of patients with symptomatic and asymptomatic carotid atherosclerosis. Carotid angioplasty and stenting is currently being compared to operation in an NIH sponsored study (CREST).[3] The aims of the study are to show equipoise between the 2 procedures. If angioplasty and stenting prove to be as safe and effective as endarterectomy, most patients will opt for a trans-femoral carotid angioplasty as opposed to an open operation. As surgeons, we need to maintain the low operative stroke and death rates that have become the nation's gold standard while at the same time reducing costs and hospital utilization to a minimum. Carotid angioplasty should not be chosen over endarterectomy because of cost issues.

For the past decade we have reduced utilization of hospital resources following carotid endarterectomy by examining the outcome of past patients in a retrospective manner. Using this retrospective data, a new protocol is established and tested prospectively. If patients do as well with the new protocol, it becomes the established protocol. We have systematically reduced hospital stay and ICU utilization in this manner. This chapter will review our past experiences in these areas as well as our current experience with same day discharge.

In the 1980s patients undergoing carotid endarterectomy had a prolonged hospital stay. Pre-operative admission for angiogram was routine and followed by an operation. Postoperative stay consisted of at least 1 day in the Intensive Care Unit for monitoring of the patient's hemodynamic status as well as their neurologic status. Their stay was then culminated with 1 or 2 days on a medical/surgical floor to insure that they were doing well. They were finally discharged home.

PREOPERATIVE CARE

As angiograms gave way to carotid duplex for pre-operative imaging, the excessive pre-operative hospital stay rapidly disappeared. Most patients currently do not require a carotid angiogram. Those patients who undergo angiography have the procedure performed as an outpatient. Thus, pre-operative stay for a routine carotid endarterectomy has effectively been eliminated and is no longer an issue.

POSTOPERATIVE CARE—ICU AND EARLY DISCHARGE

Postoperative care of these patients has likewise been reduced. Early in the 1990s several institutions, including Loyola, questioned whether or not intensive care monitoring was required for all patients following carotid endarterectomy, as the majority of patients recover uneventfully from this operation. Morasch, et al.[4] from this institution retrospectively reviewed 100 consecutive patients undergoing carotid endarterectomy in 1991 and 1992. All patients were admitted to an Intensive Care Unit. Although 44 of these patients developed some type of complication or condition such as hypertension, hypotension, arrhythmia, myocardial infarction, stroke, or postoperative hemorrhage, only 16 of these patients required ICU level intervention. We defined ICU level intervention as therapy or intervention that was not routinely administered on a medical/surgical ward, that is, intravenous vasoactive medications, anti-arrhythmics, ventilatory support, or intensive monitoring. Of those 16 patients requiring ICU level intervention, 15 were identified in the recovery room. The sixteenth patient required intravenous atropine for a functional bradyarrhythmia that was first noted and treated in the recovery room but recurred after transfer out of the recovery room. Interestingly, no patient who was weaned from intravenous antihypertensive medication or vasopressors in the recovery room required re-institution of this therapy in the ICU or during the remainder of their hospital stay.

Morasch, et al. then prospectively established a protocol in which all patients who were neurologically stable and who did not require ICU intervention were discharged directly from the recovery room to a medical/surgical floor bed. In 1996 he reported on 185 patients prospectively studied.[5] Approximately 80% of these patients were directly transferred to a floor bed after less than a 2-hour stay in the recovery room. No complication occurred in any patient that required a return to the operating room or a move to an intensive care unit. This paper then prospectively established our protocol of selective ICU usage in most patients as safe and efficacious.

Others have also established that patients who required active ICU treatment could be identified early in the postoperative period. O'Brien and Ricotta[6] from Buffalo studied 73 patients. Ten of their 13 patients who required ICU care were identified in the recovery room. Ninety percent of their 43 patients with hypertension and 3 of 4 patients with hypotension were identified within 3 hours of surgery. The majority of these patients were successfully treated in the recovery room. Most ICU patients required less than 3 hours of active treatment. These findings again supported selective use of the ICU in the postoperative period.

Currently we observe carotid endarterectomy patients in the recovery room for a varying period of time. Those patients who awake immediately and who do not require any therapy for hypotension, hypertension, bradyarrhythmias, or tachyarrhythmias, are discharged usually within an hour to a medical/surgical floor. Those patients who awake more slowly or who require some vasoactive medication utilize the recovery room for 2–3 hours before a decision is made regarding ICU level care. Other institutions have a vascular surgical floor with nurses who are trained to monitor and treat these problems. Rather than send borderline patients to an ICU, these patients are cared for on this specialized vascular surgical floor.

During the decade of the 1990s total hospital stay was also being questioned. Collier from Pittsburgh, in 1995,[7] reported on a 1-day total admission for carotid endarterectomy. Patients would enter the hospital in the morning, the operation would be performed, they would stay overnight in the hospital, and be discharged the next morning. His criteria for discharge stated that the patient needed to be neurologically and hemodynamically stable, the wound must be dry without any evidence of hematoma, and the patient must be able to eat, void, and ambulate. Using these criteria Collier was able to reduce the length of stay for his patients to 1.27 days, with only 16% of his patients requiring a length of stay greater than 1 day. Morasch and Hirko,[8] reporting statistics from this institution, showed that the total length of stay (preoperative plus postoperative days) during the 1990s was reduced from 6.18 days to 2.0 days by 1994, with a concomitant reduction in time from operation to discharge from 3.1 days to 1.24 days.

The above reduction in hospital utilization, while laudable from a cost accounting point of view, can only be justified if patient outcomes are unaffected. Holloway[9] reviewed Academic Medical Center Consortium (10 institutions) data. He assessed the effect of patient protocol changes on the outcome measures of mortality, re-admission and postoperative complication rates in over 7,000 patients who underwent carotid endarterectomy over a 6-year period (1990–1995). Holloway noted an increase in the percentage of patients with pre-operative conditions of hypertension, congestive heart failure, chronic obstructive pulmonary disease, diabetes, and a 2-year increase in the average age of the patients. The pre-operative and postoperative length of stay was halved (mean 8.8 days to 4.3 days). Despite the increase in age and severity of illness in the patient population, Holloway was unable to document any measurable changes in the outcome of care as defined by inpatient mortality, discharge disposition, 30-day readmission rates or several other measures of postoperative complications. Holloway concluded that there were no detrimental effects on patient outcome based on this reduction in perioperative length of stay or with a decreased usage of ICU. Likewise, Kaufman,[10] from Bay State Medical Center, found that 60% of his patients could be discharged on the morning after operation and 80% could be discharged on postoperative day 2. He found no significant increase in risk of complications associated with this decrease in hospital stay.

Selective ICU utilization with discharge home the morning after operation has become the norm. The safety of the above protocol has been well established nationwide. At Loyola, approximately 10% of patients require ICU care, while the postoperative stroke and death rate has remained constant at approximately 2%.

SAME DAY DISCHARGE

At Loyola we were impressed by a number of patients who on the night of operation were neurologically intact, without hematoma, eating, ambulating, and voiding. From a physiological point of view, they could easily have been discharged home. We rationalized their hospitalization stating that if they had a complication such as an acute neurologic deficit or hemorrhage into the neck, complications that required immediate return to the operating room, hospitalization was necessary. Kaufman[10] has echoed this opinion. Cardiac complications occur early in the postoperative course, usually within the first 3 hours, as well established by Morasch, et al.[4,5] as well as O'Brien and Ricotta.[6]

Thus, in order to safely discharge patients the night of operation we needed to establish when the complication of postoperative stroke or postoperative neck hematoma occurred. Sheehan, et al.[11] from this institution reviewed 835 consecutive patients undergoing carotid endarterectomy between 1988 and 1998. During this time period the operation was relatively standardized and included intraoperative post carotid endarterectomy duplex scanning. We excluded 64 patients who required prolonged hospitalization for heparinization, comorbidities, or because the operation was associated with coronary artery bypass grafting.

Sixty-two patients (8%) experienced either a neurologic deficit or neck hematoma. There were 26 (3.4%) neurologic deficits of which 19 (2.5%) were related to the operated carotid. Of these 26 patients 19 (73%) were diagnosed in the operating room or recovery room, 5 (19%) within 8 hours of operation, and 2 (7.7%) after 8 hours but in less than 24 hours (Figure 8–1). One of these patients had a hemispheric stroke that was noted during early morning rounds in the ICU. In retrospect, he had TIAs during the evening that were not appreciated. The second patient had immediate postoperative nausea and vomiting but his vertebral basilar stroke was diagnosed the morning after operation, the first time he attempted ambulation. In retrospect, he had symptoms immediately postoperatively. Thirty-six (4.7%) patients had a neck hematoma of which 23 (66%) were diagnosed in the recovery room, 11 (31%) within 8 hours, and 1 (2.7%) after 8 hours. This one patient ruptured a patch angioplasty the morning after operation, having spent a hypertensive night in the intensive care unit. Overall, 0.4% of the 771 patients had a complication occurring more than 8 hours after operation.

Armed with these statistics, we cautiously began a program of same day discharge. Patients who were up and about, eating, voiding, and had no neurologic deficit or neck hematoma were discharged 8 hours after operation. When this program was initiated in 2000 only 20% of the patients were discharged the same day. In 2001 and 2002 currently almost 40% of our patients are discharged the evening of operation (Figure 8–2). The reason for delayed discharge is multiple (Figure 8–3). The majority of the patients discharged the day after operation have their carotid endarterectomy in the afternoon and thus are not candidates for discharge at a reasonable time. Physician and patient reluctance initially were difficult to overcome but the attitudes in both populations are slowly evolving. As patients continue to do well, physicians have less

Timing of Complications

	OR/RR	< 8 hrs	> 8 hrs
NH	24 (66%)	11 (31%)	1 (2.7%)
ND	19 (73%)	5 (19%)	2 (7.6%)
Total	43	16	3

Figure 8–1. Timing of complications

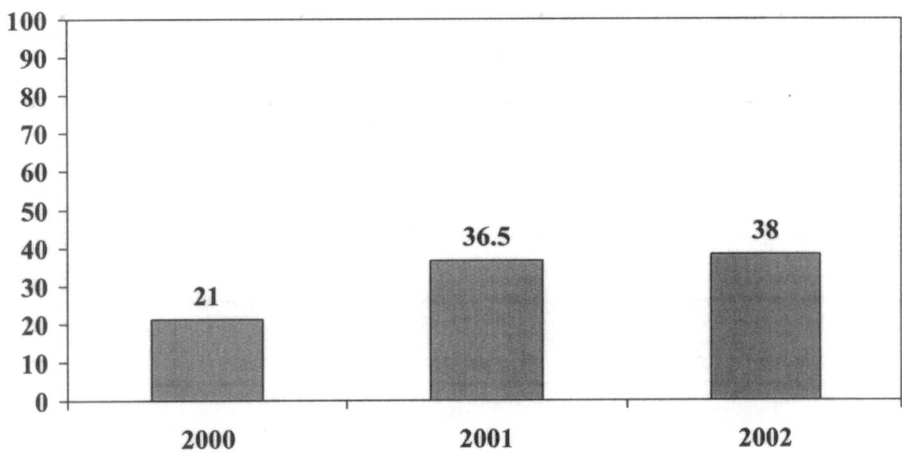

Figure 8–2. Same day discharge percentages

apprehensions regarding same day discharge, while patients' reluctance is easily overcome with appropriate preoperative counseling.

Same day discharge following carotid endarterectomy is not the norm. There will always be patients who require a night of hospitalization at a minimum. It is impractical in most settings to schedule carotid endarterectomy as only the first or second case allowing sufficient post endarterectomy observation during the same day. All of these patients are

CAROTID ENDARTERECTOMY
Delayed discharge - reasons

Discharge	2000	2001	Thru March '02	Total
Too late OR	18	17	3	38
GI	5	1	0	6
Physician Choice	16	11	3	30
Patient's Choice	4	5	1	10
GU	6	2	1	9
TIA	0	0	0	0
CVA	2	1	0	3

Figure 8–3. Carotid endarterectomy: delayed discharge reasons

elderly and the usual problems associated with age, such as cardiac disease, obstructive uropathies, and the general frailty of some of these individuals, will always be present. In our practice there are patients who live more than an hour away from the hospital, some in rural areas, and until same day discharge experience is more extensive, both the patient and the physician feel uneasy with same day discharge under these circumstances.

CONCLUSIONS

Cost containment measures are welcome as long as they do not result in an increase in either morbidity or mortality. Selective same day discharge easily fulfills these criteria. A more extensive experience, in a larger population will be necessary to prospectively prove its efficacy. Although same day discharge is well accepted by both selected patients and physicians, in 2002 it is not applicable in every patient care situation.

REFERENCES

1. North American Symptomatic Carotid Endarterectomy Trial (NASCET) Collaborators. Beneficial effect of carotid endarterectomy in symptomatic patients with high-grade carotid stenosis. *N Engl J Med*.1991; 325:445–453.

2. Executive Committee for the Asymptomatic Carotid Atherosclerosis Study (ACAS). Endarterectomy for asymptomatic carotid artery stenosis. *JAMA*. 1999; Vol 273, No. 18:1421–1428.

3. Hobson RW, Ferguson R. Stratus report on the Carotid Revascularization Endarterectomy versus Stent Trial. *Techniques in Vascular and Interventional Radiology*. 2000; 3:1–4.

4. Morasch MD, Hodgett D, Burke K, et al. Selective use of the Intensive Care Unit following carotid endarterectomy. *Ann Vasc Surg*. 1995, Vol. 9, No. 3:229–234.

5. Morasch MD, Hirko MK, Hirasa T, et al. Intensive care after carotid endarterectomy: a prospective evaluation. *J Am Coll Surg*. 1996, Vol. 183: 387–392.

6. O'Brien MS, Ricotta JJ. Conserving resources after carotid endarterectomy: Selective use of the intensive care unit. *J Vasc Surg*. 1991, Vol 14, No 6:796–802.

7. Collier PE. Are one-day admissions for carotid endarterectomy feasible? *Am J Surg*. 1995, Vol 170:140–143.

8. Morasch MD, Hirko MK, Hirasa T, et al. Intensive care after carotid endarterectomy: A prospective evaluation. *J Am Coll Surg*. 1996, Vol. 183: 387–392.

9. Holloway RG Jr., Witter DM, Mushlin AI, et al. Carotid endarterectomy trends in the patterns and outcomes of care at academic medical centers, 1990 through 1995. *Arch Neur*. 1998, Vol 55(1):25–32.

10. Kaufman JL, Frank D, Rhee SW, et al. Feasibility and safety of 1-day postoperative hospitalization for carotid endarterectomy. *Arch Surg*. 1996, Vol 131(7):751–755.

11. Sheehan MK, Baker WH, Littooy FN, et al. Timing of postcarotid complications: A guide to safe discharge planning. *J Vasc Surg*. 2001, Vol. 34, No. 1:13–16.

9

Improving Carotid Endarterectomy Outcomes

Timothy F. Kresowik, MD and
Rebecca A. Kresowik, BLS

Carotid endarterectomy (CEA) has been established as an effective procedure for stroke prevention in selected patients with symptomatic and asymptomatic carotid artery occlusive disease.[1–5] However, the therapeutic benefit of CEA over medical therapy alone is narrow especially for patients who are asymptomatic. The randomized trials that established the efficacy of CEA required participating surgeons to have an established record of performing the procedure with a low adverse outcome rate.[6,7] It should be apparent that in discussing the risk/benefit of CEA with an individual patient, the surgeon should be aware of his/her own adverse outcome rate. The benefit of CEA established in the trials should not be extrapolated to an individual surgeon unless the surgeon is achieving comparable or superior outcomes to the surgeons who participated in the trials. All surgeons should strive to continuously improve their outcomes in order to deliver the best possible care to their patients.[8]

IS THERE A NEED FOR QUALITY IMPROVEMENT FOR CEA?

Variation in outcomes of carotid endarterectomy is readily apparent from review of the published literature.[9] As part of its work as a Medicare Quality Improvement Organization (QIO, formerly known as Peer Review Organizations or PRO), the Iowa Foundation for Medical Care (IFMC) has been involved in evaluating and attempting to improve the care of Medicare patients undergoing CEA. In conjunction with other state QIOs and the Kansas City regional office of the Centers for Medicare and Medicaid Services (CMS, which was formerly known as the Health Care Financing Administration or HCFA) we evaluated the care of a random sample of Medicare patients undergoing CEA.[10]

Comprehensive medical record review of 10,561 CEA procedures from 10 different states was performed at a single abstraction center to determine indications, care processes, and outcomes. This study also included medical record review of hospital readmissions within 30 days of the procedure and identification of out-of-hospital deaths from the Medicare beneficiary files. There was significant variation in outcomes among the states (Figures 9–1 and 9–2). The observed variation in outcomes clearly indicates the need for quality improvement. The stroke or mortality rates in asymptomatic patients observed in Arkansas (6.7%) and Oklahoma (6.6%) were almost 3 times higher than the rate in Indiana (2.3%). If the observed rates in Arkansas and Oklahoma had been the surgical combined event rate in the ACAS trial, the trial certainly would not have indicated surgical benefit.

PERFORMANCE MEASUREMENT

Performance measures in health care fall into 2 main classifications: outcome measures and process measures. Outcome measures have face validity for clinicians and the general public. Outcome measures such as stroke rate or death rate are readily understood and accepted as indicators of quality by clinicians and the public. However in order to provide valid comparisons, the measures must be adjusted for baseline risk. Good risk adjustment can be complex and usually requires multiple data elements collected using uniform definitions. As an example, if one wanted to compare a surgeon's death rates following aortic aneurysm repair, it would be important to adjust for baseline cardiac

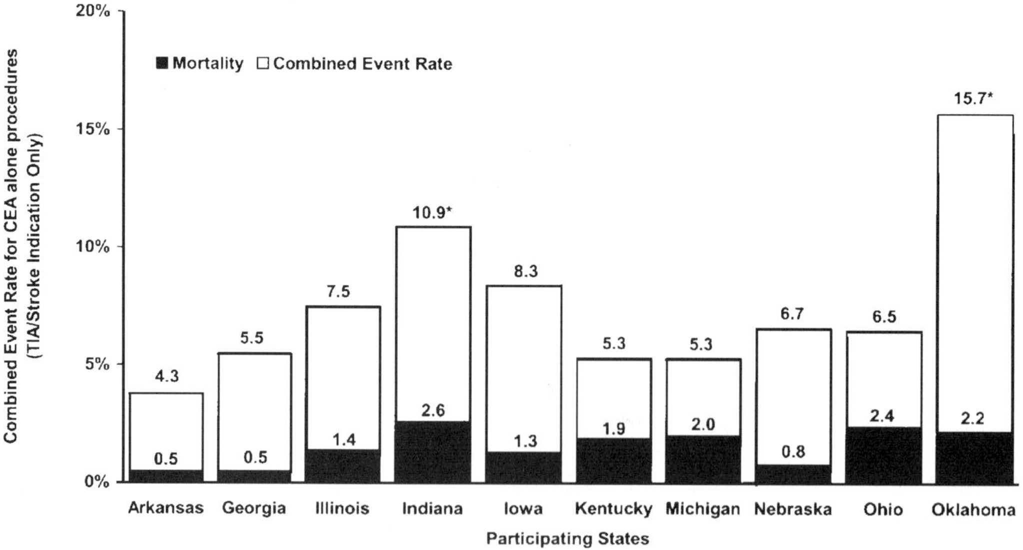

Figure 9–1. Combined event rates (30 day stroke or mortality) and mortality rates for CEA alone procedures (TIA/stroke only) by state [Arkansas (N=184), Georgia (N=218), Illinois (N=279), Indiana (N=230), Iowa (N=312), Kentucky (N=207), Michigan (N=247), Nebraska (N=240), Ohio (N=246), and Oklahoma (N=178)].
*significantly different from mean P<.05
With permission from T F Kresowik, DW Bratzler, H R Karp, et al. Multistate Utilization, Processes and Outcomes of Carotid Endarterectomy. *J Vasc Surg.* 2001:33;227–235.

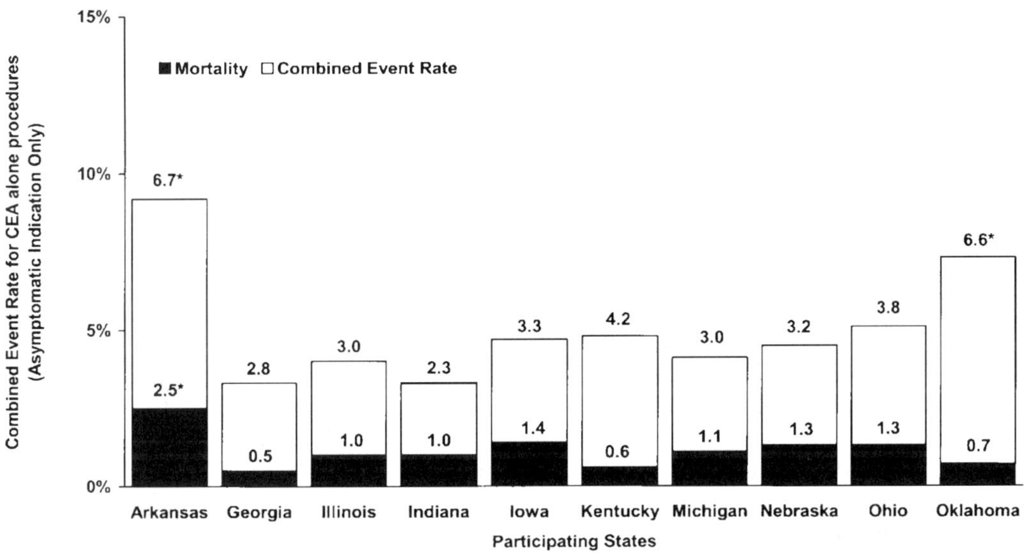

Figure 9–2. Combined event rates (30 day stroke or mortality) and mortality rates for CEA alone procedures (asymptomatic indication only) by state [Arkansas (N=284), Georgia (N=422), Illinois (N=406), Indiana (N=394), Iowa (N=512), Kentucky (N=356), Michigan (N=438, Nebraska (N=317), Ohio (N=473), and Oklahoma (N=289)]. *significantly different from mean P<.05
With permission from T F Kresowik, DW Bratzler, H R Karp, et al. Multistate Utilization, Processes and Outcomes of Carotid Endarterectomy. *J Vasc Surg.* 2001:33;227–235.

risk. There are a number of clinical risk factors and a multitude of diagnostic tests that may be used to assess cardiac risk. One could adjust for cardiac risk if consistent clinical data and uniform diagnostic testing were available for each patient. This might be possible (albeit very expensive) in an individual institution or as part of a prospective study, but it is not feasible for community wide retrospective comparisons.

If outcomes from CEA are used for comparison, it is essential that they be risk adjusted or stratified by procedural indication and for type of procedure (e.g., whether or not the procedure was performed singly or in conjunction with coronary artery bypass grafting). Comparisons are valid only if similar definitions are used for stratification or adjustment. It should be obvious that classifying patients into symptomatic and asymptomatic categories is not adequate unless clear definitions are used. If one surgeon's symptomatic patients include a large number of patients whose only symptoms are lightheadedness or dizziness and another surgeon only classifies patients as symptomatic if they meet the NASCET entry criteria (recent ipsilateral hemispheric stroke or TIA), a simple comparison of their outcomes in the symptomatic category is not valid.

In our outcome measurement projects we have used consistent, but relatively straightforward definitions. The indications for CEA were classified into 4 mutually exclusive categories. Patients were considered to have stroke as the indication for the procedure only if they had documented ipsilateral hemispheric symptoms that persisted for more than 24 hours within 90 days prior to the procedure. Similarly, patients were considered to have transient ischemic attack (TIA) as the indication only if transient (less than 24 hours) ipsilateral hemispheric symptoms occurred within 90 days prior to the procedure. Patients were considered to be asymptomatic only if there was no history at any time prior to the procedure of cerebrovascular symptoms or events in either the anterior or posterior circulations. All other patients (e.g., remote ipsilateral symptoms, global or vertebrobasilar symptoms, contralateral hemispheric symptoms) were classified in a non-specific category. These definitions were used to create relatively clean stroke, TIA and asymptomatic indication groups with high reproducibility, given the limitations of retrospective medical record review. We also stratified patients by type of procedure (CEA alone, CEA/CABG, and redo CEA).

We do not believe that it is essential to risk adjust CEA outcome data for other components of baseline medical risk such as age or coronary artery disease. Coronary artery disease risk adjustment is problematic because of the previously mentioned variation in patient assessment or screening. In addition, assessment of overall risk of operation should be part of the surgical decision-making for CEA. This is most obvious when examining outcomes in the asymptomatic indication group. We do not believe it would be appropriate to give "credit" through risk adjustment to surgeons who operate on older, sicker asymptomatic patients. The higher the medical risk, the less likely the patient will benefit from the operation. One way to improve outcomes is to select healthier patients. In the case of CEA for asymptomatic disease, this is appropriate. For other procedures (e.g., coronary artery bypass grafting), risk adjustment for baseline risk is more important because some of the patients with the highest surgical risk also have the most benefit from the operation. Improving surgical outcomes by avoiding operating on those patients would be inappropriate.

In addition to the problem of risk adjustment, case volumes adequate for valid statistical differentiation at the individual surgeon or even institutional level are often not achieved. Sample size considerations are especially important for procedural outcomes with low occurrence rates. Stroke and death following CEA are infrequent events. If one was comparing Surgeon A and Surgeon B with combined event rates (stroke or death) of 2% and 4% respectively, it appears that Surgeon A has one-half the adverse outcome rate of Surgeon B and an informed patient should choose surgeon A. If those rates actually represent 1 adverse event in 50 patients performed over the last year for Surgeon A and 2 adverse events in 50 patients performed over the last year by Surgeon B it is obvious that the rate differences are not statistically significant. Fifty CEA procedures per year is at the higher end of the typical individual volume spectrum for surgeons. The comparison becomes even more problematic if the adverse events are not of equal severity. If the 2 adverse events for Surgeon B were non-disabling strokes with complete recovery in 2 patients presenting with crescendo transient ischemic attacks and the one adverse event for Surgeon A was a fatal stroke in an asymptomatic patient, the rate comparison alone becomes even more misleading. If one attempts to stratify adverse events by categories such as death, disabling permanent stroke, temporary stroke, ipsilateral stroke etc., the sample size issue becomes critical.

Performance measurement for quality improvement (usually confidential feedback), as opposed to performance measurement for accountability or judgment (e.g., public reporting or credentialing), can have different reliability/validity thresholds. The importance of statistical significance and the need for valid risk adjustment is critical in performance measurement for accountability or judgment. On the other hand, measurement for quality improvement may not require the same degree of rigor and yet allows the individual physician to target areas in need of change.

PROCESS MEASURES

The other major category of performance measures is process measures. A process measure evaluates the performance of a given element of care. Process measures are often used in evaluation of physician performance for medical conditions. As an example, many process measures have been developed for the evaluation of care of patients presenting with acute myocardial infarction (AMI) including: administration of aspirin, administration of beta blockers and time to revascularization (e.g., initiating thrombolytic therapy or emergent angioplasty).[11] Although process measures do require some adjustment for appropriate inclusion/exclusion criteria (e.g., excluding patients with complete heart block from a beta blocker measure), the data collection requirements and complexity of inclusion/exclusion criteria are not as elaborate as would be required to risk adjust outcomes for a condition such as AMI. Another advantage of process measures is that they are usually actionable by the physician. Compliance with a measure evaluating prescription of a medical therapy in an appropriate patient is under the control of the physician. Many outcomes are more dependent on the patient's pre-existing risk profile and compliance with physician recommendations.

Good process measures have an evidence-based linkage to outcomes. If the process in question lacks that linkage, it will not be accepted as valid by the clinician. In the area of CEA, many of the care processes lack a clear association with superior outcomes. It would be inappropriate to use measures such as type of anesthesia (local vs. general), reversal of heparin, or method of cerebral perfusion monitoring as indicators of quality since the linkage between these processes and outcomes is variable in the literature. Other processes such as perioperative administration of antiplatelet therapy, use of heparin anticoagulation, and patching may be reasonable quality measures for CEA.[10,12–15] In an analysis (correcting for indication) of the multi-state CEA project, the preoperative administration of aspirin or ticlopidine (30% risk reduction), intraoperative use of heparin (51% risk reduction), and patching (27% risk reduction) were all associated with significantly lower combined event rates.[10] Significant variation in process from state-to-state was also demonstrated in this project (Figure 9–3).

CAN VOLUME BE USED AS A SURROGATE PERFORMANCE MEASURE?

One of the consequences of the lack of available measures for public accountability has been the Leapfrog Group initiative.[16] In the absence of other measures they suggested using procedural volume parameters as a surrogate measure of quality. The Leapfrog Group has recommended a hospital minimum volume of 100 CEA cases per year. Although it is hard to argue with the concept that experience is important in procedures, the evidence base for the specific volume threshold selected for CEA is lacking.[17–19] Some of the observed volume outcome relationships observed for CEA are clouded by the fact that high volume is generally associated with a higher percentage of asymptomatic and thus lower risk patients.[18–19]

Carotid endarterectomy does not require the interaction of a multi-disciplinary team to the same degree as a procedure like coronary artery bypass grafting. This makes it harder to accept the importance of hospital volume as opposed to individual surgeon volume. It seems intuitively obvious that a hospital with 20 different surgeons performing an average 5 CEA procedures each per year would not necessarily be

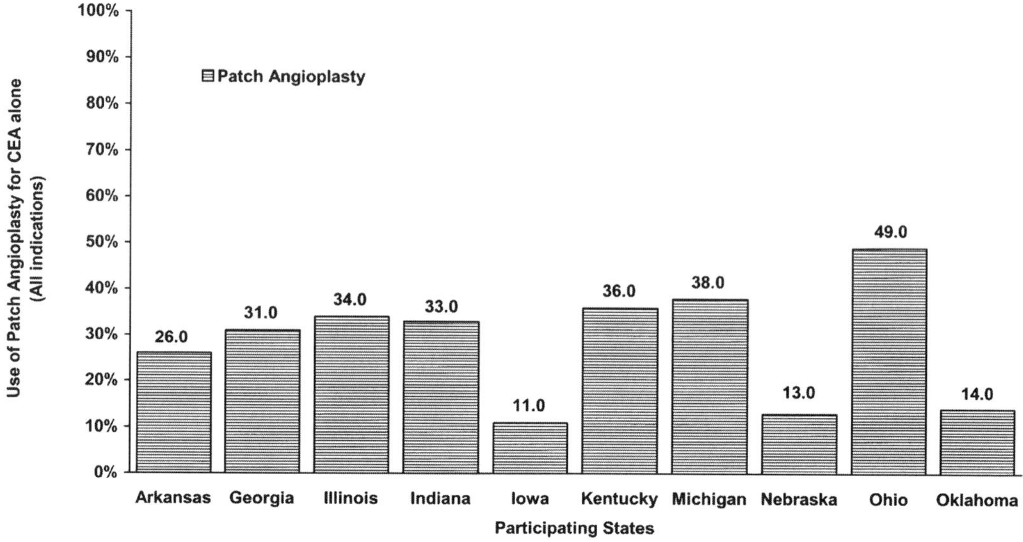

Figure 9–3. Use of patch antioplasty for CEA alone procedures (all indications) by state. With permission from T F Kresowik, DW Bratzler, H R Karp, et al. Multistate Utilization, Processes and Outcomes of Carotid Endarterectomy. *J Vasc Surg.* 2001:33;227–235.

superior to a hospital with a single surgeon performing 75 procedures per year. Annual procedure rates also do not take into account overall experience of a surgeon. A surgeon who has performed 25 procedures per year for 10 years would likely have accumulated a superior experience to one who is in their first year of practice, regardless of the overall hospital volume of the institution where they practice.

Of even greater concern are the potential unintended consequences of using volume alone as a surrogate measure of quality. The only real area for growth in performing CEA is in the asymptomatic population. If the message to surgeons is that one should only be performing CEA if one has high volumes, the pressure to perform more procedures is obvious. If that pressure translates into more asymptomatic patients undergoing operation, especially those with comorbidities who might otherwise be recommended observation, the potential for more harm than good exists. If the increased volume in the asymptomatic population is not accompanied by a low procedural adverse outcome rate, the overall population stroke morbidity may be increased.

QUALITY IMPROVEMENT

Performance measurement is an important component of quality improvement. Measurement of one's own performance and comparison to others is useful in identifying areas for improvement. Outcome and process measurements can both be useful for quality improvement purposes. An important concept in performance measure comparison is benchmarking. The term benchmark is sometimes used in different ways. We believe that the term benchmark should not be seen as synonymous with the average, but rather seen as the highest reasonably achievable performance. Maximal quality improvement does not occur if average performers are satisfied and do not seek to achieve the performance of those at the top of the curve. Perfect performance (e.g., a 0% adverse event rate) is not a reasonably achievable goal for a procedure such as CEA. Performance equal to that achieved in the randomized controlled trials (6.5% combined stroke/mortality rate for patients presenting with recent ipsilateral stroke or TIA and a 1.5% combined event rate for asymptomatic patients) is a reasonable outcome benchmark for CEA. On the other hand, 100% performance is achievable and thus a suitable benchmark for many process measures if good inclusion/exclusion criteria are used.

Quality improvement also requires understanding of the concept of system change. System change can have varying meanings depending on the situation. The system can be seen as the whole care system (e.g., the interaction of the patient with multiple physicians, other health care professionals and ancillary staff). A system may also represent the practice of an individual surgeon. Optimal performance in either concept of system is often not achieved without a protocol for delivery of care. Many of the practices in the operating room have incorporated formal protocols to optimize care and prevent errors. An example of a recent system change that has been recommended for the operating room is the preoperative marking of the operative site by the responsible surgeon in order to reduce the possibility of wrong side procedures. In addition to preventing errors of commission, the use of protocols decreases the likelihood that an important component of the care process would be inadvertently overlooked (errors of omission).

One example of the importance of system thinking specific for CEA is in the area of preoperative administration of antiplatelet therapy. Even if the surgeon is committed to 100% performance for this process measure, the lack of a formal protocol makes 100% performance unlikely. Even though many patients presenting for CEA are taking antiplatelet agents, some are not and may "slip through the cracks" unless the therapy is part of a protocol or care plan. The "system" can even work against the surgeons expressed wishes. In one institution, we found that patients were being instructed as part of the preoperative anesthesia evaluation to stop all antiplatelet medication at least 7 days prior to CEA. This recommendation originated from surgeons performing non-vascular procedures because of their concerns about hemorrhage. A formal CEA protocol that included clear instructions about preoperative antiplatelet therapy is more likely to achieve optimal results.

In our work in the state of Iowa we have shown that multi-institution performance monitoring and confidential feedback can improve the outcomes of CEA.[20] We have promoted the use of a common data collection tool for CEA processes and outcomes. Over 50% of the hospitals performing the procedure in Iowa have participated in ongoing data collection and those hospitals account for approximately 75% of the procedures performed. Hospitals receive regular comparison data without identification of other institutions. We demonstrated significant overall improvements in outcomes in participating hospitals (Figure 9–4). We have also demonstrated improvement in process measures, including patching (Figure 9–5) and antiplatelet therapy.

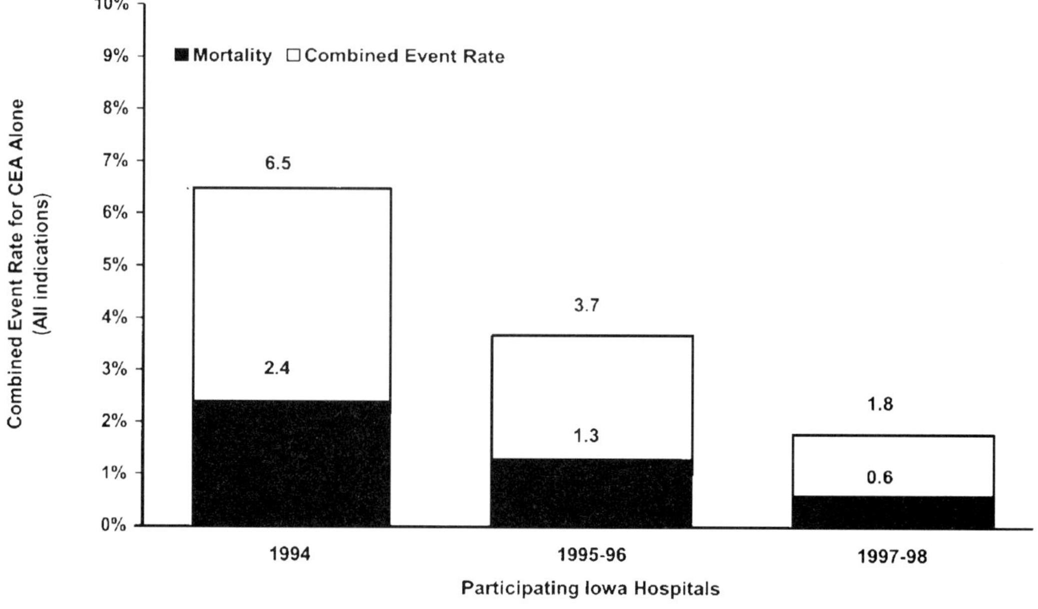

Figure 9–4. Combined event rates in participating Iowa hospitals for CEA alone procedures.

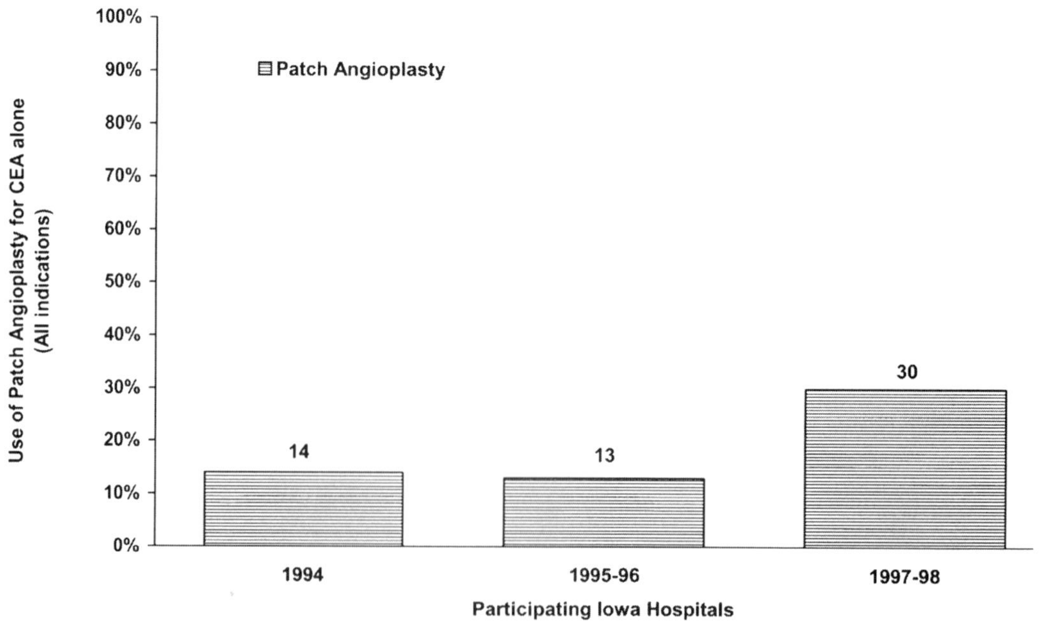

Figure 9–5. Use of patch angioplasty for CEA alone procedures (all indications) in participating Iowa hospitals.

SUMMARY

There is room for improvement in CEA performance. Participation in confidential outcome and process measurement can lead to quality improvement. Surgical volume should not be used as a surrogate for quality. Outcome measurement in CEA should include risk adjustment for the type of and indication for the procedure using standard definitions, but risk adjustment for comorbid conditions is not necessary. All surgeons performing CEA should participate in confidential outcome monitoring and strive to achieve benchmark outcomes. It is unlikely that risk adjusted outcomes from CEA will have adequate power at an individual surgeon or hospital level to be valid performance measures for public reporting. However, documented participation in standardized confidential outcome monitoring may be suitable as a publicly reported quality measure. Some process measures such as perioperative use of antiplatelet therapy and patching may have potential as accountability measures (e.g., suitable for public reporting) as well as for quality improvement. Individual surgeons should adopt protocols that include pre and post operative use of aspirin, intraoperative heparin and routine patching for CEA.

REFERENCES

1. North American Symptomatic Carotid Endarterectomy Trial Collaborators. Beneficial effect of carotid endarterectomy in symptomatic patients with high-grade carotid stenosis. *N Engl J Med*. 1991;325:445–453.
2. Mayberg MR, Wilson SE, Yatsu F, et al., for the Veterans Affairs Cooperative Studies Program 309Trialist Group. Carotid endarterectomy and prevention of cerebral ischemia in symptomatic carotid stenosis. *JAMA*. 1991;266:3289–3294.
3. Executive Committee for the Asymptomatic Carotid Atherosclerosis Study. Endarterectomy for asymptomatic carotid artery stenosis. *JAMA*. 1995;273:1421–1428.
4. European Carotid Surgery Trialists' Collaborative Group. Randomised trial of endarterectomy for recently symptomatic carotid stenosis: final results of the MRC European Carotid Surgery Trial (ECST). *Lancet*. 1998;351:1379–1387.
5. Barnett HJM, Taylor DW, Eliasziw M, et al. Benefit of carotid endarterectomy in patients with symptomatic moderate or severe stenosis. *N Engl J Med*. 1998;339:1415–1425.
6. North American Symptomatic Carotid Endarterectomy Trial. Methods, patient characteristics, and progress. *Stroke*. 1991;22:711–720.
7. The Asymptomatic Carotid Atherosclerosis Study Group. Study design for randomized prospective trial of carotid endarterectomy for asymptomatic atherosclerosis. *Stroke*. 1989;20:844–849.
8. Hertzer,NR. Presidential address: outcome assessment in vascular surgery-results mean everything. *J Vasc Surgery*. 1995;21:6–15.
9. Bratzler DW, Kresowik TF, Outcome analysis of carotid surgery, In: Loftus, CM, Kresowik TF, editors, *Carotid Artery Surgery, 1st Ed*. New York: Thieme Medical Publishers, Inc. 2000. P. 549–59.
10. T F Kresowik, D W Bratzler, H R Karp, et al. Multistate Utilization, Processes and Outcomes of Carotid Endarterectomy. *J Vasc Surg*. 2001:33;227–235.
11. Jencks SF, Cuerdon T, Burwen DR, et al. Quality of Medical Care Delivered to Medicare Beneficiaries. *JAMA*. 2000:284; 1670–1676.
12. Kretschmer G, Pratschner T, Prager M, et al. Antiplatelet treatment prolongs survival after carotid bifurcation endarterectomy: analysis of the clinical series followed by a controlled trial. *Ann Surg*. 1990;211:317–322.

13. Lindlblad B, Persson NH, Takolander R, et al. Does low-dose acetylsalicylic acid prevent stroke after carotid surgery? A double-blind, placebo-controlled randomized trial. *Stroke.* 1993;24:1125–1128.
14. Abu Rahma AF, Khan JH, Robinson PA, et al. Prospective randomized trial of carotid endarterectomy with primary closure and patch angioplasty with saphenous vein, jugular vein, and polytetrafluoroethylene: Perioperative (30-day) results. *J Vasc Surg.* 1996;24:998–1007.
15. Jackson MR, Clagett GP. Use of Vein or Synthetic Patches in Carotid Endarterectomy. In: Loftus, CM, Kresowik, TF. *Carotid Artery Surgery.* 1st Ed. New York: Thieme Medical Publishers, Inc. New York 2000. pp. 281–290.
16. Birkmeyer JD, Finlayson EV, Birkmeyer CM. Volume standards for high-risk surgical procedures: potential benefits of the Leapfrog initiative. *Surgery.* 2001;130:415–22.
17. Cebul RD, Snow RJ, Pine R, Hertzer NR, Norris DG. Indications, outcomes, and provider volumes for carotid endarterectomy. *JAMA.* 1998; 279:1282–1287.
18. Pearce WH, Parker MA, Feinglass J, Ujiki M, Manheim LM. The importance of surgeon volume and training in outcomes for vascular surgical procedures. *J Vasc Surg.* 1999; 29:768–776.
19. Birkmeyer JD, Siewers AE, Finlayson EV et al. Hospital volume and surgical mortality in the United States. *N Engl J Med.* 2002;346:1128–37.
20. Kresowik TF, Hemann RA, Grund SL, et al. Improving the outcomes of carotid endarterectomy: Results of a statewide quality improvement project. *J Vasc Surg.* 2000:31:918–926.

10

Carotid Angioplasty/Stenting: Short- and Long-Term Results

Timothy M. Sullivan, MD

Cerebrovascular accident (CVA) is the third leading cause of death in the United States, surpassed only by heart disease and malignancy.[1] Stroke accounts for 10–12% of all deaths in industrialized countries. Almost 1 in 4 men and 1 in 5 women aged 45 years can expect to have a stroke if they live to age 85. In a population of 1 million, 9 1,600 people will have a stroke each year. Only 55% of these will survive 6 months, and a third of the survivors will have significant problems caring for themselves. As our population ages, the total number of people afflicted with stroke will continue to rise unless historic stroke rates decline in the future.[2]

The etiology of stroke is multifactorial. Ischemic stroke accounts for about 80% of all first-ever strokes, while intracerebral hemorrhage and subarachnoid hemorrhage are responsible for 10% and 5%, respectively. Of those strokes which are ischemic in nature, the majority are linked to complications of atheromatous plaques. The most frequent site of such an atheroma is the carotid bifurcation. Although the prevention of stroke in the general population has largely focused on the control of hypertension, a substantial number of strokes are preventable by the identification and treatment of carotid disease, especially as our population ages.

Surgical endarterectomy of high-grade carotid lesions, both symptomatic and asymptomatic, has been identified as the treatment of choice for stroke prophylaxis in most patients when compared to "best medical therapy" (risk factor reduction and anti-platelet agents), as proven by the NASCET and ACAS studies.[3,4] Subsequently, carotid endarterectomy (CEA) has been performed in increasing numbers of patients, and now represents the most frequent surgical procedure performed by vascular surgeons. The results of this procedure have continued to improve, as exemplified by a report from Hertzer et al.[5] at the Cleveland Clinic Foundation. In a series of 2,228 consecutive isolated CEA procedures, they documented an overall stroke rate of 1.8% (1.3% for asymptomatic patients) and a mortality rate of 0.5%, for a combined stroke-mortality rate of 2.3%. Despite the proven efficacy of CEA in the prevention of ischemic stroke, great interest has been generated in carotid angioplasty/stenting as an alternative to surgical therapy. The remainder of this chapter will examine the indications, techniques, and results of this novel therapy (Figure 10–1).

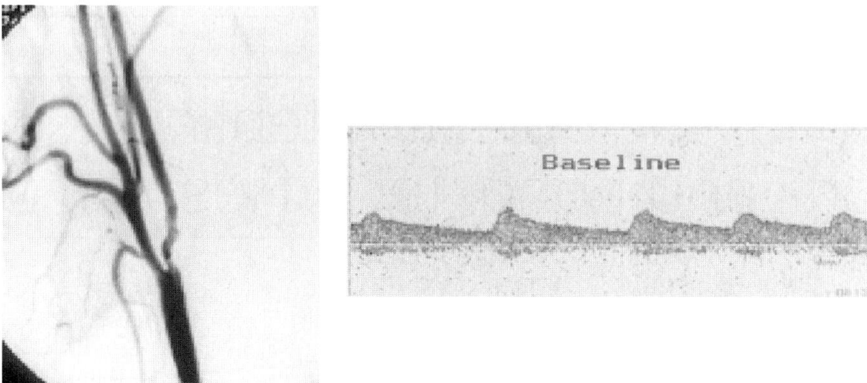

Figure 10–1A. Baseline carotid angiogram and transcranial Doppler image of the middle cerebral artery. Symptomatic left carotid stenosis. Prior radical neck dissection and radiation.

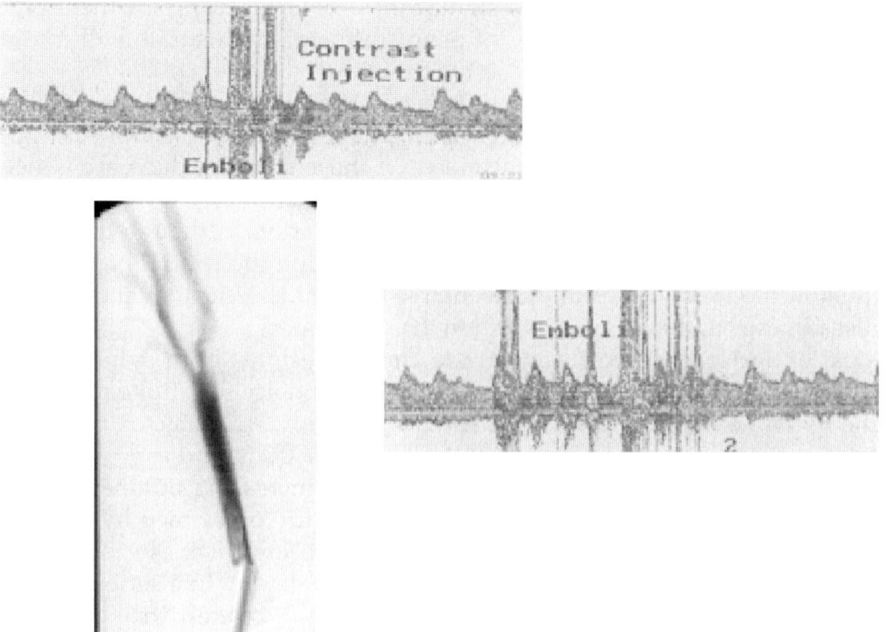

Figure 10–1B. High-intensity transient signals with contrast injection and pre-dilatation with 3 mm balloon.

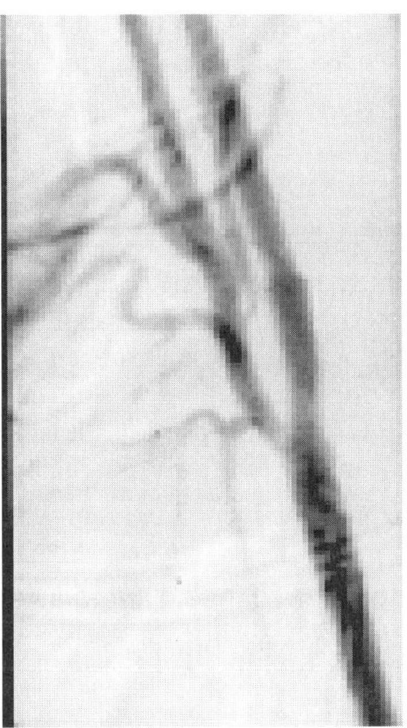

Figure 10–1C. Completion angiogram following angioplasty and placement of balloon-expandable stent.

CAROTID ANGIOPLASTY / STENTING

Indications

The indications for carotid angioplasty and stenting do not differ from those of standard surgical carotid endartectomy:

1. Asymptomatic lesions that fall within the "80–99%" range on duplex ultrasound, which correlates with an angiographic stenosis of at least 60%. Most clinical trials of carotid angioplasty/stenting in asymptomatic patients require an *angiographic* stenosis of at least 80% for study inclusion.
2. Symptomatic patients (hemispheric TIA, amaurosis fugax, or stroke with minimal residua) with at least a 70% angiographic stenosis. Patients with symptomatic, ulcerated stenoses greater than 50% may benefit from endarterectomy; this has not yet been extrapolated to carotid intervention.

Given the exemplary results of CEA, many vascular surgeons have reserved angioplasty / stenting for patients considered to be at "high-risk" for surgical therapy. Ouriel and Hertzer, et al.[6] reviewed 3061 CEA procedures performed over a 10-year period; patients were stratified into "high-risk" and "low-risk" groups based on the presence or absence of the following comorbid conditions: 1. severe coronary artery disease, 2. chronic obstructive pulmonary disease, and 3. renal disease. The composite endpoint of stroke/myocardial infarction/death was 3.8% for the entire cohort. Among the high-risk group, however, the result was 7.4%, significantly higher than those without these comorbidities (2.9%, p<0.005). The authors suggest that initial clinical evaluation of carotid angioplasty/stenting might best be performed in the group in whom CEA carries significant risk. A list of other potentially "high-risk" conditions are listed in Table 10–1. Table 10–2 lists limitations and contraindications to the technique.

Technique

As with any other surgical or interventional technique, careful pre-procedural evaluation and planning is essential to success. All patients should have a carotid duplex ultrasound from an accredited vascular laboratory confirming the presence of a high-grade stenosis, and its location with respect to the carotid bifurcation, paying careful attention to the presence of mobile atheroma or thrombus which could embolize during catheter/guidewire manipulation. Subsequently, all patients must have an arch/carotid/intracranial angiogram either as a separate study prior to the proce-

---

TABLE 10–1. POSSIBLE INDICATIONS FOR CAROTID ANGIOPLASTY IN "HIGH-RISK" PATIENTS

1. Severe cardiac disease:
   - a. requiring coronary PTA or CABG
   - b. history of congestive heart failure
2. Severe chronic obstructive pulmonary disease
   - a. requiring home oxygen
   - b. FEV-1 < 20% predicted
3. Severe chronic renal insufficiency
   - a. Serum creatinine > 3.0 mg%
   - b. Currently on dialysis
4. Prior carotid endarterectomy (restenosis)
   - a. contralateral vocal cord paralysis
5. Surgically inaccessible lesions
   - a. at or above the second cervical vertebra
   - b. inferior to the clavicle
6. Radiation-induced carotid stenosis
7. Prior ipsilateral radical neck dissection
8. Contralateral internal carotid occlusion

TABLE 10–2. LIMITATIONS OF AND CONTRAINDICATIONS TO CAROTID ANGIOPLASTY / STENTING

Inability to obtain femoral artery access

Unfavorable aortic arch anatomy

Severe tortuosity of the common carotid artery

Severely calcified / undilatable stenoses

Lesions containing fresh thrombus

Extensive stenoses (longer than 2 cm)

Critical (99+%) stenoses

Lesions adjacent to carotid artery aneurysms

Contrast-related issues:
   Chronic renal insufficiency
   Previous life-threatening contrast reaction

dure or at the time of the proposed intervention. Specific details to be gained from this complete study include tortuosity of the brachiocephalic trunks (which impacts catheter/guidewire access to the target lesion), location, character and extent of the stenosis, the presence of tandem common carotid/internal carotid lesions, the presence or absence of thrombus, and the presence of intracranial disease (occlusions, stenoses, aneurysms). It is imperative to document the status of the intracranial circulation prior to intervention, so that potential procedure-related embolic lesions can be identified and compared with the pre-angioplasty study. At the time of the diagnostic study, measurements of lesion length and diameter of the arteries proximal and distal to the lesion can be made; this will aid in the selection of an appropriate stent and protection device. Potential candidates should have a thorough cardio-pulmonary evaluation. Informed consent regarding the risks and potential benefits of the procedure, especially as they relate to alternative therapies (medical therapy, CEA) is imperative. Ideally, a team of physicians (surgeon, neurologist, interventionist) should review all case summaries and radiographic studies, and a consensus reached regarding the most appropriate therapy for each individual patient. All patients are pre-treated with aspirin and clopidogrel for several days prior to their procedure. In addition, most study protocols require both a pre- and post-procedural brain scan (CT or MRI) and a thorough, documented neurological evaluation by a certified neurologist.

Arterial access for carotid intervention is typically gained through the retrograde femoral approach. A 5-Fr sheath is placed, and a guidewire is placed under direct fluoroscopic control into the descending thoracic aorta. At this point, the patient is systemically anticoagulated with heparin (100mg/kg) to achieve an Activated Clotting Time (ACT) of greater than 250–300 seconds. The ACT is monitored during the course of the procedure to determine if additional anticoagulation is needed. The 5-Fr sheath is then exchanged for a long 7-Fr sheath through which the intervention will be performed. A 5-Fr diagnostic catheter is then advanced into the ipsilateral common carotid artery, and a selective diagnostic arteriogram of the carotid bifurcation is performed. A .035-in guidewire is then advanced into the common carotid artery to provide support for the sheath, which is advanced over the wire and catheter into the distal common carotid artery, several centimeters proximal to the target lesion. With tortuous anatomy, extra guidewire support may be necessary. This may be achieved by advancing the guidewire into the terminal branches of the external carotid artery; the target lesion should not be engaged at this point, and in fact should be avoided. The crossing guidewire/protection device, pre- and post-dilatation balloons, and the stent should be prepared by an assistant during this phase of the procedure, minimizing intervention time once the lesion has been crossed. Typically, patients are given intravenous atropine (0.5–1.0 mg) to prevent reflex bradycardia during balloon expansion and stent deployment. This may be unnecessary when treating post-endarterectomy restenoses, as the carotid bulb is typically denervated.

The lesion is then crossed with a steerable guidewire (typically .018- or .014-inch) and the protection device, if available, is deployed. With filter devices, flow through the device is confirmed with contrast injection following each phase of the procedure. For balloon-occlusion devices, *absence* of flow in the internal carotid is confirmed prior to lesion manipulation. Pre-dilation is performed with a non-compliant balloon, typically 3.5–4.0 mm in diameter. The stent is then deployed across the target lesion, and post-dilation is performed with an appropriate-sized balloon (based on pre-procedure measurement of the internal carotid artery). The guidewire is left in place until the completion angiogram is reviewed, to avoid losing access to the carotid artery in case of iatrogenic dissection. It is the author's preference not to reverse the heparin anticoagulation at the end of the procedure; a closure device is used at the arterial puncture site.

Following a brief stay in a monitored setting, patients are returned to the regular nursing floor. They are allowed to ambulate according to the status of their access site, and are typically discharged the next morning following completion of laboratory studies, carotid duplex ultrasound, neurologic evaluation and brain scan. Medical therapy includes aspirin (81 mg) and clopidogrel (75 mg) for 1 month, followed by lifetime aspirin. Follow-up duplex studies are performed at 1 month, 6 months, and every 6–12 months thereafter.

Results

The short-term result of carotid angioplasty/stenting are largely dependent upon the presence or absence of cerebral embolization. With the relatively recent addition of cerebral protection to the procedure, associated stroke risk seems to have decreased. Admittedly, however, improvements in devices and technology have created a "moving target," making evaluation of results difficult at best. Nevertheless, a reasonable summary of the procedure, as it exists today, can be created from the available literature.

A representative sample of studies/results is listed in Table 10–3. Only peer-reviewed English-language publications reporting at least 50 procedures within the last 5 years are included. In addition, several key studies deserve closer inspection.

The first peer-reviewed manuscript reporting on the results of a large cohort of patients was in 1997 by Yadav et al.[7] from the University of Alabama at Birmingham. A total of 107 patients (126 arteries) were treated; 59% were symptomatic, and many were referred from local vascular surgeons. All patients were treated with balloon-ex-

TABLE 10–3. CURRENT RESULTS OF CAROTID ANGIOPLASTY / STENTING

Author/year	n (arteries)	% asymptomatic	Cerebral protection	Stroke + death
Yadav 1997	126	41%	No	7.9%
Jordan 1997	107	36%	No	9.3%
Henry 1998	174	65%	Mixed	2.9%
Bergeron 1999	99	56%	No	2%
Wholey 2000	5,210	Not stated	Mixed	5.07%
Shawl 2000	192	39%	No	2.9%
Roubin 2001	604	48%	Mixed	7.4%
CAVATAS 2001	251	4%	No	10%
Brooks 2001	53	0%	No	0%
d'Audiffret 2001	68	70%	Mixed	5.8%
Reimers 2001	88	64%	Yes	2.3%
Paniagua 2001	69	84%	No	5.6%
Criado 2002	135	60%	Mixed	2%
Guimaraens 2002	194	8%	Yes	2.6%
Al-Mubarak 2002	164	52%	Yes	2%
Weighted average (excluding Wholey)	2,324	42%	Mixed	5.3%

pandable stents without cerebral protection. Amazingly, there were only 2 major strokes, 7 minor strokes, and 1 death at 30 days, for a combined stroke mortality (CSM) of 7.9%.

Of note, 77% of patients would not have been eligible for NASCET or ACAS (inferring that these patients were unfit for standard CEA); Jordan et al.,[8] reporting from the same institution, found that 72% of 120 CEA procedures performed during a similar time period would also have been excluded from these 2 pivotal trials.

Expanding on the UAB experience, Roubin et al. [9] have subsequently reported on patients treated at UAB and at Lenox Hill Hospital in New York. Six hundred four arteries were treated in 528 consecutive patients over a 5-year period. This included patients treated with both balloon-expandable and self-expanding stents, with and without cerebral protection devices. The overall 30-day combined stroke/mortality was 8.1% (for 528 patients), and included a 5.5% rate of minor stroke, 1.6% major stroke rate, and 1% rate of non-neurologic death. When divided into yearly intervals, the risk of stroke and death reached a maximum of 12.5% in the period ending September 1997, and fell to a minimum of 3.2% the following year. This rather dramatic change in results likely represents improvement in technology (filter devices, stents, guidewires) as well as an improved ability of the investigators to select appropriate patients for intervention.

The CAVATAS study,[10] published in June 2001, reported the results of a randomized trial of surgery *vs* angioplasty (with and without stenting) for the treatment of patients with symptomatic carotid and vertebral artery stenosis. Two hundred fifty-one patients were randomized to the endovascular arm, and 253 were randomized to the surgical arm. While the 2 procedures were essentially equivalent in their abilities to prevent (or cause, as it turned out) stroke, both treatments did so at an unacceptably high level; the combined endpoint of death or any stroke was achieved in 10% of patients in both groups. In addition, 20% of patients treated with angioplasty or stenting had severe restenosis or occlusion at 1 year. The authors conclude that endovascular techniques are better than surgery, as they avoid a neck incision and the risk of general anesthesia. Had the results from the surgical cohort approached those of the NASCET trial, however, it is likely that the trial would have been suspended in favor of surgery. This trial has several other flaws that make it essentially irrelevant in current clinical practice. It was selective and non-consecutive, and only 26% of the patients in the endovascular group had stents placed; the majority had angioplasty alone. No cerebral protection devices were used. As such, the conclusions reached are probably not applicable to current, state-of-the-art carotid angioplasty practice.

Finally, a recent report from Criado et al.[11] describes their experience with carotid angioplasty/stenting in a vascular surgery practice. During a 40-month period from 1997–2001, 135 carotid angioplasty/stent procedures were performed, largely (60%) in asymptomatic patients. The rate of complications was quite acceptable at 2%, and only one patient had a significant restenosis at 16 months mean follow-up. Perhaps more importantly, these 132 patients represent 41% of those being treated for carotid disease in their vascular/endovascular practice. While this seems extraordinarily high, it may simply be a bellweather for things to come in the practice of vascular surgery, and underscores the importance of vascular surgery's involvement in this new technology.

Proximal common carotid lesions are relatively uncommon when compared with bifurcation lesions, but may be well-treated with angioplasty and stenting (Figure 10–2). In the author's experience, most are treated via common carotid cutdown and

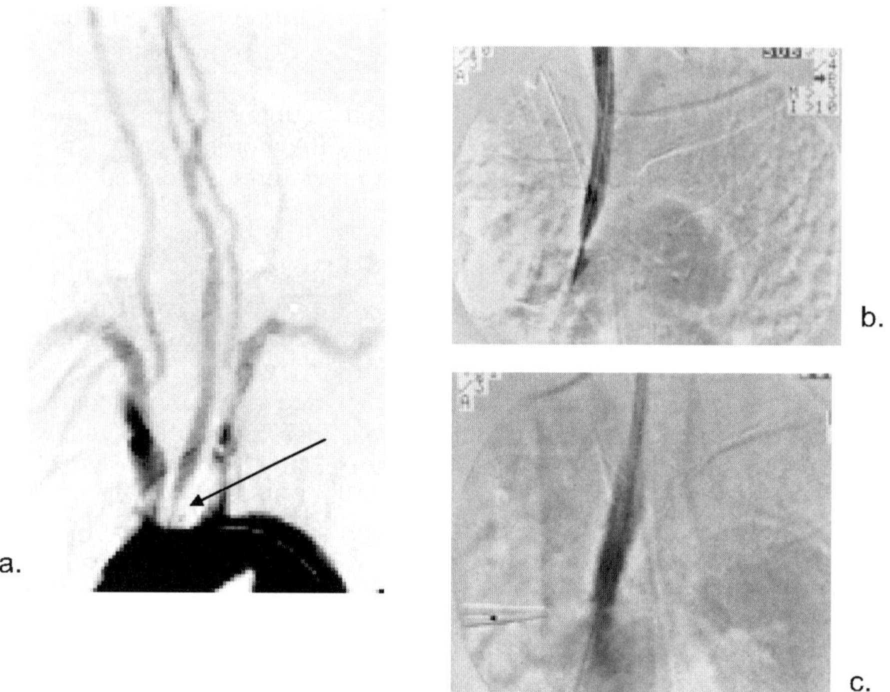

Figure 10–2. (A) Arch aortogram. High-grade symptomatic ostial left common carotid artery stenosis (arrow). **(B)** Selective carotid arteriogram performed via common carotid cutdown and retrograde access. **(C)** Completion angiogram following angioplasty and balloon-expandable stent placement.

retrograde angioplasty and placement of a balloon-expandable stent. Of 14 consecutive procedures performed at the Cleveland Clinic,[12] one was converted to carotid-subclavian transposition following an iatrogenic dissection, and 2 other procedures resulted in stroke secondary to internal carotid artery thrombosis. In both cases, which were performed in conjunction with re-do bifurcation endarterectomies, the common carotid was patent at the time of surgical re-exploration and internal carotid thrombectomy. While the carotid stent procedure was not likely implicated, caution is urged when performing these combined procedures.

Embolic stroke is the most common serious complication (Figure 10–3) reported for carotid angioplasty/stenting; its incidence may be affected by the use of cerebral protection devices. Advanced age and the presence of long or multiple lesions have been implicated as independent predictors of stroke.[13] As with most procedures, there is a significant learning curve that must be overcome.[14] Other complications have also been cited, including prolonged bradycardia and hypotension, deformation of balloon-expandable stents, stent thrombosis, and Horner's syndrome. Cerebral hyperperfusion with associated seizures and intracranial hemorrhage have also been reported. The incidence of restenosis probably ranges from 3–10% at 1 year, although restenosis rates of up to 75% have been reported following intervention for post-endarterectomy restenosis. Most patients can be safely treated with repeat angioplasty.[15–17]

Enrollment in the CREST (Carotid Revascularization Endarterectomy versus Stent Trial) has begun. This NIH-sponsored study will randomize symptomatic patients with high-grade carotid stenosis to CEA or angioplasty/stenting with a self-expanding

A

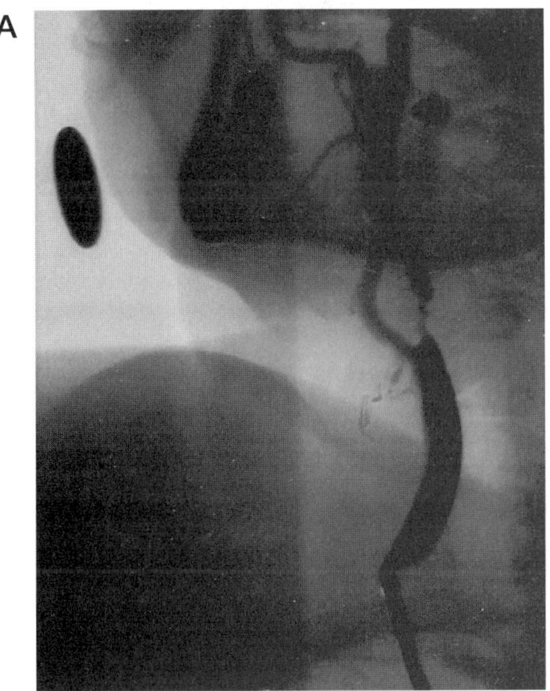

B

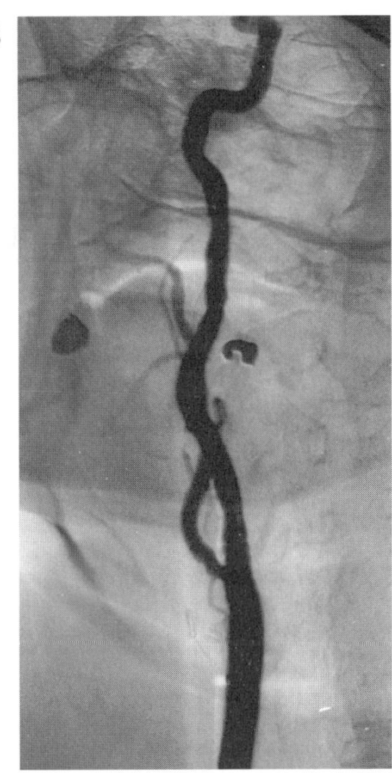

Figure 10–3. (A) Pre-procedure selective right carotid arteriogram in patient with recurrent carotid stenosis 18 months following endarterectomy with primary closure. **(B)** Completion angiogram following PTA and nitinol stent placement.

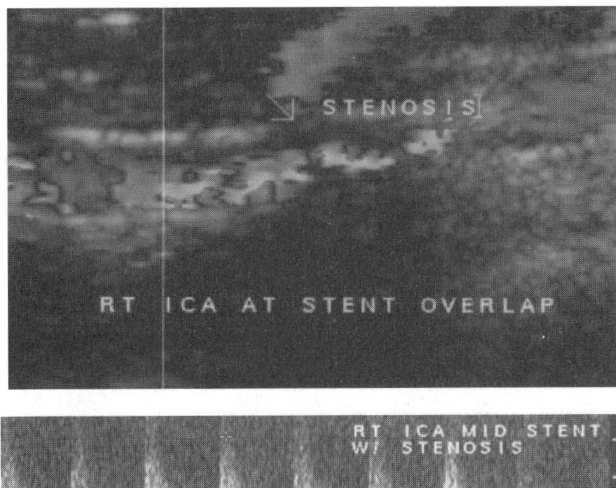

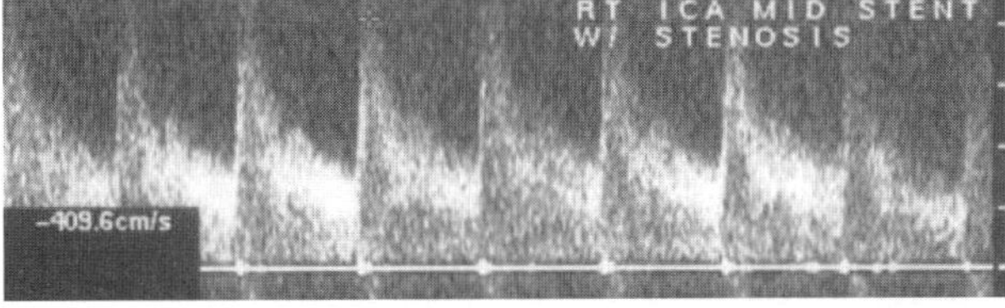

Figure 10–3C. Color duplex ultrasound 1 hour following carotid PTA/stent identifies fresh thrombus and high-grade stenosis; patient experienced right hemispheric TIA.

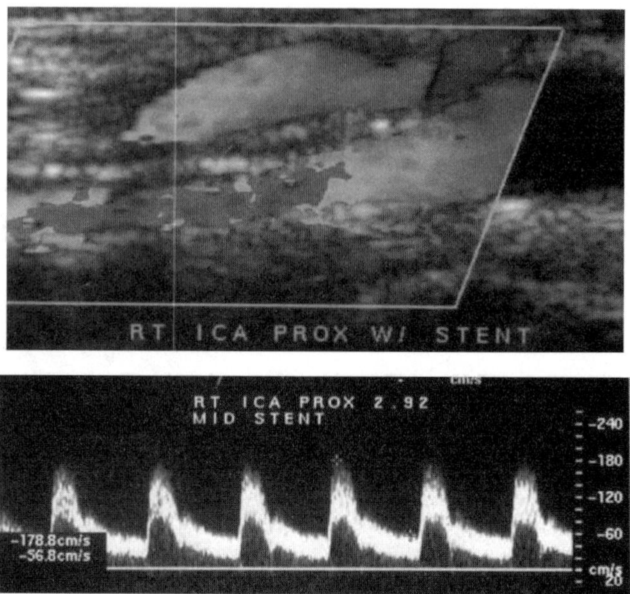

Figure 10–3D. Patient treated with heparin and 8-hour infusion of abciximab. Color duplex ultrasound 18 hours post-procedure shows resolution of thrombus/stenosis.

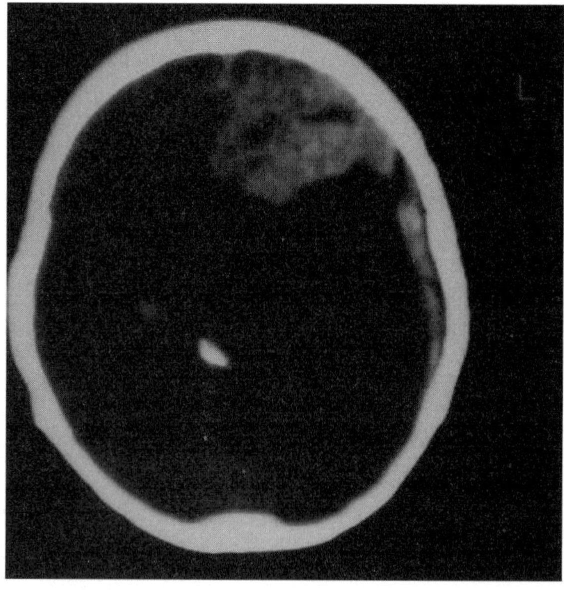

Figure 10–3E. 96 hours post-procedure. Patient suffers fatal contralateral intracranial hemorrhage.

(nitinol) stent and a cerebral protection device. Primary endpoints include stroke, myocardial infarction, and death within 30 days, and ipsilateral stroke up to 4 years. Secondary outcomes will describe differential efficacy in men vs women, contrast 30-day morbidity/mortality, examine restenosis rates of the 2 procedures, evaluate cost and quality of life, and identify subgroups at differential risk for CEA and angioplasty.[18] A parallel registry arm of the study, denoted CARESS, will run simultaneously to the parent study. In addition, a number of industry-sponsored trials of various stents and protection devices are studying the procedure in high-risk subsets.

CONCLUSIONS

Carotid angioplasty and stenting is an evolving technique which shows significant promise in the treatment of patients with carotid occlusive disease. Carotid endarterectomy remains, however, the treatment of choice for most patients with bifurcation disease, both symptomatic and asymptomatic. Certain high-risk subsets, especially those with cardiopulmonary and renal disease and those with surgically unfavorable lesions, may benefit from endovascular therapy at the present time. Carefully designed trials will hopefully answer the questions of clinical efficacy and safety.

While tremendous enthusiasm has been generated for carotid angioplasty and stenting, especially by non-surgeons, it remains an investigational/experimental procedure, and has yet to be proven equivalent or superior to carotid endarterectomy in head-to-head comparison. As noted in the American Heart Association Science Advisory[19] in 1998, we must remember the first tenet of medicine: *primum non nocere*—first, do no harm. Only through carefully-designed clinical trials with dispassionate oversight can we determine its role in the treatment of patients with carotid disease.

REFERENCES

1. U. S. Bureau of the Census, *Statistical Abstract of the United States*: 1992 (112th edition.) Washington, D.C.
2. Bonita,R Epidemiology of stroke. *Lancet*. 1992;339:342–344.
3. North American Symptomatic Carotid Endarterectomy Trial Collaborators. Beneficial effect of carotid endarterectomy in symptomatic patients with high-grade carotid stenosis. *N Eng J Med*. 1991:325;445–453.
4. Executive Committee for the Asymptomatic Carotid Atherosclerosis Study. Endarterectomy for asymptomatic carotid artery stenosis. *JAMA*. 1995;273:1421–1428.
5. Hertzer NR, O'Hara PJ, Mascha EJ, et al. Early outcome assessment for 2228 consecutive carotid endarterectomy procedures: The Cleveland Clinic experience from 1989 to 1995. *J Vasc Surg*. 1997;26:1–10.
6. Ouriel K, Hertzer NR, Beven EG, et al. Preprocedural risk stratification: Identifying an appropriate population for carotid stenting. *J Vasc Surg*. 2001;33:728–732.
7. Yadav JS, Roubin GS, Iyer S, et al. Elective stenting of the extracranial carotid arteries. *Circulation*. 1997;95:376–381.
8. Jordan WD, Schroeder BS, Fisher WK et al. A comparison of angioplasty with stenting with endarterectomy for the treatment of carotid artery stenosis. *Ann Vasc Surg*. 1997;11:2–8.
9. Roubin GS, New G, Iyer SS, et al. Immediate and late clinical outcomes of carotid artery stenting in patients with symptomatic and asymptomatic carotid artery stenosis. A 5-yr prospective analysis. *Circulation*. 2001;103:532–537.

10. CAVATAS Investigators. Endovascular versus surgical treatment in patients with carotid stenosis in the Carotid and Vertebral Artery Transluminal Angioplasty Study (CAVATAS): a randomized trial. *Lancet.* 2001;357:1729–1737.
11. Criado FJ, Lingelbach JM, Ledesma DFet al. Carotid artery stenting in a vascular surgery practice. *J Vasc Surg* 2002;35:430–434.
12. Sullivan TM, Gray BH, Bacharach JM, et al. Angioplasty and primary stenting of the subclavian, innominate, and common carotid arteries in 83 patients. *J Vasc Surg.* 1998;28: 1059–1065.
13. Mathur A, Roubin GS, Iyer SS, et al. Predictors of stroke complicating carotid artery stenting. *Circulation.* 1998;97:1239–1245.
14. Ahmadi R, Willfort A, Lang W, et al. Carotid artery stenting: effect of learning curve and intermediate-term morphologic outcome. *J Endovasc Ther.* 2001;8:539–546.
15. Chakhotura EY, Hobson RW, Goldstein J, et al. In-stent restenosis after carotid angioplasty: Incidence and management. *J Vasc Surg.* 2001;33:220–226.
16. d'Audiffret A, Desgranges P, Kobeiter H et al. Technical aspects and current results of carotid stenting. *J Vasc Surg.* 2001;33:1001–1007.
17. Leger AR, Neale M, Harris JP. Poor durability of carotid angioplasty and stenting for treatment of recurrent artery stenosis after carotid endarterectomy: an institutional experience. *J Vasc Surg.* 2001;33:1008–1014.
18. Hobson RW. Carotid angioplasty-stent: clinical experience and role for clinical trials. *J Vasc Surg.* 2001;33:S117–123.
19. Bettman MA, Katzen BT, Whisnant J, et al. AHA Science Advisory. Carotid stenting and angioplasty. *Circulation.* 1998;97:121–123.

11

Cerebral Protection Devices for Carotid Artery Stenting

Heron E. Rodriguez, MD and Mark K. Eskandari, MD

Worldwide, stroke is recognized as one of the leading causes of death and disability among the elderly. In the United States alone, 750,000 strokes occur annually, with a mortality rate exceeding 150,000 each year.[1] Atherosclerotic narrowing at the carotid bifurcation is the most common cause of large-vessel atherothrombotic stroke.[2] Since its original description in the 1950s, carotid endarterectomy (CEA) has remained the gold standard surgical treatment for severe extracranial carotid artery disease and stroke prevention.[3] This treatment option is being challenged with advances in endoluminal interventions. Even in the absence of definitive clinical evidence, carotid stenting is rapidly emerging as the minimally invasive alternative to CEA. Unregulated carotid stenting is now under the ownership of various medical specialists, of which vascular surgeons represent the minority.[4] As carotid artery stenting has taken a stronghold, new technologic advances have led to the development of mechanical distal cerebral protection devices. These devices are now being used in a number of clinical trials and registries. It makes intuitive sense that these protection devices should reduce the incidence of periprocedural stroke, however the true efficacy of many of these devices is still unknown. It is imperative that the vascular surgeon treating carotid artery pathology with carotid artery stenting be familiar with the principles and characteristics of each of the major categories of mechanical cerebral protection devices.

CEREBRAL PROTECTION DEVICES

Despite advances in extracranial stenting techniques, neurological events linked to distal intracranial embolization of particulate material have been reported to occur at prohibitive rates of 5.2% to 9.3%.[5–8] The incidence of microembolization detected by transcranial Doppler has been demonstrated to be significantly higher during carotid angioplasty and stenting than during carotid endarterectomy.[9] Furthermore, using an ex-vivo model of the carotid bifurcation, Ohki et al. demonstrated the occurrence of microembolization in each instance of carotid angioplasty and stenting.[10] Significant risk of dislodging plaque material exists throughout the entire procedure, but is critical during some steps: wire access to the branches of the aortic arch, sheath advancement into the common carotid artery, wire crossing of the stenotic lesion, balloon dilation, and stent deployment. These observations led to the notion that, in order for carotid angioplasty to have a feasible application with acceptable stroke rates, some form of distal mechanical protection needed to be developed. In 1990, Theron was the first to report the use of a "distal protection device" for the performance of a carotid angioplasty.[11] The investigators constructed a triple coaxial catheter system, which permitted temporary balloon occlusion of the distal internal carotid artery during angioplasty and stent placement in the proximal internal carotid artery. This revolutionized the concept of mechanical cerebral protection and led to the development of three main categories of cerebral protection devices: distal occlusion devices, filtration devices, and proximal occlusion devices.

The three general approaches to percutaneous cerebral protection are shown in Table 11–1. **Distal occlusion devices** employ the use of an occlusion balloon placed distal to the stenotic lesion. This temporarily halts the outflow into the distal internal carotid artery while the proximally located lesion is treated. Before deflating the distal occlusion balloon, an aspiration catheter is used to retrieve loose particulate matter trapped proximal to the balloon. **Filtration devices** use a filter with a specific pore size (measured in microns), which is placed beyond the stenotic lesion to capture embolic

TABLE 11–1. TYPES OF CEREBRAL PROTECTION DEVICES FOR CAROTID INTERVENTIONS

Type of device	Examples	Advantages	Disadvantages
Distal ICA Occlusion	• PercuSurge GuardWire™ (Medtronic AVE/PercuSurge, Sunnyvale, CA)	• Lower crossing profile • Captures particles of all size	• Possibility of local injury to ICA by balloon • Possibility of embolism via ECA branches • Possibility of embolism during lesion crossing • Inability to perform angiograms while balloon inflated • Intolerance to total ICA occlusion
Distal Filter	• MedNova NeuroShield™ (MedNova, Inc. Ireland) • AngioGuard™ (AngioGuard, Inc., Cordis, Warren, New Jersey) • EPI FilterWire™ (Embolic protection, Inc., San Carlos,CA) • AccuNet™ (Guidant Corp., Indianapolis, IN) • Interceptor™ (Medtronic Inc., Santa Rosa, CA)	• Maintenance of flow throughout the procedure • Ability to perform angiograms throughout the procedure	• Larger profiles, difficult to cross some tortuous lesions • Possibility of incomplete apposition of the filter and the arterial wall • Possibility of embolism during lesion crossing • Potential for filter thrombosis • Particles smaller than pore size may embolize
Proximal Occlusion	• ArteriA PAES™ (ArteriA, Inc. San Francisco, CA)	• Protection starts before crossing the lesion • Complete protection to ICA and ECA • Freedom for wire choice • Capture particles of all size	• Need for larger groin sheath (10 Fr) • Total arrest of antegrade flow in the protected side • Potential for arterial injury at balloon inflation sites

material during the intervention. *Proximal occlusion devices* use a balloon placed proximal to the stenotic lesion to occlude the inflow. In the presence of normal intracerebral circulation, this proximal occlusion causes reversal of flow in the distal internal carotid artery. Each category of cerebral protection has individual strengths and disadvantages. A detailed discussion of each type is offered below.

DISTAL OCCLUSION

The distal occlusion devices are currently best represented by the PercuSurge GuardWire™ (Medtronic AVE/PercuSurge, Sunnyvale, CA) (Figure 11–1).

The PercuSurge GuardWire™ is constructed as a 0.14″ hollow nitinol wire with a shapeable floppy distal tip. Proximal to the floppy tip is a compliant elastomeric polyurethane occlusion balloon with a maximal crossing profile of 0.36″ when deflated. Once the stenotic lesion is crossed with the GuardWire™, the occlusion balloon

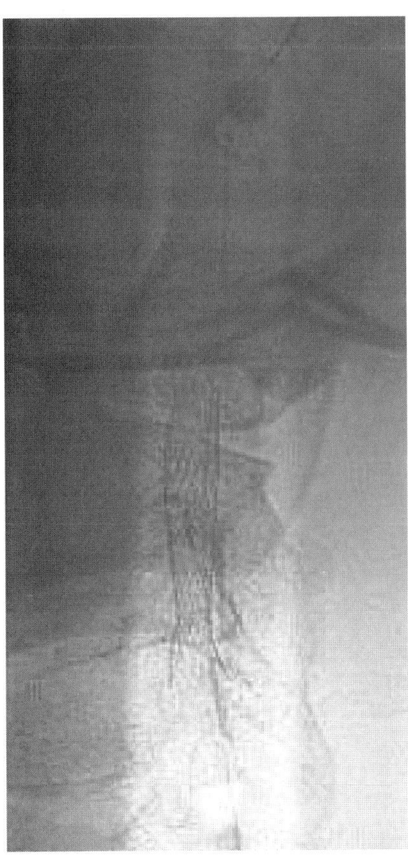

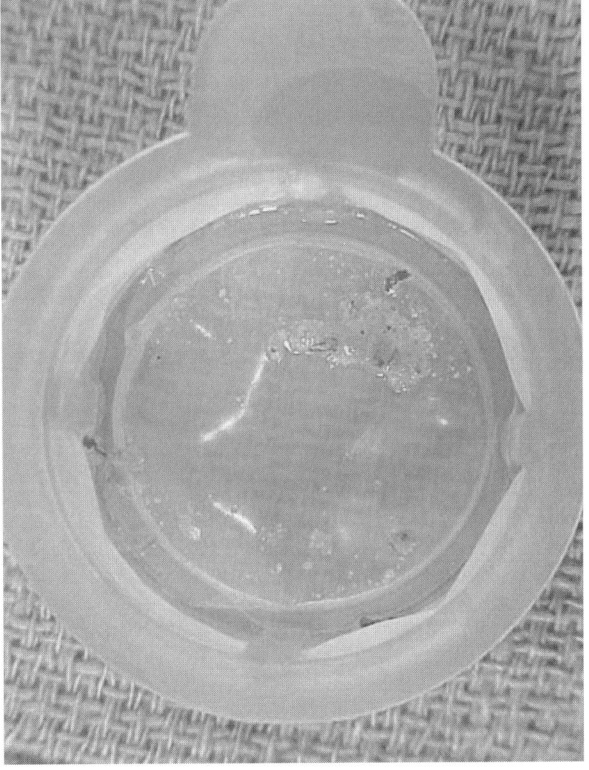

Figure 11–1A. Fluoroscopic image showing the PercuSurge distal balloon occlusion device inflated in the distal internal carotid following stent deployment and prior to aspiration of the stagnant column of blood below the occlusion balloon.

Figure 11–1B. Debris retrieved from the aspiration catheter of the PercuSurge distal balloon occlusion protection device (on a 40-micron filter membrane).

is inflated using the handheld Microseal Adaptor® and EZ Flator™ to a variable size ranging from 3 to 6 mm in diameter. The handheld system is then removed from the proximal end of the wire while the occlusion balloon remains inflated. This coaxial exchange set-up allows for over-the-wire delivery of angioplasty balloons and stent devices. Any embolic particles released during this portion of the procedure remain in the stagnant pool of blood below the occlusion balloon in the distal ICA. This column of blood is aspirated through the large bore lumen of the Export™ catheter. At the conclusion of the procedure, the occlusion balloon is deflated with the handheld device. Total occlusion times typically range from 5 to 15 minutes. Reported complications of the device include intolerance of total occlusion manifested by changes in level of consciousness, dysarthria, motor weakness, seizures, and/or convulsions. Other potential risks include cardiac arrhythmias (bradycardia and asystole), hypotension, and local trauma to the occluded segment of the distal ICA (vasospasm or dissection).

The PercuSurge GuardWire™ currently has FDA approval for use in the treatment of degenerated saphenous vein grafts following coronary artery bypass surgery. Several reports describing carotid angioplasty and stenting with cerebral protection using the PercuSurge GuardWire™ system have now been published (Table 11–2).[12–17] In 1999, Henry et al. reported their initial experience treating 53 ICA stenosis on 48 patients.[12] The immediate technical success rate was 100% with mean balloon occlusion time of 542 ± 243 seconds. One patient developed amaurosis, yielding an overall a neurologic event rate of 1.8%. More recently, they have published their mid-term results of 184 procedures performed under cerebral protection on 167 patients.[13] The technical success rate was 99.5%, mean occlusion time was 422 ± 220 seconds, and 4 patients suffered neurologic events (2.2%) for a combined 30-day stroke and death rate of 2.7%. Two other groups from Europe have reported their experience with carotid intervention using the PercuSurge GuardWire™ system. Dietz et al. published a series of 43 patients with immediate technical success rate of 93% and a combined perioperative stroke and death rate of 2.5%.[14] Tubler et al. reported a series of 54 patients treated with a technical success rate of 100%, mean occlusion time of 624 ± 240 seconds, and a perioperative neurologic event rate of 5.2%.[15] Most recently, Al-Mubarak et al. reported their results following stenting of 37 patients under cerebral protection,[16] in which one patient suffered a nondisabling stroke and another one died from conse-

TABLE 11–2. REPORTED EXPERIENCE WITH CAROTID INTERVENTION UNDER DISTAL BALLOON PROTECTION

Author	No of cases	Success rate	Combined stroke & death rate
Henry M J Endovasc Surg 1999[12]	53	100	1.8
Tubler T Circulation 2001[15]	58	100	1.7
Dietz A Stroke 2001[14]	43	93	2.5
D'Audiffret J Vasc Surg 2001[23]	15	100	0
Al-Mubarak Circulation 2001[16]	37	100	5.4
Whitlow Stroke 2002[17]	75	100	0

quences of hyperperfusion syndrome, resulting in a perioperative combined stroke and death rate of 5.4%.

This particular device offers the advantage of a low crossing profile and complete distal internal carotid protection. Disadvantages of distal occlusion devices include no protection while crossing the stenotic lesion, interruption of antegrade flow during protection, risk of local trauma to the distal ICA, risk of embolization via the ECA, limited angiogram during the procedure, and no freedom of guidewire choices.

DISTAL FILTER

The distal filter devices are best represented by MedNova NeuroShield™ (MedNova, Inc., Ireland) (Figure 11–2), AngioGuard™ (AngioGuard, Inc., Cordis, Warren, NJ) (Figure 11–3), EPI FilterWire™ (Embolic Protection, Inc., San Carlos, CA) (Figure 11–4), AccuNet™ (Guidant Corp., Indianapolis, IN), and Interceptor™ (Medtronic Inc., Santa Rosa, CA) (Figure 11–5).

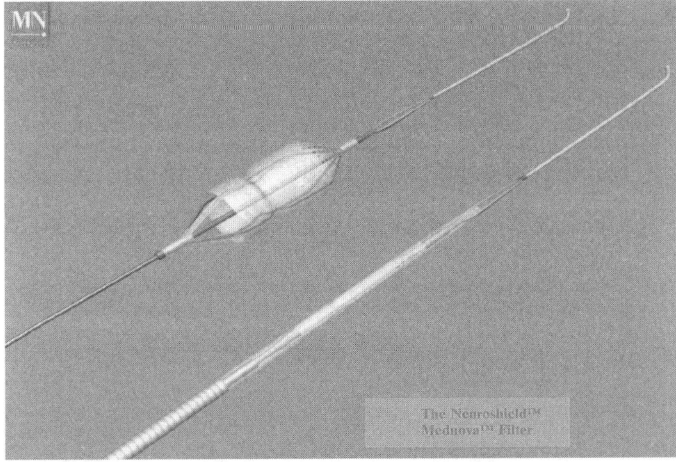

Figure 11–2. MedNova NeuroShield™ distal filter device in the deployed and undeployed states.

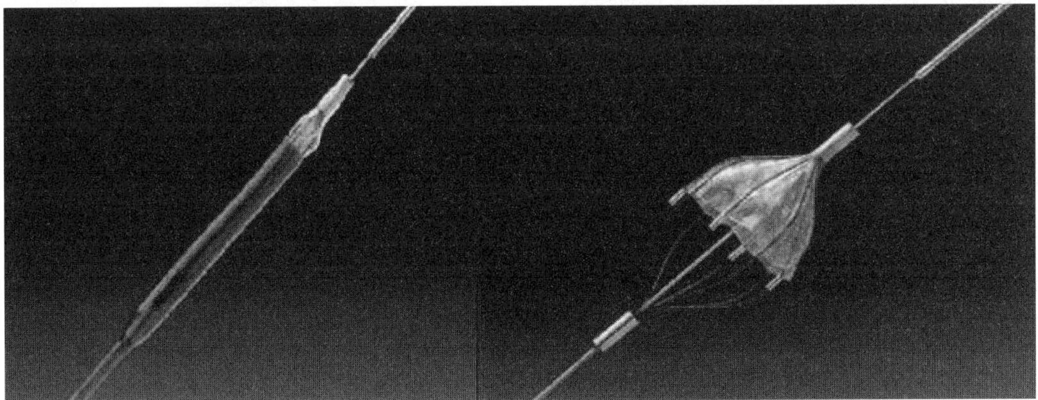

Figure 11–3. AngioGuard™ distal filter device in the deployed and undeployed states.

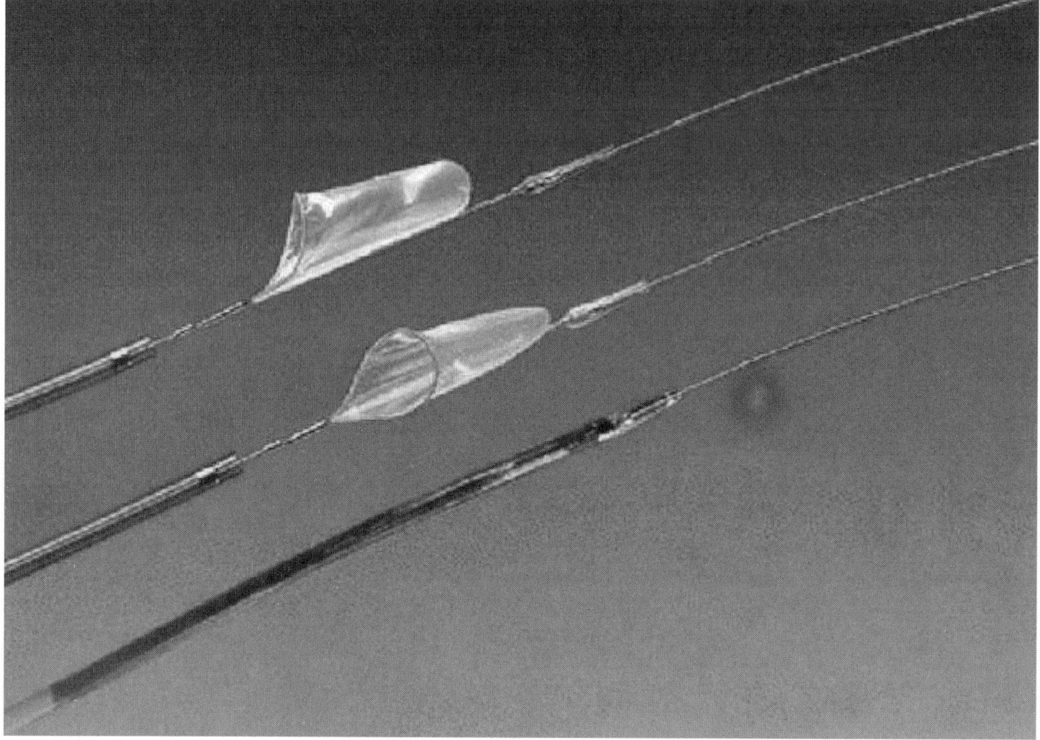

Figure 11–4. EPI FilterWire™ distal filter device in the deployed and undeployed states.

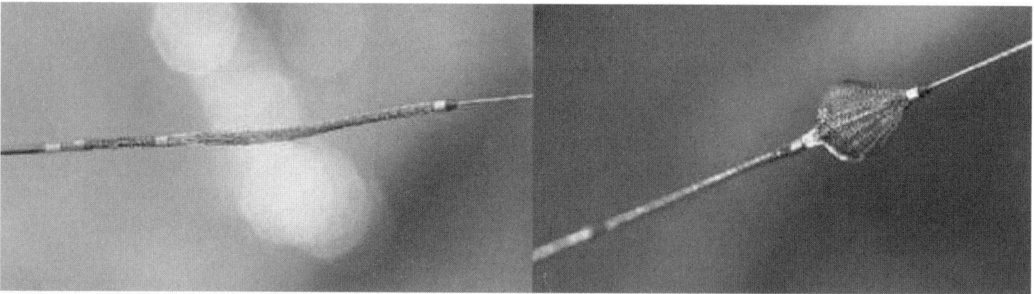

Figure 11–5. Medtronic Interceptor™ nitinol wire filter basket in the undeployed and deployed states.

The MedNova NeuroShield™ filter device is constructed on a 0.14″ wire with a distal floppy shapeable tip. The filtration element is made of a nitinol expansion system and a filter membrane with multiple laser-generated pores (100 microns in diameter) housed within a delivery catheter. Once the guidewire and delivery system cross the stenotic lesion, the delivery catheter is retracted and discarded in order to deploy the filtration system in the distal ICA. The guidewire is then used for subsequent balloon angioplasty and stent placement of the intended lesion. Ideally, the filter element is designed to conform to the vessel lumen upon deployment and capture emboli released during balloon angioplasty and stent placement of the targeted lesion. At the completion of the procedure, a retrieval catheter, passed over the wire, is used to envelop the filter system (including trapped debris) and the entire device is then removed.

The AngioGuard™ filter is similar to the MedNova™ device. It is also based on a 0.14″ guidewire design, but functions more like an umbrella. The crossing profile of the AngioGuard™ in its undeployed state is 3.2 French. The filter element consists of a nitinol wire basket and a polyurethane membrane with multiple 100-micron pores. The intended vessel sizes range from 3.0 to 7.5 mm in diameter.

A unique feature of the EPI FilterWire™ is the "fish-mouth" filter opening. The device is based on a 0.14″ guidewire system and has a crossing profile of 3.5 French. A nitinol ring supports the polyurethane "butterfly net," which theoretically provides for complete circumferential contact with the arterial wall. The ring expands to accommodate a vessel diameter range of 3.5–5.5 mm and the pore size of the membrane is 100 microns.

The AccuNet™ filter is the device being used in the carotid revascularization endarterectomy versus stent (CREST) trial and is similar in design to the AngioGuard™. The primary difference is the pore size of the polyurethane membrane, which is 120 microns.

Newest on the market is the Interceptor™. Based on a 0.14″ system, this filter device has a crossing profile of 2.9 French. The filter is made of braided nitinol with a 100-micron pore size.

Published experience using filter devices comes mainly from Europe. Jaeger et al. reported a series of 20 patients undergoing carotid angioplasty under cerebral protection using the AngioGuard™ filter.[18] Immediate technical success for the angioplasty was obtained in all 20 patients. No neurologic events occurred over a 30-day follow-up. Last year, Reimers et al. reported on a series of 88 procedures performed on 84 patients using 3 different models of filter device.[19] Forty-eight procedures were done using the AngioGuard™ filter, 30 with the NeuroShield™, and 89 with the EPI FilterWire™. One patient (1.2%) experienced a stroke and another one died from cardiac complications 7 days after the procedure (stroke and death rate of 2.2%). This year, Macdonald and colleagues reported 50 patients treated using the MedNova NeuroShield device.[20] The technical success rate was 100%. In all but one patient the filter was successfully placed distal to the lesion. The combined stroke and death rate was 6%.

In general, filters have the advantage of preservation of antegrade flow and the ability to perform angiograms throughout the entire procedure. Disadvantages of distal filter devices include no protection while crossing the stenotic lesion, larger crossing profile, possibility of missing small particles, risk of local trauma to the distal ICA, difficulties in crossing tight or tortuous lesions, risk of filter thrombosis, and no freedom of guidewire choices.

PROXIMAL OCCLUSION

Most of the technology used during carotid angioplasty has evolved from coronary interventions. The proximal occlusion protection devices are an exception. The first device of this type was designed by Juan Carlos Parodi from Argentina and is named after him (PAES™ Parodi Anti Embolism System, ArteriA, Inc., San Francisco CA). The concept behind this device relies on the same surgical principle used to measure carotid stump pressures during CEA: in the presence of a patent intracranial circulation, proximal occlusion of the CCA and the ECA causes reversal of flow into the distal ICA. The PAES™ is constructed as a 10 French guiding catheter with an occlusion balloon at the distal end, which halts antegrade flow in the common carotid artery when it is inflated. Next, an occlusion balloon is placed in the external carotid artery. The central lumen of the guiding catheter is then connected through a filter into the femoral vein and reversal of flow is established while the intervention is being performed. The stenosis in the internal carotid artery can now be crossed using the operator's choice of wire during the reversal of flow in the internal carotid artery. A multicenter trial was recently published reporting the initial experience with the PAES™.[21] Twenty-eight of 30 patients were able to tolerate the reversal of flow. No neurologic events occurred during the 30-day follow-up.

The most obvious advantage of a proximal occlusion device is that there is no need to cross the stenotic lesion prior to establishing distal cerebral protection. Another advantage is that this system does not preclude the use of additional protection devices. A combination of the PAES™ with a filter, the so-called "seat belt and air bag" technique, has been reported.[22] As with any type of occlusion device, intolerance to total carotid arrest occurs in about 10% of patients.

CONCLUSION

It appears that percutaneous carotid angioplasty and stenting is here to stay, at least in a subset of patients. Conclusive evidence is missing until multicenter prospective randomized trials employing mechanical cerebral protection devices, such as the CREST study, are completed. As manufacturers focus more attention on improving the tools necessary to perform this procedure as safely as possible, we will continue to see new and innovative ideas. The currently available protection devices in the noted series appear to reduce the periprocedural risk of neurologic events in experienced hands. Nevertheless, selection bias must be factored into the interpretation of currently published reports.

REFERENCES

1. Brott T, Bogousslavsky J. Treatment of acute ischemic stroke. *N Engl J Med.* 2000;343 (10):710–722.
2. Kistler JP, Buonanno FS, Gress DR. Carotid endarterectomy: Specific therapy based on pathophysiology. *N Engl J Med.* 1991;325(7):505–507.
3. Moore WS, Barnett JJ, Beebe HG, et al. Guidelines for carotid endarterectomy. A multidisciplinary consensus statement from the Ad Hoc Committee, American Heart Association. *Circulation.* 1995;91(2):566–579.
4. Wholey MH, Wholey M, Mathias K, et al. Global experience in cervical carotid artery stent placement. *Cathert Cardiovasc Intervent.* 2000;50(2):160–167.
5. Diethrich EB, Ndiaye M, Reid DB. Stenting in the carotid artery: Initial experience in 110 patients. *J Endovasc Surg.* 1996;3:42–62.
6. Jordan WD, Jr., Schroeder PT, Fisher WS, et al. A comparison of angioplasty with stenting versus endarterectomy for the treatment of carotid artery stenosis. *Ann Vasc Surg.* 1997;11(1):2–8.
7. Jordan WD, Jr., Voellinger DC, Fischer WS, et al. comparison of carotid angioplasty with stenting versus endarterectomy with regional anesthesia. *J Vasc Surg.* 1998;28:397–403.

8. Yadav JD, Roubin GS, Lyer S, et al. Elective stenting of the extracranial carotid arteries. *Circulation.* 1997;95:376–381.

9. Jordan WD, Voellinger DC, Doblar DD, et al. Microemboli detected by transcranial Doppler monitoring in patients during carotid angioplasty versus carotid endarterectomy. *Cardiovasc Surg.* 1999;7(1):33–38.

10. Ohki T, Marin ML, Lyon RT, et al. Ex vivo human carotid artery bifurcation stenting: Correlation of lesion characteristics with embolic potential. *J Vasc Surg.* 1998;27(3):463–471.

11. Theron JG, Courtheoux P, Alachkar F, et al. New triple coaxial catheter system for carotid angioplasty with cerebral protection. *AJNR: Am J Neuroradiol.* 1990;11:869–874.

12. Henry M, Amor M, Henry I, et al. Carotid stenting with cerebral protection: First clinical experience using the PerdcuSurge GuardWire system. *J Endovasc Surg.* 1999;6:321–331.

13. Henry M, Henry I, Klonaris C, et al. Benefits of cerebral protection during carotid stenting with the PercuSurge GuardWire system: Midterm results. *J Endovasc Ther.* 2002;9(1):1–13.

14. Dietz A, Berkefeld J, Theron JG, et al. Endovascular treatment of symptomatic carotid stenosis using stent placement. Long term follow-up of patients with a balanced surgical risk/benefit ratio. *Stroke.* 2001;32:1855–1859.

15. Tubler T, Schluter M, Dirsch O, et al. Balloon-protected carotid artery stenting. Relationship of periprocedural neurologic complications with the size of particulate debris. *Circulation.* 2001;104:2791–2796.

16. Al-Mubarak N, Roubin GS, Vitek JJ, et al. Effect of the distal-balloon protection system on microembolization during carotid stenting. *Circulation.* 2001;104:1999–2002.

17. Whitlow PL, Lylyk P, Londero H, et al. Carotid artery stenting protected with an emboli containment system. *Stroke.* 2002;33:1308–1314.

18. Jaeger H, Mathias K, Drescher R, et al. Clinical results of cerebral protection with a filter device during stent implantation of the carotid artery. *Cardiovasc Intervent Radiol.* 2001;24 (4):249–256.

19. Reimers B, Corvaja N, Moshiri S, et al. Cerebral protection with filter devices during carotid artery stenting. *Circulation.* 2001;104:12–15.

20. Macdonald S, Venables GS, Cleveland TJ, et al. Protected carotid stenting: Safety and efficacy of the MedNova NeuroShield filter. *J Vasc Surg.* 2002;35:966–972.

21. Adami CA, Scuro A, Spinamano L, et al. Use of the Parodi anti-embolism system in carotid stenting: Italian trial results. *J Endovasc Ther.* 2002;9(2):147–154.

22. Parodi JC, Schonholz C, Ferreira LM, et al. "Seat belt and air bag" technique for cerebral protection during carotid stenting. *J Endovasc Ther.* 2002;9(1):20–24.

23. D'Audiffret A, Desgranges P, Kobeiter H, et al. Technical aspects and current results of carotid stenting. *J Vasc Surg.* 2001;33(5):1001–1007.

IV

Aortic Aneurysm

12

Screening for Abdominal Aortic Aneurysm

Frank A. Lederle, MD

HISTORY OF AAA SCREENING

Schilling and colleagues reported the first screening program for abdominal aortic aneurysms (AAA) in 1966.[1] Using physical examination and lateral abdominal x-rays, they detected AAA ≥3.6 cm in 3.1% of 873 men aged 55–64.[1,2] In 1983, Cabellon and colleagues reported using ultrasound and abdominal palpation to find AAA in 7 of 73 asymptomatic patients with vascular disease.[3] There soon followed numerous similar studies and then reports of larger, community based programs. Screening for AAA with ultrasound has since been advocated by various authors and groups and debated extensively in the literature. After the several remaining large randomized trials are reported in the next few years, the place of AAA screening in the periodic health examination will be determined for the foreseeable future.

CRITERIA FOR A SCREENING TEST

Screening is an inherently appealing idea but must be undertaken with caution. The risks and costs apply to many whereas the benefits affect few, and in some instances may even be negligible compared with usual care. It has been argued that when the practitioner initiates screening procedures, there is an ethical requirement for greater certainty regarding benefit than for routine health care, in which the patient asks the practitioner for help.[4] A worthwhile screening program should meet the following criteria[5]: 1) the disease must have a significant effect on the quality or quantity of life, 2) acceptable methods of treatment must be available, 3) the disease must have an asymptomatic period during which detection and treatment significantly reduce morbidity and/or mortality, 4) treatment in the asymptomatic phase must yield a therapeutic result superior to that obtained by delaying treatment until symptoms appear, 5) tests must be available at reasonable cost to detect the condition in the asymptomatic period, 6) the incidence of the condition must be sufficient to justify the cost of screening.

Screening for AAA would appear to meet these criteria. AAA ≥3.0 cm occur in 4–8% of older men.[6, 7] Small AAA are more common than large AAA, such that with each 1 cm decrease in AAA diameter, the number of AAA that diameter or larger more than doubles (Table 12–1). Aortic aneurysm is the 15th leading cause of death in the United States,[8] and most of these deaths are due to rupture of AAA.[9] Small AAA enlarge at an average rate of 1 cm every 3 years,[10, 11] so there is usually a period of at least 5 years from the time that the abdominal aorta reaches 3 cm in diameter (the most common definition of AAA) until symptoms of rupture develop, usually after the AAA is ≥6 cm. During this period, AAA are nearly always asymptomatic and elective repair can be carried out with relatively low operative mortality of 2–5% by experienced surgeons, whereas once rupture occurs, only a fifth of patients survive.[12] The screening tests that have been proposed (ultrasound or abdominal palpation with confirmatory ultrasound) are safe, inexpensive and acceptable to patients.[13]

The great difficulty in justifying screening programs is in demonstrating that early detection improves outcome compared with usual health care in the absence of screening. Because of the many possibilities for bias, randomized trials are generally needed to make this determination. These are now becoming available for AAA screening and will be discussed below under "Effectiveness of Screening." The final criterion for screening, the cost-effectiveness of AAA screening, is also discussed below.

METHODS OF SCREENING FOR AAA

A diagnosis of asymptomatic AAA in the absence of screening would have to be "incidental," i.e. the result of a physical examination or imaging test done for reasons other than to detect AAA. The frequency of incidental diagnoses of AAA led investigators to consider screening high risk populations. Abdominal palpation was the original method of AAA detection. Few aneurysms are found by "routine" palpation of the abdomen,[14] but deliberate and careful evaluation of the aorta will detect most clinically important AAA.[15] During the exam, the patient should be supine with the abdomen relaxed and the knees raised. The examiner lays both hands on the abdomen a few centimeters cephalad of the umbilicus slightly left of center and palpates deeply to detect the aorta pulsation between the 2 index fingers. Ample skin should be included between the 2 index fingers, and it is often helpful initially to probe for one side of the aorta at a time.

The width (rather than the intensity) of the aortic pulsation determines the diagnosis; a normal aorta can often be felt strongly pulsating in thin patients or those with

TABLE 12–1. PREVALENCE OF AAA BY DIAMETER IN MALE VETERANS AGED 50–79 (N = 126196)

AAA Diam.	#AAA	%
≥ 3.0 cm	5283	4.2
≥ 4.0 cm	1644	1.3
≥ 5.0 cm	571	0.45
≥ 5.5 cm*	342	0.27
≥ 6.0 cm	212	0.17
≥ 7.0 cm	76	0.06
≥ 8.0 cm	32	0.03

*Adapted from Lederle et al.[21]

loose abdominal muscles. The aorta is normally less than an inch in diameter (2.5 cm), and aortas larger than this (after allowing for skin thickness) warrant further investigation, usually with ultrasound. Abdominal or femoral bruits or absent femoral pulses are not of much value for diagnosis of asymptomatic AAA.[14] As Osler observed, "no pulsation, however forcible, no thrill, however intense, no bruit, however loud—singly or together—justify the diagnosis of an aneurysm of the abdominal aorta, *only the presence of a palpable expansile tumour.*"[16]

The sensitivity of abdominal palpation for detecting AAA depends on both the diameter of the aneurysm and the girth of the patient. Three-fourths of AAA ≥5.0 cm in diameter are detectable by abdominal palpation whereas less than one-fourth of AAA 3.0–3.9 cm are palpable.[15] The sensitivity of palpation is also much lower in patients with an abdominal girth of more than 100 cm (a 40 inch waist) compared with thinner patients.[14,17] The sensitivity of palpation to detect AAA large enough to be considered for repair (≤5 cm) is high, especially if girth is less than 100 cm (100% in one small series of 12 cases[17]). Agreement between different examiners has been shown to be "fair to good" (kappa = .53).[17] Only about one-third of elderly men suspected of having an enlarged aorta on abdominal palpation will be found to actually have AAA. This proportion (the positive predictive value) is lower in women and young men,[15] but in any case is not of great concern because the confirmatory test is ultrasound, which is safe, accurate, and inexpensive. Thus, while abdominal palpation is not an ideal diagnostic test, it is probably more worthwhile than most other components of the physical examination, and can be a useful compromise if the patient's health plan will not cover ultrasound screening.

Various abdominal imaging procedures will accurately diagnose AAA, but the screening programs undertaken or considered to date have nearly all used ultrasound. Ultrasound is particularly useful because of its accuracy, low cost, patient acceptance, lack of radiation exposure, and general availability. The sensitivity and specificity of ultrasound for AAA are nearly 100%.[14, 18] Small portable ultrasonography equipment has increased the feasibility of mobil or temporary screening centers.

Plain radiography is a common means of incidental diagnosis of AAA and often provides early diagnostic clues to rupture, e.g. calcification, soft tissue mass, or loss of psoas or renal outlines.[19] However, plain radiography should not be used to confirm or exclude the diagnosis because many AAA will be missed due to insufficient calcification, resulting in sensitivities as low as 25%.[20] Computerized tomography, angiography, magnetic resonance imaging, and their variants are all useful for detailed preoperative evaluation of AAA, but offer no advantage over ultrasound for initial diagnosis and are more expensive. Thus, 2 methods can be recommended for AAA screening. Ultrasound is preferred when feasible, but abdominal palpation with ultrasound confirmation of positive or suggestive exams provides a reasonable alternative.

SELECTING A POPULATION FOR SCREENING

For the sake of efficiency, screening programs must target the population most likely to benefit. Considerable information has been published on factors associated with having an AAA detected at screening. The most important have been gender and age. AAA is primarily a disease of men. Numerous studies have found that men are 3–6 times as likely as women to have AAA.[6] Even after adjustment for other risk factors, men are still more than twice as likely to have AAA.[21] As result, most published population screening programs and ongoing randomized trials of screening have not included women.[22] AAA are also associated with advanced age. Prevalence increases throughout life, the result of a process of accumulation, though incidence (the rate at which new AAA develop) may peak at age 65.[23] Few develop before 50 years of age, but prevalence increases sharply after this (Figure 12–1). Screening young people yields few cases, but screening the very old is also of little value because many of those found to have AAA will not be candidates for repair or will not live long enough after repair to benefit. AAA incidence and prevalence, death rates, and screening compliance rates from several population based screening studies in England have led to the conclusion that the ideal age for AAA screening is 65,[24,25] and none of the study groups have proposed screening those over 80.

The most important criterion for defining a target population for AAA screening other than gender and age is smoking history. Smokers are more than 5 times as likely as non-smokers to have AAA at screening.[21] The excess prevalence associated with smoking accounted for 75% of all the AAA ≥4.0 cm in a veteran population.[21] The effects of age and smoking on the prevalence of AAA ≥4.0 cm are shown in Figure 12–1. Men who have never smoked have a prevalence of AAA ≥4.0 cm well below 1% regardless of age, whereas prevalence is above 2% in men over age 70 who have smoked. Thus it is reasonable to limit AAA screening to smokers and ex-smokers, but programs based on this criterion have not been reported. Non-smokers represent only about 30% of populations undergoing screening,[26] so their exclusion may not be worthwhile. However, limiting screening to current smokers is too restrictive because the majority of AAA in the population would be missed.[26]

Other moderately strong risk factors for AAA include white race, family history of AAA, coronary, cerebral or peripheral artery disease, and absence of diabetes.[21] However, strategies using these and other factors to further select a target population beyond that of men aged 65–80 have not proven worthwhile.[26,27]

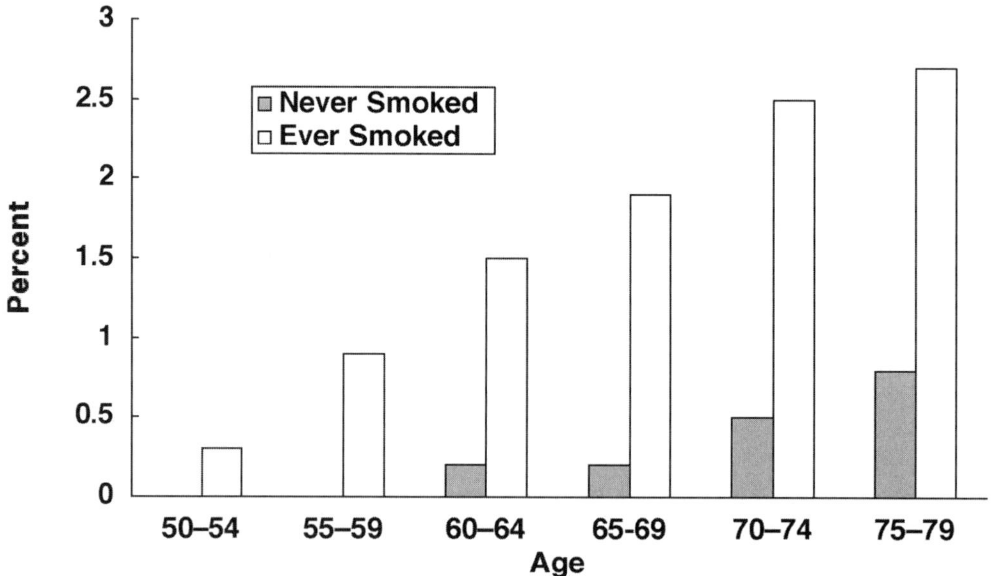

Figure 12–1. Prevalence of abdominal aortic aneurysm ≥ 4.0 cm in men by age and smoking history. Adapted from Lederle et al.[54] Reprinted from: Chesler E, ed. *Clinical Cardiology in the Elderly*. 2nd ed. Armonk, NY: Futura Publishing Company, 1999. (Permission requested.)

Effectiveness of Screening

Benefit from screening is difficult to assess because large numbers are required and ascertaining AAA-related deaths is difficult,[28] but pertinent data are rapidly becoming available. Two non-randomized community-based studies from England have reported beneficial results from AAA screening of older men. One reported significant reductions in AAA-related deaths in men in the age group offered screening (65–73 years old) that was not seen in other men in the district, based on a total of 83 AAA-related deaths.[29] The other reported a significant reduction in rupture rate in men after being invited for screening compared with before being invited.[30] Of concern in the latter study, 1) those considered unfit for surgery (and who may be more prone to rupture)[31] appear to have been included in the control group and 2) the outcome did not include deaths from elective surgery.

Two randomized trials of AAA screening have been reported. In a study from Chichester UK that included 9,342 women and 6,433 men, no benefit was seen in women, but AAA screening and elective repair resulted in a 55% reduction in AAA ruptures in men.[32] The associated 41% reduction in AAA-related deaths (from 17 to 10) did not reach statistical significance, however. There were no operative deaths in 33 elective repairs in this study and repair was offered only for AAA ≥6 cm or rapid growth; 2 factors important to the success of the program but unlikely to be replicated in general practice. In a second randomized trial of 12,658 men reported from Denmark, inpatient AAA-related deaths were significantly reduced in the screening group, from 19 to 6.[33] Unfortunately, outcome ascertainment was incomplete as no information was collected on outpatient deaths. The findings of these trials are suggestive of a benefit from screening, but the number of AAA-related deaths was very small. Several more randomized trials of AAA screening with ultrasound in older men are currently underway,[24] and their findings will be crucial to determining the effectiveness of screening for AAA.

REPEAT SCREENING

The studies discussed above describe the results of one-time screening programs. A related issue is whether screening should be repeated at specified intervals. Limited information is available on the yield of repeat screening. In one study, 2,622 veterans who had aortic diameters <3.0 cm by ultrasound at age 50–79 underwent repeat ultrasound after 4 years.[34] Of these, 58 (2.2%) had aortic diameters ≥3.0 cm (meeting the usual definition of AAA), of which 3 were ≥4.0 cm. Because of the low yield and small diameters of the AAA detected, repeat screening at 4 years was not considered worthwhile. In another study, 223 men with aortic diameters <2.6 cm by ultrasound at age 65 were rescreened after 5 and 12 years.[25] Six had aortic diameters (3.0 cm at repeat screening, but because of their age, none were considered likely to ever require elective repair. Based on these studies, it appears that screening, if implemented, need only be one-time. As noted above, the ideal time for one-time screening appears to be at age 65.

COST EFFECTIVENESS

Most of the total cost of an ultrasound screening program is generated by treatment of the AAA detected, with only about 15% coming from the screening program *per se*.[35]

The benefit of screening would therefore appear to be closely linked to the benefit of treatment because if repairing an AAA is worthwhile, then spending an additional 15% to detect it is probably also worthwhile.

At least 6 cost effectiveness models of ultrasound screening for AAA have been published for men over age 60.[35, 36] One concluded that screening did more harm than good; the others found screening to be beneficial, with costs per year of life saved ranging from $2,000 to $41,550. In addition, the previously mentioned Danish randomized trial found that ultrasound screening prevented AAA-related deaths at a cost of only about $1000 per year of life saved.[33] Cost effectiveness ratios up to $40,000 per year of life saved are consistent with currently funded programs and those under $20,000 are considered to be "very attractive,"[35] so screening for AAA looks very promising in this regard. Screening with abdominal palpation and confirmatory ultrasound was also considered in one of the studies and was calculated to be more cost effective than screening with ultrasound.[37]

Most of the 6 cost effectiveness studies based on models assumed that all AAA ≥4.0 cm would be repaired. However, 2 recent randomized trials found no reduction in mortality from repair of asymptomatic AAA smaller than 5.5 cm,[10, 11] and the strategy of surveillance with repair reserved for AAA ≥5.5 cm is less costly than repairing all AAA ≥4.0 cm.[38] Revised cost effectiveness models incorporating surveillance to 5.5 cm would be expected to show improved cost-effectiveness.

MISCELLANEOUS CONCERNS REGARDING SCREENING

Screening will identify many small AAA that are unlikely to rupture in the patient's lifetime. Adverse consequences for these patients include 1) needless worry and 2) risk from unnecessary procedures. The limited data available on the possible adverse psychological effects of screening suggest that false positive results may be associated with depression[39] and with increased anxiety that persists even after further testing rules out the disease.[40] Regarding AAA screening in particular, a report of no difference in anxiety and depression scores between screened and unscreened subjects is encouraging,[41] but may not be reliable because the groups were small and dissimilar (the unscreened group had fewer married men). Another study reported that anxiety levels were lower one month after AAA screening than immediately before screening regardless of whether AAA was detected, but baseline anxiety levels (from before the patient was invited) were not obtained.[42]

More concerning for those with small AAA detected at screening is the risk from unnecessary procedures. Despite the results of the 2 trials demonstrating that survival is not improved by elective repair of AAA smaller than 5.5 cm even in good operative candidates,[10,11] the inclination to repair smaller AAA remains strong in the United States. Following publication of the UK trial, several editorials endorsed elective repair of AAA smaller than 5.5 cm under various circumstances, contrary to the study's conclusions.[43,44] Patient anxiety regarding a "u-boat in the belly"[45] also leads to repair of small AAA. AAA are most common in the oldest and sickest patients who are least likely to benefit from repair even if their AAA is larger than 5.5 cm. The operative mortality for elective AAA repair is higher in both the U.S. and the U.K in general than it was in the randomized trials from those countries.[46,47]

The incentive to repair small AAA may be increased by the option of endovascular repair. The combined effects of endograft manufacturers seeking return on the their research and development investment, radiologists seeking to expand into the market of AAA repair, and vascular surgeons resisting that expansion, all favor repair of smaller AAA since these make up the great majority of AAA. Elective AAA repair causes about 2,000 deaths per year in the U.S., compared with 9,000 for AAA rupture.[9] If screening resulted in a large number of elective repair procedures in patients whose AAA would not have ruptured, overall AAA-related mortality could potentially increase.

CURRENT RECOMMENDATIONS

The Vascular Surgery Society of the United Kingdom has recommended a national ultrasound screening program for AAA,[48] and a review of the periodic physical examination found abdominal palpation for AAA to be one of the few maneuvers that could be recommended for older men.[49] The Canadian Task Force on the Periodic Health Examination[50] and the U.S. Preventive Services Task Forces (USPSTF)[51] each gave AAA screening a "C" rating (poor evidence to include or exclude from the periodic health examination). The Canadian Task Force report noted that abdominal palpation of men over age 60 was "prudent" and that ultrasound "could be considered" in obese or high risk patients. These recommendations were issued before publication of the studies cited above under "Evidence for Screening." The USPSTF plans to reconsider their AAA recommendation after the remaining ongoing randomized trials report their findings (Russell Harris, M.D., 2001).

Current practice

Screening for AAA remains uncommon in usual practice in the United States, partly reflecting lack of endorsement by the USPSTF. Merenstein et al. interviewed medical directors of 10 health plans and found that none covered routine ultrasound screening for AAA.[52] Legs For Life®, a program developed by the Society of Cardiovascular & Interventional Radiology and sponsored by several endovascular graft manufacturers, added AAA screening to its national screening week for peripheral vascular disease in 2001. Approximately 50 of the 400 Legs For Life® sites in the United States offered AAA screening with ultrasound in 2001. Eligible subjects were over age 60 with 2 of the following 3 risk factors: male gender, history of smoking, and family history of AAA. The AAA screening program is expected to expand to nearly all Legs For Life® sites in the next few years.

Long term success of a screening program depends on the willingness of the target group to attend. Acceptance rates for AAA screening invitations have been reported for a number of investigational programs. Community screening programs using letters sent by the patients' general practitioner have reported acceptance rates of about 75%.[7, 30, 53] Acceptance rates are higher at age 65 than in more elderly patients.[30, 53] A lower acceptance rate of 30% was observed when letters were sent to veterans from physicians whom they did not know.[54]

AFTER THE SCREENING TEST

The success of a screening program is largely dependent on how patients are managed after the screening test. For those who test negative, being actively informed of the negative results is more reassuring than telling the patient beforehand that "no news is good news."[39] Patients with a pulsatile mass on physical examination should have confirmatory ultrasound. For patients who have AAA on screening or confirmatory ultrasound, the first consideration is whether to recommend elective repair. As noted earlier, 2 randomized trials have demonstrated that survival is not improved by elective repair of AAA <5.5 cm even in good operative candidates. Therefore, asymptomatic AAA should be considered for repair when they are ≥5.5 cm in good surgical candidates, and repair should be further deferred in patients with high operative risk until the risk of rupture outweighs that risk in the opinion of the attending vascular surgeon. For most patients with AAA detected at screening, the management plan will be periodic imaging surveillance of the AAA until the AAA diameter crosses that patient's threshold for elective repair. The patient and family must be educated that periodic follow-up is essential to the patient's safety. Patients with unrepaired AAA who are potential operative candidates should have AAA measurement, usually with ultrasound, annually until the AAA is within 1 cm of the threshold for repair, and then every 6 months afterwards until the AAA is repaired. Variations in AAA measurement of 0.5 cm or more are not uncommon, and this should be taken into account in management decisions.[55]

COMMENTS

The continued high mortality from ruptured AAA reflects the fact that many AAA remain undetected during the years required for the AAA to enlarge to the point of rupture. At the same time, many small AAA that are detected incidentally and may never have ruptured are repaired, and operative mortality remains 2–8% in the U.S. Both scenarios contribute to aortic aneurysm's remaining the fifteenth leading cause of death in the US.[8] The public health would clearly be better served by the policy employed in Chichester UK, whereby men are screened with ultrasound once at age 65 and elective repair is undertaken when an AAA attains a diameter of 6.0 cm or greater.[32] Despite the appeal of the Chichester policy, a firm recommendation for AAA screening must await the completion of the ongoing randomized trials. If these trials demonstrate a benefit from screening, as is likely based on the trials already reported, recommendations from the influential Canadian and U.S. Task Forces should soon follow, and will in turn be followed by local health system guidelines and performance measures, at which point the era of widespread population screening for AAA will have begun. If screening is accompanied by prudent criteria for elective repair, the mortality associated with AAA may at last be reduced.

REFERENCES

1. Schilling FJ, Hempel HF, Becker WH, et al. Asymptomatic aortic aneurysms detected on the abdominal roentgenogram. *Circulation.* 1966;33(Suppl 3):209.
2. Schilling FJ, Christakis G, Hempel HH, et al. The natural history of abdominal aortic and iliac atherosclerosis as detected by lateral abdominal roentgenograms in 2663 males. *J Chronic Dis.* 1974;27:37–45.
3. Cabellon S, Moncrief CL, Pierre DR, et al. Incidence of abdominal aortic aneurysms in patients with atheromatous arterial disease. *Am J Surg.* 1983;146:575–576.

4. Cochrane AL, Holland WW. Validation of screening procedures. *Br Med Bull.* 1971;27 (1):3–8.

5. Frame PS, Carlson SJ. A critical review of periodic health screening using specific screening criteria. Part 1: Selected diseases of respiratory, cardiovascular, and central nervous systems. *J Fam Pract.* 1975;2:29–36.

6. Lederle FA, Johnson GR, Wilson SE, for the Aneurysm Detection and Management Veterans Affairs Cooperative Study. Abdominal aortic aneurysm in women. *J Vasc Surg.* 2001;34:122–126.

7. Boll AP, Verbeek AL, van de Lisdonk EH, et al. High prevalence of abdominal aortic aneurysm in a primary care screening programme. *Br J Surg.* 1998;85:1090–1094.

8. Hoyert DL, Arias E, Smith BL, et al. Deaths: final data for 1999. *National Vital Statistics Reports* 2001;49:1–113.

9. Gillum RF. Epidemiology of aortic aneurysm in the united states. *J Clin Epidemiol.* 1995; 48:1289–1298.

10. The UK Small Aneurysm Trial Participants. Mortality results for randomised controlled trial of early elective surgery or ultrasonographic surveillance for small abdominal aortic aneurysms. *Lancet.* 1998;352:1649–1655.

11. Lederle FA, Wilson SE, Johnson GR, et al., for the Aneurysm Detection and Management (ADAM) Veterans Affairs Cooperative Study Group. Immediate repair compared with surveillance of small abdominal aortic aneurysms. *N Engl J Med.* 2002;346:1437–1444.

12. Adam DJ, Mohan IV, Stuart WP, et al. Community and hospital outcome from ruptured abdominal aortic aneurysm within the catchment area of a regional vascular surgical service. *J Vasc Surg.* 1999;30:922–928.

13. Lindholt JS, Juul S, Henneberg EW, et al. Is screening for abdominal aortic aneurysm acceptable to the population? Selection and recruitment to hospital-based mass screening for abdominal aortic aneurysm. *J Public Health Med.* 1998;20:211–217.

14. Lederle FA, Walker JM, Reinke DB. Selective screening for abdominal aortic aneurysms with physical examination and ultrasound. *Arch Intern Med.* 1988;148:1753–1756.

15. Lederle FA, Simel DL. The Rational Clinical Examination. Does this patient have abdominal aortic aneurysm? *JAMA.* 1999;281:77–82.

16. Osler W. Aneurysm of the abdominal aorta. *Lancet* 1905;1089–96.

17. Fink HA, Lederle FA, Roth CS, et al. The accuracy of physical examination to detect abdominal aortic aneurysm. *Arch Intern Med.* 2000;160:833–836.

18. Nusbaum JW, Freimanis AK, Thomford NR. Echography in the diagnosis of abdominal aortic aneurysm. *Arch Surg.* 1971; 102:385–388.

19. Loughran CF. A review of the plain abdominal radiograph in acute rupture of abdominal aortic aneurysms. *Clin Radiol.* 1986;37:383–387.

20. Roberts A, Johnson N, Royle J, et al. The diagnosis of abdominal aortic aneurysms. *Aust N Z J Surg.* 1974;44:360–362.

21. Lederle FA, Johnson GR, Wilson SE, et al., and the ADAM VA Cooperative Study Investigators. The Aneurysm Detection and Management Study screening program: validation cohort and final results. *Arch Intern Med.* 2000;160:1425–430.

22. Collaborative Aneurysm Screening Study Group (CASS Group). A comparative study of the prevalence of abdominal aortic aneurysms in the United Kingdom, Denmark, and Australia. *J Med Screening.* 2001; 8:46–50.

23. Vardulaki KA, Prevost TC, Walker NM, et al. Incidence among men of asymptomatic abdominal aortic aneurysms: estimates from 500 screen detected cases. *J Med Screen.* 1999;6:50–54.

24. Scott RA, Vardulaki KA, Walker NM, et al. The long-term benefits of a single scan for abdominal aortic aneurysm (AAA) at age 65. *Eur J Vasc Endovasc Surg.* 2001;21:535–540.

25. Crow P, Shaw E, Earnshaw JJ, et al. A single normal ultrasonographic scan at age 65 years rules out significant aneurysm disease for life in men. *Br J Surg.* 2001 Jul;88(7):941–944.

26. Spencer CA, Jamrozik K, Norman PE, et al. The potential for a selective screening strategy for abdominal aortic aneurysm. *J Med Screen.* 2000;7:209–211.

27. Lindholt JS, Henneberg EW, Fasting H, et al. Mass or high-risk screening for abdominal aortic aneurysm. *Br J Surg.* 1997;84:40–42.
28. Lederle FA. Screening for snipers: the burden of proof. *J Clin Epidemiol* 1990;43:101–4.
29. Heather BP, Poskitt KR, Earnshaw JJ, et al. Population screening reduces mortality rate from aortic aneurysm in men. *Br J Surg.* 2000;87:750–753.
30. Wilmink TB, Quick CR, Hubbard CS, Day NE. The influence of screening on the incidence of ruptured abdominal aortic aneurysms. *J Vasc Surg.* 1999 Aug;30(2):203–208.
31. Lederle FA, Johnson GR, Wilson SE, et al. Rupture rate of large abdominal aortic aneurysms in patients unfit for or refusing elective repair; results of a prospective Veterans Affairs Cooperative Study. *JAMA.* 2002;287:2968–2972.
32. Scott RA, Wilson NM, Ashton HA, et al. Influence of screening on the incidence of ruptured abdominal aortic aneurysm: 5-year results of a randomized controlled study. *Br J Surg.* 1995;82:1066–70.
33. Lindholt JS, Juul S, Fasting H, et al. Hospital costs and benefits of screening for abdominal aortic aneurysms. Results from a randomised population screening trial. *Eur J Vasc Endovasc Surg.* 2002;23:55–60.
34. Lederle FA, Johnson GR, Wilson SE, et al., and the ADAM VA Cooperative Study Investigators. Yield of repeated screening for abdominal aortic aneurysm after a four-year interval. *Arch Intern Med.* 2000;160:1117–1121.
35. Lederle FA. Looking for asymptomatic abdominal aortic aneurysms. *J Gen Intern Med.* 1996;11:774–775.
36. Pentikainen TJ, Sipila T, Rissanen P, et al. Cost-effectiveness of targeted screening for abdominal aortic aneurysm. Monte Carlo-based estimates. *Int J Technol Assess Health Care.* 2000 Winter;16(1):22–34.
37. Frame PS, Fryback DG, Patterson C. Screening for abdominal aortic aneurysm in men ages 60 to 80 years: a cost-effectiveness analysis. *Ann Intern Med.* 1993;119:411–416.
38. UK Small Aneurysm Trial Participants. Health service costs and quality of life for early elective surgery or ultrasonographic surveillance for small abdominal aortic aneurysms. *Lancet.* 1998;352:1656–1660.
39. Marteau TM. Psychological costs of screening. *Br Med J.* 1989;299:527.
40. Stewart-Brown S, Farmer A. Screening could seriously damage your health. *Br Med J.* 1997;314:533–534.
41. Khaira HS, Herbert LM, Crowson MC. Screening for abdominal aortic aneurysms does not increase psychological morbidity. *Ann R Coll Surg Engl.* 1998;80:341–342.
42. Lucarotti ME, Heather BP, Shaw E, et al. Psychological morbidity associated with abdominal aortic aneurysm screening. *Eur J Vasc Endovasc Surg.* 1997;14:499–501.
43. Pretre R, Turina MI. Facts, at last, on management of small infrarenal aortic aneurysms. *Lancet.* 1998;352:1642–1643.
44. Cronenwett JL, Johnston KW. The United Kingdom Small Aneurysm Trial: implications for surgical treatment of abdominal aortic aneurysms. *J Vasc Surg.* 1999;29:191–194.
45. Santiago F. Screening for abdominal aortic aneurysms: the U-boat in the belly. *JAMA.* 1987;258:1732.
46. Bayly PJ, Matthews JN, Dobson PM, et al. In-hospital mortality from abdominal aortic surgery in Great Britain and Ireland: Vascular Anaesthesia Society audit. *Br J Surg.* 2001;88:687–692.
47. Birkmeyer JD, Siewers AE, Finlayson EV, et al. Hospital volume and surgical mortality in the United States. *N Engl J Med.* 2002;346:1128–1137.
48. Harris PL. Reducing the mortality from abdominal aortic aneurysms: need for a national screening programme. *Br Med J.* 1992;305:697–699.
49. Oboler SK, LaForce FM. The periodic physical examination in asymptomatic adults. *Ann Intern Med.* 1989;110:214–226.
50. Canadian Task Force on the Periodic Health Examination. Periodic health examination, 1991 update: 5. Screening for abdominal aortic aneurysm. *Can Med Assoc J.* 1991;145:783–789.

51. U.S. Preventive Services Task Force. *Guide to Clinical Preventive Services, 2nd ed.* Baltimore: Williams & Wilkins, 1996, Ch. 6.
52. Merenstein D, Rabinowitz H, Louis DZ. Health care plan decisions regarding preventive services. *Arch Fam Med.* 1999;8:354–356.
53. Khoo DE, Ashton H, Scott RA. Is screening once at age 65 an effective method for detection of abdominal aortic aneurysms? *J Med Screen.* 1994;1:223–225.
54. Lederle FA, Johnson GR, Wilson SE, et al., for the Aneurysm Detection and Management (ADAM) Veterans Affairs Cooperative Study Group. Prevalence and associations of abdominal aortic aneurysm detected through screening. *Ann Intern Med.* 1997;126:441–449.
55. Lederle FA, Wilson SE, Johnson GR, et al., for the Abdominal Aortic Aneurysm Detection and Management Veterans Administration Cooperative Study Group. Variability in measurement of abdominal aortic aneurysms. *J Vasc Surg.* 1995;21:945–952.

13

Functional Outcome after Open Repair of Abdominal Aortic Aneurysms

Lloyd M. Taylor, Jr., MD, Gregory J. Landry, MD, and Gregory L. Moneta, MD

Few conditions in medicine seem more ideally suited to prophylactic surgical treatment than abdominal aortic aneurysms (AAA). Physicians and patients alike can readily visualize the risk of sudden painful premature death implicit in a large pulsating abdominal tumor. Effective surgery is widely available, and has been performed with success for at least 50 years. This fact, coupled with the frequency with which ruptured aneurysm is encountered in daily practice (it is the fifteenth leading cause of death in the USA)[1] would seem to leave little room for analysis. Indeed, few physicians hesitate to recommend repair upon discovery of AAA, and few patients hesitate to accept.

Given this situation, it is perhaps surprising to reflect upon what little objective information is available concerning the AAA natural history and treatment outcomes. For AAA in general, many basic facts regarding natural history remain unknown. Although several cross sectional studies have documented the prevalence of AAA, the associated risk of rupture was not documented by prospective studies until very recently. The recently reported UK small aneurysm study, and the US Veteran's Administration ADAM study both have finally shown that the actual prospectively documented risk of rupture for AAA less than 5.5 cm in greatest diameter is exceedingly small, actually less than 1%/year.[2,3] Interestingly, prior to these carefully conducted trials, many published reports suggested rupture rates ranging from 5–15% for small aneurysms.[4,5] At present the belief that the rupture risk for AAA larger than 5.5 cm is greater than for small aneurysms is widespread, and not without some justification. But we just don't know. There has never been a prospective study, and given the prevailing belief, there may never be.

In contrast to our general lack of information regarding natural history, the basics regarding surgical treatment of AAA are well documented. Elective repair carries general operative mortality of 1–5% in large series from selected centers, higher when conglomerate results are examined.[6] Factors increasing mortality are also well known and include advanced age, cardiac and pulmonary dysfunction, and, especially, chronic renal insufficiency.[7] Indeed, if AAA produced distressing symptoms, and if successful surgery resulted in relief of these symptoms, we would need little more knowledge.

Herein lies the problem with AAA surgery. In fact, AAA almost never produce symptoms. The benefit of surgery (if there is one) lies in prevention of premature death from AAA rupture. Given that the procedure is entirely prophylactic, other factors resulting from surgical repair become much more important. This is especially true of the functional outcome following AAA repair. For example, if AAA repair results in the need for postoperative nursing home confinement in a patient who was previously living independently, is this a reasonable cost for the prophylactic benefit of the procedure?

During the past decade, the question of functional outcome after AAA repair has become even more important, because of the advent of endovascular AAA repair. This procedure, now widely performed, is preferred by many surgeons and patients because of the perception that successful AAA repair by endovascular methods is followed by less functional deficit, and quicker recovery than is conventional repair. Since it is now widely known that performance of endovascular AAA repair does not entirely eliminate the risk of aneurysm rupture,[8] a legitimate question is whether the presumed improved functional outcome of endovascular repair is worth the residual risk of AAA rupture following this procedure.

In this chapter we will briefly review currently available information about functional outcome after standard open AAA repair. Sadly, the task is not a large one. Information has been reported from only one randomized trial, and there are few prospective studies. The same is true for retrospective reviews. And to date, only a single study has compared functional outcome after standard open AAA repair to that following endovascular AAA repair. Perhaps this should not be too surprising. The history of surgery includes many examples of procedures introduced and widely performed, with comprehensive evaluation of the relevance of the procedure to overall health status performed only many years after introduction.

PREOPERATIVE FUNCTIONAL STATUS OF PATIENTS WITH AAA

The mean age of patients undergoing AAA repair in cumulative series is about 75 years. Obviously, this is an age range when many individuals already have significant co-existing medical problems, and significant functional impairment. In addition, this is an age when many individuals can be expected to have decreasing functional status, as a normal consequence of diseases and conditions associated with aging. In a prospective study of 454 patients undergoing AAA repair, total hip arthroplasty, and lung cancer surgery, Mangione and colleagues[9] used the SF-36 score[10] and found that preoperative AAA patients had significantly greater role limitations from physical or emotional problems, and significantly poorer mental health scores when compared to a population-based sample. The AAA patients' overall health scores were comparable to those of the other groups. That some of the emotional/mental health problems associated with AAA patients might be directly attributable to their knowledge of the AAA was suggested by a study by Lindholt and coworkers.[11] They found that elderly men found to have AAA in a screening program had a 5–7% reduction in quality of life scores mostly related to perception of poor health and emotional distress, when compared to a control group in whom no AAA was found. Interestingly, the difference was eliminated by successful AAA surgery.

In our own retrospective study of 154 patients undergoing AAA repair,[12] all were ambulatory preoperatively and none were living in a nursing home/assisted care preoperatively. More than 90% were driving and more than 90% were shopping and traveling preoperatively.

RECOVERY AFTER OPEN AAA REPAIR

As expected, open repair of AAA results in an immediate decrease in functional status and quality of life. In a prospective study of 59 patients undergoing AAA repair, Perkins and colleagues[13] found significant decreases in the SF-36 components measuring social function, pain, mental health, physical function, and physical role limitation. These changes were maximal at 6 weeks postoperatively, and had resolved to preoperative levels by 3–6 months postoperatively. Similar findings were noted by Mangione and colleagues.[9] Their 95 patients undergoing AAA repair had significant negative changes in physical role limitation, vitality, physical function, and social function. SF-36 scores in these areas had largely returned to preoperative levels by 6 months postoperatively, levels which were comparable to a population-based control group. The postoperative improvement was maintained at 12 months postoperatively.

The UK Small Aneurysm Trial prospectively evaluated health related quality of life in 1,090 patients randomized to early surgery or surveillance.[14] In the overall assessment of quality of life as measured by the SF-36, there were no significant differences between the randomized groups after 12 months, emphasizing that the decrease in function/quality of life resulting from surgery was transient. However the early surgery group did show a significant improvement in the health perception subscore, confirming the finding of Lindholt and coworkers,[11] that knowledge of the presence of AAA has a negative effect on mental health, that can be improved by surgery. Interestingly, the surveillance group in the UK small aneurysm trial demonstrated significant but slight worsening in physical functioning, role functioning, social functioning, and bodily pain scores emphasizing that the AAA patient group consists of elderly individuals, and that decreasing functional status over time is expected in this setting, and is not always the result of the particular medical condition we are studying, or its treatment.

These aggregate results describing the outcome of AAA surgery indicate that, on average, open surgical repair of AAA is not associated with lasting functional deficit. That the average result does not always apply to each individual patient was emphasized in our study of functional outcome after open AAA repair in 154 patients.[12] In response to a specific questionnaire, 64% of patients reported that they had experienced a "full recovery" from surgery, with a mean time to recovery of 3.9 months. The patients who stated that they had not fully recovered from the operation had a mean followup period of 34 months. All patients appeared to have a clear understanding of why the AAA operations had been performed. Despite this, 18% of patients stated that they would not have agreed to have the surgery if they had been able to forsee the difficulty of the recovery process. As is logical, patients who did not report full recovery, and patients who said they would not have had the operation, had they known what was involved, were slightly older, were more likely to have had urgent operations, and had more preoperative coexisting disease, longer ICU/hospital stays, and more postoperative complications (Table 13–1).

Postoperatively, 17 patients (11%) were discharged from hospital to a nursing home, for a mean stay of 3.7 months. At last followup (median 25 months) 9% of patients were in nursing homes, or assisted living facilities. Other functional characteristics are compared preoperativly and at last followup in Table 13–2.

Of course, these results must be interpreted with perspective. The study group consisted of patients referred to a University Service, many presumably because of a perception of increased operative risk. Their postoperative outcome may not be generalizable to the population of patients at large with AAA. Also, the study was without controls. It is not possible to determine what portion of the documented decline in functional status was the result of the AAA surgery, and what portion represents the general decline in functional status expected in patients of advanced age.

TABLE 13–1. DEMOGRAPHIC DATA ON GROUP AS A WHOLE, THOSE WHO STATED THEY DID NOT HAVE COMPLETE RECOVERY, AND THOSE WHO STATED THEY WOULD HAVE NOT UNDERGONE AAA REPAIR KNOWING THE RECOVERY PROCESS.

Parameter	All Patients n = 154	Not Fully Recoverd n = 28	Repair Not Again n = 16
Age	68.7 yrs	70.7 yrs	69.7 yrs
Urgent Operations	9.7 %	27.6 %	12.5 % (p = 0.88)
Pre-op CAD	59.7	58.6	62.5
Pre-op Stroke	15.6	13.7	25.0
Pre-op HTN	57.1	65.5	50.0
Pre-op CRI	20.7	31.0	37.5
Pre-op Tobacco	55.8	58.6	75.0
Pre-op Claudication	12.3	10.3	12.5
Prev. Leg Bypass	6.5	6.9	6.2
Prev. CABG	12.9	6.9	12.5
Prev CEA	9.1	10.3	12.5
Pre-op Steriod Use	9.7	6.9	6.2
Prev. DM	12.9	3.4	6.2
Prev. COPD	27.9	41.4	50.0
Male	75.9	75.9	62.5
Female	24.0	24.1	37.5
Complication	24.7	37.9	43.8 (p = 0.067)
Pre-op Walking	100	100	100
Time in SNF			
Median	23.5 days	61 days	61 days
Mean	230 days	296 days	296 days
Time in ICU			
Median	3 days	3 days	5 days
Mean	4.52 days	4.58 days	6.31 days
Aneurysm Size			
Median	6.0 cm	6.0 cm	5.1 cm
Mean	6.24 cm	6.12 cm	5.65 cm

Key: CAD = coronary artery disease; HTN = hypertension; CRI = chronic renal insufficiency as defined as creatiine ≥1.5 mg/dl; Pre-op = preoperative; CABG = coronary artery bypass grafting; DM = diabetes mellitus, either type I or II; SNF = skilled nursing facility; COPD = chronic obstructive pulmonary disease (From Williamson et al. *J Vasc Surg.* 2001;33:913-920, with permission)

TABLE 13–2. FUNCTIONAL OUTCOME AFTER OPEN AAA REPAIR*

Characteristic	Preoperative Per Cent	At Last Followup
Live in Care Center	0%	9%
Ambulatory	100%	67%
Travel (ever)	>90%	52%
Drive a car	>90%	72%
Employed	9%	8%
Ever leave the house	>90%	78%
Go shopping	>90%	61%

*data from Williamson et al. *J Vasc Surg.* 2001;33:913–920

COMPARISON OF FUNCTIONAL OUTCOME AFTER ENDOVASCULAR REPAIR AND OPEN REPAIR

Lloyd and colleagues[15] prospectively studied 82 AAA patients (34 endovascular and 48 open) with respect to quality of life (SF-36) and cognitive function (various psychometric tests). The study was not randomized, but there were no significant differences in cognitive function or in quality of life between the 2 groups preoperatively. At 6 months postoperatively the SF-36 scores had deteriorated significantly in the areas of physical function and vitality when compared to preoperative values. There were no significant differences between the endovascular and open repair groups in any of the scales from the SF-36 form. Similarly, although patients cognitive function was slightly worse on the visual search task at 6 months postoperatively, when compared to preoperatively, there were no differences detected between the open and endovascular groups.

This study was small, and non randomized, and only examined outcomes at a single point in time (6 months) postoperatively. Nevertheless, it serves to illustrate that the automatic assumption that functional outcome will be better following a less invasive endovascular repair may well be open to question.

CONCLUSIONS

Perhaps the most striking fact about our knowledge of AAA treatment outcomes is how little we really know. This is true for the central issue of whether AAA surgery is helpful or harmful in terms of preventing premature death. It is also true for our knowledge of the specific issue of functional outcome after treatment. Those prospective studies which have been performed appear to confirm that knowledge of the presence of AAA produces a measurable decrement in patients' mental health, and that successful repair of AAA eliminates this decrement. Studies also show that, in general, open AAA surgery is associated with a temporary decrease in functional status/quality of life which returns to preoperative levels within 3 to 6 months postoperatively. That this generality is not always the case is illustrated by our own study, in which a minority of patients stated that they had never fully recovered from surgery, and/or required nursing home placement, and/or stated that they would not have the procedure again. These undesirable functional outcomes were associated with preoperative advanced age and comorbid conditions, and with complicated procedures, and prolonged hospital stays, emphasizing that 2 very important parts of avoiding poor postoperative functional outcomes are careful preoperative selection of patients, and uncomplicated surgery. The only study reported to date appears to show that functional outcomes after endovascular AAA repair are similar to those achieved with open repair. Hopefully, increasing attention to functional outcome studies in future will allow us to accumulate additional data to more appropriately determine the best role of AAA repair, whether open or endovascular, for our patients.

REFERENCES

1. Cronenwett JL, Krupski WC, Rutherford RB. Abdominal aortic and iliac aneurysms. chapt in Rutherford RB, (ed) *Vascular Surgery, 5th Ed.* W.B. Saunders, Philadelphia, 2000;1246.
2. The UK Small Aneurysm Trial Participants. Mortality results for randomised controlled trial of early elective surgery or ultrasonographic surveillance for small abdominal aortic aneurysms. *Lancet.* 1998;352:1649–1655.
3. Lederle FA, Wilson SE, Johnson GR, et al. Immediate repair compared with surveillance of small abdominal aortic aneurysms. *NEJM.* 2002;346:1437–1444.
4. Darling RC, Messina CR, Brewster DC, et al. Autopsy study of unoperated aortic aneurysms. *Circulation.* 1977;56(Suppl 2):161–164.
5. Szilagyi DE, Elliott JP, Smith RF. Clinical fate of the patient with asymptomatic abdominal aortic aneurysm and unfit for surgical treatment. *Arch Surg.* 1972;104:600–606.
6. Taylor LM Jr. Porter JM. Basic data relating to clinical decision making for abdominal aortic aneurysms. *Ann Vasc Surg.* 1987;1:502–504.
7. Hollier LH, Taylor LM, Jr., Ochsner J. Recommended Indications for Operative Treatment of Abdominal Aortic Aneurysms. *J Vasc Surg.* 1992; 15:1046–1056.
8. Bernhard VM, Mitchell RS, Matsumura JS, et al. Ruptured abdominal aortic aneurysm after endovascular repair. *J Vasc Surg.* 2002;35:1155–1162.
9. Mangione CM, Goldman L, Orav J, et al. Health-Related quality of life after elective surgery. *J Gen Intern Med.* 1997;12:686–697.
10. Stewart AL, Hays RD, Ware JE. The MOS short-form general health survey: reliability and validity in a patient population. *Med Care.* 1988;26:724–35.
11. Lindholt JS, Vammen S, Fasting H, et al. Psychological consequences of screening for abdominal aortic aneurysm and conservative treatment of small abdominal aortic aneurysms. *Eur J Vasc Endovasc Surg.* 2000;20:79–83.
12. Williamson WK, Nicoloff AD, Taylor LM Jr., et al. Functional outcome after open repair of abdominal aortic aneurysm. *J Vasc Surg.* 2001;33:913–920.
13. Perkins JTM, Magee TR, Hands LJ, Collin J, et al. Prospective evaluation of quality of life after conventional abdominal aortic aneurysm surgery. *Eur J Vasc Endovasc Surg.* 1998;16: 203–207.
14. The UK Small Aneurysm Trial Participants. Health service costs and quality of life for early elective surgery or ultrasonographic surveillance for small abdominal aortic aneurysms. *Lancet.* 1998;352:1656–1660.
15. Lloyd AJ, Bell PRF, Thompson MM. Comparison of cognitive function and quality of life after endovascular or conventional aortic aneurysm repair. *Br J Surg.* 2000;87:443–447.

14

Treatment of Ruptured
Aortoiliac Aneurysms by
Endovascular Approaches

*Frank J. Veith, MD, Takao Ohki, MD, PhD, and
Evan C. Lipsitz, MD*

Standard open surgical treatment for ruptured abdominal aortoiliac aneurysms (AAAs) has achieved some favorable individual results but continues to be associated with substantial morbidity and an in-hospital mortality which ranges from 35–70%.[1–9] All efforts to improve these poor results have not changed this outlook significantly.

Beginning in 1994, we have evaluated the possibility that endovascular grafts coupled with other interventional techniques might help to improve the treatment outcomes of ruptured AAAs.[10] Although we first used these grafts and techniques in a selected group of high-risk patients in whom pretreatment computerized tomographic (CT) scans could be obtained, we presently believe that they should be applied more widely to treat most patients with ruptured AAAs. The present chapter describes our experience to date with the use of endovascular grafts and other catheter-based techniques to treat ruptured AAAs.

The less invasive nature of endovascular treatment of ruptured AAAs offers many potential advantages. However, selection of the appropriate graft for each patient requires complex measurements of aneurysmal and adjacent arterial lengths and diameters. These measurements are usually based on high quality contrast CT scans and arteriography which take time which may not be available in the ruptured AAA setting. Moreover, it may not be possible to have available a stock of grafts suitable for most patients. A second obstacle to the use of endovascular grafts was that standard surgical practice mandated early proximal aortic control, and it was thought that that could be achieved most rapidly and most effectively by laparotomy with placement of a supraceliac or infrarenal aortic clamp.[11]

MONTEFIORE ENDOVASCULAR GRAFTING SYSTEM (MEGS)[*]

Since 1993, we have utilized a derivative of the original Parodi endograft[12] to treat aortic and aortoiliac aneurysms. This MEGS graft,[*] which is used in an aortofemoral configuration, is comprised of a large proximal Palmaz balloon expandable stent affixed to a long tulip shaped PTFE graft (Figure 14–1).[13] This graft fits most AAA patients since the proximal diameter can vary between 20 and 28 mm depending on the inflation pressure applied to the deployment balloon, and the excess graft length can be cut off and tailored appropriately before the distal graft is sutured to the graft introduction site within the common femoral artery (Figure 14–2).

Details of graft fabrication are as follows: The graft is constructed by suturing a Palmaz stent (P4010 or P5010, Cordis, Warren, NJ) to a standard ePTFE graft (6 mm x 40 cm, Impra, Tempe, AZ). This stent-graft combination is then mounted onto a large angioplasty balloon (Maxi LD 25 mm x 4 cm, Cordis) and inserted into a 16-Fr sheath (Cook Inc., Bloomington, IN). An occluder device (for occlusion of the opposite common iliac artery) is constructed by attaching a Palmaz stent (P308 or P4014) to an ePTFE graft that is closed at one end by ligatures. This occluder device is also mounted onto an angioplasty balloon and inserted into either a 12- or a 16-Fr sheath. These devices are prefabricated and are kept sterile for emergent use.

Having this graft sterilized and available has the potential for eliminating the need for preoperative measurement and fabricating or procuring a suitable graft for use in the urgent ruptured aneurysm setting.

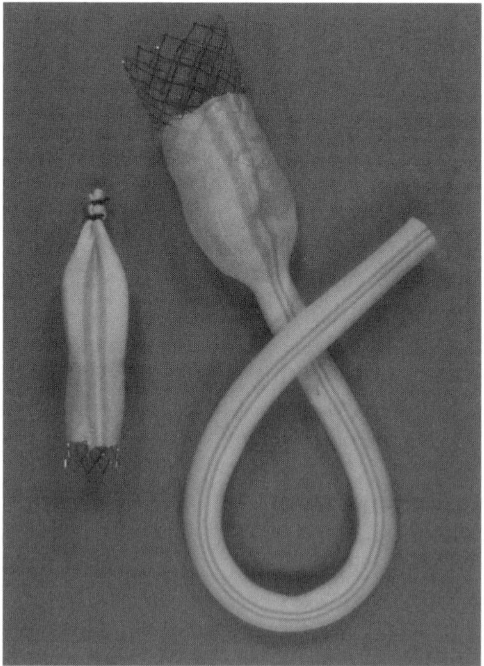

Figure 14–1. MEGS graft. A large Palmaz stent is attached to the PTFE graft. The occluder device is shown on the left.

---

*To be commercialized as the Vascular Innovation Parodi Graft, Vascular Innovation, Inc.

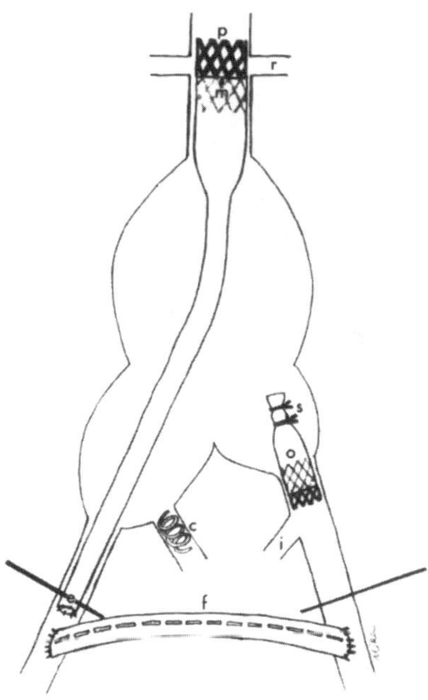

Figure 14–2. Schematic drawing illustrating deployment of the MEGS graft. This graft is fixed within the proximal neck with a large Palmaz stent (p). The cranial end of the graft is denoted by a metallic marker (m) attached to the graft. The bare portion of the stent is deployed across the orifice of the renal arteries so that the graft is implanted immediately below the renal arteries (r). An endoluminal anastomosis (e) is performed at the distal end of the endograft. The occluder device (o) is deployed in the contralateral common iliac artery to preserve at least one internal iliac artery (i). c, embolization coil; f, femorofemoral bypass; s, sutures to occlude the end of the occluder.

EARLY EXPERIENCE WITH ENDOVASCULAR TREATMENT OF RUPTURED AAAS

Because of our access to the MEGS graft, on April 21, 1994, we had a patient with a ruptured abdominal aorta and all the clinical sequellae thereof, i.e., severe abdominal pain, hypotension, and a large pulsatile abdominal mass. Because the patient had had a total cystectomy and ileal bladder, and because he had severe symptomatic coronary artery disease, he was deemed unsuitable for an open repair of his ruptured aortic aneurysm. He, therefore, underwent a MEGS endovascular graft repair of his ruptured aortic aneurysm along with placement of a right common iliac artery occluder and a femorofemoral bypass (Figure 14–3).[10] The patient did well following this procedure until he died from cardiac disease 3 years later. To our knowledge this was the first endovascular graft repair of a ruptured aortic aneurysm, although another early case had been reported by Yusuf, Hopkinson, et al.[14]

Following our experience with our first successful case we performed similar operations on another 11 patients with ruptured aortoiliac aneurysms.[13] All these patients had major contraindications to open operation with serious medical comorbidities (e.g., coincident major myocardial infarction, chronic obstructive pulmonary disease (COPD) requiring home oxygen therapy), or surgical problems (e.g., abdominal infection or massive recurrent incisional hernias). All 12 of these first patients had been stable enough to undergo preoperative CT scanning to confirm the aneurysmal rupture. In all 12 of these original patients, the ruptured aneurysm was successfully

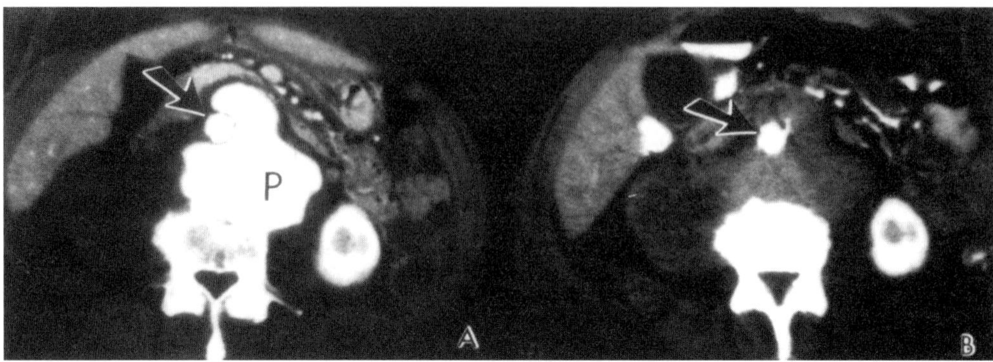

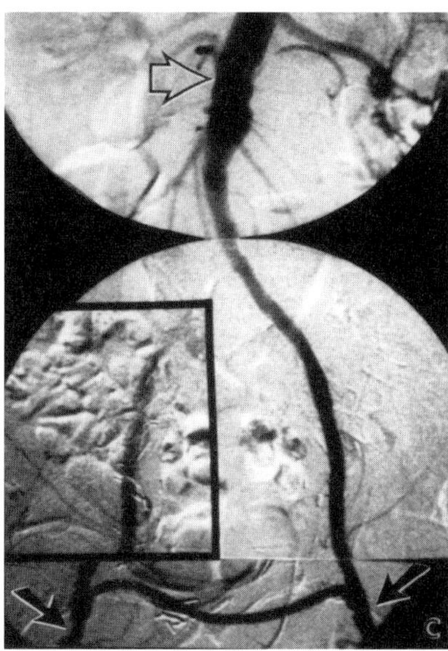

Figure 14–3. Transfemoral repair of a rupture of the distal aorta. **(A)** A spiral CT scan demonstrates extravasation of contrast material from the aorta (arrow) into a large, partially clot-filled pseudoaneurysm (P). **(B)** A spiral CT scan performed after transfemoral insertion of an endovascular graft demonstrates that the pseudoaneurysm is excluded and vascular continuity within the lumen of the aorta (arrow) is preserved. **(C)** A postoperative transfemoral arteriogram at 1 week demonstrates vascular continuity between the aorta (open arrow) and the common femoral arteries (arrows). The inset shows flow up the external iliac artery to the right hypogastric artery. An occluder has been placed in the right common iliac artery. (Reproduced with permission.[10])

excluded by the endovascular graft. Moreover, only 2 of the patients died within 2 months of the procedure, yielding only a 17% operative mortality.

HYPOTHESIS REGARDING ENDOVASCULAR TREATMENT OF RUPTURED AAAS AND CURRENT MANAGEMENT PLAN

This low operative mortality prompted us to speculate that all ruptured AAAs should be treated endovascularly.[15] Such an approach might lead to better outcomes than were currently being achieved with open repair. In 1996, we therefore adopted the following treatment plan. All patients with a *presumed diagnosis* of a ruptured AAA were taken immediately to the operating room. A presumed diagnosis of ruptured AAA was made if 2 or more elements of the diagnostic triad were present; namely syncope, abdominal or back pain, and a known or palpable AAA.[11] In the operating room, with preparation for fluoroscopy of the patient from the neck to the knees, via a brachial or femoral puncture under local anesthesia a wire was placed in the supraceliac aorta. Using this guidewire a catheter was placed to visualize the abdominal aorta and iliac arteries angiographically. This angiogram, which was best performed with a power injector, allowed a determination of whether or not an endovascular graft repair of the ruptured AAA was possible on the basis of aortic neck and iliac artery anatomy (Table 14–1). If not, a standard repair was carried out.

TECHNIQUE OF ENDOVASCULAR REPAIR.

If an endovascular graft repair was deemed feasible, the following technical steps were employed using local or general anesthesia to perform the bilateral open exposures of the femoral arteries. Either before or after deployment of the MEGS graft, coil embolization of the hypogastric artery ipsilateral to the side of graft insertion was performed. The MEGS graft delivery system was inserted into the aorta over a superstiff wire placed in the upper thoracic aorta. Once the graft was inserted into the proximal aneurysm neck, the delivery sheath was retracted. To confirm appropriate positioning in regard to the renal arteries, a repeat angiogram was performed using the catheter introduced via the brachial or contralateral femoral artery. Inflation of the deployment balloon expanded the stent and fixed the graft within the proximal neck. By varying the inflation pressure, the MEGS graft could accommodate a wide range of proximal neck diameters ranging from 18 to 28 mm (Figure 14–4). In each case, the length of the graft was 40 cm so that the distal end of the graft always emerged from the introduction arteriotomy site (Figure 14–5A). The graft was then cut to the appropriate length and hand-sewn endoluminally within the common femoral or distal external iliac artery (Figure 14–5B).

The occluder device was then placed in the opposite common iliac artery in an effort to preserve at least one hypogastric artery. In addition, a femorofemoral bypass was performed (Figures 14–2, 14–6, and 14–7).

CONTROL OF BLEEDING AND BLOOD PRESSURE: RESTRICTED RESUSCITATION, HYPOTENSIVE HEMOSTASIS, AND PROXIMAL BALLOON CONTROL

As already noted, it is widely believed that with ruptured AAAs, it is necessary to perform immediate laparotomy to permit clamp control of the aorta proximal to the aneurysm. With major arterial bleeding in other circumstances, however, restricted fluid resuscitation and withholding blood transfusions have been shown to decrease

TABLE 14–1. EXCLUSION CRITERIA FOR ENDOVASCULAR REPAIR

Proximal neck diameter larger than 28 mm

Pararenal AAAs (neck length shorter than 12 mm)

Bilateral, iliac artery occlusions

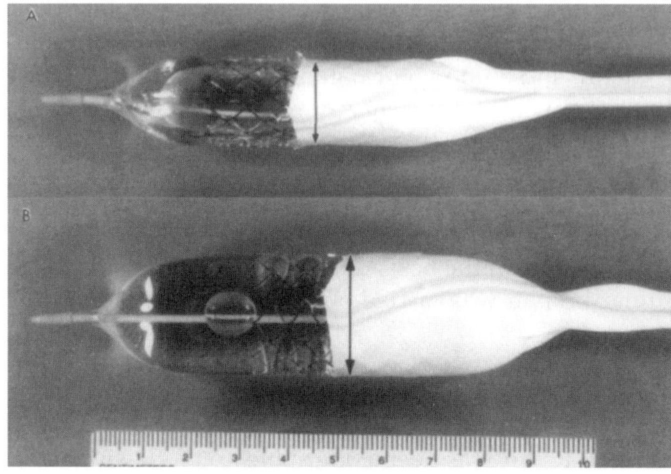

Figure 14–4. Method for customizing the proximal stent diameter of the MEGS graft intraoperatively. **(A)** When the deployment balloon is inflated to 2 ATM, the stent is expanded to 20 mm in diameter (small arrow). **(B)** Due to the compliant nature of the balloon, at 6 ATM of inflation pressure the stent is expanded to 28 mm (large arrows). (Reproduced with permission.[13])

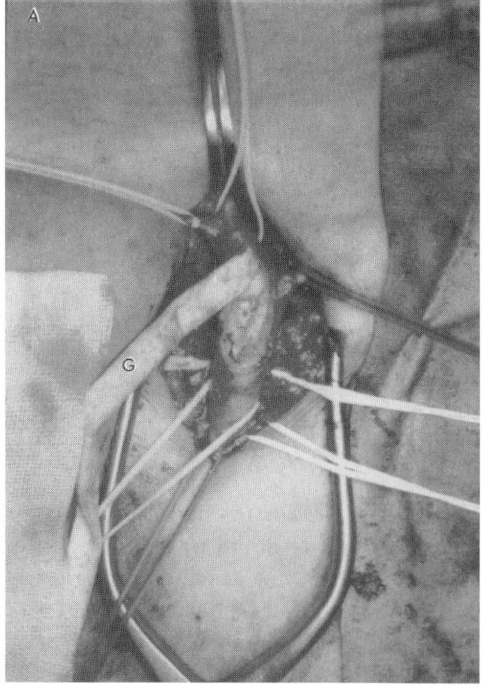
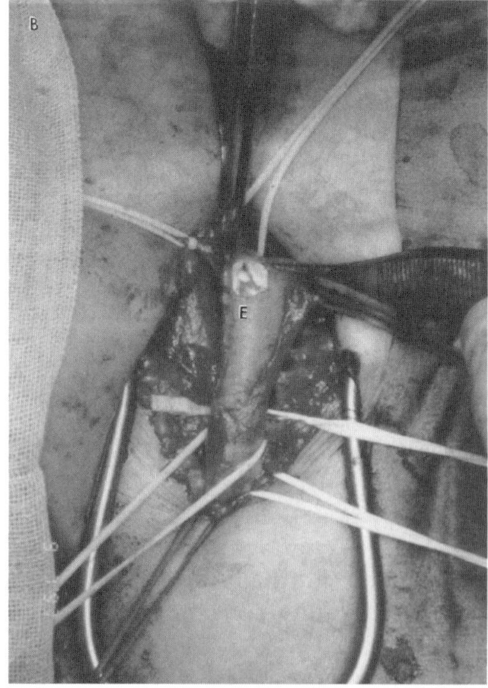

Figure 14–5. Method for customizing the length of the MEGS graft intraoperatively. **(A)** In each case, the endograft is made long enough so that the distal end of the graft (G) emerges from the arteriotomy site. **(B)** The graft is cut to the appropriate length as it emerges from the femoral artery and an endoluminal anastomosis (E) is carried out. (Reproduced with permission.[13])

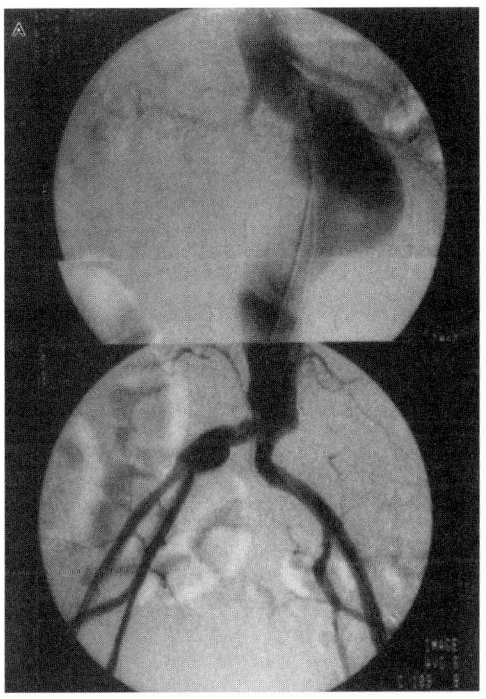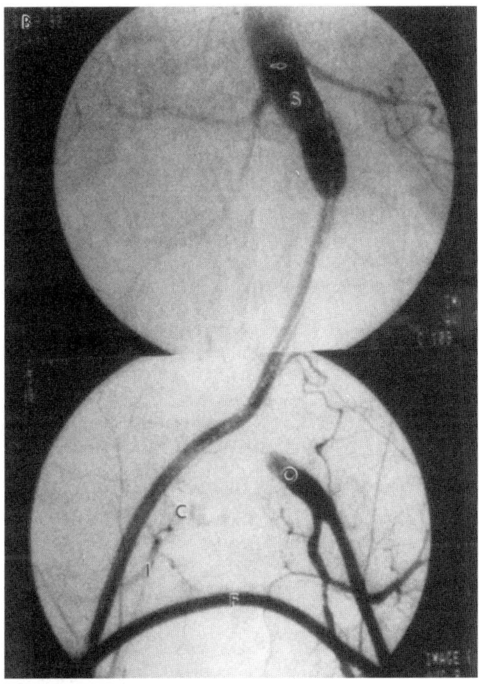

Figure 14–6. Intraoperative angiogram of the patient described in Figure 14–7. **(A)** Preoperative angiogram reveals a large AAA and a small right common iliac aneurysm. Because the blood pressure was low, no extravasation was noted on this arteriogram. **(B)** Completion angiogram. The AAA is completely excluded with no evidence of an endoleak. The bare portion of the proximal stent (S) is placed above the renal arteries, and the cranial end of the graft, which is denoted by the gold marker (arrow), is placed immediately below the renal arteries. The right internal iliac artery is opacified by retrograde flow. C, embolization coils; O, occluder device; F, femorofemoral bypass. (Reproduced with permission.[13])

blood loss and improve outcomes.[16–19] Restriction of fluid resuscitation has also been advocated in the preoperative management of ruptured aneurysms.[3] We also believe that restriction of fluid resuscitation and blood transfusion in the ruptured AAA setting is not only desirable but mandatory. If the blood pressure is in the 50–70 mm Hg range, that is acceptable. If the patient is moving and talking, no fluids should be given. This should continue when the patient is first in the operating room being prepared for treatment and having a catheter and guidewire placed in the pararenal aorta under local anesthesia via either a brachial or femoral puncture.

Patients with ruptured AAAs frequently deteriorate with induction of anesthesia. If that occurs and the blood pressure falls below 50–70 mm Hg or is unobtainable, administration of fluid and blood become necessary. We believe such deterioration warrants proximal balloon control and have used this technique selectively in our current management plan for ruptured aneurysms.

PROXIMAL BALLOON CONTROL

If and when patients deteriorate before, during or after induction of anesthesia, a larger size (14-Fr) hemostatic sheath is inserted over the previously placed guidewire

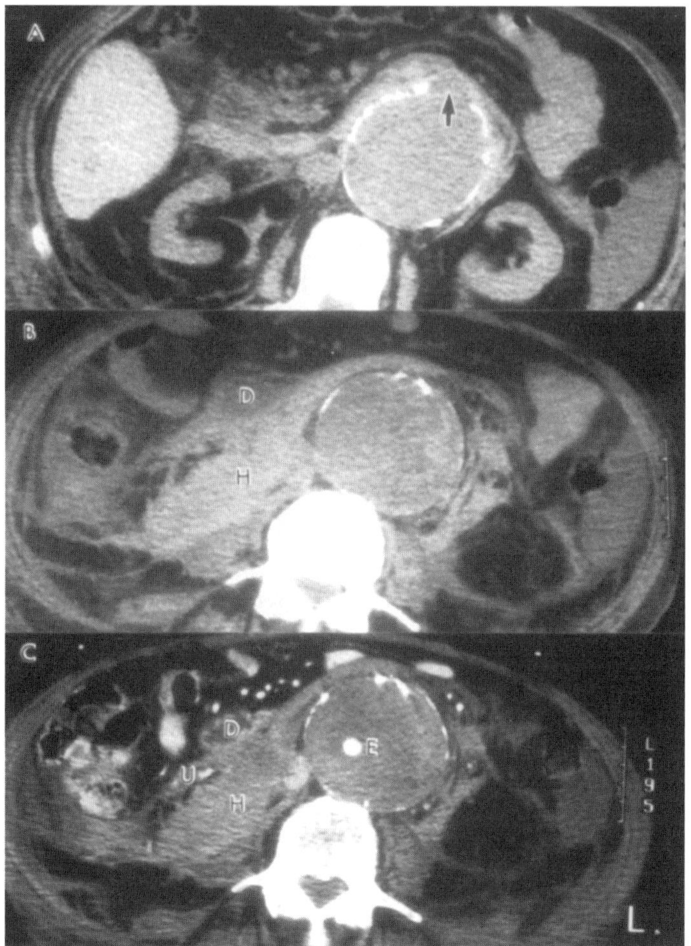

Figure 14–7. CT scan images of a ruptured AAA. This 71-year-old male was admitted to another hospital for medical treatment of his pneumonia secondary to chemotherapy for leukemia. His other comorbid diseases included severe COPD requiring home oxygen and congestive heart failure with an ejection fraction of 25%. The patient experienced a sudden onset of severe abdominal pain with CT scan evidence of a ruptured AAA. Due to his coexisting diseases, standard repair was deemed prohibitively risky and he was transferred to our institution. On arrival, his systolic blood pressure was 75 mm Hg and his hematocrit was 18%. **(A)** Preoperative CT scan reveals a possible rupture site (arrow) in the AAA. **(B)** Preoperative CT scan showing the more distal portion of the AAA. The AAA measures 7.5 cm in diameter. In addition, a large hematoma (H) can be seen in the right retroperitoneal space with displacement of the duodenum (D). **(C)** Postoperative contrast CT scan. Contrast is confined within the endograft (E) with evidence of complete aneurysmal exclusion. The ureter, which is displaced by the large hematoma, is visualized. Despite his comorbid conditions, he was extubated 6 hours following the procedure and was able to eat on the second postoperative day. (Reproduced with permission.[13])

in either the brachial or femoral artery. Keeping the wire in place a 33 or 40 mm compliant (latex) balloon is inserted through the sheath and inflated with dilute contrast under fluoroscopic control in either the suprarenal (Figure 14–8), pararenal or infrarenal aorta (depending on the length of the infrarenal neck). With the balloon inflated, the remainder of the procedure is conducted as rapidly as possible to minimize the duration of visceral and renal ischemia. If the infrarenal neck is too short for an endovascular repair, open infrarenal control is obtained and a standard AAA repair per-

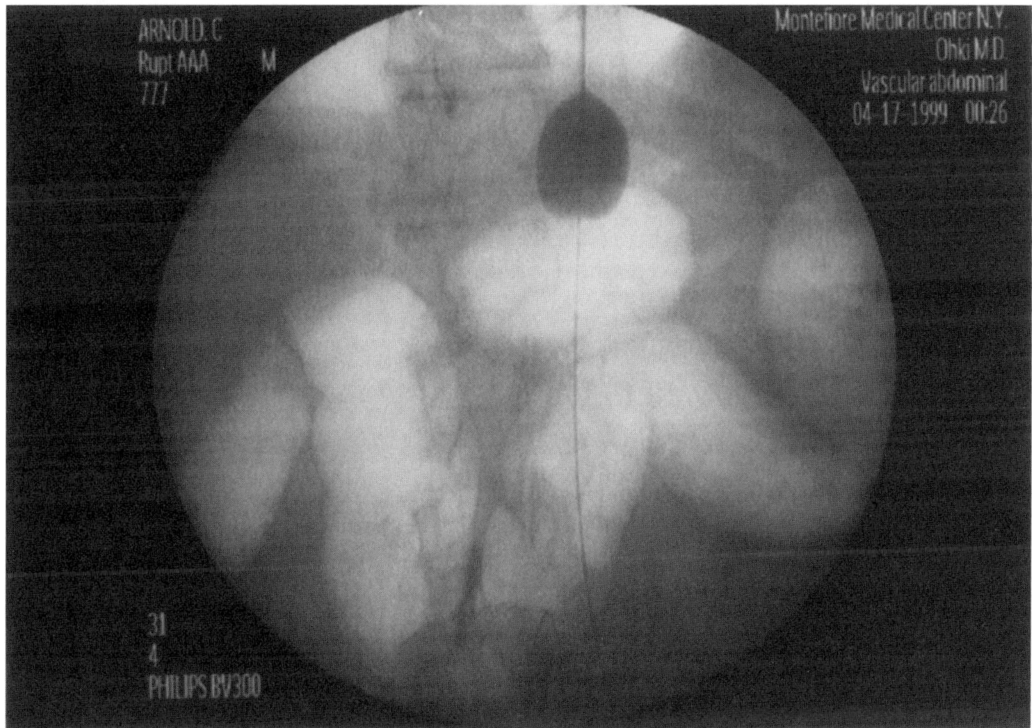

Figure 14–8. Fluoroscopic view of a proximal occlusion balloon introduced through the brachial artery.

formed. If the infrarenal neck is long enough, an infrarenal balloon should replace the more proximal balloon as soon as possible, and then the endograft placed in a deliberate fashion, although the supraceliac balloon may have to be reinflated during the graft deployment when any infrarenal balloon must be removed.

RESULTS

To date, we have treated 32 patients with ruptured aortoiliac aneurysms using endovascular techniques.[14] Included are the 12 original patients already described and another 20 patients treated according to our current management plan. Of these 32 patients, 6 were deemed unsuitable for endovascular treatment because of their aortic neck or iliac anatomy. All 6 underwent open repair, only 2 required inflation of the proximal balloon. All 6 survived for more than 2 months after operation.

Of the remaining 26 patients who received an endovascular graft, 18 had the graft* inserted without the need for proximal balloon control. Only 8 required balloon control. In all 26 patients, the graft was deployed successfully and completely excluded

---

*One patient received an AneuRx modular bifurcated graft.

the ruptured aneurysm. There were no significant endoleaks and all surviving patients became and remained asymptomatic. Three of the 26 patients died during the 30 days after their procedure, but all 3 had serious medical comorbidities (2 coincident major myocardial infarctions, 1 oxygen dependent COPD). Thus, in this entire series of 32 ruptured AAAs, there was a procedural mortality of only 9.4%.

Two patients receiving endovascular grafts required evacuation of a large retroperitoneal hematoma for abdominal compartment syndrome. In one of these patients the decompression was required immediately after graft placement; in the other it was required 7 days later. Two groin wound infections required drainage but healed without graft involvement.

ADVANTAGES OF ENDOVASCULAR REPAIR

Among the advantages of endovascular repair of ruptured aneurysms are the ability to obtain proximal control without general anesthesia, the ability to deploy the graft from a remote access site, reduced blood loss, and minimizing hypothermia by eliminating laparotomy.

Proximal Control without General Anesthesia

Patients with ruptured AAAs may be severely hypotensive. However, some patients may remain normotensive and stable, and many patients may have their blood pressure stabilized at a nonlethal level. The latter state is due to sympathetically mediated vasoconstriction in response to hypotension. It is not uncommon for this vasoconstriction to be released during the induction of general anesthesia, which results in a sudden drop in blood pressure. Therefore, a relatively stable patient may become severely hypotensive, mandating urgent application of a proximal aortic clamp. However, a guidewire can be inserted in the upper abdominal or lower thoracic aorta through a percutaneous puncture under local anesthesia, while maintaining the vasoconstriction. Once the guidewire is inserted in the aorta, the patient can then safely undergo induction of general anesthesia because proximal control can be rapidly and safely obtained by an occlusion balloon placed over the previously inserted guidewire.

Deployment of Graft from a Remote Access Site

Endovascular grafts can be inserted and deployed through a remote access site, thereby obviating the need for laparotomy and, more importantly, eliminating the technical difficulties that may be encountered when performing a standard repair in the rupture setting. With the associated bleeding, the anatomy of the retroperitoneal structures is often distorted and obscured by a large hematoma, which may lead to inadvertent injury of the inferior vena cava, the left renal vein or its genital branches, the duodenum, or other surrounding structures. These iatrogenic injuries have been the cause of significant operative morbidity and mortality following standard open surgery for ruptured aneurysms. In contrast, endograft repair is performed within the arterial tree, which is unaffected by extravasated blood or previous operative scarring. Thus, the technical difficulty encountered when treating a ruptured aneurysm with an endograft is similar to that for elective cases. Moreover, this approach completely eliminates the risk of inadvertent injury to surrounding structures.

Reduced Blood Loss

In our experience, endovascular repair for ruptured AAA was accomplished with a relatively small amount of additional blood loss (800 ml) compared with that which occurs during open, ruptured AAA repair. This advantage is more important in patients with ruptured aneurysms because these patients have already lost a significant amount of blood following rupture, and coagulopathy or disseminated intravascular coagulation secondary to further blood loss can be devastating complications. There are several reasons why this limited blood loss was possible, including the maintenance of the tamponade effect within the retroperitoneum. In addition, back-bleeding from the iliac and lumbar arteries and bleeding from the anastomotic suture lines and from iatrogenic venous injuries can be eliminated.

Minimizing Hypothermia

Hypothermia secondary to poor perfusion and laparotomy can exacerbate coagulopathy, which is one of the causes of mortality following open surgical repair. Endovascular graft repair can minimize the extent of hypothermia by avoiding laparotomy.

CONCLUSION

The relatively low mortality rate (9.4%) in our group of patients was encouraging, particularly because many were high-risk patients who were not surgical candidates. Our results as well as those of others[12,14,19–21] show that endograft repair of ruptured AAAs is feasible and effective in selected cases. However, before the widespread use of this technique is adopted, further experience by other groups will be required using our graft or others to treat ruptured AAAs. Nevertheless, we believe that endovascular grafts represent a potentially better way to treat this entity since previous open surgical methods have had a persistently high morbidity and mortality. Moreover, we believe that the use of fluoroscopic techniques to facilitate the placement of proximal occlusion balloons, an old idea,[23–26] will make this endovascular adjunct a practical and valuable one, even if an endovascular graft procedure is not possible and an open repair is required. And finally, we believe that hypotensive hemostasis or restricted fluid resuscitation will prove valuable in the ruptured AAA setting and will become the standard of care for this entity leading to improved treatment outcomes.

REFERENCES

1. Ernst CB. Abdominal aortic aneurysms. *N Engl J Med.* 1993;328:1167–1172.
2. Ouriel K, Geary K, Green RM, et al. Factors determining survival after ruptured aortic aneurysm: the hospital, the surgeon, and the patient. *J Vasc Surg.* 1990;11:493–496.
3. Crawford ES. Ruptured abdominal aortic aneurysm: an editorial. *J Vasc Surg.* 1991;13:348–350.
4. Johansen K, Kohler TR, Nicholls SC, et al. Ruptured abdominal aortic aneurysm: the Harborview experience. *J Vasc Surg.* 1991;13:240–247.
5. Gloviczki P, Pairolero PC, Mucha P. Ruptured abdominal aortic aneurysms: repair should not be denied. *J Vasc Surg.* 1992;15:851–859.
6. Marty-Ane CH, Alric P, Picot MC, et al. Ruptured abdominal aortic aneurysm: influence of intraoperative management on surgical outcome. *J Vasc Surg.* 1995;22:780–786.

7. Darling RC, Cordero JA, Chang BB. Advances in the surgical repair of ruptured abdominal aortic aneurysms. *Cardiovasc Surg.* 1996;4:720–723.

8. Dardik A, Burleyson GP, Bowman H, et al. Surgical repair of ruptured abdominal aortic aneurysms in the state of Maryland: factors influencing outcome among 527 recent cases. *J Vasc Surg.* 1998;28:413–423.

9. Noel AA, Gloviczki P, Cherry KJ, et al. Ruptured abdominal aortic aneurysms: The excessive mortality rate of conventional repair. *J Vasc Surg.* 2001;34:41–46.

10. Marin ML, Veith FJ, Cynamon J, et al. Initial experience with transluminally placed endovascular grafts for the treatment of complex vascular lesions. *Ann Surg.* 1995;222:1–17.

11. Veith FJ. Emergency abdominal aortic aneurysm surgery. *Compr Ther.* 1992;18:25–29.

12. Parodi JC, Palmaz JC, Barone HD. Transfemoral intraluminal graft implantation for abdominal aortic aneurysms. *Ann Vasc Surg.* 1991;5:491–499.

13. Ohki T, Veith FJ, Sanchez LA, et al. Endovascular graft repair of ruptured aorto-iliac aneurysms. *J Am Coll Surg.* 1999;189:102–113.

14. Yusuf SW, Whitaker SC, Chuter TA, et al. Emergency endovascular repair of leaking aortic aneurysm. *Lancet.* 1994;344:1645.

15. Ohki T, Veith FJ. Endovascular grafts and other image guided catheter based adjuncts to improve the treatment of ruptured aortoiliac aneurysms. *Ann Surg.* 2000;232:466–479.

16. Andresen AFR. Results of treatment of massive gastric hemorrhage. *Am J Digest Dis.* 1939;6:641–650.

17. Andresen AFR. Management of gastric hemorrhage. *NY State J Med.* 1948;48:603–611.

18. Shaftan GW, Chiu CJ, Dennis C, Harris B. Fundamentals of physiologic control of arterial hemorrhage. *Surg.* 1968:58:851–856.

19. Bickell WH, Wall MJ Jr, Pepe PE, et al. Immediate versus delayed fluid resuscitation for hypotensive patients with penetrating torso injuries. *N Engl J Med.* 1994;331:1105–1109.

20. Yusuf SW, Whitaker SC, Chuter TAM, et al. Early results of endovascular aortic aneurysm surgery with aortouniiliac graft, contralateral iliac occlusion, and femorofemoral bypass. *J Vasc Surg.* 1997;25:165–172.

21. Yusuf SW, Hopkinson BR. It is feasible to treat contained aortic aneurysm rupture by stent-graft combination? In: Greenhalgh RM, ed. *Indications in Vascular and Endovascular Surgery.* London: WB Saunders; 1998:153–165.

22. Greenberg RK, Srivastava SD, Ouriel K, et al. An endoluminal method of hemorrhage control and repair of ruptured abdominal aortic aneurysms. *J Endovasc Ther.* 2000;7:1–7.

23. Hughes LCCW. Use of an intra-aortic balloon catheter tamponade for controlling intra-abdominal hemorrhage in man. *Surgery.* 1954;36:65–68.

24. Hesse FG, Kletschka HD. Rupture of abdominal aortic aneurysm: control of hemorrhage by intraluminal balloon tamponade. *Ann Surg.* 1962;155:320–322.

25. Anastacio CN, Ochsner EC. Use of Fogarty catheter tamponade for ruptured abdominal aortic aneurysms. *Am J Roentgenol.* 1977;128:31–33.

26. Hyde GL, Sullivan DM. Fogarty catheter tamponade of ruptured abdominal aortic aneurysms. *Surg Gynecol Obstet.* 1982;154:197–199.

15

Infected Aortic Aneurysm

Kenneth J. Cherry, Jr., MD

Aortic graft infections remain a risk to patients undergoing aortic reconstruction, and their treatment a challenge to vascular surgeons. Mycotic aneurysms pose similar risks. Historically, loss of limb(s) and life were high. The first operation used routinely and with some predictable success was excision of the infected aortic graft, closure of the wounds, re-prepping and draping, and construction of an axillofemoral graft. Not surprisingly, the prolonged periods of pelvic and limb ischemia attendant to that operation were marked by high morbidity and mortality. Mortality rates were in the order of 50 to 70% and amputation rates high.[1] Infection of the aorta itself at the proximal site of graft excision and aortic oversewing resulted in aortic stump blow out in over 20% of patients.

Wylie and colleagues at UCSF proposed in situ reconstruction using autogenous saphenous vein or arterial grafts usually from the patient's ileofemoral system as an alternative to graft excision and extra-anatomic reconstruction.[2] That same group and others were also proponents for the rational juxtaposition of the component parts of axillary grafting, namely, *axillofemoral reconstruction first* followed by a *staged* excision of the infected graft.[3–5] These innovations, particularly extracavitary, or ex situ, prosthetic reconstruction preceding staged excision, succeeded in lowering mortality rates from 60% to 20%.[1] Limb loss, however, has continued to be an issue. Amputation rates for axillofemoral grafting for infection range in multiple series from 11% to 29%, averaging 21%.[1,4,6–8] In a group of patients we followed, 33% of survivors eventually lost an extremity, and 15% of survivors suffered late deaths from problems attendant to failing grafts and limb ischemia. (Cherry KJ, Kreps JT, Pairolero PC, O'Brien PC, Hallett JW, Glovizcki P, Ballard DJ. Abdominal aortic graft infections: Management and long-term outcome 1989, unpublished study)

In the midst of these developments was a report from the Texas Heart Institute by Walker and colleagues, detailing in situ reconstruction of infected infrarenal grafts with prosthetics.[9] In that series of 23 patients, limb salvage was 100%. Autogenous coverage of the graft with omentum or muscle was beneficial in that group to a statistically significant degree. The presence of an abscess, on the other hand, was associated statistically with poor outcome.

Current techniques to treat aortic graft infections and mycotic aneurysms include ex situ reconstruction with staged excision, in situ reconstruction with superficial femoral vein, in situ reconstruction with rifampin-bonded prosthetics, in situ reconstruction with cryopreserved aortic allografts, endovascular repair, and other less commonly utilized modalities such as ex situ retroperitoneal bypass.[10]

ENDOVASCULAR GRAFTING

Arterial-enteric fistulas have been reported following placement of endografts in both the aortic and iliac positions.[11,12] On the other hand, endografts have been used for aorto-enteric fistulas planned as either temporary or definitive treatment.[13–15] There are not enough data to condemn or recommend their use in the treatment of arterial graft infections. Anecdotally, we, as well as others, have patients for whom this modality has been life saving in acutely ill, very high-risk patients, for whom operation is not possible or not likely to be of benefit. The incidence of infections with aorto-iliac endografts and the role of endografts in treating infections remain to be delineated.

CRYOPRESERVED AORTIC ALLOGRAFTS

Cryopreserved aortic allografts are theoretically an attractive means of replacing infected grafts or mycotic aortic aneurysms. Their reported use in the thoracic and suprarenal aortas is encouraging.[16–17] Centers in Europe have been leading proponents of the use of cryopreserved allografts with initial good results in short to medium follow-up.[18–20] Freshly preserved and cryopreserved allografts may still have unacceptably high rates of aneurysmal and stenotic complications because of degeneration of the medial layer.[21,22]

The report from the United States Cryopreserved Aortic Registry by Noel et al. reported a 30-day mortality of 13% and an overall mortality of 25%.[23] There was a 5% amputation rate and a graft-related complications rate of 25%. Two patients (4%) died of graft complications. Those authors felt that their data failed to justify the preferential use of cryopreserved aortic allografts. The recent proscription of cryopreserved tissue by the U.S. FDA will delay resolution of the questions concerning cryopreserved tissue.

EX SITU (EXTRA ANATOMIC: AXILLOFEMORAL) GRAFTING

For most vascular surgeons, extra-anatomic grafting followed by staged excision of the infected graft remains the first choice in the treatment of infected aortic grafts and infrarenal mycotic aneurysms. In a review of multiple institutional experiences, we found that the mortality was 20%, the reinfection rate 22%, and the amputation rate 20%.[1,4,6–8] It is this latter figure which vascular surgeons have found most disturbing and which has, in part, impelled basic and clinical research into in situ reconstruction.

Nonetheless, axillofemoral grafting remains an excellent choice for many, if not most, patients. Patients with infrarenal mycotic aneurysm or with infected grafts confined to the abdomen, done usually for aneurysmal disease, with straight or aortoiliac grafts, are excellent candidates for axillofemoral grafting. The groins are free of infection, allowing anastomosis to the common femoral arteries. Further, any intra-abdominal abscesses are avoided with this technique. Severe femoropopliteal occlusive disease in such patients, however, mitigates against graft patency and successful limb salvage. Although a few reports claim patency for axillofemoral grafting nearly equivalent to that of in-line aortofemoral grafting in elective situations,[24-26] most authors report and most vascular surgeons feel that axillofemoral graft is hemodynamically inferior to aortofemoral bypass grafting with reduced patency and limb salvage.[27,28] Infection, of course, complicates the issue and the presence of infrainguinal occlusive disease compounds it further.

Patients with infected aortofemoral bypass grafts are also treated by this modality. The involvement of the common femoral area necessitates construction of the distal anastomosis in less hemodynamically advantageous sites beyond the infected groins. This, undoubtedly, contributes to the 20% amputation rate in these patients. It is a less appealing operation for these patients than it is for those whose grafts are confined to the abdomen. It may be necessary because of intra-abdominal abscess, presence of virulent organisms such as methicillin-resistant Staphylococcus aureus or Pseudomonas, and the absence of suitable superficial femoral vein to allow for autogenous reconstruction. One technique that may hold some promise to allow anastomosis to the common femoral artery as opposed to less advantageous sites, such as the distal profunda femoris artery, superficial femoral artery or the popliteal artery, is preliminary incision and drainage of the infected groins with aggressive local debridement and the institution of suction irrigation systems some days prior to embarking on a formal reconstruction for the infected graft. This mechanical and antibiotic cleansing of the groins may allow a better milieu to avoid reinfection for grafts placed in the area.

Whether an aortic graft is infected locally in one limb, e.g., at the groin anastomosis, or is infected in its entirety is of vital importance. Partial graft excision has been recognized as a very reasonable way to manage graft infections in those patients for whom total graft excision is not necessary. In many cases, it is preferred to total graft resection, especially for very early infections or for late indolent cases of Staphylococcus epidermidis in which the groins only are involved. This is especially true in high-risk patients. We have used a combination of computed tomographic scans and neutrophil-specific white cell scans to determine as much as possible preoperatively the extent of graft infection. Operative exploration is, of course, the ultimate test for well-incorporated, noninfected graft.

Further, patients with very poor cardiac status are probably better treated by axillofemoral grafting followed by excision even if the femoral arteries are involved in the infectious process. Axillofemoral grafting followed by excision places less stress on the heart than aortic clamping and direct in-line reconstruction. Outflow in these patients is often compromised as detailed above, with distal anastomoses of necessity performed to vessels beyond the groin. The tradeoff in these patients for a reduced cardiac morbidity is perhaps a marked reduction in limb salvage.

Mortality remains at about 20% due to a combination of sepsis, graft reinfection and aortic stump blow out. Aortic stump blow out remains a major problem although is reported much less frequently than in the past. This reduction in aortic stump blow out may reflect better patient selection.

Although most series report reinfection rates that average around 22%, there are exceptions to this. Henke and associates from the University of Louisville reported no recurrent graft infections in an experience dating back to 1985.[29] Reinfection of axillofemoral grafting may be treated by contralateral axillofemoral grafting, autogenous reconstructions, or combinations thereof.

IN SITU RECONSTRUCTION

Hayes and colleagues from the Leicester Royal Infirmary used rifampin-bonded grafts in 11 patients treated from 1992 through 1997 their mortality was 18% and limb salvage 100%. The 2 deaths occurred in one patient with E. coli infection and another with both methicillin-resistant Staphylococcus aureus and candida. These authors cared for patients with the full gamut of aortic infections. There were 4 aortic-enteric fistulas with hemorrhage, 3 retroperitoneal abscesses, 2 graft occlusions, 1 perigraft fluid collection, and 1 ruptured suprarenal false aneurysm. Those patients who died were unusual in that both presented with acute infections occurring 2 months after their initial operations. Both presented in extremis.[30]

Prompted by the experience at the Texas Heart Institute with its impressive limb salvage, surgeons at the Mayo Clinic in Rochester presented a series of patients reconstructed with in situ prosthetic grafts, some of which were soaked in rifampin.[31] The mortality was 9%, reinfection rate 21%, and limb salvage 100%. As in the earlier report from Houston, the authors found a statistically significant advantage with the use of autogenous coverage of the graft.

There were no operative or late amputations and primary graft patency was 86% at 5 years.

There were 5 reinfections. All 5 reinfections occurred in patients who originally had aortofemoral bypass grafting for aortoiliac occlusive disease. The association with aortofemoral grafting was not statistically significant; neither was the association with abscess versus fistula, although only 1 patient presenting with a fistula developed reinfection. Only 1 of the 9 patients treated with the rifampin-bonded graft developed reinfection. Only 2 of 19 patients who had full 360 degree coverage of the graft developed reinfection, and that was significant. None of the reinfections were fatal; they were treated by a variety of methods, including autogenous reconstruction. Just as the group from Leicester had, we found the poorest initial presentation to be patients with hemorrhagic aorto-enteric fistulas.

Bandyk and associates at the University of South Florida have been leaders in proposing the use of in situ rifampin-bonded prosthetic graft replacement for infected grafts and in determining which subset of patients may be treated by that technique.[32,33] In June 2001, they reported 27 patients treated with in situ rifampin-bonded grafts for 22 prosthetic infections and 5 mycotic or primary infections.[32] All prosthetic infections were "low grade" infections with Staphylococcus epidermidis, Staphylococcus aureus and Streptococcus. Mortality was 8%. A patient with a salmonella mycotic AAA and another with methicillin-resistant Staphylococcus aureus died. The amputation rate was 0% and the reinfection rate 8%. They recommended that in situ prosthetic grafts be offered to patients with "low grade Staphylococcus aureus and Staphylococcus epidermidis, biofilm infection and Gram positive infection involving the aorta at sites that precluded conventional management." A later paper from that same group detailed a cumulative experience over 10 years with prosthetic infections treated by a variety of methods.[33] They found in situ grafting applicable to 64% of their patients but had modified their recommendations to patients with localized Staphylococcus epidermidis infection only. They felt that a biofilm infection of the entire graft was a contraindication to this technique. They further felt that the more conventional ex situ, or axillofemoral, reconstruction should be offered to patients with sepsis, false aneurysms or fistulas.

Our group would differ slightly in its patient selection recommendations. First, none of our patients had Staphylococcus aureus or Pseudomonas infections, and we are loathe to use this technique if those virulent bacteria are known or thought to be causative agents. In over 30% of our patients, we were unable to identify the causative bacteria. However, if the bacteria are known to be Staphylococcus aureus or Pseudomonas, we feel remote ex situ reconstruction is preferable to in situ repair; we have not made a distinction between "low level" Staphylococcus aureus and more active strains, but treat all Staphylococcus aureus as an aggressive infection. The Tampa group discontinues antibiotics after 2 months. We have maintained life-long suppressive doses in those patients able to tolerate it.

We feel patients with aorto-enteric fistulas without abscess are well treated by this technique in distinction to both the Leicester and Tampa groups. Admittedly, patients with fistulas presenting with overwhelming sepsis or hemorrhage are poorly handled by all techniques. Nonetheless, in-line prosthetic grafting offers the most rapid opportunity to repair the fistula, remove the infected graft, and restore blood flow to the pelvis and lower extremities in a timely manner. Furthermore, our recurrences, with one exception, did not occur in patients presenting with fistulas.

We feel that patients with intra-abdominal abscesses and virulent strains of bacteria are poorly treated with this technique. Patients with aortofemoral grafts are also more likely to have recurrence. Full length 360-degree autogenous coverage down to and including the groin anastomoses provides protection.

It is our feeling that in situ prosthetic grafting is the treatment of choice for the very highest risk patients, that is those presenting with exsanguination from aorto-duodenal fistulas. Much less time is required with this technique to control the bleeding and to replace the infected graft. Flow can be restored to the pelvis and limbs in a much more expeditious manner. Aortic stump blow out is obviated although the problem of false aneurysm and the subsequent rupture at the proximal anastomosis remains an analogous complication.[9] Nonetheless, this high-risk group of patients is poorly treated by femoral vein reconstruction, as documented by Clagett et al.[34] Likewise, control of the hemorrhage and repair of the fistula and abdominal closure followed by axillofemoral reconstruction is a poor choice in these patients, with lengthy ischemia of the pelvis and lower extremities. Patients who develop reinfection of an in situ prosthetic may be subsequently treated in a less urgent setting.

AUTOGENOUS RECONSTRUCTION

Improving on the techniques of autogenous reconstruction, Clagett and associates from Dallas reported excellent results with autogenous in situ reconstruction of the aorta using superficial femoral veins.[34] The mortality in their patients was 10%, reinfection rate 0% and limb salvage 95%. The patients who lost extremities in that study did so because of distal disease. Patients with aorto-enteric fistulas tended to do less well than others in their series. The time required to harvest and repair the superficial femoral veins and construct an aortic conduit with them mitigated against the use of this "long and arduous operation" in unstable patients with fistulas presenting with hemorrhage or overwhelming sepsis.

Superficial femoral veins have more utility than harvested and endarterectomized superficial femoral arteries or saphenous veins as autogenous conduits: the conduits are more predictably of adequate caliber and length. It is a time-consuming procedure and not all patients are candidates for it, either because of old thrombosis with stenotic veins or co-morbidities. However, in patients with recurrent infections that have been unresponsive to standard techniques, it is certainly the procedure of choice for patients with full-length aortofemoral graft infections, those known to have virulent organisms, those who have abscesses, and who are stable. It is not the preferred technique in patients presenting with exsanguination, as there is simply not the time available to allow use of this approach.

SUMMARY

Ex situ grafting and excision of infection grafts continues to be the most commonly performed operation for infected grafts in this country. Limb salvage, however, continues to be a problem with this technique. The in-line reconstructions, rifampin-bonded prosthetics and superficial femoral vein conduits provide more predictable graft patency and limb salvage. The summaries presented above of the various techniques and materials available to treat aortic graft infection and mycotic aneurysms are presented as a guide to the relative strengths and weaknesses of each and to an interpretation of current indications and contraindications. It is not possible to compare different reports in a direct manner, as different subsets of patients with varying spectra of bacteria or clinical presentation had been treated by these modalities. In general ex situ grafting reports encompass patients from all risk categories, whereas reports concerning in situ prosthetics detail, for the most part, selected subsets of patients. As an example, in our report on in situ prosthetics, there were no cases of Staphylococcus aureus or Pseudomonas infection. In the multicenter study of cryopreserved aortic allografts, 52% of people had Staphylococcus aureus, which may well have preordained some of the results.

In spite of these reservations, we feel, as do Bandyk et al., that in situ reconstruction may be anticipated to be applicable to the plurality, if not the majority, of patients. It is our first choice if the criteria presented are met; the rationale for that preference is the apparent reduction in operative mortality, similar rates of reinfection compared to axillofemoral grafting, the avoidance of aortic stump blowout, but most of all, the great improvement in limb salvage. Careful patient selection is absolutely necessary if acceptable results are to be anticipated. We reserve in situ reconstruction with the deep veins of the thigh to recurrent cases or patients for whom the other techniques are not suited. It remains the best option in providing ultimate cure of graft infection.

REFERENCES

1. Curl RG, Ricotta JJ. Total prosthetic graft excision and extra-anatomic bypass. In: Calligaro KD, Veith FJ, eds. *Management of infection arterial grafts.* St. Louis: Quality Medical Publishing; 1994:82–94.
2. Ehrenfeld WK, Wilbur BG, Olcott CN, et al.: Autogenous tissue reconstruction in the management of infected prosthetic grafts. *Surgery.* 1979;85:82.
3. Trout HH, Kozloff L, Giordano JM: Priority of revascularization in patients with graft enteric fistulas, infected arteries, or infected arterial prostheses. *Ann Surg.* 1984;199:669.
4. O'Hara PJ, Hertzer NR, Beven EG, Krajewsi LP. Surgical management of infection abdominal aortic grafts: review of a 25-year experience. *J Vasc Surg.* 1986;3:725–731.

5. Reilly LM, Stoney RJ, Goldstone J, et al. Improved management of aortic graft infection: The influence of operation sequence and staging. *J Vasc Surg.* 1987;5:421.
6. Reilly LM, Altman H, Lusby RJ, et al. Late results following surgical management of vascular graft infection. *J Vasc Surg.* 1984;1:36–44.
7. Yeager RA, Moneta GL, Taylor LM, et al. Inproving survival and limb salvage in patients with aortic graft infection. *Am J Surg.* 1990;159:466–469
8. Quinones-Baldrich JW, Jernandez JJ, Moore WS. Long-term results following surgical management of aortic graft infection. *Arch Surg.* 1997;14(suppl A):102–107.
9. Walker EW, Cooley DA, Duncan JM, et al. The management of aortoduodenal fistula by in situ replacement of the infected abdominal aortic graft. *Ann Surg.* 1987;205:727–732.
10. Darling RC, Resnikoff M, Kreienberg PB, et al. Alternative approach for management of infected aortic grafts. *J Vasc Surg.* 1997;25:106–112.
11. Deiparine MK, Ballard JL, Taylor FC, Chase DR. Endovascular stent infection. *J Vasc Surg.* 1996;23:529–533.
12. D'Othée BJ, Soula P, Otal P, et al. Aortoduodenal fistula after endovascular stent-graft of an abdominal aortic aneurysm. *J Vasc Surg.* 2000;31:190–195.
13. Deshpande A, Lovelock M, Mossop P, et al. Endovascular repair of an aortoenteric fistula in a high-risk patient. *J Endovasc Surg.* 1999;6:379–384.
14. Chuter TAM, Lukaszewicz GC, Reilly LM, et al. Endovascular repair of a presumed aortoenteric fistula: late failure due to recurrent infection. *J Endovasc Ther.* 2000;7:240–244.
15. Eskandari MK, Makaroun MS, Abu-Elmagd KM, Billiar TR. Endovascular repair of an aortodudenal fistula. *J Endovasc Ther.* 2000;7:328–332.
16. Vogt PR, Turina MI. Management of infected aortic grafts: development of less invasive surgery using cryopreserved homografts. *Ann Thorac Surg.* 1999;67:1986–1989.
17. Müller BT, Wegener OR, Grabitz K, et al. Mycotic aneurysms of the thoracic and abdominal aorta and iliac arteries: Experience with anatomic and extra-anatomic repair in 33 cases. *J Vasc Surg.* 2001;33:106–113.
18. Vogt PR, Pfammatter T, Schlumpf R, et al. In situ repair of aortobronchial aortoesophgeal, and aortoenteric fistulae with cryopreserved aortic homografts. *J Vasc Surg.* 1997;26:11–17.
19. Vogt RP, Brunner-La Rocca HP, Carrel T, et al. Cryopreserved arterial allografts in the treatment of major vascular infection: a comparison with conventional surgical techniques. *J Thorac Cardiovasc Surg.* 1998;116:965–972.
20. Lesèche G, Castier Y, Petit MD, et al. Long-term results of cryopreserved arterial allograft reconstruction in infected prosthetic grafts and mycotic aneurysms of the abdominal aorta. *J Vasc Surg.* 2001;34:616–622.
21. De Gama AD, Sarmento C, Vieira T, do CG. The use of arterial allografts for vascular reconstruction in patients receiving immunosuppression for organ transplantation. *J Vasc Surg.* 1994;20:271–278.
22. Koskas F, Plissonnier D, Bahnini A, et al. In situ arterial allografting for aortoiliac graft infection: a 6-year experience. *Cardiovasc Surg.* 1996;4:495–459.
23. Noel AA, Gloviczki P, Cherry KJ Jr, et al. Abdominal aortic reconstruction in infected fields: early results of the United States Cryopreserved Aortic Allograft Registry. *J Vasc Surg.* 2002;35:847–852.
24. Harris EJ Jr, Taylor LM Jr, McConnell DB, et al. Clinical results of axillobifemoral bypass using externally supported polytetrafluoroethylene. *J Vasc Surg.* 1990;12:416–421.
25. El-Massry S, Saad E, Sauvage LR, et al. Axillofemoral bypass with externally supported, knitted Dacron grafts: A follow-up throgh twelve years. *J Vasc Surg.* 1993;17:107–115.
26. Passman MA, Taylor LM Jr, Moneta GL, et al. Comparison of axillofemoral and aortofemoral bypass for aortoiliac occlusive disease. *J Vasc Surg.* 1996;23:263–271.
27. Kalman PG, Hosang M, Cina C, et al. Current indications for axillounifemoral and axillobifemoral bypass grafts. *J Vasc Surg.* 1987;5:828–832.
28. Schneider JR, McDaniel MD, Walsh DB, et al. Axillofemoral bypass: Outcome and hemodynamic results in high-risk patients. *J Vasc Surg.* 1992;15:952–963.
29. Henke PK, Bergamini TM, Rose SM, Richardson JD. Current options in prosthetic vascular graft infection. *Amer Surg.* 1998;64:39–45.

30. Hayes PD, Nasim A, London NJM, et al. In situ replacement of infected aortic grafts with rifampin-bonded prostheses: The Leicester experience (1992 to 1998). *J Vasc Surg.* 1999;30:92–98.
31. Young RM, Cherry KJ Jr, Davis PM, et al. The results of in situ prosthetic replacement for infected aortic grafts. *Amer J Surg.* 1999;178:136–140.
32. Bandyk DF, Novotney ML, Johnson BL, et al. Use of rifampin-soaked gelatin-sealed polyester grafts for in situ treatment of primary aortic and vascular prosthetic infections. *J Surg Res.* 2001;95:44–49.
33. Bandyk DF, Novotney ML, Back MR, et al. Expanded application of in situ replacement for prosthetic graft infection. *J Vasc Surg.* 2001;34:411–420.
34. Clagett GP, Valentine RJ, Hagino RT. Autogenous aortoiliac/femoral reconstruction from superficial femoral-popliteal veins: feasibility and durability. *J Vasc Surg.* 1997;25:255–266.

V

Aortic Endovascular Graft

16

Selection and Choice of Endovascular Grafts for Abdominal Aortic Aneurysm

Richard M. Green, MD

The decision to recommend endovascular aneurysm repair (EVAR) and then to choose a specific device is critical to the individual patient, the surgeon, and the evolution of endovascular care. Bad choices result in bad results and discredit an evolving technology that is already under attack.[1] Some already claim that EVAR is a "failed experiment."[2] Midterm results with early technology clearly show that devices may fail, that secondary interventions are often required, and protection from rupture is not absolute. The *in vivo* stresses on these devices far exceed anything that could have been anticipated from bench testing. This should not come as a great surprise since there are no animal models that accurately duplicate the clinical condition. On the other hand, many surgeons and patients have an unrealistically favorable impression about the results of conventional repair. Although no one would deny that at this time conventional repair remains the most reliable method of managing AAA,[3] surgeons and patients underestimate the risks particularly when there are significant medical co-morbidities.

ASSESSING THE RISK OF CONVENTIONAL TREATMENT

It is inappropriate for any surgeon to quote a mortality rate to a patient that is not based on his/her own results. Reciting the mortality rate as one's own from a center of excellence, from a multi-center trial or a population-based study is problematic. Single-center studies exceeding 100 patients report the most favorable results (mortality rates of 0 to 3.7%). Operative mortality rates from multi-institutional series of greater than 300 patients are higher ranging from 3.6% to 4.9%. Population-based studies report still higher mortality rates ranging from 6% to 7.3%. Patients randomized to operation in the UK Small Aneurysm Trial had a 30-day mortality rate of 5.8%. A much lower rate was predicted (2%) during study design.[4]

In 1992, the Society for Vascular Surgery/International Society for Cardiovascular Surgery defined age, cardiac function, pulmonary function, and renal function as the predictors of medical risk for elective aneurysm repair.[5] Other factors are now known to affect mortality rates, namely the experience of the surgeon and the hospital. Dardik et al. reviewed all patients undergoing elective aneurysm repair in the state of Maryland between 1990 and 1995.[6] There were 2,335 operations performed by 219 surgeons in 46 hospitals and the in-hospital overall mortality rate was 3.5%. A multivariate analysis of these data showed that patient age (0.0002), low hospital volume (0.039), and very low volume surgeons (0.01) were independent variables of mortality. Specifically, patients older than 80 years had a mortality rate of 7.3% after aneurysm repair as compared to a rate of 2.2% for patients less than 65 years. Furthermore, the mortality rates for hospitals with high volumes (>50 during study period) and surgeons with very high volumes (>100 during study period) were roughly one-half the rates of hospitals and surgeons with little experience in aneurysm repair. Data from the National Inpatient Sample on 16,540 patients undergoing elective conventional AAA repair between 1994 and 1996 indicate an in-hospital mortality rate of 4.2% and an overall complication rate of 32.4%.[7] None of these figures include the long-term problems of graft thrombosis, infection, anastomotic aneurysms, sexual dysfunction, incisional hernias and bowel obstructions from adhesions.[8]

Steyerberg et al. have identified 7 factors that predict surgical death rates after AAA repair.[9] The information provided after a thorough meta-analysis of multiple series allows each surgeon to predict the mortality rate for any given patient using surgeon and hospital specific data. The factors that are included in the analysis are the average mortality rate for the hospital for a minimum of 25–50 similar procedures by the surgeon plus points for renal insufficiency (Cr >1.8mg-dl), congestive heart failure, EKG ischemia, FEV1<1 liter, older age and female gender. A score is tabulated (Table 16–1) and

TABLE 16–1. RISK CALCULATION OF MORTALITY FOLLOWING AAA RESECTION (AFTER STEYERBERG ET AL.[9]).

Center specific average operative mortality rates

%	3	4	5	6	8	12
Score	–5	–2	0	+2	+5	+10

Individual prognostic factors

Age (yr)	60	70	80	
Score	–4	0	+4	
Gender	Female			
Score	+4			
Cardiac co-morbidity	MI	CHF	ECG:ischemia	
Score	+3	+8	+8	
Renal co-morbidity (Cr>1.8)	Impairment			
Score	+12			
Pulmonary co-morbidity	Impairment			
Score	+7			

Estimated Individual Operative Mortality Rate

Sum score	(5)	0	5	10	15	20	25	30	35	40
Mortality rate %	1	2	3	5	8	12	19	28	39	51

a risk calculated. For instance, an 80-year-old woman with a 6 cm AAA, a past history of CHF, and a creatinine of 2.2 mg-dl would have a specific mortality rate approaching 20% (assuming the surgeon has an operative mortality rate of 4%).[10] If this analysis is valid and there is no reason to think otherwise, the benefits of EVAR done in similar high risk patients is evident already.

EARLY RESULTS OF EVAR

It is now well documented that EVAR can be performed safely with a variety of devices in patients with suitable anatomy. Technical success in well over 98% of patients is achievable with proper patient selection.[11,12] These patients have documented benefits that include decreased ICU utilization, decreased blood loss, shorter hospitalizations, and recovery times.[13] In addition, EVAR does not interfere with male potency.

The concern about EVAR relates to what happens after implantation. This is really a half full, half empty proposition. Despite the device failures, endoleaks, remodeling, etc., EVAR has prevented rupture in 98–99% and prevented growth in 85–90% of patients treated over the 6–8 years of clinical usage.[14] On the other hand, long-term efficacy is achieved at the price of a significant re-intervention rate. Many of these problems have occurred with devices that have already been withdrawn and the FDA is actively monitoring adverse events in the US IDE trials and PMA surveillance periods. Nonetheless, to anoint EVAR as the gold standard for AAA repair will require an acceptance of palliation rather than cure. This is not a new concept for vascular surgeons with other clinical problems and has gained wide acceptance among patients and doctors in other areas such as coronary angioplasty and stenting.

SELECTION FOR PATIENTS FOR EVAR

The selection of patients appropriate for EVAR is largely anatomical. The availability of a product that fits a patient's anatomy ultimately dictates the applicability of EVAR. No single device will accommodate every patient with an AAA and ideally no device should be used outside of its recommended anatomic guidelines. A relatively small number of patients will be anatomically suitable for EVAR if only the 2 approved devices are considered. As of July 2001, the FDA had reviewed 36 IDE applications for endovascular devices.[15] At the time of this writing 2 devices have received approval for commercial usage and at least 2 other approvals are anticipated during 2002–3. It is important to recognize that patient and device selection are not the only variables that affect outcome. There are also operator and procedure factors that are critical to success (Table 16–2).

TABLE 16–2. ERRORS IN SELECTION OF PATIENTS AND DEVICES

Poor proximal anatomy	Short or conical necks
	Extensive plaque in neck
	Marked angulation (>60 degrees)
	Large accessory renal arteries
Poor access anatomy	Occlusive disease with tortuosity
	Aneurysms extending to hypogastric arteries
Operator errors	Oversizing
	Undersizing
	Inaccurate placement

The issue of whether endografts should be largely limited to those patients at high risk for conventional repair or utilized for all anatomically suitable patients with AAA is unresolved. Most centers with active endovascular programs suggest open repair for young, healthy patients and EVAR for older, sicker patients. One of the major assumptions of the EVAR for large AAA (>5.5 cm in diameter) in patients unfit for open repair philosophy has been that these patients will quickly rupture and die if not treated. Conway and colleagues from Cardiff, Wales examined this hypothesis.[16] They prospectively maintained a registry of 106 patients with AAA >5.5 cm in diameter over a 10-year period that were turned down for elective repair. The mean age of the study population was 78.4 years. The actuarial survival rates for the 106 patients at 1, 2, and 3 years was 54%, 40%, and 17%. They concluded that the risk of dying from the AAA versus the risk of dying from a non-AAA cause was not different as long as the AAA was less than 6 cm. As the size of the AAA increased, an increased risk of death from rupture was noted. The largest cohort in this series was a group of 31 patients who refused operation. Twenty of these patients died, 12 secondary to their AAAs.

Selecting patients with poor anatomy or significant medical co-morbidities may not be the proper approach to EVAR as the former will result in more device-related problems and the latter a shorter life expectancy. Those patients who met the size criteria for operation in the UK Small Aneurysm Trial but were medically unfit had a mortality rate of 22% at 10 months and 50% at 2 years.[17] Buth et al. analyzed EUROSTAR data and found that patients unfit for open AAA repair had higher morbidity and mortality rates after EVAR when compared to patients with normal operative risk.[18] These older, sicker patients who underwent EVAR had a cumulative survival of 58% at 3 years suggesting limited advantage for repair in this high risk group of patients. They concluded that a patient must have a life expectancy of at least one year before any meaningful benefit in life expectancy after EVAR could be realized.

There is a natural temptation to lower the threshold for aneurysm repair with EVAR because of the reduced morbidity and mortality rates of the lesser procedure. Certainly EVAR is more readily accepted by patients. Mathematical models (Markov) have been created to examine whether the optimal diameter for elective aneurysm repair in average and high-risk patients should be different for the 2 treatment modalities.[19] Assumptions were made from published reports and were as follows: the annual rupture rates for infrarenal aortic aneurysms <4cm, 4.5 cm, 5.5 cm, and 6.5 cm were 0%, 1%, 11%, and 26% respectively; the mortality rates were 1% for EVAR and 3.5% for conventional repair (age 70 years); the immediate conversion rate from EVAR to open repair was 5% and was 1% per year thereafter. The benefit of EVAR increased with increasing patient age and disappeared with procedural mortality rates exceeding 3.5% and long-term endovascular grafts failure rates exceeding 6% per year. The benefits were small however and these authors concluded that lowering the threshold for EVAR was not justified except for patients >80 years in poor health where the data supported reducing the diameter threshold from 8.1 cm to 5.7 cm. The Aneurysm Detection and Management (ADAM) Veterans Affairs Cooperative Study Group recently published the results of its randomized trial.[20] There was no survival benefit for immediate operation in AAA <5.4 cm despite a low operative mortality rate of less than 3%. At this time there are no data that support lowering the threshold for AAA repair with EVAR and the ADAM data along with the UK Small Aneurysm Trial may actually raise the size threshold for AAA repair of any type.

ANATOMIC CONSIDERATIONS

Important anatomic factors that affect device selection include the diameter, length, shape, and angulation of the infrarenal neck, any involvement of the common iliac arteries with either aneurysmal or occlusive disease, occlusive disease or marked tortuosity of the ilio-femoral access vessels, or intrinsically small iliac arteries. It is critical that the device fit the patient's anatomy as opposed to making a patient fit a specific device. Anatomic factors are best evaluated with thin-cut (3 mm) CT scans. Reformatted spiral CT scans can be used to accurately measure lengths and angles that are more difficult to assess with standard imaging. These reformatted axial studies have drastically reduced the need for arteriography in the evaluation of a patient for EVAR. Magnetic resonance imaging can be utilized when patients have renal insufficiency and these datasets can be reformatted (Figure 16–1). IVUS is helpful for assessing access anatomy during the startup phase of a program but quickly becomes unnecessary as the operators gain experience.

Stable fixation is the key to long-term durability. The ability of a device to maintain its position over time is dependent on the balance between the displacement and the stabilizing forces. The displacement forces on the proximal attachment site are related to the diameter and curvature of the aorta. Increasing angulation of the proximal neck is associated with significant Type I endoleaks and migration. Stabilization factors include the radial force upon the proximal and distal attachment sites from stents, columnar support and penetrating components such as hooks and barbs. As the angulation increases, the attachment area must lengthen. A length of 15 mm is sufficient in

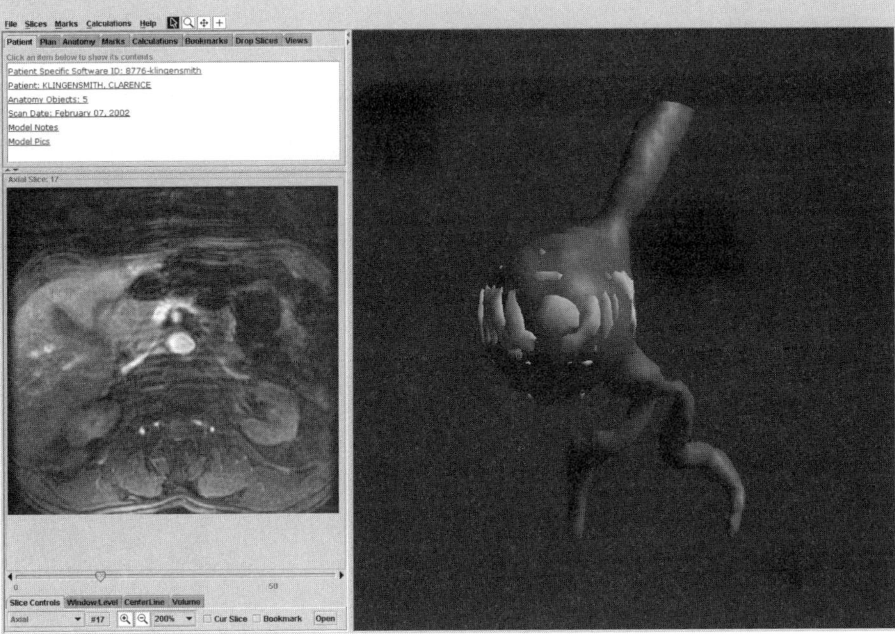

Figure 16–1. Measurement of diameters and lengths without angiography. The image shown here is from a magnetic resonance dataset in a patient with renal insufficiency. This has become our image of choice in the work-up of a patient for a possible endograft. This image was prepared by Medical Media Systems (MMS), 12 Commerce Ave., West Lebanon, NH 03784.

the absence of proximal angulation. Patients that fall in the 30 and 60 degree range are not anatomically ideal and should receive an endograft only when other options are even less desirable. Greenberg at al examined EVAR in 55 patients with short proximal necks (<15mm) using the Talent graft.[21] 13 of these patients had necks less than 10 mm. Endoleaks were more frequent in patients with larger aneurysms and were not correlated with the length of the proximal neck. Further validation and longer follow-up periods will be required, however, before EVAR for short necks can be recommended. An unexplained finding in this series was a striking increase in the proximal neck diameter of 0.9 mm over 30 days. These grafts were all oversized as a matter of policy and are designed with self-expanding stents. Data from Juan Parodi suggest that dilatation of the proximal neck does not happen to the same degree when balloon-expandable proximal attachments are used. He found that after 5 years that there was no dilatation of the proximal anastomoses in his original series of patients.[22]

Achieving a permanent seal at an attachment site is dependent upon the apposition of graft material to a segment of the normal vessel. Devices are designed to function in cylindrical vessels and may not achieve a satisfactory seal in a conical vessel. The CT image in Figure 16–2 shows a conical neck in a patient with an expanding aneurysm. This anatomic configuration is not ideal for EVAR. If a patient like this is too high risk for open repair and a Type I endoleak occurs, deploying a large balloon expandable stent may in the short term provide an adequate seal. This should be done with caution when there is disease involving the renal arteries. We stent significant renal artery ostial lesions prior to endograft deployment especially if a device with a supra-renal stent is utilized.

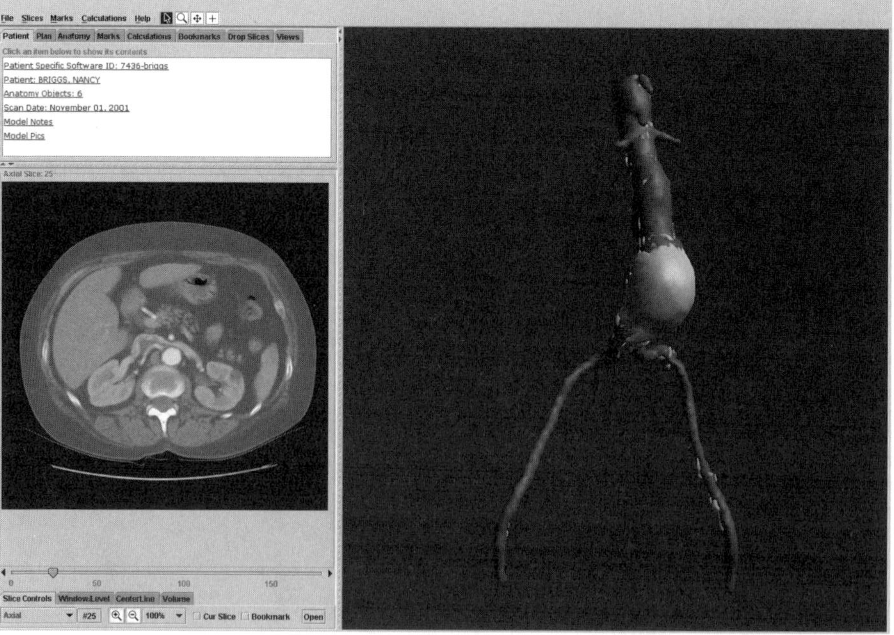

Figure 16–2. MMS image in an 82 year old man with an enlarging AAA and significant coronary artery disease. The conical shape of this neck makes this case a poor choice for EVAR but the medical risk and the enlarging AAA offset the anatomical consideration. If a Type I endoleak results, a large balloon-expandable stent can be used just below the renal arteries with a good chance of controlling the problem at least in the short-term.

Heavily calcified, narrow aortic bifurcations (Figure 16–3) may not provide sufficient room for a bifurcated graft and limb compression and graft thrombosis may occur. Alternatively, the contralateral limb may be difficult to deploy. For this reason, maintaining wire access to the sac is critical prior to cannulation of the contralateral iliac limb. Once both limbs have been deployed, the distal aorta can be dilated with angioplasty balloons in the iliac limbs. Modular, fully supported devices are easier to deploy in a narrow aortic bifurcation. Two limbs up to 16 mm each can fit into a 20 mm aorta depending on the degree of angulation. It should be noted that the long-body modular designs are not ideal in this setting and if for other reasons one must be used the body should be left shorter than usual. Unibody bifurcated devices are particularly difficult to manipulate when the aortic bifurcation is small and severely calcified. The availability of an aorto-uni-iliac device will be a useful tool in this setting.

The iliac arteries must be of sufficient diameter to allow access to the aneurysm yet still provide suitable deployment sites within the size ranges of the available devices. The combination of significant calcification and tortuosity is a relative contraindication to EVAR with the commercially approved devices. The distal attachment sites should not interfere with the existing internal iliac arteries and there should be a landing zone at least 2 cm in length. Iliac vessels greater than 20 mm can be excluded by deploying the device into the external iliac artery and occluding the ipsilateral hypogastric artery. This technique is not without risk. Review of our own experience with hypogastric embolization is not encouraging. We found that 39% of our patents had complications directly attributable to interruption of internal iliac artery flow. Buttock, thigh, and

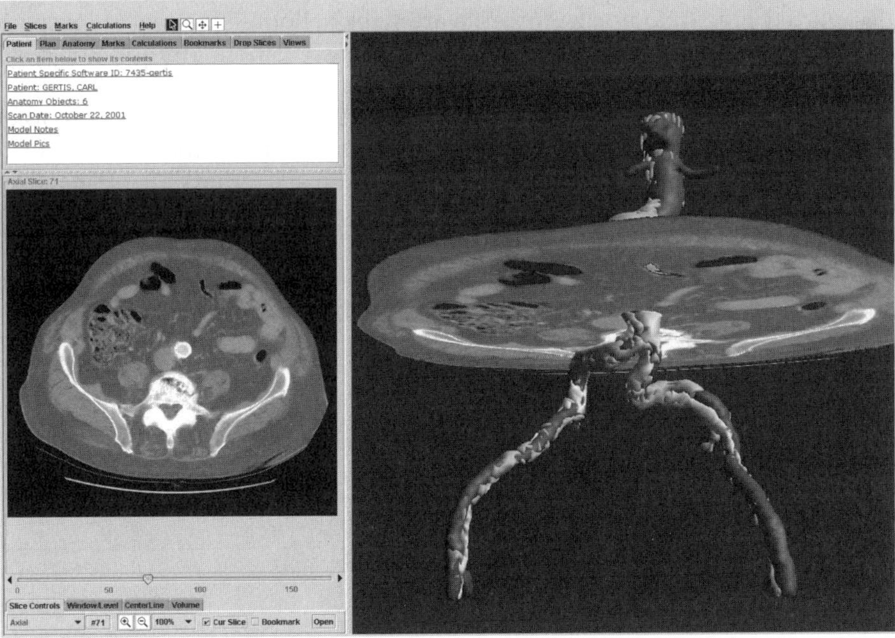

Figure 16–3. The narrow calcified aortic bifurcation can present problems with both difficult deployments and compression of the iliac limbs. Maintaining wire access to the sac is critical prior to cannulation of the contralateral iliac limb. Once both limbs have been deployed, the distal aorta can be dilated with angioplasty balloons in the iliac limbs. Two limbs up to 16 mm each can fit into a 20 mm aorta depending on the degree of angulation.

pelvic claudication or ischemia was the major morbidity and occurred in 30% of patients. Bilateral hypogastric occlusion should be avoided.[23] We now consider direct surgical reconstruction of iliac anatomy to preserve hypogastric artery flow and have performed this procedure in selected cases rather than sacrifice both hypogastric arteries. As the size of the aneurysm increases and the medical co-morbidities worsen, one may be justified in offering endovascular repair including those patients with anatomically less favorable situations provided that an experienced team is on hand to deal with any untoward events (Table 16–3). When only a single device is available, the likelihood of anatomic suitability falls to 20%.[24]

DESIGN CONSIDERATIONS

The relevant time span for an endograft is the patient's life expectancy. Pre-clinical bench testing that required over 40 million heart beats has not proved a sufficient stress as every one of the devices has exhibited structural failure after implantation. Product design must cope with segmental variations in the type and intensity of the stress based on a patient's anatomy. We now have the luxury of assessing the performance of a variety of device designs *in vivo*. Many of us were impressed early in our experience that tortuous vessels could be straightened and devices deployed. Altering the anatomy to fit a device may not be a good idea. Much important data not previously available will allow engineers to design devices that actually fit the anatomic variables of a given patient.

Many concepts have been developed and implemented almost on an *a priori* basis (Table 16–4). There are unibody and component devices. There are fully supported and unsupported grafts. Some attachments are with balloon-expandable stents, others are with self-expanding stents. Some stents are barbed, others are not. Some devices allow for partial deployment and movement prior to engagement, others do not. Some have longer common trunks than others. Some grafts are made of polyester, others are made of polytetrafluorethylene. Some stents are stainless steel, others are made of nitinol. Some stents are attached to the graft fabric by sutures, others are attached chemically. Some devices cross the renal arteries with uncovered stents, others do not. Some

TABLE 16–3. SUGGESTIONS FOR DEALING WITH ANATOMIC DIFFICULTIES

Anatomic factor	Suggestion	Preference
Short proximal neck	Suprarenal fixation	Zenith, Talent
Small Iliacs	Use smallest most flexible delivery system or create common iliac conduit	Excluder
Bilateral iliac artery Aneurysms	Do not sacrifice both internal iliac arteries. Create external to internal iliac bypass prn	None
Neck angulation	Do not use suprarenal fixation. Use most flexible graft. Be careful using AneuRx when removing delivery system	Ancure, Excluder
Iliac tortuosity	Depending on the level of calcification the vessels may straighten with stiff wire. Use most flexible delivery	Excluder, Zenith
Narrow aortic bifurcation	Be certain not to lose guidewire access to sac. Use kissing balloon dilatation once graft is deployed or use aorto-uniiliac system	Ancure Aorto-uniiliac system

TABLE 16–4. DEVICE CHARACTERISTICS

	Design	Fixation	Problems	Advantages
AneuRx[1] Main body 20–28mm; limbs 12–16 mm	Polyester, modular fully supported device with metal rings sutured to fabric	Radial force from self-expanding stents.	It may be difficult is disengage obturator and runners when proximal aorta is angulated	Simple deployment- Can use aortic extension to "bell-bottom" large iliac
Ancure[2] Main body up to 26 mm, iliac limbs to 13- no oversizing	Unibody, flexible non-supported polyester	Active fixation with balloon-expandable proximal stent with hooks that penetrate aorta.	Unsupported limbs may require stents. Complicated deployment.	Also configured as aorto-uniilac device. Can accommodate tortuous anatomy and contoured aortic necks.
Talent[3] Main body up to 32 mm with limbs up to 20 mm. Each graft is customized	Modular, fully supported polyester with suprarenal stent fixation	Self-expanding without hooks or barbs	Delivery system is prone to kinking in tortuous anatomy and unsheathing device can be problematic	Simple deployment, excellent customer service. Can accommodate large and short proximal neck
Excluder[4] Main body 20–28.5 mm; limbs taper from 16 mm anywhere to 10 mm	Exoskeleton of nitinol with PTFE graft material without sutures. Modular.	Self-expanding and fully supported. Can be configured as both cylinder and tapered graft.	Deployment less controlled than with devices that allow for some adjustments after upper stents released	Flexible delivery reduces chance of access vessel injury. Flexible, supported limbs likely to reduce incidence of occlusion.
Zenith[5] Main body size up to 30 mm and limbs up to 20 mm	Modular exoskeleton of stainless steel self-expanding stents with a barbed suprarenal stent.	Radial force and suprarenal barbs. Main body designed to terminate 15 mm from aortic bifurcation.	More difficult deployment sequence to master because of the need to recapture the cap holding the suprarenal stent.	Excellent quality delivery system in setting of access vessel tortuosity.

[1]Medtronic AVE
[2]Guidant Corp.
[3]Medtronic AVE
[4]W.L. Gore & Associates, Flagstaff, Arizona
[5]Cook, Bloomington, Indiana

of these design factors may ultimately prove superior others but at this time conclusions are conjectural and individual preferences are based on operator bias and device availability.

Modular systems offer flexibility in the size and length of the iliac attachments but have the disadvantage of component separation (Type III endoleak). Unibody constructs cannot develop Type III endoleaks and have a lower risk of distal attachment migration. The disadvantage of the unsupported unibody design is an increased risk of twisting and/or kinking during deployment and compression from stenotic iliac artery lesions. The pull-out force increases in a proportional relationship to the number of barbs and/or hooks and whether a balloon-expandable or a self-expanding stent is utilized. There does not appear to be any significant adverse effects of suprarenal fixation.[25] There is however a problem with suprarenal stent fixation when there is angulation of the suprarenal aorta. Opposing angulations can result in displacement of the sealing stent and a Type I endoleak. There are some preliminary data that suggest that Type II endoleaks are less frequent with devices whose main body is both long and supported as compared to shorter body configurations.[26] Another advantage of the long-bodied graft is the potential to straddle the aortic bifurcation, provide greater longitudinal support and therefore less of a tendency to migrate. Some of the characteristics of the approved and soon to be approved devices (probably) are listed in Table 16–2. I have included some of the issues related to each graft largely based upon my own bias. Each of these grafts appears to successfully and safely provide protection against AAA rupture.

CONCLUSIONS

The decision to recommend one type of aneurysm repair over another varies from institution to institution and is governed by a number of factors including anatomy, medical co-morbidity, operator skills, and access to the devices. Since most patients, if given a choice, would opt for the less invasive procedure, the fundamental question each of us must ask is how to select those most suitable for EVAR given the limited long-term data available. There is compelling evidence that in properly selected patients, EVAR appears to be comparable to conventional repair using rupture and death as endpoints within the first year following deployment. One only has to discharge a patient with a symptomatic AAA on home oxygen on the second post-operative day to appreciate the giant step forward endoluminal therapy has made.

Despite the concerns about long-term efficacy, it is now appropriate to offer EVAR to anatomically suitable patients with significant medical co-morbidities and/or hostile abdomens. A truly informed opinion however requires each of us to examine our results with both techniques in both healthy and compromised patients. The decision to liberalize the usage of EVAR should only occur when results are superior to the other choices including observation.

The choice of devices is limited now but will expand. That will allow the surgeon to fit the device to the patient and not vice versa. Some patients will require suprarenal fixation, some will not. Others will require small insertion sheaths, others will not. Some patients will require supported iliac limbs, others will not. I anticipate that adjusting to the patient's anatomy will lessen the stresses on the devices and improve long-term performance.

REFERENCES

1. Ohki T, Veith FJ, Lipsitz R, et al. Increasing incidence of mid- and long-term complications after endovascular graft repair of AAAs: A word of caution based on an 8-year experience with 212 cases. *Ann Surg.* 2001.
2. Collins J, Murie JA. Endovascular treatment of abdominal aortic aneurysms:a failed experiment. *Brit J Surg.* 2001;88:1281–1282.
3. May J, White GH, Yu W, et al. Concurrent comparison of endoluminal versus open repair in the treatment of abdominal aortic aneurysms: Analysis of 303 patients by life table method. *J Vasc Surg.* 1998;27:213–221.
4. The UK Small Aneurysm Trial: design, methods, and progress. The UK Small Aneurysm Trial participants. *Eur J Vasc Endovasc Surg.* 1995;9:42–48.
5. Hollier LH, Taylor LM Jr, Ochsner J. Recommended indications for operative treatment of abdominal aortic aneurysms. *J Vasc Surg.* 1992;15:1046–1056.

6. Dardik A, Lin JW, Gordon TA, Williams M, Perler B. Results of elective abdominal aortic aneurysm repair in the 1990s: a population based alaysis of 2335 cases. *J Vasc Surg.* 1999;30: 985–995.

7. Huber TS, Wang J, Derrow DE, et al. Experience in the United States with intact abdominal aortic aneurysm repair. *J Vasc Surg.* 2001;33:304–311.

8. Hallett JW Jr, Marshall DM, Petterson TM, et al. Graft-related complications after abdominal aortic aneurysm repair: Reassurance from a 36 year population-based experience. *J Vasc Surg.* 1997;25:277.

9. Steyerberg EW, Kievit J, Otterloo JC, et al. Perioperative mortality of elective abdominal aortic aneurysm: A clinical prediction rule based on literature and individual patient data. *Archives Int Med.* 1995;155:1998–2004.

10. Hallett JW Jr. What are the realistic expectations for standard open abdominal anrtic aneurysm repair in contemporary practice: The gold standard. *Vascular Surgery 2002: New approaches to old problems.* Department of Continuing Education, Harvard Medical School, Boston Mass May 9–11, 2002.

11. Zarins CK, White RA, Schwarten D, et al. AneuRx stent graft versus open surgical repair of abdominal aortic aneurysms: Multicenter prospective clinical trial. *J Vasc Surg.* 1999;29: 292–308.

12. Moore W, Kashyap V, Vescer C, et al. Abdominal aortic aneurysm: A 6-year comparison of endovascular versus transabdominal repair. *Ann Surg.* 1999;230:298–306.

13. Brewster DC, Geller SC, Kaufman JA, et al. Initial experience with endovascular aneurysm repair: Comparison of early results with conventional open repair. *J Vasc Surg.* 1998;27:992–1005.

14. Brewster DC. Do current results of endovascular AAA repair justify more widespread use? *Vascular Surgery 2002: New approaches to old problems.* Department of Continuing Education, Harvard Medical School, Boston, Mass May 9–11, 2002.

15. Sapirstein W, Chandeeysson P, Wentz C. The Food and Drug Administration approval of endovascular grafts for abdominal aortic aneurysm: An 18-month retrospective. *J Vasc Surg.* 2001;34:180–183.

16. Conway KP, Byrne J, Townsend M, Lane IF. Prognosis of patients turned down for conventional abdominal aortic aneurysm repair in the endovascular and sonographic era: Szilagyi revisited? *J Vasc Surg.* 2001;33:752–757.

17. The UK Small Aneurysm Trial P:articipants. Results for randomised controlled trial of early elective surgery or ultrasonic surveillance for small abdominal aortic aneurysms. *Lancet.* 1998, 352:1649–1660.

18. Buth J, van Marrewijk CJ, Harris P, et al. Outcome of endovascular abdominal aortic aneurysm repair in patients with conditions considered unfil for an open procedure: A report on the EUROSTAR experience. *J Vasc Surg.* 2002;35:211–221.

19. Finlayson S, Birkmeyer J, Fillinger M, Cronenwett J. Should endovascular surgery lower the threshold for repair of abdominal aortic aneurysms? *J Vasc Surg.* 1999;29:973–985.

20. Lederle FA, Wilson SE, Johnson GR, et al. Immediate repair compared with surveillance of small abdominal aortic aneurysms. *NEJM* 2002;346:1437–1444.

21. Greenberg R, Fairman R, Srivastava S, et al. Endovascular grafting in patients with short proximal necks: an analysis of short-term results. *Cardiovasc Surg.* 2000;8:350–354.

22. Personal communication. Dr. Juan Parodi, Buenos Aires, Argentina.

23. Leyden S, Sternbach Y, Green RM. Clinical implications of internal iliac artery embolization in endovascular repair of aortoiliac aneurysms. *Ann Vasc Surg.* 2001;15(5):539–43.

24. Treiman GS, Lawrence PF, Edwards WH, et al. An assessment of the current applicability of the EVT endovascular graft for treatment of patients with an infrarenal abdominal aortic aneurysm. *J Vasc Surg* 1999;30:68–75.

25. Greenberg RK, Lawrence-Brown M, Bhandari M, et al. An update of the Zenith endovascular graft for abdominal aortic aneurysms: initial implantation and mid-term follow-up data. *J Vasc Surg* 2001;33:S157–64.

26. Fairman RM, Velazquez OC, Carpenter JP, Baum RA. How are Type II endoleaks related to graft design. Presented at the VEITH Symposium, New York City, November 2001.

17

Will Endovascular Aneurysm Repair Survive the Test of Time?

David C. Brewster, MD

Standard operative repair of abdominal aortic aneurysm (AAA), with the goal of preventing aneurysm rupture and thereby potentially prolonging patient survival, is well documented as a very effective and durable method of treatment which can be performed with highly acceptable morbidity and mortality rates in many experienced centers. Nonetheless, the risk of operation may be considerably higher (5–10% mortality) in numerous population-based reports, and high-risk patients are often denied surgical repair due to presumed hazards of the procedure. Convalescence commonly requires a prolonged period of many months, and some older or frail patients never quite regain their preoperative baseline status. In addition, standard repair represents a significant expense. Hence, the possibility that a less invasive method of treatment might reduce risks, provide much quicker patient recovery and other patient benefits, and possibly achieve cost savings by reduced duration of stay and decrease use of hospital resources has tremendous appeal to patients and physicians alike, and has generated considerable enthusiasm in the development and use of such devices.

Endoluminal repair of an AAA is achieved by exclusion of the aneurysm from the circulation by means of a prosthetic graft inserted from a remote site, guided to the desired location intraluminally under radiologic control, and then secured there by an expandable stent attachment system. The development and application of this method of AAA repair is a logical growth of the intense interest in minimally-invasive treatment modalities in general, the tremendous growth in balloon angioplasty, stenting, and other catheter-based interventions, and ever increasing constraints on costs and reimbursement.

Since its initial clinical description by Parodi and associates in 1991, endovascular AAA repair has been eagerly accepted and utilized with rapidly increasing frequency in a growing number of centers within recent years. In September 1999, 2 devices were granted FDA approval, and several additional endografts have completed clinical trials and will likely become available for commercial distribution within the near future.

Some advocates of endoluminal AAA repair have proposed more widespread use of the technique, suggesting that it should be regarded as the preferred therapy of choice for all AAA patients with suitable anatomy. In addition, some have suggested the possible advantages of endograft treatment of "small" AAA at an earlier stage as a possible strategy to reduce the incidence of AAA rupture. However, while the feasibility and early efficacy of this method of repair have been clearly demonstrated, uncertainty remains regarding its long-term effectiveness and proper role in the management of patients with AAA. Dilemmas in this regard have been highlighted recently by an FDA alert which has been widely circulated, expressing their concerns about reports of device problems and AAA ruptures after endograft repair. In particular, considerable debate continues in regard to whether or not younger, good-risk patients should undergo endoluminal repair, or if they are instead better served by conventional open surgical repair.

Early Results

Widespread experience reported in many clinical trials and published series have documented that endovascular AAA repair can be performed safely in almost all patients with suitable anatomy.[1–7] Technical implant success is now 98–99% in most experienced centers with current second-generation devices and with the now better-defined patient selection. Although estimates vary, about 50–60% of patients with infrarenal AAA have suitable anatomy for consideration of endograft repair.

Because of the dramatically less invasive nature of endoluminal repair, morbidity and mortality are less than with conventional surgical repair. In addition, clear-cut benefits in terms of diminished blood loss and transfusion requirements, shorter procedure times, decreased ICU utilization, and dramatically reduced hospital duration of stay have been well documented. Recovery time is also reduced, occurring usually within 1–2 weeks in contrast to the 2–3 months commonly required for open operation.[2,7]

Midterm Results

While no true long-term follow-up data are yet available, endoluminal repair has been performed for 6–8 years in many centers worldwide. Thus fairly extensive and reliable outcome data for mid-term follow-up periods are becoming available.[8–11] One must realize, however, that this may be somewhat misleading as these "long-term" data tend to emphasize early experience with first-generation devices.

In aggregate, midterm experience with endoluminal AAA repair remains generally favorable. As compared to the known natural history of AAA in the 5–6 cm range (11% *annual* rupture risk, 10% expansion *per year*),[12] successful endograft implantation has prevented rupture in 98–99% of patients and prevented AAA growth (or achieved actual AAA shrinkage) in 85–90% of patients.

Nonetheless, accumulating midterm experience has documented several potential problem areas, thereby emphasizing the debate as to whether endoluminal repair is less reliable and durable than conventional open operation.[9,13] In other words, will endovascular repair survive the test of time? This question, in turn, impacts on the issue of whether or not use of endovascular AAA repair should be more widespread and if it is appropriate to recommend it to younger, good-risk patients who are otherwise fit candidates for standard open graft repair.

AREAS OF CONCERN

Endoleak

Failure to totally exclude the AAA from continued perfusion and pressurization, as defined by "endoleak" observed on post-implant surveillance computed tomography, remains a potential shortcoming of endoluminal repair. Although incidences of endoleak vary appreciably from series to series, the incidence of early endoleak at discharge after endograft implantation is in the range of 20–30%.[14] While the majority of these are Type II branch leaks generally felt to be of less clinical significance, and recognizing that over one-half of early leaks will seal spontaneously within several months of ongoing follow-up, nonetheless endoleaks may persist in 10–15% of patients. In addition, late secondary endoleak may develop in another 5–10% of patients.[15]

While the overall impact and significance of endoleaks is a complex issue, several series have demonstrated that they are associated with the risk of continued AAA expansion and even potential rupture in a small percentage of patients.[16]

Device Failures

As duration of follow-up extends to longer time intervals, the observed incidence of structural device failures is becoming increasingly apparent.[17] These can represent breakage of metallic stent components or hooks, erosion of the graft wall with actual holes, junctional separation of modular components, late endoleaks due to graft migration at proximal or distal attachment sites, or similar problems.

It is also being recognized that mechanical stresses secondary to morphologic changes in the AAA sac over time may be extreme and lead to deformation of the indwelling endograft with resultant graft failure or endoleak by a variety of end-stage mechanisms.[18] I have termed this the "paradox of success," that is, problems occurring due to the very goal of a successful procedure: AAA sac exclusion and shrinkage.

Re-Interventions

Due to various problems arising during later follow-up intervals, re-interventions of one sort or another have been required in 10–30% of patients in most series.[19] This re-intervention rate appears to be a cumulative incidence, steadily increasing as follow-up intervals extend to longer time frames. In the large Eurostar registry, the incidence is approximately 10% per year, and within 4 years, one-third of Eurostar patients have undergone some form of secondary intervention. While many re-intervention procedures can be successfully performed with various catheter-based interventions, this is still a marked contrast to the infrequent need for reoperation or other re-intervention following standard open operative repair.

Late Conversions

A more major, clinically significant re-intervention is the need for endograft explant and conversion to standard open graft implantation. Such procedures are usually necessary for various late problems including persistent endoleak with continued AAA expansion, AAA enlargement despite no demonstrable endoleak ("endotension"), graft migration (with or without endoleak), device failure (holes, kinks, stent fractures, limb occlusions, etc.), endograft infection, and the most serious late problem: AAA rupture after endoluminal repair.

Many series, including the Eurostar registry experience, indicate an annual conversion rate risk of approximately 1–2% per year.[20] Because late conversions are often technically difficult and more extensive procedures than primary open operation, morbidity and mortality are greater, with mortality rates of 10–20% in several reports.[21]

AAA Rupture

The ultimate failure after endoluminal repair is the occurrence of rupture despite a seemingly technically successful endovascular repair. While infrequent, this is not a negligible risk, with approximately a 1% cumulative risk of rupture per year as evidenced by AneuRx experience, Eurostar data, and other reports in the literature.[16,19,21–23] Type I or III endoleaks appear to be a common feature of post endograft ruptures, due to poor initial patient selection, or later device migration, junctional component separation, or a variety of other failure modes.[23]

Cost-Effectiveness

Cost-consciousness is an important topic. Due to its significantly reduced ICU utilization and shortened hospital stay, endoluminal repair at first glance seems a cost-saving approach. However, use of preoperative imaging studies is often more extensive than for standard operative repair, and the device itself is quite expensive. Further, the continued need for careful follow-up and ongoing surveillance by computed tomography and other investigations to ensure durable AAA exclusion adds to the overall procedure costs. These and related issues require analysis. However, it seems clear that, at present, endovascular repair is more costly than standard operation, with any cost-savings more than offset by extremely high costs of the devices.[24,25] Cost differentials may become more disparate if more extensive late radiographic follow-up surveillance becomes necessary, as seems likely as more late follow-up problems are recognized. Given current economic pressures facing medicine today, such cost issues may make widespread acceptance of AAA endograft repair unlikely.

OVERVIEW

Endoluminal AAA repair has clearly been a major advance of particular benefit to elderly, high-risk patients. In addition to increased morbidity and mortality, a significant number of these patients may never completely regain their functional status after open surgical AAA repair.[26] In such patients who were previously denied AAA repair, endograft repair seems clearly the procedure of choice if they have appropriate anatomy. However, it should be recognized that the actual definition of "high-risk" is open to some debate and has not been well defined in the literature.

In addition, the less invasive nature of the procedure seems particularly well suited and advantageous in AAA patients with a "hostile abdomen" due to a variety of factors such as multiple prior operations, stomas of varying types and location, etc.[27] Finally, endoluminal repair may be beneficial in the management of AAA patients with other unusual, technically challenging problems such as para-anastomotic pseudoaneurysms complicating previous aortic graft procedures, AAA in the presence of a horseshoe kidney, or in the patients with prior renal transplants.

Because of concerns related to durability of the devices and long-term reliability of the repair, in my opinion more widespread use of endografts to repair small (<4.5–5.0 cm) AAA cannot, at least at this time, be supported. Similarly, because endoleak, graft migration, and other failure modes of endoluminal repair are more frequent in patients with adverse anatomy, this procedure should not be utilized over aggressively in patients who do not have well defined, appropriate aneurysmal anatomic features. This is particularly true in very high-risk patients, as the need for conversion in these circumstances is likely to be associated with excessive morbidity and mortality. One cannot over-emphasize the importance of proper and appropriate patient selection.

Whether or not the procedure should be recommended to younger, good-risk patients remains unclear.[28] Given current technology, the increasing evidence of problems related to device durability, and the not insignificant incidence of persistent endoleak and its potential implications for continued AAA rupture risk, standard open repair still seems best for such patients. It is mandatory, in my opinion, that vascular surgeons properly inform patients of options, risks, potential benefits, and shortcomings of both open and endoluminal repair, so that they may make a truly informed decision. This decision most often represents a trade off: less certainty of repair and reduced durability in return for less invasive therapy with quicker recovery and reduced morbidity and mortality. In our own 7-year experience with endoluminal repair of 362 primary infrarenal AAA, clinical failures (procedural death, early or late conversion, post implant rupture, or AAA sac growth >5 mm despite endovascular treatment) was noted in 8.3% of patients, and reinterventions required in 10.7%. These results suggested to us that endovascular repair provides good results and many benefits for most properly selected patients, but is not as durable as standard open repair.[29]

Even when appropriately informed, many patients may still opt for less invasive repair. Patient interest and demand for less-invasive treatment, as well as societal pressures propelling quicker, more simplified and less costly procedures will surely accelerate. Recognition of such forces serves to re-emphasize the need for continued scientific scrutiny and evaluation of endograft repair. In this regard, the potential value of a central registry of these devices rather than unrestricted distribution and usage without appropriate accumulation of outcome data is obvious.

In conclusion, it must be recognized that current opinions and concerns regarding the question of whether endovascular AAA repair will stand the test of time may well be altered by future advances in technology. It is clear that many series to date are dominated by outcome results of early first-generation endografts.[30] Third and fourth generation devices will likely overcome many prior limitations and complications, although this premise remains to be established by further study.

REFERENCES

1. Blum U, Voshage G, Lammer J, et al. Endoluminal stent-grafts for infrarenal abdominal aortic aneurysm. *N Engl J Med.* 1997;336:13–20.
2. Brewster DC, Geller SC, Kaufman JA, et al. Initial experience with endovascular aneurysm repair: Comparison of early results with conventional open repair. *J Vasc Surg.* 1998;27:992–1005.

3. May J, White GH, Yu W, et al. Concurrent comparison of endoluminal versus open repair in the treatment of abdominal aortic aneurysms: Analysis of 303 patients by Life-table method. *J Vasc Surg.*1998;27:213–221.

4. Moore W, Kashyap V, Vescer C, et al. Abdominal aortic aneurysm: A 6-year comparison of endovascular versus transabdominal repair. *Ann Surg.* 1999;230:298–306.

5. Zarins CK, White RA, Schwarten D, et al. AneuRx stent graft versus open surgical repair of abdominal aortic aneurysms: Multicenter prospective clinical trial. *J Vasc Surg.* 1999;29:292–308

6. Moore WS, Brewster DC, Bernhard VM, for the EVT/Guidant Investigators. Aorto-uni-iliac endograft for complex aortoiliac aneurysms compared with tube/bifurcation endografts: Results of the EVT/Guidant trials. *J Vasc Surg.* 2001;33:S11–20.

7. Matsumura JS, Brewster DC, Makaroun MS, et al., for the Excluder Bifurcated Endoprosthesis Investigators. A multicenter controlled clinical trial of open versus endovascular treatment of abdominal aortic aneurysms. Presented at the 56th Annual Meeting of the Society of Vascular Surgery, Boston, MA. *J Vasc Surg.* (in press).

8. Becquemin J, Bourriez A, D'Audiffret A, et al. Mid-term results of endovascular versus open repair for abdominal aortic aneurysm in patients anatomically suitable for endovascular repair. *Eur J Vasc Endovasc Surg.* 2000;19:656–661.

9. Holzenbein TJ, Kretschner G, Thurnher S, et al. Mid-term durability of abdominal aortic aneurysm endograft repair: A word of caution. *J Vasc Surg.* 2001;33:S46–54.

10. Zarins CK, White RA, Moll FL, Crabtree T, Bloch DA, Hodgson KJ, et al. The AneuRx stent graft: Four-year results and worldwide experience 2000. *J Vasc Surg.* 2001;33:S135–145.

11. Bush RL, Lumsden AB, Dodson TF, et al. Mid-term results after endovascular repair of the abdominal aortic aneurysm. *J Vasc Surg.* 2001;33:S70–76.

12. Finlayson SRG, Birkmeyer JD, Fillinger MF, et al. Should endovascular surgery lower the threshold for repair of abdominal aortic aneurysms? *J Vasc Surg.* 1999;29:973–985.

13. Ohki T, Veith FJ, Shaw P, Lipsitz E, et al. Increasing incidence of midterm and long-term complications after endovascular graft repair of abdominal aortic aneurysms: A note of caution based on a 9-year experience. *Ann Surg.* 2001;234:323–335.

14. Schurink GW, Aarts NJ, van Bockel JH. Endoleak after stent-graft treatment of abdominal aortic aneurysm: A meta-analysis of clinical studies. *Br J Surg.* 1999;86:581–7.

15. Buth J, Laheij RJF, and Eurostar collaborators. Early complications and endoleaks after endovascular abdominal aortic aneurysm repair: Report of a multicenter study. *J Vasc Surg.* 2000;31:134–46.

16. Matsumura JS, Moore WS. Clinical consequences of periprosthetic leak after endovascular repair of abdominal aortic aneurysms. *J Vasc Surg.* 1998;27:606–613.

17. Beebe HG, Cronenwett JL, Katzen BT, et al. Results of an aortic endograft trial: Impact of device failure beyond 12 months. *J Vasc Surg.* 2001;33:S55–63.

18. Harris P, Brennan J, Martin J, et al. Longitudinal aneurysm shrinkage following endovascular aortic aneurysm repair: a source of intermediate and late complications. *J Endovasc Surg.* 1999;6:11–16.

19. Laheij R, Buth J, Harris P, Moll F, et al., on behalf of the Eurostar Collaborators. Need for secondary interventions after endovascular repair of abdominal aortic aneurysm: Intermediate-term follow-up results of a European Collaborative Registry (EUROSTAR). *Br J Surg.* 2000;87:1666–73.

20. Cuypers Ph, Buth J, Harris PL, et al. Realistic expectations for patients with stent-graft treatment of abdominal aortic aneurysm. Results of a European Multicentre Registry. *Eur J Vasc Endovasc Surg.* 1999;17:507–16.

21. Harris PL, Vallabhaneri SR, Desgranges P, et al. Incidence and risk factors of late rupture, conversion, and death after endovascular repair of infrarenal aortic aneurysms: The Eurostar experience. *J Vasc Surg.* 2000;32:739–49.

22. Zarins CK, White RA, Fogarty TJ. Aneurysm rupture after endovascular repair using the AneuRx stent graft. *J Vasc Surg.* 2000;31:960–970.

23. Bernhard VM, Mitchell RS, Matsumura JS, et al. Ruptured abdominal aortic aneurysm after endovascular repair. *J Vasc Surg.* 2002;35:1155–1162.

24. Clair DG, Gray B, O'Hara PJ, Ouriel K, et al. An evaluation of the costs to health care institutions of endovascular aortic aneurysm repair. *J Vasc Surg.* 2000;32:148–152.
25. Sternbergh WC 3rd, Money SR. Hospital cost of endovascular versus open repair of abdominal aortic aneurysms: a multicenter study. *J Vasc Surg.* 2000;31:237–244.
26. Williamson WK, Nicoloff AD, Taylor LM Jr, et al. Functional outcome after open repair of abdominal aortic aneurysm. *J Vasc Surg.* 2001; 33:913–20.
27. Chuter TAM, Reilly LM, Faruqi RM, et al. Endovascular aneurysm repair on high-risk patients. *J Vasc Surg.* 2000;31:122–33.
28. Brewster DC. Presidential address: What would you do if it was your father? Reflections on endovascular abdominal aortic aneurysm repair. *J Vasc Surg.* 2001;33:1139–47.
29. Dattilo JB, Brewster DC, Fan CM, et al. Clinical failures of endovascular abdominal aortic aneurysm repair: Incidence, causes and management.
30. May J, White GH, Waugh Ret al. Improved survival after endoluminal repair with second-generation prostheses compared with open repair in the treatment of abdominal aortic aneurysms: A 5-year concurrent comparison using life-table method. *J Vasc Surg.* 2001;33: S21–6.

18

Endovascular Approach to
Thoracic and
Thoracoabdominal Aneurysms

Nicholas J. Morrissey, MD and Larry H. Hollier, MD

INTRODUCTION

Thoracic and thoracoabdominal aneurysms generally affect elderly patients with significant comorbidities. As a result, open repair of these lesions continues to result in high morbidity and mortality rates in spite of numerous advances in operative and perioperative care. Since the introduction of endovascular stent graft (EVSG) repair of abdominal aortic aneurysms (AAA) by Parodi in 1991[1] there has been tremendous interest in the application of such techniques to all types of arterial pathology. Endovascular repair of AAA has become an accepted practice and numerous devices have been approved or are undergoing trials in the US. The development of endovascular techniques for thoracic and thoracoabdominal aneurysms (TAA) has proceeded more slowly. A number of obstacles to successful endografting of TAA must be overcome in order for this technology to be widely applicable. The relative infrequency of TAA when compared to AAA may also explain the slower pace of endovascular technology for these lesions. Until thoracic stent-grafts are fully developed, the best approach to TAA may involve a combined open and endovascular procedure.

EARLY EXPERIENCE

Numerous reports of endovascular repair of small descending thoracic aortic lesions using "home-made" devices have been published.[2-6] The earliest large series of endovascular repair of descending thoracic aneurysms was reported by Dake and colleagues in 1997.[7] They repaired descending thoracic aneurysms in 108 patients with a stent-graft. The device was "home-made" and consisted of self expanding "Z" stents covered with a woven Dacron graft. The device was delivered through a 27 French sheath. All patients were considered too high risk for open repair. This series revealed a number of important issues related to thoracic stent-grafting. The larger diameter, longer devices designed for thoracic placement require larger sheaths which can be difficult to pass through femoral and iliac vessels. Because of this, the use of larger more proximal vessels (common iliac, aorta) for device introduction was needed in 41 patients. There were 10 procedure related deaths. Four were due to device complications and 2 were due to stroke from wire manipulation in the arch. The other 6 were due to comorbidities. Four cases of paraplegia occurred after stent-graft deployment and 4 patients suffered stroke. There were 6 attachment site endoleaks. Overall, this series was encouraging since it demonstrated the safety and efficacy of endovascular techniques for TAA in high risk patients. Greenberg and colleagues reported their results in 25 patients with descending thoracic lesions treated with stent-grafts.[8] Once again, these were high-risk patients including a number with ruptured aneurysms. There were 5 perioperative deaths related to rupture and massive embolization. These authors suggested that shorter proximal and distal neck lengths predicted type I endoleaks, and paraplegia was associated with longer device length. Currently, trials of a number of commercially made devices are underway in the US (Figure 18–1).

HYBRID PROCEDURES

With proximal and distal neck challenges making most TAA and all thoracoabdominal aneurysms unacceptable for endovascular repair, one strategy is to perform combined open and endovascular procedures in an effort to minimize the insult to the patient. As devices with side branches are developed, the problem of dealing with major branches will be addressed. Until the technology is fully developed, combined procedures offer the most promising option for some patients.

The simplest hybrid procedure involves performing a subclavian to carotid transposition on the left through a supraclavicular incision. This allows the subclavian orifice to be covered with the device, thus lengthening the proximal aortic neck by as much as 15 mm (Figure 18–2). Such a maneuver allows TAA with short proximal necks to be treated with EVSG. We have performed this procedure in 6 patients and all have had successful EVSG of their thoracic lesion. If the aneurysm extends further

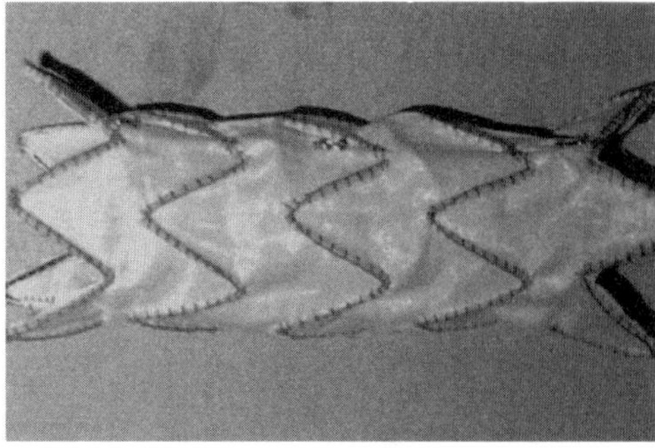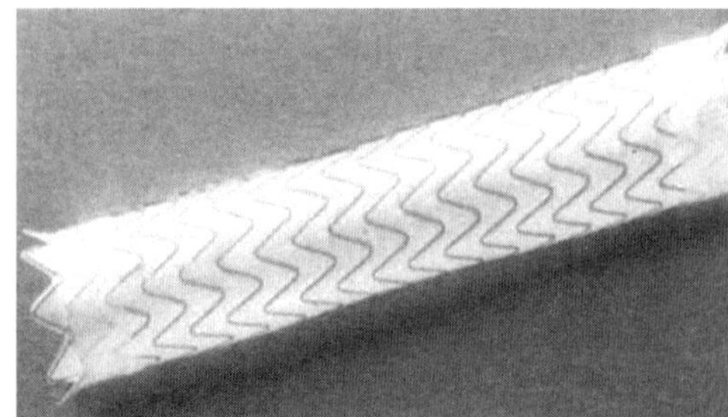

Figure 18–1. (A) Talent™ Thoracic stent graft. (World Medical/Medtronic, Sunrise Fl.) **(B)** Gore Excluder™ Thoracic stent-graft (W.L. Gore and Associates, Flagstaff, Arizona.)

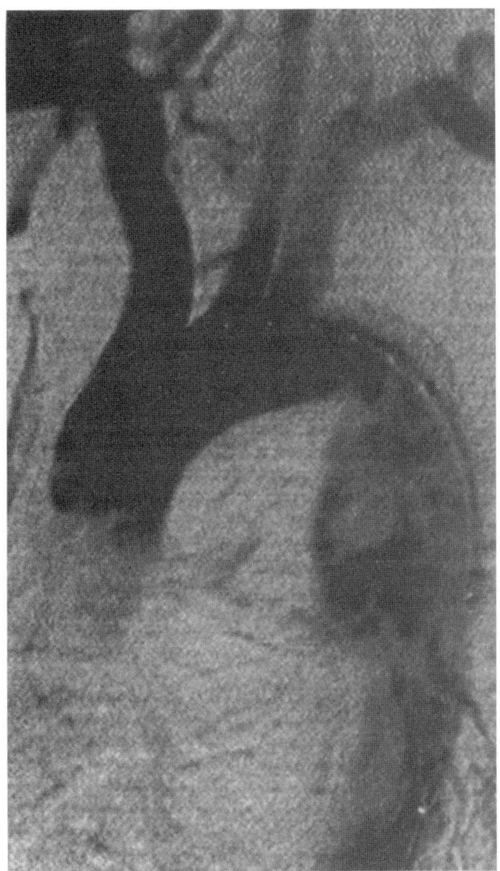 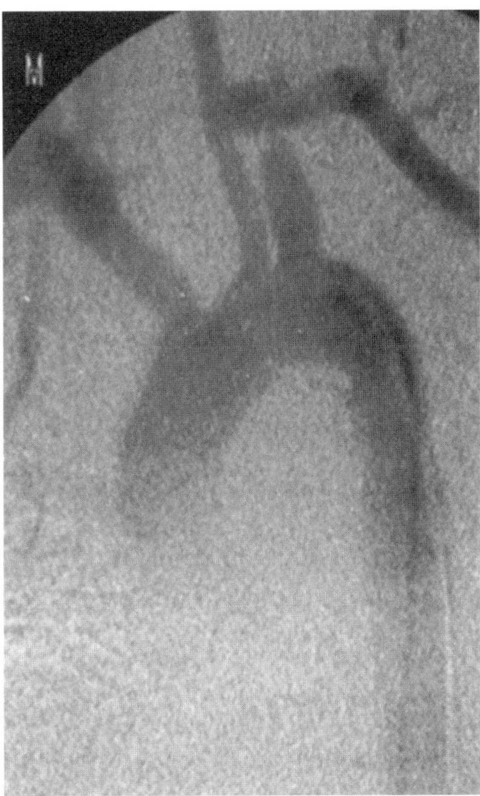

Figure 18–2 (A) and (B). Subclavian to carotid transposition performed via supraclavicular approach provides additional length of normal aorta for stent graft deployment while maintaining perfusion to the left subclavian

proximal along the arch, it is possible to revascularize 1 or all of the arch vessels with a graft taken off the ascending aorta. This can be done via median sternotomy and a stent graft can be placed across the aneurysm at the same time or at a later procedure (Figure 18–3A, 3B). In our experience, this has been done twice and both lesions were successfully treated. Importantly, a 2-stage open procedure requiring sternotomy and thoracotomy can be replaced with sternotomy and endovascular repair. Another option for aneurysms involving the arch and descending thoracic aorta is to perform the first stage of a standard elephant trunk repair via median sternotomy. Metallic clips are left on the end of the graft as it is placed into the descending aorta (Figure 18–4A, 4B). At a second stage, the distal end of the elephant trunk graft is accessed with a wire and an endovascular device is deployed in the descending aorta, excluding the lesion (Figure 18–5A, 5B). We have attempted this combined procedure in 6 patients. Both stages were completed in 5 patients. Two patients had persistent endoleaks and 1 of these died 8 months postoperatively secondary to aneurysm rupture. There were no procedure related deaths. While our initial experience is small, it continues to expand. Although the data are not yet powerful enough to demonstrate significant improvement in morbidity and mortality, we believe that minimizing the invasiveness of aneurysm repair in this population of patients should be beneficial.

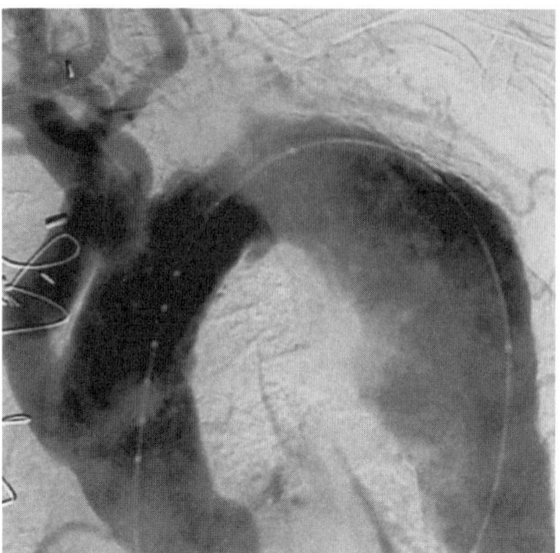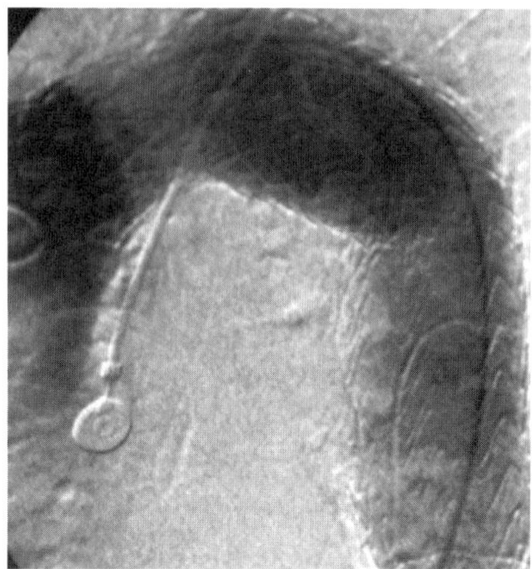

Figure 18–3. (A) Transposition of arch vessels to the ascending aorta. (B) Endovascular stent-graft placed in distal arch and descending aorta to exclude aneurysm.

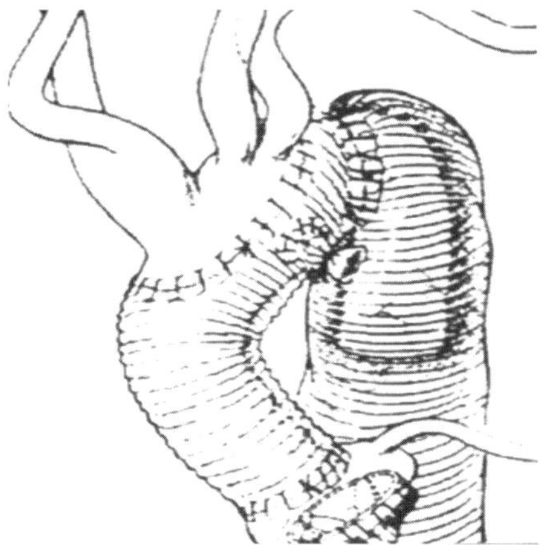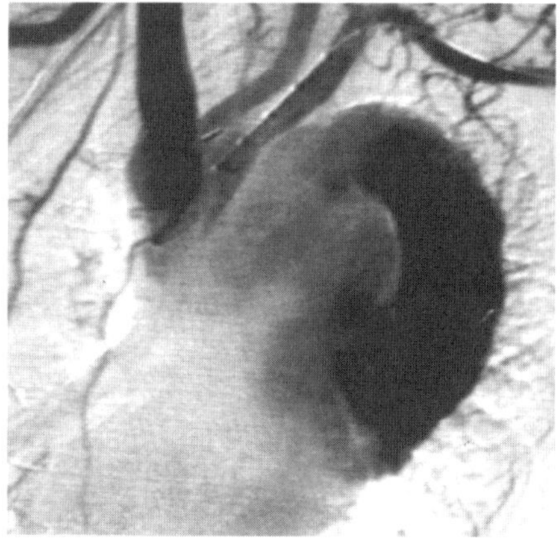

Figure 18–4. (A) Diagram and (B) angiogram of first stage elephant trunk repair for arch and descending thoracic aortic aneurysm. Note clips marking distal end of graft in (B). This allows identification of the cannulation site for later stent-graft placement.

For thoracoabdominal aneurysms involving part or all of the visceral segment branch vessel technology offers hope for complete endovascular approach to these lesions. Given the high morbidity and mortality associated with open repair of TAAA, endovascular repair may result in less morbidity and may provide a treatment option for patients too ill to undergo open repair. One report of a multi-branched device has been published by Chuter and colleagues.[9] The aneurysm was successfully excluded, however the patient developed paraplegia. The authors suggested that coverage of a long segment of normal aorta with graft may increase the risk of paraplegia. Until branch vessel devices are improved, the option of performing a combined open and endovascular procedure may result in lower morbidity for selected patients. It is possible to revascularize 1 or more of the visceral vessels (celiac, SMA, renal) via an open

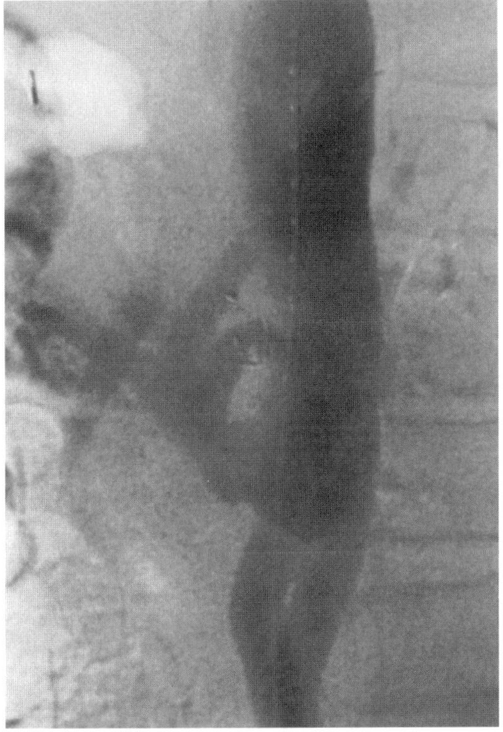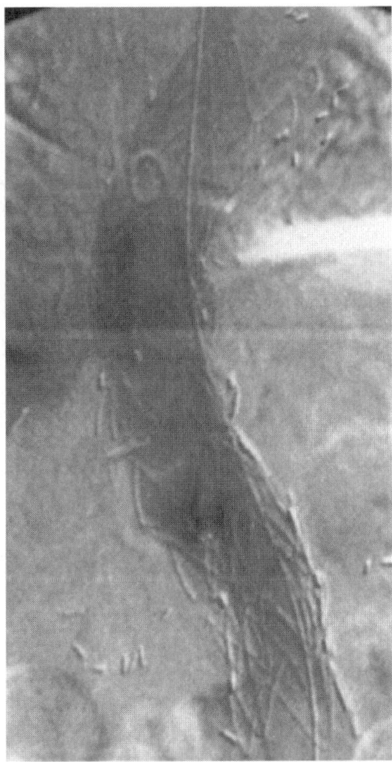

Figure 18–5. **(A)** Catheter access of elephant trunk graft. **(B)** Endovascular exclusion of descending thoracic aneurysm to complete repair without need for thoracotomy.

approach thus moving their origins off of the aneurysmal aorta. A stent graft can then be placed to cover the involved segment. While there is a significant physiological insult resulting from open revascularization, a thoracoabdominal incision can be avoided with this approach. We have attempted this in 4 cases and completed both stages in 3. On patient died from rupture of the aneurysm after unsuccessful attempt to pass the endovascular device (Figure 18–6).

PARAPLEGIA

The complication most frequently discussed in the TAAA literature is neurologic dysfunction related to spinal cord ischemia.[10,11] Early series of open repair reported paraplegia rates of 16%–30%. Factors associated with increased risk of paraplegia are length of involved aorta, duration of cross-clamp, and perioperative hypotension.[12] Although EVSG of TAA involves no aortic clamping, long segments of thoracic aorta can be covered without the option of intercostal artery reimplantation. Paraplegia after EVSG of TAAs occurs in 1%–5% of cases and may be related to previous infrarenal aortic replacement as well as the length of aorta covered by stent-graft.[7,8,13] We have had 3 cases of neurologic dysfunction in 53 endovascular TAA repairs.[13] In 2 of these cases, cerebrospinal fluid drainage instituted promptly successfully reversed the deficit. Interestingly, paraplegia occurred in a delayed fashion in 2 cases, with patients developing neurologic symptoms more than 6 weeks after endovascular TAA repair.

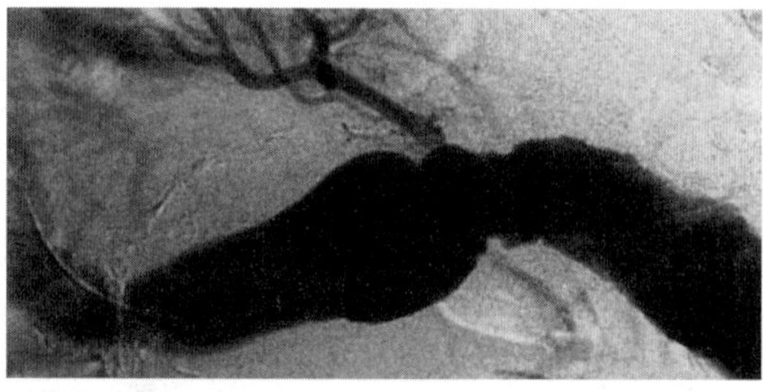

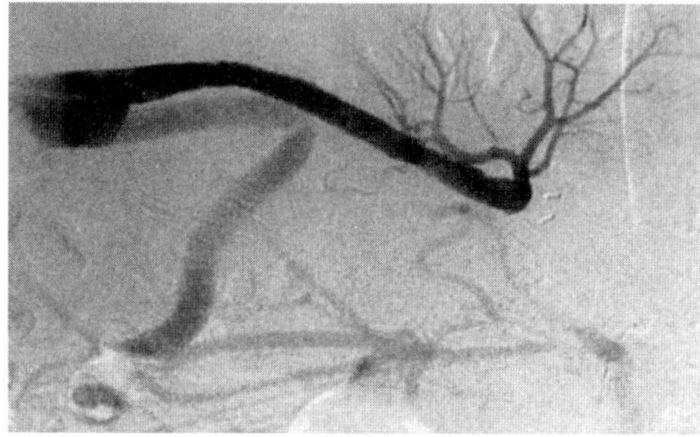

Figure 18–6. (A) Large type IV thoracoabdominal aortic aneurysm with left renal, celiac and SMA occlusion. **(B)** Revascularization of right renal artery and SMA with bifurcated graft. The patient died from aneurysm rupture following unsuccessful attempt at stent-graft placement.

Neurologic dysfunction appears to be associated with previous infrarenal aortic replacement. We have instituted a policy of draining cerebrospinal fluid perioperatively in TAA stent-graft patients who have had previous infrarenal aortic repair. The CSF drain is removed on day 2 or 3 if the patient remains neurologically intact.

It is unclear why a number of patients develop neurologic dysfunction so long after TAA repair, however it seems likely that the spinal cord circulation is delicately balanced following extensive coverage of intercostals and lumbar arteries. Small physiologic insults at remote times may result in sufficient decrease in spinal cord perfusion to result in infarction. Important collateral circulation may be provided by the vertebral, subclavian and hypogastric arteries. Immediate institution of CSF drainage may reverse the neurologic dysfunction in certain cases. The lack of mesenteric ischemia/reperfusion in endovascular TAA repair may also favor lower rates of paraplegia since this factor has been associated with higher rates of paraplegia.[14,15]

SUMMARY

Endovascular repair of thoracic and thoracoabdominal aneurysms presents a number of unique challenges. Device delivery sheaths may be too large for femoral or iliac access vessels and the angle of the aortic arch can make device passage and deployment difficult. As with AAA, short proximal and distal necks can prohibit simple endografting for many thoracic and thoracoabdominal lesions. The development of devices with branches to maintain flow to vital vessels while covering aneurysmal aorta should greatly improve thoracic stent graft techniques. In the interim, creative combination of open and endovascular techniques can allow treatment of complex lesions with less invasive procedures. The unique problem of paraplegia may actually be reduced in endovascular TAA repair, although large series data have not yet been reported. Importantly, replaced infrarenal aorta and longer length of covered normal aorta may be important predictors pf paraplegia risk.

REFERENCES

1. Parodi JC, Palmaz JC, Barone HD. Transfemoral intraluminal graft implantation for abdominal aortic aneurysms. *Ann Vasc Surg.* 1991;5:491–499.
2. Kato N, Dake MD, Miller DC, et al. Traumatic thoracic aortic aneurysm: treatment with endovascular stent-grafts. *Radiology.* 1997;205:657–662.
3. Lobato AC, Quick RC, Phillips B, et al. Immediate endovascular repair for descending thoracic aortic transection secondary to blunt trauma. *J Endovasc Ther.* 2000;7:16–20.
4. Desgranes P, Mialhe C, Cavillon A, et al. Endovascular repair of posttraumatic thoracic pseudoaneurysm with a stent-graft. *Am J Roentgenol.* 1997;169:1743–1745.
5. Deshpande A, Mossop P, Gurry J, et al. Treatment of traumatic false aneurysm of the thoracic aortawith endoluminal grafts. *J Endovasc Surg.* 1998;5:120–125.
6. Murgo S, Golzarian J. The use of endovascular stents in the treatment of penetrating ulcers of the thoracic aorta. *J Vasc Surg.* 2000;31:1078.
7. Dake MD, Miller DC, Mitchell RS, et al. The first generation of endovascular stent-grafts for patients with aneurysms of the descending thoracic aorta. *J Thorac Cardiovasc Surg.* 1998;116:689–703.
8. Greenberg R, Resch T, Nyman U, et al. Endovascular repair of descending thoracic aortic aneurysms: an early experience with intermediate term follow-up. *J Vasc Surg.* 2000;31: 147–156
9. Chuter TA, Gordon RL, Reilly LM, et al. An endovascular system for thoracoabdominal aneurysm repair. *J Endovasc Ther.* 2001;8:25–33.
10. Safi HJ, Miller CC. Spinal cord protection in descending thoracic and thoracoabdominal aortic repair. *Ann Thorac Surg.* 1999;67:1937–1939.
11. Safi HJ, Miller CC, Subramaniam MH, et al.Thoracic and thoracoabdominal aortic aneurysm repair using cardiopulmonary bypass, profound hypothermia and circulatory arrest via left side of the chest incision. *J Vasc Surg.* 1998;28:591–598.
12. Crawford ES, Crawford JL, Safi HJ, et al. Thoracoabdominal aortic aneurysms: preoperative and intraoperative factors determining immediate and long-term results of operations in 605 patients. *J Vasc Surg.* 1986;3:389–404.
13. Gravereaux EC,Faries PL,Burks JA, et al. Risk of spinal cord ischemia after endograft repair of thoracic aortic aneurysms. *J Vasc Surg.* 2001;34:997–1003.
14. Vermeulen EG, Blankensteijn JD, van Urk H. Is organ ischemia a determinant of outcome of operations for suprarenal aortic aneurysms. *Eur J Surg.* 1999;165:441–445.
15. Morrissey NJ, Kantonen I, Liu H, et al. Effect of mesenteric ischemia/reperfusion on spinal cord injury following transient aortic occlusion in a rabbit model. *J Endovasc Ther.* 9,Suppl II:44–50.

19

Technical Tips for Endovascular Abdominal Aortic Aneurysm Repair

S. William Stavropoulos, MD and
Jeffrey P. Carpenter, MD

Significant progress has been made in endovascular abdominal aortic aneurysm repair (EVAR) since the initial homemade devices were first deployed. Despite this, stent graft technology remains in flux as the materials and delivery platforms continue to undergo refinements. This chapter is intended to highlight some of the technical aspects of placing stent grafts. We will examine pre-procedure imaging, patient selection, arterial access, device placement, and post-deployment imaging. Most of what is covered in this chapter will apply to placement of any stent graft, however, when appropriate, differences between the specific devices will be highlighted.

PRE-PROCEDURE IMAGING AND PATIENT SELECTION

The most critical step in EVAR is patient selection and planning prior to stent graft placement. When being considered for EVAR, all patients should undergo computed tomography angiography (CTA) along with 3D-reformations of the CT data. The CTA yields images, which can be used to plan the entire procedure in most instances. This includes centerline measurements needed for length and diameter determination, even in patients with significant iliac and aortic tortuosity. It is now only the exceptional patient, who requires a traditional catheter based contrast angiogram prior to stent graft placement.[1] The unenhanced CT provides important information about the location and extent of calcification, which may preclude successful endograft placement or suggest the need for preliminary angioplasty to provide a suitable access route for the endograft.

The important pre-procedure diameter measurements are the diameter of the infrarenal aortic neck, aneurysm diameter, and diameter of the common and external iliac arteries. The important length measurements are proximal neck, the distance from the lowest renal artery to the aortic bifurcation, and the distance from the lowest renal artery to each iliac bifurcation. Because many stent grafts are self-expanding and rely on friction to create a proximal and distal seal, it is important to oversize the graft diameter by 10–20%. As experience from the Eurostar registry has shown, oversizing guards against the hazard of continued expansion of the aneurysm neck with the potential for loss of seal.[2] Conversely, oversizing a length measurement should not be done. A limb that is too short, can always be extended; however, if the device is too long the options are limited and a hypogastric artery may be inadvertently covered unnecessarily. Tube grafts should be avoided owing to the observation of continued dilatation of the distal aorta leading to late distal leakage with these devices.[3]

Strict attention should be given to the aortic bifurcation. A small or narrow bifurcation can make it difficult to place a bifurcated device. If stent graft limbs are placed in a narrow bifurcation this can lead to decreased flow and eventual thrombosis of a limb. If a stent graft is going to be placed in a patient with a narrow aortic bifurcation, an unsupported graft should be considered, because it may conform better to the narrow bifurcation. However, even unsupported grafts can have a limb occlude when placed in a patient with a narrow aortic bifurcation (Figure 19–1). Alternatively, an aortouniiliac graft with a femoral-femoral bypass can be placed in patients with narrow bifurcations. Bifurcated grafts should be placed into narrow bifurcations with "kissing" technique, deploying both limbs simultaneously. If in this circumstance limbs are deployed sequentially, access to the sac may be lost owing to complete coverage of the access route by the first limb and the operator may be unable to deploy the second limb.

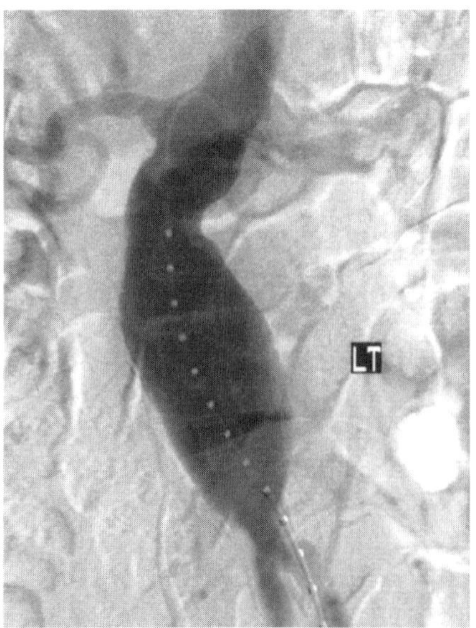

Figure 19–1A. Pre-procedure angiogram shows patient with a narrow aortic bifurcation

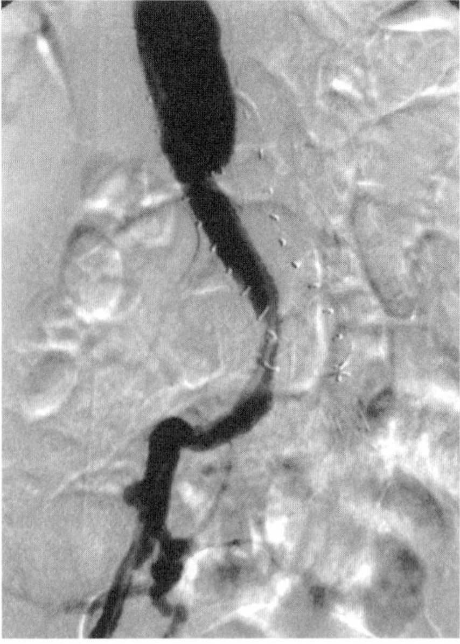

Figure 19–1B. Left limb of unsupported stent graft was occluded on post-procedure angiogram.

Once iliac diameter measurements are made, consideration should be given to iliac artery tortuosity. Stiff wires, such as the Luderquist wire (Cook Inc, Bloomington, IN) straighten all but the most tortuous iliac arteries. In patients with tortuous iliac arteries, the least tortuous artery should be used for delivery of the main body of the graft if possible. Calcified iliac arteries can also present problems during stent graft placement. A non-calcified artery can accommodate a larger device than a calcified artery. Calcified iliac arteries are less forgiving and can rupture with less force than a similar noncalcified artery. Predilatation of calcific lesions can be advantageous. In addition, liberal use of sheaths, which often can negotiate calcified vessels with greater ease than device delivery systems, should be employed. Calcified, tortuous iliac arteries can be especially problematic regardless of the actual diameter measurements of the iliac arteries.

AORTIC NECKS

It is important to characterize the infrarenal aortic neck before EVAR. Infrarenal necks can be divided into simple and complex. Complex proximal necks are those that are short, angulated, trapezoidal in shape, ulcerated, or calcified (Figure 19–2). Most grafts have a suggested minimum neck length requirement of 15 mm length. If the neck is shorter than this or there is concern about a proximal seal, a device with suprarenal fixation is beneficial. Early data shows no increase incidence of renal artery stenosis or occlusion with the suprarenal fixation devices.[4] Zenith (Cook, Inc), Talent (World Medical Manufacturing Corp, Sunrise FL), and Endologix (Endogix, Irvine, CA) are the stent

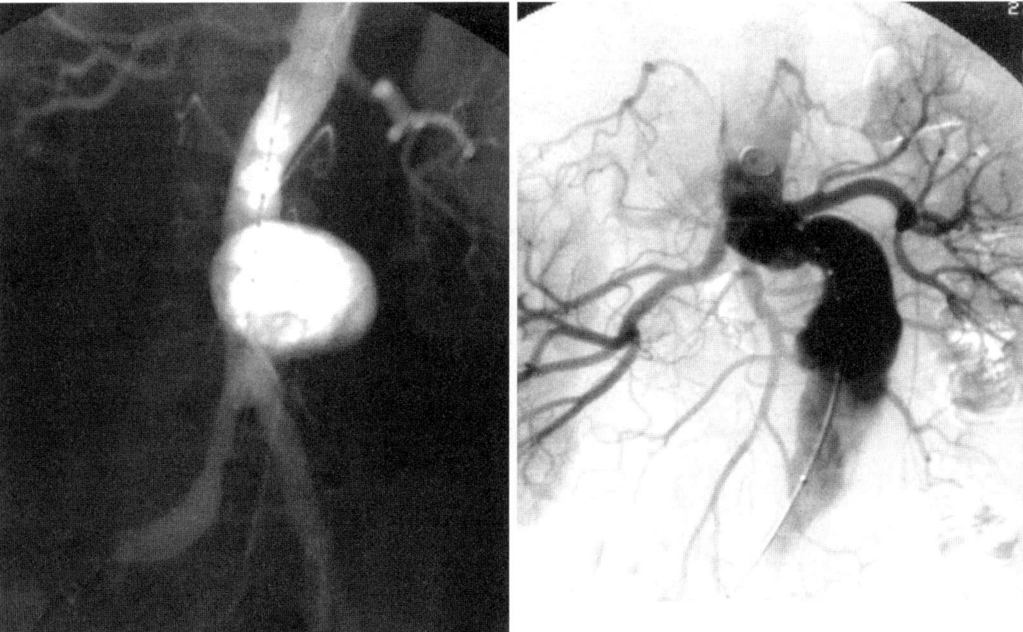

Figure 19–2A. Simple proximal neck seen on AP aortogram. The neck is long and not angled.

Figure 19–2B. Angled proximal neck seen on AP aortogram.

grafts currently available employing suprarenal fixation. Angled necks can also be problematic and the angle of the proximal aortic neck should be carefully evaluated. Patients with trapezoidal or conical shaped necks are also at increased risk for a type I endoleak and late device migration (Figure 19–3). Necks with these shapes may benefit from a suprarenal fixation scheme as well to provide a secure proximal attachment and anchoring point. Necks angled greater than 45 degrees are associated with an increased difficulty deploying the graft and obtaining a proximal seal.[5,6] Grafts with high radial force, which can straighten tortuous necks may be advantageous in this circumstance.

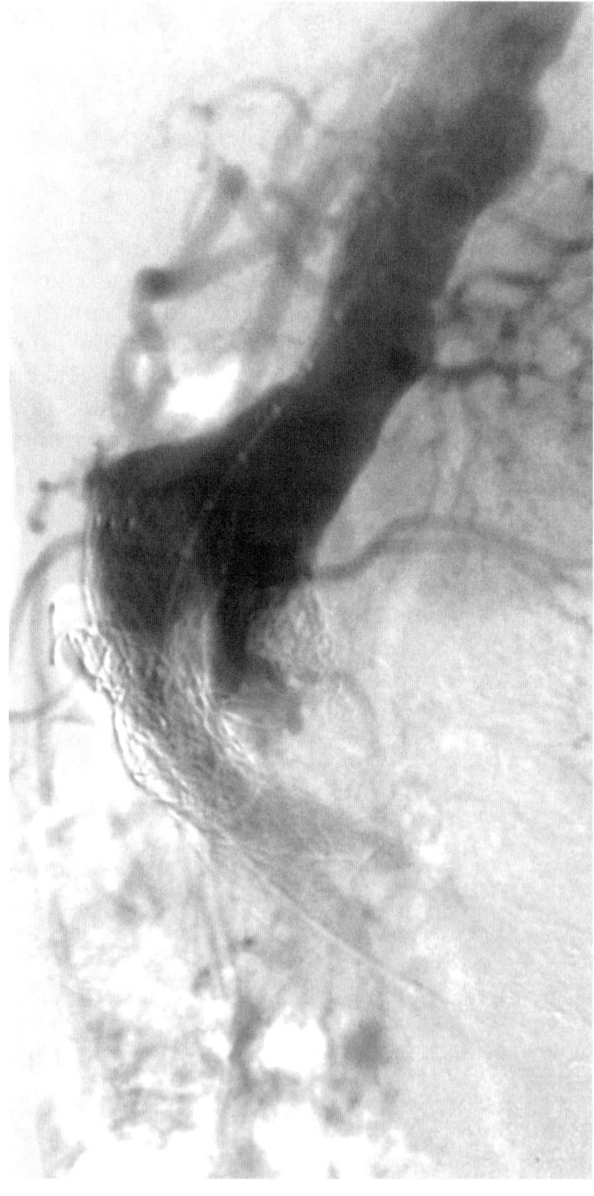

Figure 19–3. Lateral aortogram shows migration of stent graft into the sac in the patient with a trapezoidal proximal neck. This occurred 6 months after stent graft placement.

INTERNAL ILIAC ARTERY EMBOLIZATION

Embolization of the internal iliac artery is useful in the presence of a common iliac artery which is sufficiently aneurysmal such that it is necessary to attach the distal limb in the external iliac artery. Embolizing the internal iliac artery in these patients decreases the risk of a type II endoleak from retrograde blood flow of the internal iliac artery into the aneurysmal common iliac artery and aorta. Although some authors[7,8] advocate the safety of embolizing both internal iliac arteries, we do not advocate sacrifice of bilateral internal iliac arteries because of the risk of buttock claudication as well as bowel ischemia.[9-11] This is especially true in patients who have had prior bowel resection. In patients with bilateral common iliac artery aneurysms other options include placement of an aortouniiliac device or using an aortic cuff to flare the common iliac artery landing zone. This "bell-bottom" approach preserves hypogastric flow while accepting a large common iliac artery seal zone.[12]

Using proper technique for internal iliac artery embolization is essential to decrease the incidence of complications. It is very important to embolize above the internal iliac artery bifurcation. This decreases the risk of distal vessel embolization and subsequent ischemic complications. The most common endovascular approach to the internal iliac artery is a contralateral approach. However, in patients with abdominal aortic aneurysms approaching the internal iliac artery from a contralateral approach can be quite difficult and risky. Therefore, during EVAR we prefer to approach the internal iliac artery from an ipsilateral approach using a Simmons catheter (Cook, Inc). Coils are the embolic agent of choice. We have used detachable balloons, however, these are more expensive and less reliable.[13] Particulate agents such as gelfoam, PVA, or calibrated microspheres should never be used during embolization of internal iliac artery for this application as they place the patient at risk for colonic ischemia, claudication and even paraplegia as they lodge in the distal circulation.

PREOPERATIVE BRANCH VESSEL EMBOLIZATION

Because of the risk of type II endoleaks following EVAR, it has been proposed that the inferior mesenteric artery (IMA) and/or lumbar arteries be preoperatively embolized. We do not advocate doing this in the vast majority of cases because it is quite difficult, it is associated with significant risk to the patient, and is unnecessary. Searching for inferior mesenteric arteries or lumbar arteries in an aneurysmal aorta can be quite difficult and time consuming. In addition, because the sac is filled with thrombus, manipulating catheters and guidewires places the patient at significant risk for distal embolization of clot. Most importantly, however, embolization of the IMA or lumbar is really unnecessary because the majority of patients with patent inferior mesenteric arteries preoperatively do not develop an endoleak.[14,15] Predicting which patients would benefit from preoperative embolization is not possible at this time.

ACCESS

Obtaining and maintaining arterial access during EVAR is of critical importance. In all currently available devices, the body of the stent graft must be placed through a surgically exposed femoral artery. There are 3 devices—Ancure (Guidant Corp, Menlo

Park, CA), Excluder (W. L. Gore & Associates, Flagstaff, AZ), and Endologix—which have contralateral limbs with a diameter of 12 French or smaller. These can be placed using percutaneous access for the contralateral limbs. Another method to allow a percutaneous approach for the contralateral limb is by using a Perclose device.[16] The Perclose can be inserted before the contralateral limb is placed in the artery, allowing for percutaneous closure of the common femoral artery.

The inadequacy of access vessels remains a significant limitation for EVAR. In a recent evaluation of patients rejected for endovascular aneurysm repair it was noted that 47% of those patients where disqualified on the basis of poor access arteries due to occlusive disease, with an additional 10% not qualifying because of tortuosity of the iliac arteries.[17] Techniques to deal with these problems include straightening of arterial tortuosity with stiff guidewires, placing aortouniiliac stent grafts, and the use arterial conduits.

Most cases of iliac tortosisity can be managed by the placement of a stiff guidewire such as a Lunderquist wire. Prior to inserting this wire the floppy tip is reshaped to form a curve. This decreases the chance of the tip of the wire entering one of the branch vessels of the aorta (particularly the carotid) and facilitates its passage into the ascending portion of the thoracic aorta. In addition, we mark the position of the distal tip of the wire on the outer drape so that the position of the wire is known without having to repeatedly image over the chest.

More severe iliac tortuoisity can be managed by surgical techniques. Straightening of the arteries involves blunt dissection of the artery into the retroperitoneum from a femoral approach and pulling on the distal vessel to remove redundancy. This technique is effective in the external iliac artery but does not relieve tortuosity in the more immobile common iliac artery. This is also not very effective for calcified vessels. Aortouniiliac devices are useful in patients with one acceptable iliac artery and one very diseased artery. Arterial conduits are bypass grafts, which attach to arteries proximal to the diseased segment of the iliac artery. These conduits require full control of the vessel, usually the common iliac artery, similar to that which would be obtained for a surgical anastomosis. The device is introduced via the conduit into the patient's native circulation beyond the point of significant occlusive disease. The conduit may be abandoned or used as a bypass at the completion of the procedure.

An alternative technique, which we have employed in 18 patients is that of direct puncture of the aorta or iliac arteries with placement of a large sheath to facilitate delivery of a stent graft without the use of arterial conduits.[18] Hemostasis is achieved by placement of pursestring sutures at the cannulation site, similar to placement of aortic cannulas for cardiopulmonary bypass. This technique involves exposing the surface of the distal common iliac artery via a limited flank incision (Figure 19–4). The common iliac is visualized in the base of the exposure and is cannulated distal to the landing zone of the ipsilateral iliac limb. Circumferential control of the artery is unnecessary. A hemostatic sheath large enough to accommodate the stent graft is placed over a stiff wire using the tapered dilator of the sheath to enlarge the puncture site. Device delivery then proceeds through the hemostatic valve of the sheath. Sheath removal follows removal of the device delivery system. The tourniquets holding the purse string sutures are removed and the sutures are held securely as the sheath is pulled from the access artery. While an assistant holds the outer purse string, the surgeon is able to tie the inner purse string under tension free and hemostatic conditions. The outer purse string is then tied and the repair can be oversewn if necessary. Closure of the incision can proceed in the standard fashion.

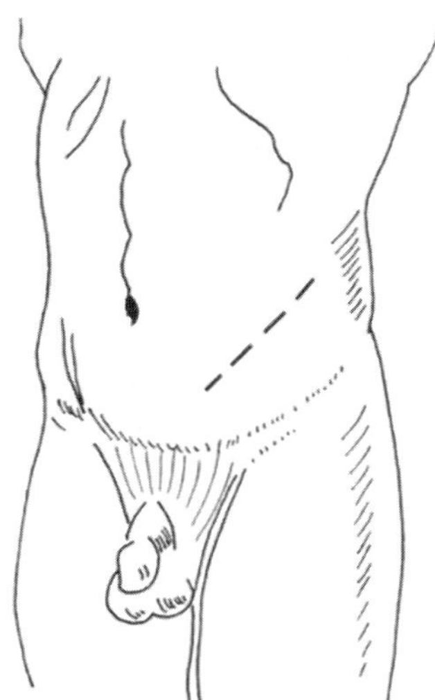

Figure 19–4A. Incision placement for retroperitoneal exposure of the common iliac artery or distal aorta. Only the surface of the access vessel needs to be exposed.

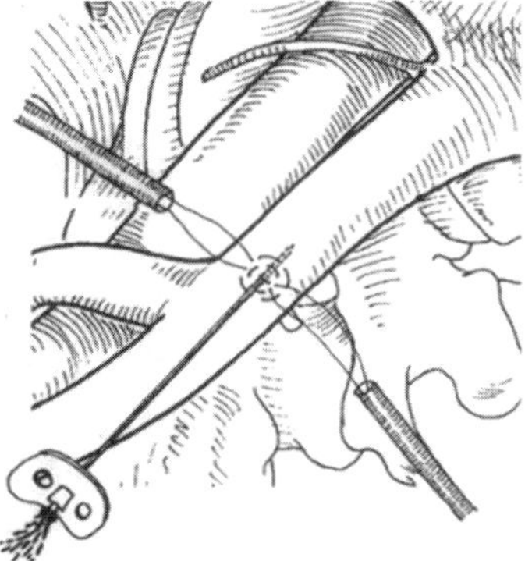

Figure 19–4B. Placement of a double purse-string suture in the access vessel. Each of the concentric purse-strings is constructed of 2-0 polypropylene sutures initiated on opposite sides of the vessel and held by rubber tourniquets. The artery is punctured in the center of the purse-string and a guidewire inserted and manipulated into the proximal aorta.

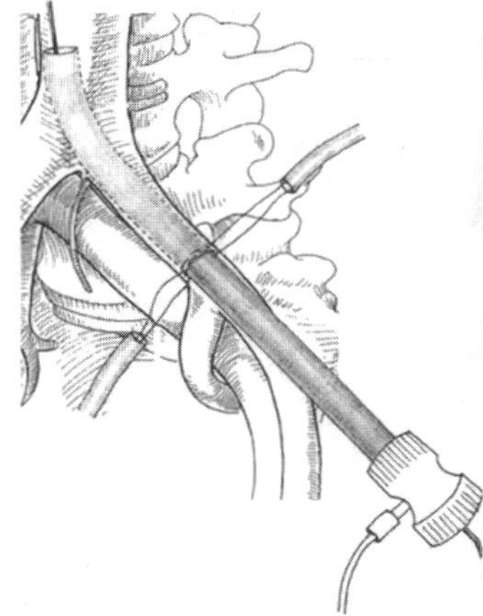

Figure 19–4C. Sheath placement. The sheath with its tapered dilator is placed over the stiff wire and fluoroscopically guided into the common iliac artery or aorta. The tourniquets can be used to control any puncture site bleeding around the sheath. All further exchanges occur through the sheath with its hemostatic valve. Sheath removal is accomplished with simultaneous traction on both purse-string sutures to relieve tension on the puncture and maintain hemostasis while the sutures are sequentially tied.

Figure 19–4. Direct sheath placement into the aorta or iliac arteries to facilitate EVAR.

UPPER EXTREMITY ACCESS

Although upper extremity arterial access is not routinely needed, it is important to have the left arm accessible for the rare case in which access to the left brachial artery is needed. guide wires placed from the arm can be snared from the femoral approach to obtain through and through brachio-femoral access.[19] This can be helpful if there is significant resistance to placing the body of stent graft in the abdominal aorta due to occlusive disease or tortuosity. If through and through wire access is obtained, measures to avoid damage to the left axillary and subclavian arteries must be taken. These arteries should be protected with a catheter over the wire to distribute the force of traction on the wire transmitted to the arterial wall. Excessive downward force on the wire can damage the vessel, even if it is protected with a catheter.

DEVICE PLACEMENT

Imaging during EVAR is a critical issue. Although an endovascular suite with operating room anesthesia and sterility and a ceiling-mounted C-arm is ideal, adequate imaging for EVAR can be obtained using a portable C-arm. This C-arm needs to be capable of doing digital subtraction angiography and road mapping. Other necessary equipment includes a power injector and a fluoroscopic table without seams, allowing head to toe imaging. Hand injections during stent graft placement are not adequate. Some surgeons advocate the placement of catheters in renal arteries as a way to accurately determine a level of the renal arties, as well as, to decrease the amount of contrast used during the procedure. In our experience the use of a road map shows the level of the renal arteries adequately. In addition, using road maps also decreases the amount of contrast during the procedure as well as the dose of radiation to both patient and surgeon. Many aneurysm necks are angulated anteriorly. An estimate of this angulation can be made from review of the reformatted CT angiogram. Cranio-caudal angle correction of the c-arm gantry angle can provide a greatly expanded view of the aneurysm neck, facilitating precise placement of stent grafts at the level of the renal arteries. The foreshortening of the AP view without this angle correction can led to an radiographic appearance of accurate placement of the graft, which in fact is significantly caudad to the renal artery origins. This can be critical in patients with short aneurysm necks.

In many cases, cannulating the opening of the contralateral limb of a modular bifurcated self expanding graft can be one of the most challenging and time consuming aspects of the procedure. The standard technique involves manipulating a guidewire through the open end of the contralateral limb with an angled catheter. If initial attempts are unsuccessful, the contralateral limb can be entered in an antegrade fashion by going over the bifurcation of the graft from the ipsilateral side using a reverse curve catheter such as a Simmons. A wire can then be placed through the Simmons catheter that can be snared and pulled thorough a sheath in the contralateral common femoral artery. Alternatively, access from the left brachial artery may be used to obtain access into the contralateral limb opening.

Another simple technique for accessing the contralateral limb involves use of a tip deflecting wire. The Disposable Reuter Tip Deflecting Wire (Cook Inc.) has a diameter of 0.035 in and is 110 cm long. The curve radius of the deflecting portion of the wire is 10 mm (Figure 19–5). The tip of the deflecting wire is placed just inferior to the open-

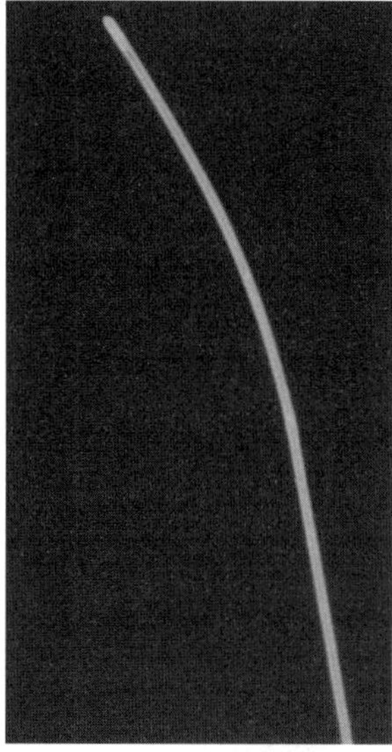

Figure 19-5A. Tip deflecting wire in the straight position.

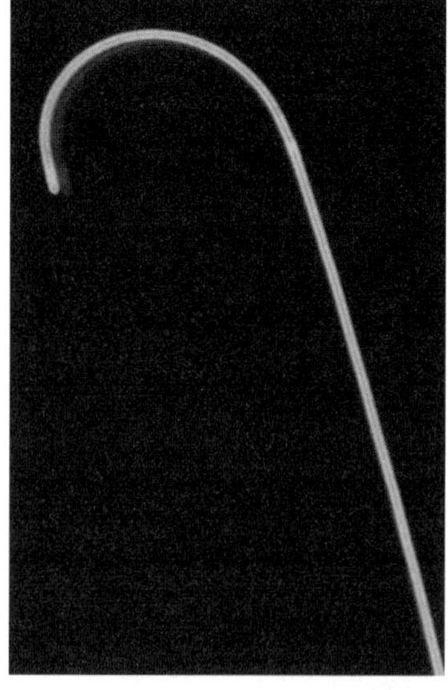

Figure 19–5B Tip deflecting wire with tip deflected.

ing of the contralateral limb and an angled catheter, such as an MPA catheter (Cook, Inc), is placed over the wire so the tip of the catheter is approximately 5 cm proximal to the tip of the DTDW. The DTDW is then deflected and the MPA catheter is fed off the wire into the contralateral limb opening. Once access to the contralateral limb with the MPA catheter in confirmed, the DTDW can be advanced into the body of the graft and the catheter can be advanced over this wire. The deflecting wire can then be removed and a stiff wire can be placed through the MPA catheter.

Once the contralateral limb has been accessed, it is important to confirm placement of the catheter in the body of the graft. Inadvertent placement of the contralateral limb outside the body of the graft may require open conversion. Confirmation that the contralateral limb has been accessed is obtained by exchanging the angled catheter used to cannulate the contralateral limb for a pigtail catheter. The pigtail catheter is placed in the proximal main body portion of the stent graft and is rotated. If the pigtail catheter moves feely when rotated, the catheter is within the stent graft. If the pigtail catheter does not move freely when rotated, the catheter is within the aneurysm, outside the stent graft. Additional attempts to cannulate the contralateral limb should then be made.

RENAL ARTERY COVERAGE

During EVAR, the covered portion of the graft may inadvertently obstruct 1 or both of the renal arteries. If both renal arteries are completely covered, attempts to drag the stent graft down should be made. This can be accomplished by inflating an angioplasty balloon in the main body portion of the graft just above the flow divider. If the balloon diameter is larger than the iliac limb diameter but smaller than the main body graft diameter, the balloon will be free to move in the main body but will not pass through the iliac limb when downward traction is applied. This enables the operator to pull the main body caudad. Alternatively, placement of a guidewire across the flow divider, exiting both femoral arteries allows the operator to pull the graft down by applying traction to the transfemoral wire. If a renal artery is only partially covered, a balloon mounted stent can be used to keep the vessel patent. The stent should be placed in the renal artery with 1–2 mm of the stent extending into the aorta, pushing the stent graft clear of the ostium. This generally supplies enough force to keep the affected renal artery patent.

ANEURX STENT GRAFT

The AneuRx (Medtronic Corp, Minneapolis, MN) device contains 6 runners on the outside of the graft. Occasionally these can be difficult to withdraw. Forceful withdrawl results in caudad migration of the graft. If difficulty is encountered when withdrawing the runners, the surgeon should first ensure that the stent graft has been fully deployed. If the stent graft has been fully deployed, 2 techniques can be used to assist in withdrawing the runners. One technique involves placing a 16 French sheath in the contralateral groin and using the sheath and/or a balloon placed through the sheath to provide support to the graft while the runners are removed. The sheath tip can be used to stabilize the graft as it supports the contralateral stub limb, or a balloon can be inflated partly in the sheath and partly in the stub limb, providing great columnar force to resist downward migration during delivery system withdrawl. A second technique involves first deploying the contralateral limb before withdrawl of the main body delivery system. A balloon can then be advanced into the contralateral gate to support the graft and allow for more forceful efforts at withdrawing the runners.

Placing the contralateral limb through the contralateral stub limb opening can be difficult with the AneuRx system. The blunt profile of the limb delivery system may not pass easily into the stub limb orifice. Preliminary balloon dilatation of the stub limb may remedy this. Alternatively, a 16 French sheath can be placed through the stub limb opening into the main body of the graft. The contralateral limb can then easily be placed through the sheath. The sheath can then be withdrawn and the contralateral limb will be in proper position, ready to be deployed.

Balloon dilation of the proximal portion of the AneuRx is usually not necessary after placement. If the proximal seal is not achieved and balloon dilation at this level is necessary, it is important to use a low pressure balloon (not more than 2 atmospheres of pressure) and to keep the balloon within the stent graft if at all possible. This decreases the risk of aortic rupture.

When deploying the AneuRx it is important to begin deployment proximal to the intended landing site. A partially deployed AneuRx can be pulled down into the correct position, but if it is deployed too low, it is quite difficult to push this device cephalad.

ANCURE STENT GRAFT

The Ancure stent graft is an unsupported, unibody device with characteristics that can create unique challenges during deployment. Occasionally, the contralateral pull-wire can become caught on the proximal attachment hooks. If this occurs, the operator controlling the pull-wire should immediately stop pulling on the wire. Occasionally, simply pushing upward on the wire may free it from the hooks. If this is not successful, an 8 French guide catheter can be placed over the wire and advanced so it is above the superior hooks. The catheter and wire can then be manipulated in order to free the wire.

The Ancure device is unsupported, therefore there is an increased tendency for the limbs to become narrowed or kinked.[20,21] The risk of limb thrombosis when this happens greatly increases. Because of this, careful attention must be paid to the limbs of the Ancure on the completion angiogram. If there is any evidence that the Ancure limbs are narrowed, a self-expanding stent should be placed to support the limbs (Figure 19–6).

WHEN IS THE OPERATION OVER?

After the stent graft has been placed, a final angiogram is done to look for an endoleak. Stiff guide wires should be removed prior to performing the final angiogram. This enables the graft to take a more natural position in the aorta and more accurately simulates how the device will look once the patient is off the operating room table. Oblique as well as AP completion views should be obtained. During the completion angiogram access across the graft from both groins should be maintained with either a catheter or floppy wire in the event additional interventions are deemed necessary. On the final angiogram the flush catheter should be placed just above the renal arteries. Flow in both renal arteries should be assessed to ensure they were not covered or in-

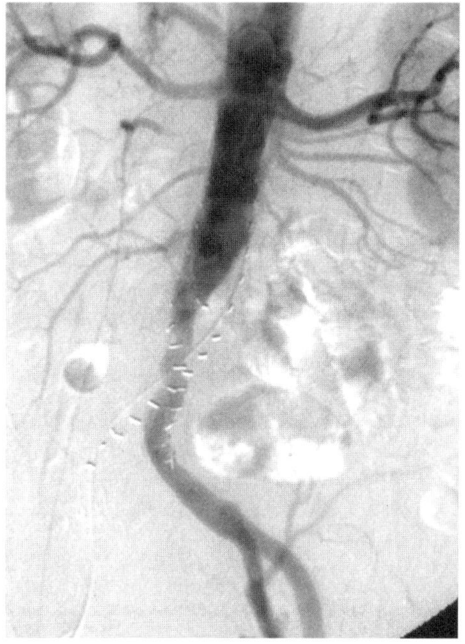

Figure 19–6A. Immediate post-deployment AP angiogram shows stenosis of right limb of Ancure graft resulting in limb occlusion

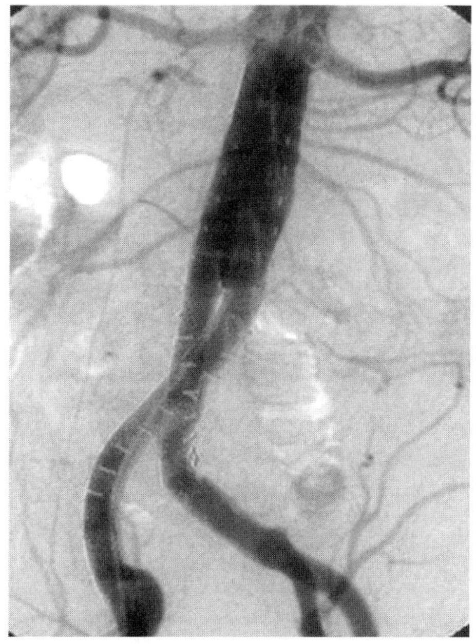

Figure 19–6B. Bilateral self-expanding stents were placed in the Ancure limbs resulting in patent limbs bilaterally

jured during the procedure. The operator should look carefully for endoleaks. Type I and type III endoleaks should be repaired immediately and the patient should not leave the operating room with a type I or type III endoleak[22] (Figure 19–7). These leaks usually require the placement of extension cuffs or additional balloon dilatation to secure the seal zone. In angulated vessels, the leak may be due to tortuosity with poor attachment of the graft to the vessel wall. This may be remedied with the placement of a stent within the graft to increase the radial force and securely appose the graft to the wall. Type II endoleaks represent flow into the sac from collateral vessels, and can be seen on the intraoperative angiogram. Some type II leaks seen immediately after stent graft placement thrombose spontaneously without therapy, after heparin reversal.[23] Therefore, patients with type II leaks do not receive treatment at the time of stent graft placement. Decisions on treatment of type II endoleaks are made after the 30 day postoperative CT scan. A type IV endoleak should be diagnosed only after the other types of endoleak have been completely excluded (Figure 19–8). Type IV endoleaks are due to porosity in the graft material and no therapy is needed.[24] These endoleaks resolve following reversal of anticoagulation.

RADIATION SAFETY

Radiation safety in the operating room setting is a topic that has received little attention to date. Distance from the x-ray tube, shielding of the beam, and fluoroscopy time are the 3 factors physicians can control to limit their amount of radiation exposure. Nobody would consider doing a fluoroscopic procedure without wearing a lead apron, how-

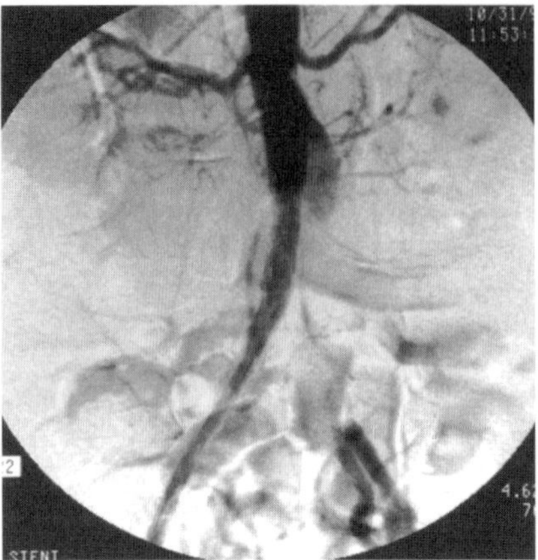

Figure 19–7A. Immediate post-deployment AP angiogram shows type 1 endoleak from inadequate seal at proximal neck in this patient who has had an aortouniiliac stent graft placed.

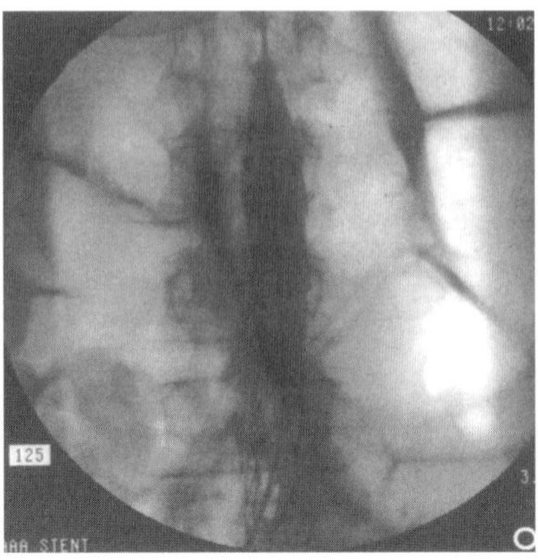

Figure 19–7B. Balloon angioplasty of proximal neck of stent graft.

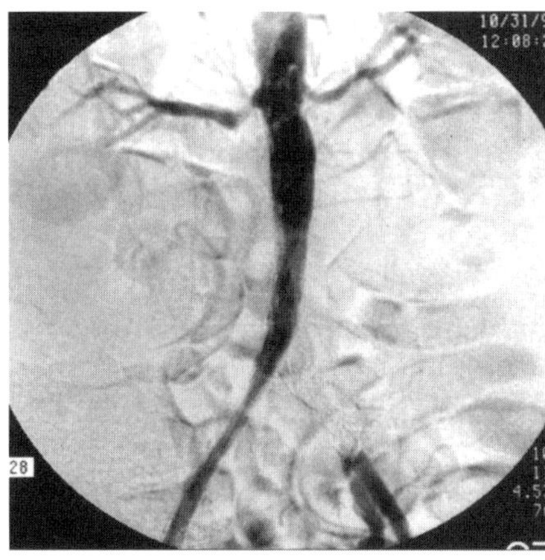

Figure 19–7C. Angiogram after angioplasty shows no proximal type 1 endoleak.

ever, many physicians are still resistant to the idea of wearing lead glasses. The lens of the eye is a radiosensitive part of the body and anyone who does a significant amount of work with ionizing radiation is at risk for developing premature cataracts. Wearing lead glasses can decrease the radiation exposure to the eye up to 70%.[25]

Ceiling mounted radiation shields are present in every interventional radiology suite, but rarely are seen in the operating room setting. New endovascular suites should be built with ceiling mounted lead shields, which would provide an additional barrier of protection for the surgeon.

The amount of scatter radiation absorbed by the surgeon can be greatly reduced by stepping away from the patient and x-ray tube whenever possible.[25–27] This is particularly important during angiographic runs when large amounts of radiation are emitted. These runs are almost always done with a power injector, and it is rarely necessary to stand immediately adjacent to a patient or the x-ray tube.

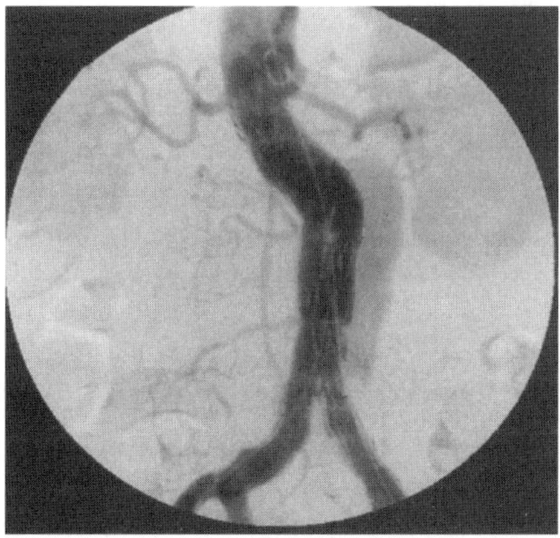

Figure 19–8. Type IV endoleak seen on AP view of immediate post-procedure angiogram.

CONCLUSION

Endovascular stent grafts for the treatment of AAA have progressed a great deal since the initial home made devices were deployed. However, this technology is still in its infancy. Technical aspects of this procedure will continue to progress as new materials and new devices are developed. Currently, the differences between the current devices are quite small when compared with the limitations of the entire technology.

The fundamental lesson we have learned is that the majority of the procedure should be completed in the office before the patient ever arrives in the operating room. This is accomplished through careful patient selection and meticulous pre-procedure imaging. Both anatomic and device related problems should be anticipated before entering the operating room. Once in the operating room, EVAR should be performed by physicians who possess a full complement of surgical and endovascular skills. We feel this is best accomplished in an environment where collaboration between specialties is encouraged. This evolving technology requires that physicians who perform EVAR learn the intricacies of each device before placing them. It is important to know the limitations of the device being used, to anticipate problems, and to be prepared to handle potential complications.

REFERENCES

1. Beebe HG, Kritpracha B, Serres S, et al. Endograft planning without preoperative arteriography: a clinical feasibility study. *J Endovasc Ther.* 2000;7:8–15.
2. Mohan IV, Laheij RJ, Harris PL. Risk factors for endoleak and the evidence for stent-graft oversizing in patients undergoing endovascular aneurysm repair. *Eur J Vasc Endovasc Surg.* 2001;21:344–349.
3. Faries PL, Briggs VL, Rhee JY, et al. Failure of endovascular aortoaortic tube grafts: a plea for preferential us of bifurcated grafts. *J Vasc Surg.* 2002;35:868–873.
4. Morrissey NJ, Faries PL, Teodorescu V, et al. Transrenal bare stents in endovascular treatment of abdominal aortic aneurysms. *J Invasive Cardiol.* 2002;14:36–40.
5. Adelman MA, Rockman CB, Lamparello PJ, et al. Endovascular abdominal aortic aneurysm (AAA) repair since the FDA approval. Are we going too far? *J Cardiovasc Surg.* 2002;43:359–367.

6. Sternbergh WC 3rd, Carter G, York JW, et al. Aortic neck angulation predicts adverse outcome with endovascular abdominal aortic aneurysm repair. *J Vasc Surg.* 2002;35:482–486.

7. Mehta M, Veith FJ, Ohki T, et al. Unilateral and bilateral hypogastric artery interruption during aortoiliac aneurysm repair in 154 patients: A relatively innocuous procedure. *J Vasc Surg.* 2001;33:27–32.

8. Halloul Z, Burger T. Grote R, et al. Sequential coil embolization of bilateral internal iliac artery aneurysms prior to endovascular abdominal aortic aneurysm repair. *J Endovasc Ther.* 2001;8:87–92.

9. Lyden SP, Sternbach Y, Waldman DL. Clinical implications of internal iliac artery embolization in endovascular repair of aortoiliac aneurysm. *Ann Vasc Surg.* 2001;15:539–543.

10. Soulen MC, Fairman RM, Baum RA. Embolization of the internal iliac artery: still more to learn. *J Vasc Interv Radiol.* 2000;11:543–545.

11. Criado FJ, Wellons E, Barker CF, et al. Safety of coil embolization of the internal iliac artery in endovascular grafting of abdominal aortic aneurysms. *J Vasc Surg.* 2000;32:684–688.

12. Kritpracha B, Pigott JP, Russell TE, et al. Bell-bottom aortoiliac endografts: an alternative that preserves pelvic blood flow. *J Vas Surg.* 2002;35:874–881.

13. Chong A, Soulen MC, Shlansky-Goldberg RD, et al. Balloon embolization of the internal iliac artery prior to aneurysm endografting. *J Vasc Intervent Radiol.* 2001;12:637–639.

14. Velazquez OC, Criado FJ, Carpenter JP, et al. Relationship between preoperative patency of the IMA and subsequent occurrence of Type II endoleak in patients undergoing endovascular repair of abdominal aortic aneurysms. *J Vasc Surg.* 2000;32:777–788.

15. Walker SR, Halliday K, Yusuf SW, et al. A study on the patency of the inferior mesenteric and lumbar arteries in the incidence of endoleak following endovascular repair of infrarenal aortic aneurysms. *Clin Radiol.* 1998;53:593–595.

16. Rachel ES, Bergamini TM, Kinney EV, et al. Percutaneous endovascular abdominal aortic aneurysm repair. *Ann Vasc Surg.* 2002;16:43–49.

17. Carpenter JP, Baum RA, Barker CF, et al. Impact of exclusion criteria on patient selection for endovascular abdominal aortic aneurysm repair. *J Vasc Surg.* 2001; 34:1050–1054.

18. Carpenter JP. Delivery of endovascular grafts by direct sheath placement into the aorta or iliac arteries. *AnnVasc Surg.* 2002 (In Press)

19. Criado FJ, Wilson EP, Abul-Khoudoud O, et al. Brachial artery catheterization to facilitate endovascular grafting of AAA: Safety and rationale. *J Vasc Surg.* 2000;32:1137–1141.

20. Baum RA, Shetty SK, Carpenter JP, et al. Limb kinking in supported and unsupported abdominal aortic stent-grafts. *J Vasc Interv Radiol.* 2000;11:1165–1171.

21. Carpenter JP, Neschis DG, Fairman RM, et al. Failure of endovascular AAA graft limbs. *J Vasc Surg.* 2001;33:296–303.

22. Veith FJ, Baum RA, Ohki T, et al. Nature and significance of endoleaks and endotension: summary of opinions expressed at an international conference. *J Vasc Surg.* 2002;35:1029–1035.

23. Baum RA, Carpenter JP, Golden MA, et al. Treatment of type 2 endoleaks after endovascular repair of abdominal aortic aneurysms: comparison of transarterial and translumbar techniques. *J Vasc Surg.* 2002;35:23–29.

24. White GH, May J, Waugh RC, et al. Type III and type IV endoleak: toward a complete definition of blood flow in the sac after endoluminal AAA repair. *J Endovasc Surg.* 1998;5:305–309.

25. Bushberg JT, Seibert JA, Leidholdt EM, et al. Radiation Protection. In: Bushberg JT, Seibert JA, Leidholdt EM, Boone JM eds. *The Essential Physics of Medical Imaging.* Baltimore: Williams and Wilkins; 1994:583–632.

26. Marx MV, Niklason L, and Mauger EA. Occupational radiation exposure to interventional radiologists: a prospective study. *J Vasc Interv Radiol.* 1992;3:597–606.

27. Ito H, Hosoya T, Eguchi Y, et al. Analysis of radiation scatter during angiographic procedures: evaluation of a phantom model and a modified radiation protection system. *J Vasc Interv Radiol.* 1999;10:1343–1350.

20

Endovascular Grafting with Suprarenal Stenting

Roy K. Greenberg, MD

The medical community has readily accepted the treatment of abdominal aortic aneurysms with endovascular devices. The obvious advantages over conventional surgical management relates to the diminished morbidity and mortality associated with a minimally invasive repair. However, one of the disadvantages of the less invasive technique pertains to the stability and durability of the device over time. The positional stability of an endoprosthesis, with respect to the native arterial vasculature, is dependent upon the forces exerted by the device on the surrounding anatomy as well as the displacement forces exerted on the device during the course of the patient's life time. Although a great deal of thought has gone into defining displacement forces experienced by an endovascular graft, to date, there is an absence of accurate *in vivo* or *in vitro* data. Consequently, design engineers have attempted to balance the desire for additional fixation force, within the constraints of device deliverability, required flexibility, and the strength or durability of the native vessels. Additional confounding information includes a lack of knowledge regarding the precise extent of the aneurismal disease. Although a proximal neck may be of a diameter small enough to place an endovascular prosthesis, the stability of each proximal neck varies. Subjective descriptions of suspect proximal necks include those that have a conical or reverse conical shape, necks that harbor thrombus within them, and short length necks. A significant number of proximal neck dilations following open or endovascular surery have been reported[1,2] and most surgeons have evaluated patients with aneurysms that have formed proximal to surgically implanted grafts. These conditions likely represent further degeneration of the immediate infrarenal neck and force one to question the stability and durability of this region of the aorta. Aneurysms of the visceral aortic segment are considerably more rare, and thus this more proximal segment of the aorta is thought to represent a region of greater stability, and is thus more desirable for the fixation of an implantable prosthesis. Extensions of early endograft iterations into the suprarenal aorta were intended to increase the fixation of the proximal portion of the endovascular prosthesis providing greater fixation force in a more stable segment of the arterial tree.

DEVICE OPTIONS AND PATIENT SELECTION

There are currently 3 devices utilized that utilize suprarenal fixation to provide additional fixation force for endografts utilized to treat infrarenal abdominal aortic aneurysms. The Talent (Medtronic) and Zenith (Cook) grafts are still in their US pivotal trials but commercially available elsewhere in the world. Cordis has recently initiated a trial on a third device, the Quantum LP, which also utilizes an uncovered suprarenal stent. The Talent prosthesis is constructed from nitinol wireforms 0.5 mm thick formed into serpentine shaped stents attached to a Dacron fabric. A single wireform approximately 15 mm in length is located at the proximal portion of the implant and attached to the graft material with sutures. A total of 5 apices are formed on the suprarenal stent, thus 10 struts have the potential to cross the renal ostia. The proximal portion of the graft material is identified during deployment by fluoroscopically identifying 2 figure-of-8 markers. The intent is to place the fabric as close to the renals as possible in the immediate infrarenal aorta. The Zenith device is constructed with stainless steel Z-stents that vary in length. The uncovered suprarenal portion is 26mm long is attached with sutures to the Dacron graft material. The wire thickness of the suprarenal component is 0.018 inches. A total of 10–12 apices are formed by the Z-stent, the variation is dependent upon the aortic diameter. Therefore 20–24 wireforms could potentially cross the renal ostia. A barb, approximately 5 mm long and 0.009 inches in diameter, is soldered to every other wireform with the intent of increasing the force required to dislodge the prosthesis. The proximal aspect of the graft material is visualized during implantation by the location of 4 gold markers. Placement of the graft material is intended in the immediate infrarenal position. The suprarenal component of the Zenith device is released using a delivery mechanism separate from that deploying the graft material. The barbs and suprarenal stent are constrained within a top cap. After the Dacron graft has been deployed and properly positioned, the top cap is advanced allowing engagement of the barbs within the suprarenal aortic wall. The Quantum LP is constructed out of nitinol and Dacron. It has a series of wireforms that extend approximately 25 mm above the graft material that are circumferentially bound at the superior aspect by a nitinol ring that is intended to extend into the suprarenal aorta in a manner similar to the other devices. The number of struts is between 12–16 depending on the aortic size, and the width of each strut is 0.01 inches. The cell distance between the struts is 0.27 inches. The suprarenal component is deployed prior to any of the graft material deployment using a simple sheath pull-back mechanism.

PATIENT SELECTION ISSUES FOR PROSTHESES
WITH SUPRARENAL EXTENSION

Patient selection is critical to successful endovascular grafting regardless of the endograft utilized. However, there are some specific factors that deserve mention when considering the use of a suprarenal stent. When present, aortic angulation is most commonly located immediately below the renal arteries or within the aneurysmal segment. However, a subset of patients will have significant angulation of their suprarenal aorta as well. Attention must be directed towards an assessment of the vectors that describe the direction of angulation. If the suprarenal and infrarenal aorta are angled in the same direction, suprarenal stenting is not typically a problem. However, if the vectors oppose each other, the angulation on the suprarenal component may compromise the seal required in the infrarenal aorta by preventing circumferential wall apposition of the sealing stent (see Figure 20–1). Therefore, in the setting of steep, opposing angles, the use of a suprarenal stent would not be advisable. An additional complication can arise when there is a significant diameter discrepancy between the infrarenal and suprarenal aorta. Normal arteries decrease in size as one moves in a distal direction however; a large percentage of patients with aneurysmal disease have infrarenal necks that are larger in diameter than the visceral aortic segment. Although this implies that the aortic tissue within the infrarenal aorta is not entirely healthy and may be prone to dilation, it is often used as a region to seal allowing the implantation of an endovascular prosthesis immediately below the renal arteries. The durability of such a practice is unknown. Significant diameter discrepancies can also have the effect of creating a "teepee" within the proximal portion of the endograft; again potentially compromising the seal in the infrarenal position, warranting additional caution for the use of these types of stentgrafts in patients with this anatomy. Despite anatomical concerns, stentgrafts with suprarenal extensions have been used in complex situations with respect to angulation or diameter discrepancies. In these circumstances, the addition of a balloon expandable stent can help one to achieve a seal. However, caution should be exercised due to the force that is required to overcome the inherent anatomy, and the lack of preclinical testing of devices used in conjunction with these stents.

FIXATION ISSUES

The intent of utilizing the suprarenal aorta is largely to add fixation force to the prosthesis, in an effort to prevent distal migration. The suprarenal component of a device provides a portion of the fixation force for a device. Fixation as a whole can be calculated by summarizing the radial forces of the proximal sealing stent (and the suprarenal stent if one is present), columnar forces, the additional forces opposing displacement from hooks and or barbs, any participation of tissue ingrowth. All of these must be viewed within the context of any arterial angulation. Calculating these forces is a complex problem and must be independently assessed for each patient's anatomy

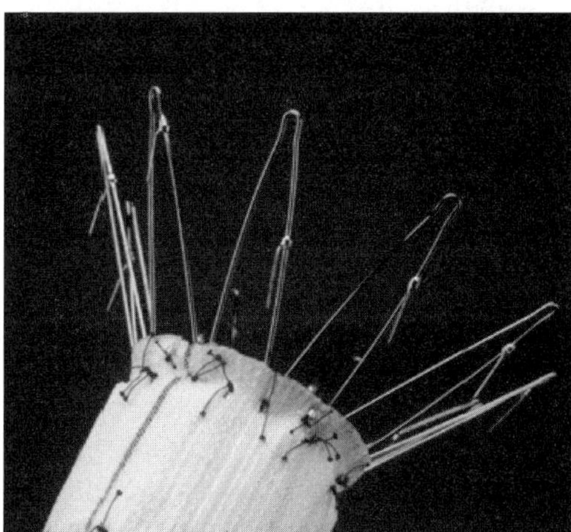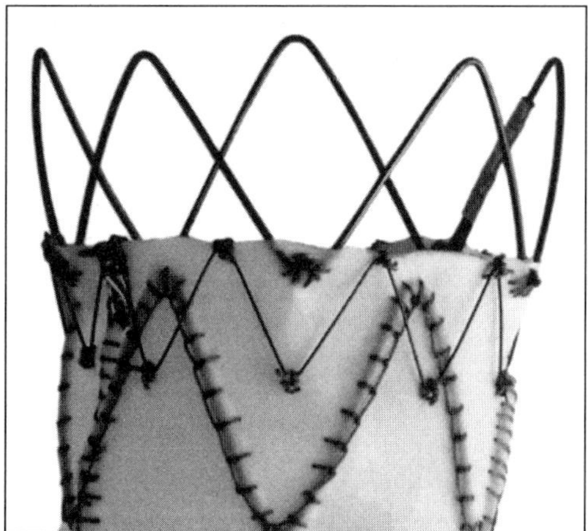

Figure 20–1. The Suprarenal component of the Zenith graft **(A)** and the Talent graft **(B)** are depicted here.

and each type of prosthesis. Superficially, it would appear that the more force applied the better. However when the forces exceed the durability of the aortic tissue significant problems can arise. It is clear that the presence of a suprarenal stent will add some radial force to the overall stabilization forces. However, the suprarenal components of all 3 devices vary considerably, some relying on the radial force applied by serpentine stents (Talent), others with a greater degree of straight struts forming a ring of radial force above the renals (Quantum LP), and some allowing each strut to function relatively independently and used as a mechanism to deliver barbs into the stabile portion of the aorta (Zenith).

RENAL ARTERY ISSUES

Among the several concerns regarding the use of the suprarenal aorta for fixation of infrarenal grafts is their effect on the renal arteries. Regardless of the prosthesis design, a portion of the structure must traverse the aortic segment containing the renal ostia. Obviously, if none of the struts cross a renal ostium, it would be hard to postulate renal complications. However, this is rarely the case with any of the devices. If one were to assume a 26 mm diameter aorta at the level of 2 renal ostia, each 6 mm in diameter, the chance of a Zenith device wireform crossing any portion of the renal artery is quite high. However, the chance of a strut actually traversing the center of the ostium is approximately 7%. Were this to occur, one must question the effect of a 0.018-in wire crossing a 6 mm renal ostium. This has been studied in preclinical (animal) and clinical studies and postulata to have no effect on renal function. The Malmo group demonstrated the safety of crossing the renal arteries in a porcine model,[3] and this was corroborated by the work of Whitebread.[4] Nuclear radiographic evaluation of renal function pre and post endovascular repair with a suprarenal device was shown to be unaffected over a short-term follow-up period by the Nottingham group.[5] Additionally, number of clinical series have also failed to elicit renal problems attributable to suprarenal stenting techniques.[3,6–8] However, were a renal artery problem to arise, it could be classified as a new stenosis, exacerbation of a pre-existing stenosis, or obstruction as a result of the prosthesis itself. All of these issues beg the question as to whether treatment of such lesions are possible, and whether some problems (such as denovo stenoses) are better handled prior to placement of the endovascular graft. We retrospectively evaluated our series of renal artery intervention in the setting of devices with suprarenal fixation and found, in a relatively small series of patients, that it is quite feasible to address the problem prior to, or following, the placement of the aortic prosthesis.[9] However, attention should be directed towards the timing of a planned intervention on a renal artery in a patient that is to undergo stentgraft placement with suprarenal fixation.

RENAL ARTERY INTERVENTIONS

The indications for renal artery interventions have been controversial for a great deal of time. The addition of stentgrafts with suprarenal fixation confuses matters further, with respect to the need for an intervention, the timing of the intervention, and the technique utilized. Historically, accepted indications for intervention in the setting of renal artery stenoses have been the presence of hypertension refractory to traditional medical therapy or evidence of renal insufficiency. Additionally, some feel that tight renal artery stenoses have a significant incidence of progression over time, that ultimately deteriorates renal function.[10,11] The presence of a device utilizing suprarenal fixation changes things in 2 ways. First the chance of a strut crossing the center of a tight renal artery stenosis is nearly the same of a strut traversing the center of a 6 mm artery. However, the effect of a wireform 0.018 inches in diameter crossing a renal artery with a 1 mm lumen may be dramatically different than the same strut traversing a normal renal artery. Secondly, once a stent graft with suprarenal fixation is in place, there exists a potential to make renal artery interventions more complex. Therefore, some physicians will treat a tight renal artery stenosis, even in the absence of a specific clinical indication, other than the perceived need to treat an aneurysm with a stentgraft inclusive of a suprarenal component. Clearly, this practice must be justified with respect to the risk of complications during the placement of a renal artery stent, the potential for restenosis, and the need to treat the aneurysm with a particular type of prosthesis. The argument to intervene on the renal arteries without clinical indications is obviously flawed without long-term data defining its benefit in the setting of suprarenal fixation however; clinical situations arise where the physician feels that the benefit of an early intervention will outweighs the risk potential difficulties later. In these circumstances, the physician may choose to intervene on the renal artery to simplify any renal interventions prior to the placement of a stentgrafts with suprarenal fixation. It must be emphasized that this issue has not been thoroughly investigated, and no definitive conclusion as to the safety of such a practice is advocated.

When placing a renal artery stent, most interventionalists utilize balloon expandable devices, in an effort to achieve a high radial force within a calcified stenosis coupled with extremely accurate device placement. The majority of renal occlusive disease is ostial in nature, and more accurately is described as aortic plaque impinging on the renal ostium. It has been common practice to place most of the stent within the renal artery, but intentionally leave a portion of the stent extending into the aorta, to ensure adequate treatment of the aortic component of the blockage. This practice can be quite dangerous when used in conjunction with a suprarenal stentgraft. Any significant protrusion in the region of the suprarenal stent may have the effect of distorting the device away from the aortic wall preventing a proper seal, and thus the technical aspects of performing renal artery stenting must be carefully addressed.

There are 3 options, with respect to the timing of elective renal interventions and endovascular grafting. Renal procedures may be performed prior to, during or subsequent to the placement of the aortic endoprosthesis. If one desires to place a renal artery stent prior to the endografting procedure, extreme accuracy is necessary to properly treat the ostial disease without allowing the stent to protrude any significant distance into the aortic lumen. Stents extending into the aortic lumen have the potential to push the suprarenal component of the endograft away from the aortic wall, which may also offset the infrarenal sealing stent causing an undo amount aortic wall tension in the region surrounding the renal stent, or preclude the sealing stent from adequate wall apposition. Alternatively, the renal stent can be deployed at the same time as the endovascular prosthesis implantation. The stent can be placed through the contralateral limb of a device (see Figure 20–2) during the deployment of the endograft, or immediately following the deployment of the aortic device. Depending on the type of endograft, this method of renal artery stenting may allow for a greater margin of error with respect to the amount of the stent that is allowed to protrude into the aorta, primarily because it is placed after the suprarenal component, and therefore will

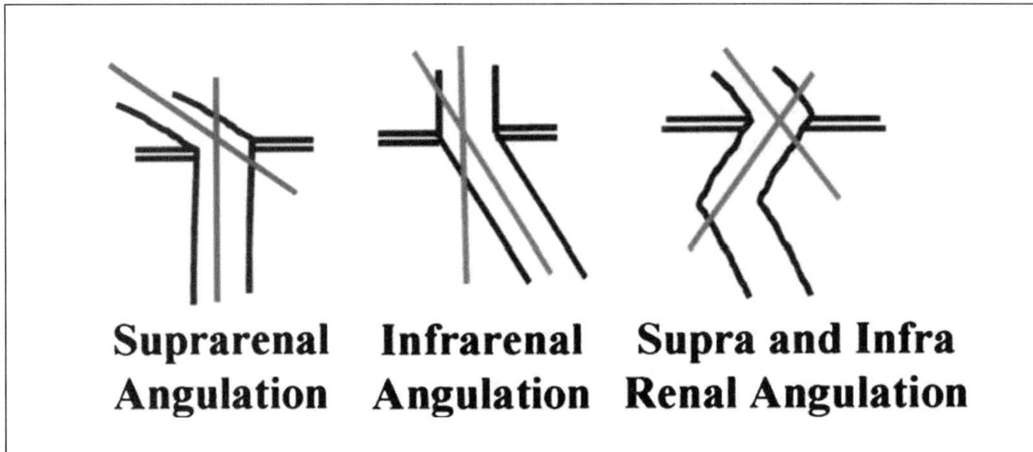

Figure 20–2. Stent placement.

not push the aortic prosthesis away from the aortic wall. Finally, renal stents can be placed following the endograft implantation. In most cases, the placement of a renal stent after a stentgraft with suprarenal extension is no different than the standard renal stent placement. However, should one of the suprarenal struts significantly cross or impinge access to a renal ostium, technical challenges can be encountered. In this circumstance, smaller, more flexible (0.014 in) systems are desirable. Frequently the brachial approach simplifies the access to the renal artery when used in conjunction with an angled catheter, rather than a hooked catheter that can be more difficult to manipulate within the struts of the fixation segment.

FOLLOW-UP

Although the follow-up algorithms for endografts with and without suprarenal components have been similar in the US prospective trials, some subtle differences should be recognized. The standard of care in our institution includes post-procedural CT and 4 view abdominal flat plates (AP, lateral, and bilateral obliques) within 30 days, at 6, 12, and 24 months. Yearly studies are performed but the cross-sectional imaging study may be substituted with an ultrasound provided the aneurysm is behaving as predicted. It is clear that if renal interventions were performed in conjunction with the aneurysm repair, an effort must be made to evaluate the flow within the respective renal artery as well. We now utilize duplex ultrasonography for this purpose at 6, 12, and 24 months. Additionally, an assessment of the creatinine level at each of the follow-up visit is used to monitor renal function.

The evaluation of migration of a device with a suprarenal extension can be quite difficult. It is nearly impossible to delineate the proximal aspect of the graft material on a CT scan. The technique that we have developed to assess movement at the proximal neck level requires knowledge regarding the position of the proximal aspect of the suprarenal stent, the superior mesenteric artery, the lowest renal artery, and the point that the metallic portion of the stentgraft is fully visualized (360-degree strut visualization). Using this method, downward (or upward) migration can be detected with respect to the vascular anatomy that is believed to be static (superior mesenteric artery). This can also be used to define any angulation of the proximal component, where one may see the distance between the uppermost portion of the suprarenal component remain stable while the full circle of stent struts may be noted to be more proximal or distal to its original position. Although this does not represent a perfect method for measuring migration, it is far more complete than any assessment of abdominal flat plate radiographs, or simpler algorithms designed to only measure the most proximal device component over time.

EXPLANTING DEVICES WITH SUPRARENAL STENTS

Devices with suprarenal components have the potential to be more complicated to explant than pure infrarenal devices. In all cases (grafts with infrarenal and suprarenal fixation), we prepare for the placement of a supraceliac clamp either from a retroperitoneal or transperitoneal approach. The choice of the incision largely depends on the need for access to the right renal or right iliac arteries. In our experience of explanting the suprarenal components of one Zenith and one Talent device at The Cleveland Clinic, the suprarenal segments have been well incorporated within the aortic tissue. This adds an aspect of challenge to the procedure. Caution must be exercised around the renal ostia, as tearing of the intima in this region can create renal artery dissections. Alternatively, if there is significant tissue incorporation, the graft can be transected immediately below the suprarenal stent and the proximal anastomosis of the repair can incorporate the uncovered portion of the suprarenal stent within the suture line. Some authors have advocated pulling the suprarenal component out, or cinching it down with umbilical tape in an attempt to constrict the stent allowing one to pull the barbs (with the Zenith device) out of the aorta rather than force the barbs to bend or the aorta to tear. A well-planned operation with attention to detail in the region of the renal arteries is paramount to success.

CONCLUSIONS

Suprarenal stenting is a safe and effective means of increasing the fixation force of endovascular prosthesis. The presence of a suprarenal stent will likely improve the long-term durability of the device, and it may also increase the accuracy of deployment. The timing and indications for the treatment of renal artery stenoses in the setting of suprarenal stenting remain controversial. The effect of the suprarenal component on renal function appears to be minimal if any at all. Despite the added security of a suprarenal stent, follow-up must be meticulous; attention has to be consciously directed at the assessment of migration, and renal flow in the setting of renal artery stenoses.

REFERENCES

1. Illig K, Green R, Ouriel K, Riggs P, Bartos S, DeWeese J. Fate of the proximal aortic cuff: implications for endovascular aneurysm repair. *J Vasc Surg.* 1997;26(3):492–499.
2. Sonnesson B, Resch T, Lanne T, Ivancev K. The fate of the infrarenal aortic neck after open aneurysm surgery. *J Vasc Surg.* 1998;28(5):889–894.

3. Malina M, Brunkwall J, Ivancev K, Lindh M, Lindblad B, Risberg B. Renal arteries covered by aortic stents: clinical experience from endovascular grafting of aortic aneurysms. *Eur J Vasc Endovasc Surg.* 1997;14(2):109–113.
4. Whitbread T, Birch P, Rogers S, Beard J, Gaines P. The effect of placing an aortic wallstent across the renal artery origins in an animal model. *Eur J Endovasc Surg.* 1997;13:154–158.
5. Maclerewicz J, Walker S, Vincent R, Wastie M, Elamrasy N, Hopkinson BR. Vascular surgical society of Great Britian and Ireland: perioperative renal function following endovascular repair of abdominal aortic aneurysm with suprarenal and infrarenal stents. *Br J Surg.* 1999;86(5):69.
6. Criado F, Fry P. The Talent endolumnial stent-graft system: technical success and acute clinical outcome: report of a collective internationl experience. *J Endovasc Surg.* 1998;5:1–9.
7. Greenberg R, Lawrence-Brown M, Bhandari G, Hartley D, Stelter W, Umschied T, et al. An update on the Zenith endovacsular graft for abdominal aortic aneurysms: initial implantation and mid-term follow-up data. *J Vasc Surg.* 2001;2(33):S157–S165.
8. Marin M, Veith F. Endovascular stents and stented grafts for the treatment of aneurysms and other arterial lesions. *Adv Surg.* 1996;29:93–109.
9. Scovell S, Greenberg R, Clair D, Srivastava S, Ouriel K. *Feasibility of Renal Artery Stenting in Patients Undergoing Endovascular Aneurysm Repaid with Suprarenal Fixation.* 2002. Ref Type: Unpublished Work
10. Hansen K, Thomason R, Craven T, Fuller S, Keith D, Appel R, et al. Surgical management of dialysis-dependent ischemic nephropathy. *J Vasc Surg.* 1995;21:197–211.
11. Tollefson D, Ernst C. Natural history of atherosclerotic renal artery stenosis associated with aortic disease. *J Vasc Surg.* 1991;14:327–331.

VI

Issues in
Vascular Surgery

21

Competency in Vascular Surgery

Norman R. Hertzer, MD

While he was the editor of the *New England Journal of Medicine,* Arnold Relman wrote in 1988 that the medical care system in the United States had undergone 2 revolutions since World War II and was about to enter another.[1] He described the first of these as the Era of Expansion, which was distinguished by rapid growth in the number of hospitals and physicians, a national commitment to the funding of important clinical and basic research, and the passage of Medicare and Medicaid legislation to guarantee additional millions of Americans their access to modern health care. The second revolution was termed the Era of Cost Containment—or the Revolt of the Payers—and has been marked by fiscal constraints on the part of insurance companies, state agencies, and the federal government. This era has witnessed regulatory restrictions on hospital construction, capitations in hospital charges on the basis of diagnosis-related groups, and reductions in reimbursement for many specialists, primarily surgeons, through the resource-based relative value scale. Relman called the third revolution the Era of Assessment and Accountability, and predicted that it would feature a demand for uniformity in treatments and outcomes on the part of those who receive health care and those who pay for it.

In response to these observations, Epstein[2] pointed out several factors underlying what has become a sustained interest in outcome assessment: 1) the need for cost containment by payers; 2) an increasingly competitive medical marketplace, in which insurers first may have concentrated only on price but have begun to search for ways to measure quality in order to satisfy their beneficiaries; 3) an explosion in medical technology that conceivably could lead to unnecessary complications for certain treatment interventions; 4) the geographic differences in utilization that have been reported for some of these interventions, which raise the question of whether they might be abused in high-use areas as well as underutilized for appropriate patients in low-use areas. As an example of the growing concern with both price and quality among buyers, the Leapfrog Group, a consortium of over a hundred Fortune 500 companies that provide health care plans for approximately 30 million employees and their dependents, soon will require hospitals to meet volume standards for 5 high-risk surgical procedures.[3] Of interest to vascular surgeons, 2 of these procedures are abdominal aortic aneurysm repair and carotid endarterectomy.

Competency in vascular surgery undoubtedly will come under even closer scrutiny in the future than it has in the past. Beyond the traditional expectations of patients and their families for expert care, payers now are discovering that anything less than expert care often is more expensive because it may be associated with inappropriate management and higher complication rates. This ultimately should work to the advantage of surgeons who truly are competent in the field of vascular surgery, but they must be prepared to demonstrate their competency by virtue of their training and/or experience, and, most importantly, by the documentation of their own results. In this regard, the American Board of Medical Specialties (ABMS) also has concluded that the knowledge of personal surgical outcomes is an indispensable component of ongoing self-assessment, and has instructed its member boards to make the submission of outcome data a requirement for recertification.[4] The American Board of Surgery (ABS) has announced that it intends to begin this process with its current Sub-board of Vascular Surgery.[5]

TRAINING AND EXPERIENCE

Veith[6] and Stanley[7] proposed and defended the concept of an independent Board of Vascular Surgery in their presidential addresses to the Society for Vascular Surgery (SVS) in 1996 and in 1997. After an open discussion of this matter at their annual business meetings in 2001, the members of the SVS and the American Association for Vascular Surgery (AAVS) voted in favor of petitioning the ABMS for independent board status. The advocates for this approach maintained that the breadth of vascular surgery clearly qualifies it as a recognizable specialty—especially with the addition of a growing array of endovascular techniques—and that a separate board and residency review committee are necessary to govern the certification of its diplomates and the structure of its training programs. Perhaps the most persuasive argument for abandoning the present system, however, was the underlying conviction that surgeons who have received dedicated training in vascular surgery can be expected to have the best results.

This conviction seems even more defensible today than when it first was offered as a reason for sub-certification in vascular surgery 30 years ago. Although Kempczinski et al.[8] found in 1986 that general surgeons and self-designated vascular surgeons had similar stroke and mortality rates after carotid endarterectomy (CEA) in Cincinnati, the vascular surgeons in this survey were defined merely by their membership in regional or national vascular societies. Recent studies, using either the ABS vascular certificate or the completion of a vascular surgical fellowship as their criteria for designation as a vascular surgeon, suggest that vascular surgeons do have significantly better outcomes than general surgeons with respect to the combined stroke and mortality rate for CEA[9] and the mortality rate for abdominal aortic aneurysm (AAA) repair.[9,10]

Furthermore, the number of general surgeons who can claim a large personal experience with vascular surgery in the absence of formal training almost certainly has declined since the ABS began to offer the Certificate of Special (now Added) Qualifications in Vascular Surgery in 1982.[11] According to data that were collected by the ABS from 1995 to 1997, 2,434 applicants for recertification in general surgery performed an average of 398 operations annually, including 39 that were related to vascular surgery.[12] Urban general surgeons were responsible for significantly more vascular procedures (mean, 59 per year) than were those from rural areas (mean, 25 per year; P<0.05), but over half (56%) of all of these procedures were done for dialysis access (Figure 21–1). Other major operations for peripheral arterial disease (e.g., lower extremity revascularization), cerebrovascular disease, and aortic aneurysms represented only about 5% and 2.5% of the annual caseload for urban and rural general surgeons, respectively. Collectively, however, general surgeons still perform a substantial volume of vascular surgery despite their low individual caseloads. In another review of ABS data, Hobson[13] found that general surgeons were responsible for approximately 25% of the major vascular operations and for nearly 65% of the dialysis access procedures that were done by surgeons who applied for recertification in either vascular surgery or general surgery in 1995 (Table 21–1).

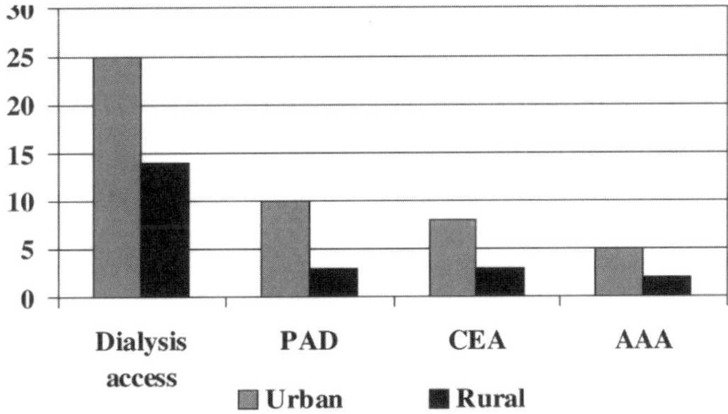

Figure 21–1. Mean annual number of dialysis access, peripheral arterial disease (PAD), carotid endarterectomy (CEA), and abdominal aortic aneurysm (AAA) procedures that were performed by 2,434 urban and rural general surgeons who applied for recertification by the American Board of Surgery from 1995 to 1997.[12]

TABLE 21–1. ANNUAL CASELOAD FOR 177 VASCULAR SURGEONS AND 685 GENERAL SURGEONS WHO APPLIED FOR RECERTIFICATION BY THE AMERICAN BOARD OF SURGERY IN 1995.[13]

Annual Caseload	Group 1 (n = 87)	Group 2 (n = 90)	Group 3 (n = 685)
All procedures	274*	352*	381*
Vascular procedures	197* (81%)	192* (55%)	41* (12%)
Total vascular Procedures	17,139	17,280	28,085
Carotid Endarterectomy	34* 2958†	32* 2880†	3* 2055†
Infrainguinal Revascularization	37* 3393†	31* 2790†	3* 2055†
Elective abdominal aortic aneurysm repair	11* 957†	10* 900†	1* 685†
Dialysis access	38* 3306†	51* 4590†	20* 13,700†

Group 1: Certified vascular surgeons applying for recertification in vascular surgery
Group 2: Certified vascular surgeons applying for recertification in general surgery
Group 3: Certified general surgeons applying for recertification in general surgery
*Mean
†Total

On the basis of a questionnaire that was mailed to members of the SVS, the AAVS, and several regional vascular societies, Stanley et al.[14] estimated that board-certified vascular surgeons performed about 40% of the CEAs, 35% of the AAA repairs, and 30% of the dialysis access procedures that were done in the U.S. in the mid-1990s. The 1996 Medicare data in the *Dartmouth Atlas of Vascular Health Care* confirm the relative accuracy of these estimates (Figure 21–2), but they also illustrate the eclecticism of vascular surgery with respect to those who practice at least parts of it.[14] According to the *Atlas*, 39% of the major vascular surgery (i.e., CEA, AAA repair, lower extremity revascularization) in the U.S. is performed by vascular surgeons and 29% by general surgeons. The remaining 32% is done by cardiothoracic surgeons (29%) or by neurosurgeons (3%), neither of these 2 specialty groups having any investment whatsoever in the current controversy between the SVS/AAVS and the ABS regarding the establishment of an American Board of Vascular Surgery. The only unifying principle among all of these surgical disciplines is that outcomes are the most reliable indication of competency in vascular surgery, no matter who performs it. As the data in the *Dartmouth Atlas* again reveal, the incidence of serious complications following major vascular surgery is inversely related to the experience of individual surgeons with specific operations, *irrespective of their specialty designations.*

THE VOLUME/OUTCOME RELATIONSHIP

No credible initiative concerning competency in vascular surgery can afford to ignore the inverse relationship between case volume and complication rates that already has been well documented both for hospitals and for surgeons.[16] As long ago as 1979, Luft et al.[17] questioned whether vascular surgery should be regionalized to centers in which a minimum of 200 operations were done each year, citing postoperative mortality rates that were nearly 50% higher for AAA repair and other vascular procedures in hospitals having lower volumes. Ten years later, Fisher et al.[18] investigated the outcomes of CEA for Medicare beneficiaries in several New England states and discovered that high stroke and mortality rates correlated as closely with low hospital

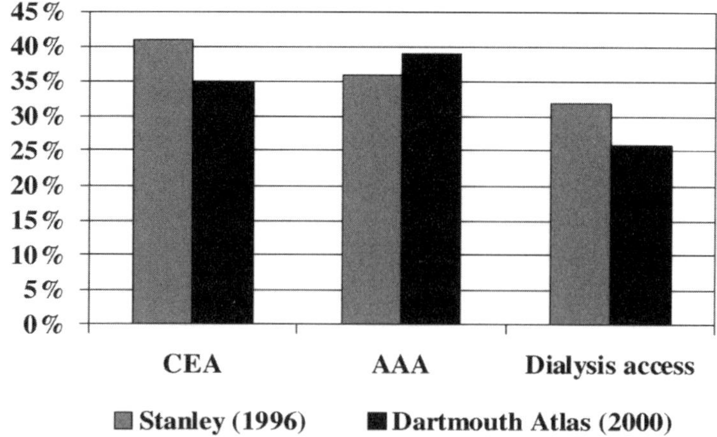

Figure 21–2. Estimated proportions of the carotid endarterectomy (CEA), abdominal aortic aneurysm (AAA), and dialysis access procedures that are performed by board-certified vascular surgeons in the United States according to Stanley et al.[14] and the *Dartmouth Atlas of Vascular Health Care.*[15]

volume as with advanced patient age. During the past decade, other statewide and/or Medicare audits have substantiated that hospital volume continues to be inversely related to the stroke and/or mortality rates for CEA (Georgia,[19] Maryland,[20] New York,[21] Ohio[22]) and to the mortality rate for AAA repair (New York,[23] Michigan,[24] California[25]). The volume/outcome relationship has been studied less extensively for lower extremity revascularization, possibly because such a wide variety of treatment options are available for patients who require it. Nevertheless, Ebaugh et al.[26] found that its mortality rate in Illinois was lowest at hospitals having additional capabilities in vascular surgery, such as a cardiac surgical service, an accredited vascular laboratory, and training programs in either general surgery or vascular surgery. Finally, in a report that serves as an important reference for the Leapfrog initiative, Dudley et al.[27] estimated that over 600 deaths might have been prevented in California in 1997 if certain high-risk patients-including those who underwent CEA or AAA repair-had been treated strictly at high-volume hospitals.

Table 21–2 contains data from several sources in which significant volume/outcome relationships also have been demonstrated for surgeons who perform vascular

TABLE 21–2. SURGEON VOLUME AND OUTCOME RELATIONSHIPS FOR CAROTID ENDARTERECTOMY, THE REPAIR OF NON-RUPTURED ABDOMINAL AORTIC ANEURYSMS, AND LOWER EXTREMITY REVASCULARIZATION.

Study Population (years)	Operative outcome measure(s)	High-volume surgeons (%)	Low-volume surgeons (%)	P-value
Carotid endarterectomy				
Tennessee Statewide[28] (1979–1988)	A. Stroke B. Death	16/772 (2.1) 9/772 (1.2)	203/5067 (4.0) 130/5067 (2.6)	0.008 0.02
Pennsylvania Medicare[29] (1989–1992)	Death	28/2384 (1.2)	85/3273 (2.6)	<0.005
Connecticut Statewide[30] (1985–1991)	Combined stroke and/or death	Odds ratio 1.0	Odds ratio 2.5	0.002
New York Statewide[21] (1990–1995)	Death	281/25,584 (1.1)	50/2623 (1.9)	<0.05
Toronto, Ontario[31] (1994–1996)	Combined stroke and/or death	53/980 (5.4)	7/38 (18)	0.0019
Abdominal aortic aneurysm repair				
New York Statewide[23] (1985–1987)	Death	76/1232 (6.2)	96/1019 (9.4)	<0.05
Maryland Statewide[32] (1990–1995)	Death	13/344 (3.8)	7/71 (9.9)	0.01
Lower extremity revascularization				
Northeastern Ohio[33] (1978–1981)	Amputation	10/388 · (2.6%)	29/313 (9.3%)	<0.001
Finland[34] (1991–1994)	Amputation	Odds ratio 1.0	Odds ratio 1.8	0.01

surgery in the U.S. and elsewhere.[21,23,28–34] At least 3 additional observations have been common to these and similar studies. First, about half of the low-volume surgeons in some series have been responsible for only 1 or 2 major vascular procedures per year.[23,28–30,32] Second, the hospital charges and length of stay tend to be higher for low-volume surgeons.[28–30,32] Third, the highest complication rates appear to occur in the setting of low-volume surgeons operating in low-volume hospitals.[21–23] In 1987, Luft and his associates[35] revisited his analysis of the inverse relationship between hospital volumes and complication rates on the basis of whether it might be related either to practice-makes-perfect (Do busy hospitals become good?) or to selective-referral patterns (Do good hospitals become busy?), and concluded that both of these were contributing factors. The same issues certainly seem to apply to individual practitioners.

PROSPECTIVE OUTCOME ASSESSMENT

In an attempt to bring objectivity to the hospital credentialing process for surgeons who seek to obtain or retain privileges in vascular surgery, an ad hoc committee of the SVS and the North American Chapter of the International Society for Cardiovascular Surgery (now AAVS) proposed in 1989 that continuous audits of surgeon-specific complication rates for CEA, AAA repair, and lower extremity revascularization should be conducted at every hospital in which vascular surgery is performed.[36] This proposal contained a number of measures that were designed to keep the credentialing process open to experienced surgeons who had not received training in accredited vascular programs, as well as to provide a sufficient amount of preoperative risk stratification that would accommodate most patient populations. The recommendations of this committee generated a flurry of early inquiries from hospital administrators, but it seems unlikely that many hospitals ever put them into place on a permanent basis. A recent development in the area of board certification may rekindle the notion of personal outcome assessment once again, however.

In response to a growing interest in treatment outcomes on the part of the public and payers alike, the ABMS has reached several important conclusions that promise to influence the future recertification process for every medical and surgical discipline in the U.S.[4] The most fundamental of these conclusions is that the competence implied by board certification should be *maintained* by a lifelong commitment to learning and self-assessment, not merely recertified on the basis of a passing grade on a written examination every few years. Although examinations undoubtedly will continue to play a role in the maintenance of certification by the 10 surgical boards that are represented on the ABMS, the current directive to these boards is to find a meaningful way for their diplomates to demonstrate competence by blending a sustained program of postgraduate education with an ongoing appraisal of their own surgical results. In order to comply with this mandate, the ABS has announced that it soon will require the submission of postoperative outcome data by surgeons who apply for subspecialty recertification in vascular surgery, pediatric surgery, or surgical oncology. In vascular surgery, these data will include the 30-day stroke and mortality rates for CEA in symptomatic and asymptomatic patients, the 30-day mortality rates for open and endovascular repair of infrarenal AAAs, and the 30-day mortality and amputation rates for infrainguinal revascularization (vein and synthetic) in patients with either claudication or advanced ischemia.[5]

The recognition that continued certification in a specialty field somehow should be linked to results is long overdue, but the new ABMS policy and the ABS response to it will have to be refined before any conclusions can be reached regarding their relevance to competency in vascular surgery. First, there presently is no stipulation for the accuracy of outcome data that are submitted by a candidate for recertification in any specialty field to be validated by an impartial third party, such as the chief of service at the hospital in which the candidate practices. Furthermore, citing the heterogeneity of general surgery, the ABS initially has exempted candidates for recertification in general surgery from submitting any outcome data at all, an exemption that obviously includes data for the vascular procedures that they perform. In addition, the results for the substantial volume of vascular surgery that currently is done in the U.S. by cardiothoracic surgeons and neurosurgeons will be captured only if their respective boards happen to choose certain procedures—AAA repair and CEA, for instance—as index cases for outcome assessment in their own requirements for recertification. In summary, board-certified vascular surgeons may be the only candidates for recertification in any discipline who will be asked to pursue self-assessment specifically on the basis of their outcomes in vascular surgery. According to the information that already is available from the *Dartmouth Atlas* and from previous ABS recertification files, this approach will fail to encourage surgeon self-assessment for approximately 60% of all major vascular procedures and for a likely majority of those that are done by low-volume practitioners.[11–13, 15]

The most reliable way to measure and ultimately to enhance competency in vascular surgery is to document local results for individual hospitals and surgeons.[5] In a prospective study of 14 hospitals in Iowa, Kresowik et al.[37] found that an ongoing audit of CEA outcomes and an objective analysis of the processes that could be used to improve them were associated with a significant ($P<0.05$) reduction in the postoperative stroke and mortality rate from 6.5% in 1994 to 1.8% in 1998. The importance of outcome assessment also is well illustrated by a recent Medicare demonstration project in which CEA probably can be viewed as a proxy for all types of major vascular surgery.[38] In this retrospective survey, the medical records were audited for a total of 10,561 CEAs that were performed in 10 states (Arkansas, Georgia, Illinois, Indiana, Iowa, Kentucky, Michigan, Nebraska, Ohio, Oklahoma) from June 1995 through May 1996. The utilization rates (per 10,000 Medicare beneficiaries) and the complication rates for CEA varied widely from one state to another, both of these representing surrogate measures of competency. In 6 states (Figure 21–3) the combined stroke and mortality rate for symptomatic patients exceeded the surgical risk in the North American Carotid Endarterectomy Trial (NASCET),[39] and in 9 states (Figure 21–4) the combined stroke and mortality rate for asymptomatic patients exceeded the surgical risk in the Asymptomatic Carotid Atherosclerosis Study (ACAS).[40]

If the NASCET and the ACAS had been conducted only at these hospitals and by these surgeons, their conclusions—and the merit of carotid surgery—might have been interpreted entirely differently. Just as importantly, did the patients in these states know what the risk of their operations would be? Did the surgeons? Competency in vascular surgery must be determined at every hospital in which it is performed, and it will continue to be an elusive target as long as questions like these remain unanswered.

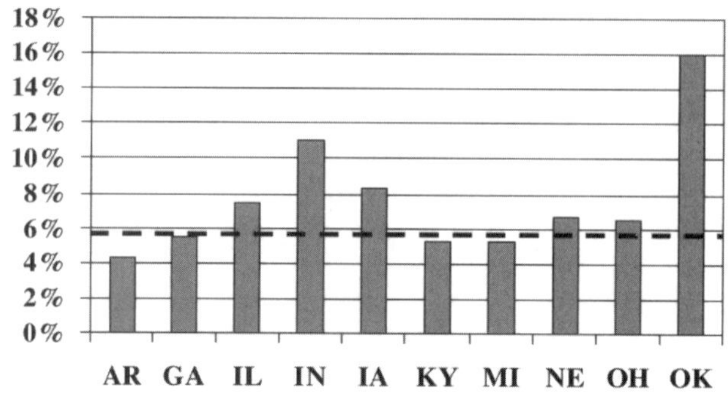

Figure 21–3. The 30-day combined stroke and mortality (CSM) rates after carotid endarterectomy for symptomatic patients in 10 states.[38] The dotted line represents the CSM (5.8%) for the surgical cohort (70% to 99% stenosis) of the North American Carotid Endarterectomy Trial.[39] (Adapted with permission from: Kresowik TF, Bratzler D, Karp HR, Hemann RA, Hendel ME, Grund SL, Brenton M, Ellerbeck EF, Nilasena DS. Multistate utilization, processes, and outcomes of carotid endarterectomy. *J Vasc Surg.* 2001;33:227–35.)

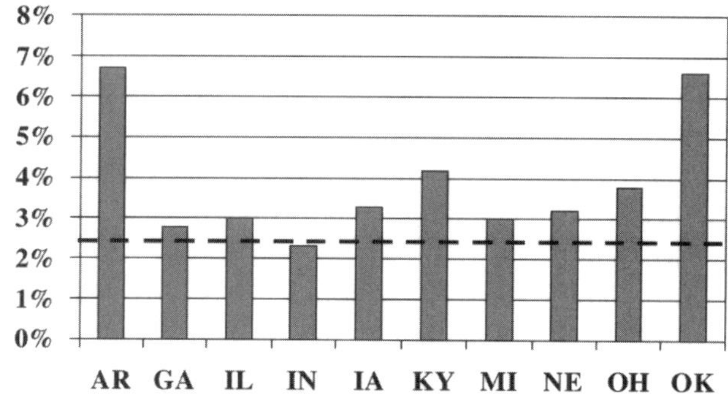

Figure 21–4. The 30-day combined stroke and mortality (CSM) rates after carotid endarterectomy for asymptomatic patients in 10 states.[38] The dotted line represents the CSM (2.3%) for the surgical cohort of the Asymptomatic Carotid Atherosclerosis Study.[40] (Adapted with permission from: Kresowik TF, Bratzler D, Karp HR, Hemann RA, Hendel ME, Grund SL, Brenton M, Ellerbeck EF, Nilasena DS. Multistate utilization, processes, and outcomes of carotid endarterectomy. *J Vasc Surg.* 2001;33:227–35.)

REFERENCES

1. Relman AS. Assessment and accountability. The third revolution in medical care. *N Engl J Med.* 1988;319:1221–2.
2. Epstein AM. The outcomes movement-will it get us to where we want to go? *N Engl J Med.* 1990;323:266–70.
3. Birkmeyer JD, Finlayson EVA, Birkmeyer CM. Volume standards for high-risk surgical procedures: Potential benefits of the Leapfrog initiative. *Surgery.* 2001;130:415–22.
4. Nahrwold DL. The competence movement. *Bull Am Coll Surg.* 2000;85:14–8.
5. Hertzer NR. Outcome assessment: A new approach to the maintenance of board certification in vascular surgery. *J Vasc Surg.* 2001;34:371–3.
6. Veith FJ. Presidential address: Charles Darwin and vascular surgery. *J Vasc Surg.* 1997;25: 8–18.

7. Stanley JC. Presidential address: The American Board of Vascular Surgery. *J Vasc Surg.* 1998;27:195–202.
8. Kempczinski RF, Brott TG, Labutta RJ. The influence of surgical specialty and caseload on the results of carotid endarterectomy. *J Vasc Surg.* 1986;3:916.
9. Pearce WH, Parker MA, Feinglass J, Ujiki M, Manheim LM. The importance of surgeon volume and training in outcomes for vascular surgical procedures. *J Vasc Surg.* 1999;29:768–78.
10. Tu JV, Austin PC, Johnston KW. The influence of surgical specialty training on the outcomes of elective abdominal aortic aneurysm surgery. *J Vasc Surg.* 2001;33:447–52.
11. Wheeler HB. Myth and reality in general surgery. *Bull Am Coll Surg.* 1993;78:21–7.
12. Ritchie WP Jr, Rhodes RS, Blester TW. Work loads and practice patterns of general surgeons in the United States, 1995-1997. A report from the American Board of Surgery. *Ann Surg.* 1999;230:533–43.
13. Hobson RW II. Presidential address: Practice patterns in vascular surgery-Implications for the certification and training of vascular surgeons. *J Vasc Surg.* 1997;26:905–912.
14. Stanley JC, Barnes RW, Ernst CB, et al. Vascular surgery in the United States: Workforce issues. Report of the Society for Vascular Surgery and the International Society for Cardiovascular Surgery, North American Chapter, Committee on Workforce Issues. *J Vasc Surg.* 1996;23:172–81.
15. Cronenwett JL, Birkmeyer JD. The Dartmouth atlas of vascular health care. Chicago: AHA Press; 2000.
16. Hertzer NR. Presidential address: Outcome assessment in vascular surgery—Results mean everything. *J Vasc Surg.* 1995;21:6–15.
17. Luft HS, Bunker JP, Enthoven AC. Should operations be regionalized? The empirical relation between surgical volume and mortality. *N Engl J Med.* 1979;301:1364–9.
18. Fisher ES, Malenka DJ, Solomon NA, et al. Risk of carotid endarterectomy in the elderly. *Am J Public Health.* 1989;79:1617–20.
19. Karp HR, Flanders D, Shipp CC, et al. Carotid endarterectomy among Medicare beneficiaries. A statewide evaluation of appropriateness and outcome. *Stroke.* 1998;29:46–52.
20. Perler BA, Dardik A, Burleyson GP, et al. Influence of age and hospital volume on the results of carotid endarterectomy: A statewide analysis of 9918 cases. *J Vasc Surg.* 1998;27:25–33.
21. Hannan EL, Popp J, Tranmer B, et al. Relationship between provider volume and mortality for carotid endarterectomies in New York State. *Stroke.* 1998;29:2292–7.
22. Cebul RD, Snow RJ, Pine R, et al. Indications, outcomes, and provider volumes for carotid endarterectomy. *JAMA.* 1998;279:1282–87.
23. Hannan EL, Kilburn H Jr, O'Donnell JF, et al. A longitudinal analysis of the relationship between in-hospital mortality in New York State and the volume of abdominal aortic aneurysm surgeries performed. *Health Serv Res.* 1992;27:517–42.
24. Katz, DJ, Stanley JC, Zelenock GB. Operative mortality rates for intact and ruptured abdominal aortic aneurysms in Michigan: An eleven-year statewide experience. *J Vasc Surg.* 1994;19:804–17.
25. Manheim LM, Sohn MW, Feinglass J, et al. Hospital vascular surgery volume and procedure mortality rates in California, 1982–1994. *J Vasc Surg.* 1998;28:45–58.
26. Ebaugh JL, Feinglass J, Pearce WH. The effect of hospital vascular operation capability on outcomes of lower extremity arterial bypass graft procedures. *Surgery.* 2001;130:561–9.
27. Dudley RA, Johansen KL, Brand R, et al. Selective referral to high-volume hospitals. Estimating potentially avoidable deaths. *JAMA.* 2000;283:1159–66.
28. Edwards WH, Morris JA Jr, Jenkins JM, et al. evaluating quality, cost-effective health care. Vascular database predicated on hospital discharge abstracts. *Ann Surg.* 1991;213:433–9.
29. Segal HE, Rummel L, Wu B. The utility of PRO data on surgical volume: The example of carotid endarterectomy. *Qual Rev Bull.* 1993;19:152–7.
30. Ruby ST, Robinson D, Lynch JT, Mark H. Outcome analysis of carotid endarterectomy in Connecticut: The impact of volume and specialty. *Ann Vasc Surg.* 1996;10:22–26.
31. Kucey DS, Bowyer B, Iron K, et al. for the University of Toronto Carotid Study Group. Determinants of outcome after carotid endarterectomy. *J Vasc Surg.* 1998;28:1051–8.

32. Dardik A, Lin JW, Gordon TA, et al. Results of elective abdominal aortic aneurysm repair in the 1990s: A population-based analysis of 2335 cases. *J Vasc Surg.* 1999;30:985–95.
33. Hertzer NR, Avellone JC, Farrell CJ, et al. The risk of vascular surgery in a metropolitan community. With observations on surgeon experience and hospital size. *J Vasc Surg.* 1984;1: 13–21.
34. Kantonen I, Lepäntalo M, Luther M, et al. and the Finnvasc Study Group. Factors affecting the results of surgery for chronic critical leg ischemia-a nationwide survey. *J Vasc Surg.* 1998;27:940–7.
35. Luft HS, Hunt SS, Maerki SC. The volume-outcome relationship: practice-makes-perfect or selective-referral patterns? *Health Serv Res.* 1987;22:157–82.
36. Moore WS, Treiman RL, Hertzer NR, et al. Guidelines for hospital privileges in vascular surgery. *J Vasc Surg.* 1989;10:678–82.
37. Kresowik TF, Hemann RA, Grund SL, et al. Improving the outcomes of carotid endarterectomy: Results of a statewide quality improvement project. *J Vasc Surg.* 2000;31:918–26.
38. Kresowik TF, Bratzler D, Karp HR, et al. Multistate utilization, processes, and outcomes of carotid endarterectomy. *J Vasc Surg.* 2001;33:227–35.
39. North American Symptomatic Carotid Endarterectomy Trial Collaborators. Beneficial effect of carotid endarterectomy in symptomatic patients with high-grade carotid stenosis. *N Engl J Med.* 1991;325:445–53.
40. Executive Committee for the Asymptomatic Carotid Atherosclerosis Study. Endarterectomy for asymptomatic carotid artery stenosis. *JAMA.* 1995;273:1421–28.

22

Information Dissemination by Internet

Joseph R. Schneider, MD, PhD

Nearly everyone in the developed world now has contact with computers and the Internet. Thus, most readers of this chapter will have used electronic mail or the World Wide Web in their non-professional life and this is also increasingly true of medical professional life. This presentation assumes basic familiarity with the Internet and some of its common applications including electronic mail and World Wide Web browsers. Readers interested in a more basic introduction to these concepts will find many articles and books on the subject. There are relatively few specific literature citations in this chapter. However, I have tried to provide a sample of the literature pertinent to this topic including several articles not cited in the text that are nevertheless listed in the Bibliography as well as a small sample of pertinent World Wide Web pages in the Appendix. For readers interested in a basic introduction to the Internet and its available resources with emphasis on surgery and vascular surgery, may I suggest our previous article on the topic.[1] Readers interested in a more detailed practical discussion of some of the historical and technical aspects of the Internet, problems with the current Internet and the Next Generation Internet and Internet II are advised to read the excellent article by Feied.[2]

WHAT CAN THE INTERNET DO FOR US AND OUR PATIENTS?

The Internet provides an extraordinarily powerful medium for the transfer of information. The organization and utilization of this information is difficult and particularly so for medicine. Smithline and Christenson in their excellent review have posed an ambitious set of requirements for clinical medicine and the Internet to "get along":

"Does the Internet help or hinder the physician in his or her daily work? Does it fulfill the promise of increased efficiency, increased knowledge, and less wasted time? Does it leapfrog quality so far forward that no one would consider practicing without it? And does it do this in ways that make it easy to integrate new tools into the physician's daily flow of work? One answer is clear: if the Internet does not fulfill the last promise, we will never get to see if it can fulfill the other promises—because physicians will not use it."[3]

The answers to these questions are not yet certain. However, each of us is capable of learning to use the Internet (and our patients already have). The genie is out of the bottle and there can be no doubt that the computer and the Internet will be increasingly essential to management of in-patients and out-patients, their medical records, registration, billing and collection, and to continuing medical education and life long learning.

ELECTRONIC MAIL

Electronic mail is a potential way for medical practitioners to communicate with each other and with patients. The advantage is that messages can be sent and received at the convenience of the user. However, it is easier (and less expensive) to compose and send an e-mail letter than to write and mail a paper note and e-mail has undoubtedly increased the amount of mail that each of us receives. Many physicians fear that giving their e-mail addresses to patients will mean the patients will deluge them with e-mail and never come to the office. Furthermore, many physicians are concerned about liability and are reluctant to send off a brief spontaneous message that provides something in writing to a patient. A telephone conversation is subject to some interpretation, whereas a written e-mail record is less so. Certainly, the pre-printed information and instruction sheets we often provide to patients may be easily e-mailed to patients. E-mail is an increasingly useful way to communicate with colleagues for both clinical and academic information. E-mail messages may include text or image files including audio and video and any other documents that might otherwise be part of the patient's "chart." Files may be broadcast to multiple e-mail recipients, but it is generally more efficient to make these available via a Web page (see below) for recipients interested in the contents of these files.

WORLD WIDE WEB

The World Wide Web, often abbreviated as "the Web," is the nearly all-purpose tool for individuals to obtain and provide information essentially in real time. The World Wide Web is perhaps the "second revolution" of the personal computer era because it has made publication of, access to, and use of information orders of magnitude easier, faster, and more comprehensive than ever before. One need only have the uniform resource locator (URL, the "address" of the information on the Internet). Organizations seem to find new ways every day to make use of the Web for internal and external information distribution. Patients often come to the office carrying information they have obtained over the Web. Business to consumer (B2C) sites (see appended brief list at the end of this article) are provided by universities, commercial, government, and other entities with an interest in providing information to and, often, obtaining information from "consumers" of health services. These are generally peer reviewed and physicians can usually trust that the information is reliable to the point of suggesting them to their patients. Sites provided by health care providers may integrate information and service, for example, a multispecialty clinic might provide information on a specific disease or complaint and then offer a list of specialists with expertise in the area of the consumer's inquiry.

THE WORLD WIDE WEB FOR PATIENTS

Several of these B2C (patient oriented) sites are listed in the appendix at the end of this article. These sites often have advertising, occasionally to the point of obscuring the path to the information sought by the practitioner or patient (as an example of what I would consider excessive advertising, see *www.drkoop.com*). These sites often have links to other useful sites. For example, HealthWeb links to VascularWeb through its surgery hot link. Some "consumers" may not feel they have received adequate or specific enough information from the available online site, so many sites also invite questions that lead to an individual response.

The Web has been used to help patients manage their own health and illness.[4] The baby boomers approaching retirement have been part of an unprecedented era of activism, consumerism, education, and prosperity and they are computer and Web savvy.[5] Indeed, this consumerism and growing dissatisfaction with "Managed Care" may ultimately force "Managed Care" to evolve or become extinct.[6] WellMed and LifeMasters[7] purport to help patients make more informed decisions about their own care. Some employers or insurance companies may contract with Web-based services to provide health decision making information to their subscribers. Subimo is an example of the latter. There is a growing presence of resources to provide what might be called a virtual doctor encounter.[8] Providers can charge for such virtual consultations. Patients need to have the judgment to separate the truly urgent problem that requires a direct exchange with a physician or a trip to the office or hospital from those that can be managed using these virtual consultations. Consumers can also examine the outcomes for selected procedures for hospitals (and in some cases in some states for individual practitioners) using resources such as HealthGrades. The Leapfrog Group (*www.leapfroggroup.org*) including employers such as Boeing and Ford Motor Company are clearly interested in this type of hospital outcome information. One interesting variation is the use of the Web for patient entry of their own medical information.[9] Patients may be asked by physicians or other health entities to enter some of their own demographic and health history using a Web interface as part of an electronic medical record implementation.

THE WORLD WIDE WEB FOR PHYSICIANS

Information specifically targeted at physicians falls into the business to business (B2B) category of Web sites. These may represent a higher level of the information in the B2C sites described above, such as finding a specialist. However, there are many other physician activities for which the Internet provides great promise.

Many sites, especially those sponsored by providers or payors, also integrate clinical and business activities. A provider or group might provide a physician finder or might even suggest individuals from their organization with specific expertise in an area of questioning by the consumer. Development of these sites is time and resource consuming and return on investment is difficult to measure. However, it is another way to "tell your story" in this new medium and there is little doubt this type of activity will be viewed as key by large provider groups and payors.

Physicians and patients have to deal with an increasingly complex set of requirements to determine eligibility and to collect for services provided to beneficiaries. Insurers are rapidly moving these functions to the Web so that office staff can determine immediately without any phone calls whether a potential patient is eligible for evaluation and other services. Authorization for services such as consultations and surgery that must be pre-approved may also be given, for example, by a primary care physician or requested, for example, by a vascular surgeon using the Web. MedUnite was created by a consortium of several health insurers to provide paperless insurance functions such as eligibility determination and claims submission. Waiting on the telephone for these authorizations and eligibility determinations take much of our office staff's time and this holds the promise of saving nearly all of this time.

Practice management functions such as scheduling, billing, claims management, and accounts receivable can now be performed using computer resources within an office or institution, increasingly using a Local Area Network (LAN) and the client-server relationship so effective for other "Distributed Computing Environments," or alternatively using software that is available over the Internet through an Application Service Provider (ASP). In the latter case, the software and potentially even the data are maintained on a server remote from the physician office. The office needs only an adequate personal computer/work station, an Internet connection, and the appropriate browser (along with a service contract with the ASP). This saves the individual physician or group office the trouble of choosing and maintaining the software and local network that would otherwise be required for these functions. While there are potential economies to be realized using this approach, there is also the greater potential for "down time" if one's Internet connection is not working 100% of the time. This general approach of having a fairly simple computer with most applications accessed via the Internet has long been predicted to dominate home use, but these predictions have thus far failed to be fulfilled in home use, probably because the vast majority of software used at home is relatively inexpensive anyway.

Electronic prescribing has great potential as well. The software can be configured to check for drug interactions, can suggest doses, alternative medications, can provide cost information, and an integrated solution can also check to see if a specific medication is listed in the patient's provider's formulary. Prescriptions can be "written" by the physician with a wireless device such as a PDA (*vide infra*) and can be transmitted as soon as they are written. One would expect fewer errors and the prescription would arrive at the pharmacy (via the Internet) well before the patient.

ELECTRONIC MEDICAL RECORDS

The electronic medical record (EMR) is the Holy Grail of medical informatics. The company that can integrate all the various elements of the record including in-patient, out-patient, laboratory, demographic, and insurance information will have done a great service for physicians and patients and will likely be rewarded financially. Many of the EMR solutions involve the Internet to varying extents. Some maintain both applications and data at remote sites accessed via the Internet, a type of ASP as mentioned above. Other solutions link portions of the record stored locally in the hospital or physician office (history and physical exam, outpatient encounters, etc.) with laboratory and other test data that may be provided using the Internet. Most EMR implementations have been disappointing in the past, but progress is being made and some institutions have made the transition to a complete EMR. A potential benefit of the EMR is that the systems can be (and hopefully are) configured to prompt physicians when abnormal results are obtained, when health maintenance activities are due, and they may even alert physicians that a proposed test may not be appropriate (and, therefore, may not be reimbursed) in the clinical situation. Literature suggests that the EMR improves compliance with health maintenance protocols such as vaccination and improves patient outcomes as well. Despite the failures in the past, this is clearly in our future.

WIRELESS COMMUNICATION AND PERSONAL DIGITAL ASSISTANTS

An increasing number of physicians now use Personal Digital Assistants (PDAs) in their daily work. I have found my PDA to be of great value because of the immediate access to the more than 1,200 (and still increasing) addresses and phone numbers of professional colleagues and other individuals and organizations that I have recorded as well as the daily schedule function on my PDA. I have also found the prescription drug information utility ePocrates, available at no charge to physicians at *www.ePocrates.com* which resides on my PDA, to be very helpful. Radio frequency (RF) wireless networks may allow a pocket sized hand held device to behave like a computer on a hard-wired network. For example, large wireless devices have been in use at patient bedsides at Evanston Hospital for several years and have become an alternative way to both enter and review vital signs, intake and output records, and laboratory results at the patient's bedside. However, the potential for PDAs and similar hand-held wireless devices is to provide much more in the way of timely and efficient availability of individual patient information.[10] A physician may see a patient in the office or other setting and her PDA or other wireless device may contain or have immediate access to all of the patient's pertinent information. Information such as laboratory test results, radiology reports, etc. can be updated instantly from the wireless network as long as she is within the range of the wireless network. The physician may enter her encounter note (she may be able to dictate her note with immediate electronic transcription). She may enter her orders including outpatient prescriptions and may also enter her CPT codes. These may be "uploaded" via the same wireless network and the orders and charge codes routed appropriately. The physician has continuously up to date information on the patient and the organization has continuously up to date orders and charge capture. Testing of small community-wide wireless networks is underway at the time of this writing.[11] Wireless devices are now produced that combine the function of a PDA and wireless telephone and have access to the Internet for e-mail and the Web. There is every reason to think that physicians will use devices like these and their successors in the immediate future to provide constant access to the Internet for both individual patient related information and the other generally available Internet resources. If I may make one bold prediction in this chapter, this is it: This is how we will practice within 5 years.

IMAGES AND OTHER "NON-TEXT" INFORMATION

Medicine in general and vascular surgery in particular are increasingly dependent on images. All new imaging technologies are inherently digital and even plain radiography is increasingly done without film. Consequently, more than 80% of all images generated in modern radiology departments start as digital images and would never have to be filmed if digital image files were available to physician "consumers" of those images. An increasing number of radiology departments are now "filmless" and use some version of electronic archiving of images using Picture Archiving and Communications Systems (PACS). Appropriate computer equipment must be available in adequate numbers and locations to allow physicians to review images to make this approach practical, but most current personal computers have adequate power and monitor resolution to allow review of these images with adequate resolution in the office or even at home. These images are frequently transmitted over Intranets within health care systems and can be transmitted anywhere in the world using the Internet. Clearly this has great value both for patient care and for academic activity.

Audio and video files may also be sent or made available on the Internet. This can and is even being done in "real time" as "Web casts."[12] Audio and video conferences can obviate the need for travel and the use of the Internet precludes the need for a dedicated single purpose (and, therefore, very expensive on a per use basis) medium to transmit such audio and video information. Individuals register for such conferences (and probably pay a fee) just as they would for a conference they would previously have traveled to see. They then "log on" at the appropriate time using the URL for the conference and generally with a password and may "attend" the conference in their office or home. Two-way interaction is possible since virtually all personal computers are now provided with a microphone and video cameras can be added for less than US$100. Thus, a participant can truly participate despite being physically remote from other participants.

SECURITY OF PATIENT INFORMATION ON THE INTERNET

Information transferred over the Internet is inherently insecure. The increasing availability of information has raised new questions about privacy and other security matters, questions which will only become more difficult as patient information becomes more available and traffic in this information increases on the Internet. Improved security is provided by a number of approaches, such as encryption of information or by preventing access to the Internet at large by using internal "Intranets" with security "fire walls," requiring people attempting access to sensitive information to provide a security code or some other evidence that they are entitled to access. Indeed, the Health Insurance Portability and Accountability Act (HIPAA) will be implemented as of April 2003 and will require several levels of security including some unique identifier of the individual, eg. with a unique electronic "key fob" or a method such as bioauthentication, e.g., electronic finger print scan or "retina" scan (I believe the latter have all actually been scans of the iris thus far), for access to confidential electronic patient information. Each new approach to security provides a new challenge to "hackers" and others interested in gaining access to information, for whatever reason. We will need to be increasingly more careful about how we manage confidential patient information as the Internet becomes our communication channel. More availability means more risk of loss of security. HIPAA will not be the last law to address this topic during the practice lifetime of most people reading this chapter.

ACCESS TO LITERATURE SEARCHES

Most of our careers in medicine began when literature searches required searching through 1 of roughly 25 volumes of roughly 1,000 pages each of citations for each year in order to find a few articles pertinent to a subject of interest. This required physical presence in the medical library, which was also required in most cases to be able to locate the journals of interest if one were fortunate enough to have that journal in that library's collection. Now, such searches can be conducted in much less time and with much more comprehensive results at home or at any personal computer or workstation with an Internet connection and a Web browser. The entire Medline and many other databases can be searched by topic, author, journal, title, text words, and other "switches." The search can also be performed for any year or years of interest. For example, when I use the Ovid software, available through the Galter Health Sciences Library of Northwestern University, I can search the entire Medline database from 1966 through the present. Furthermore, I can view at least the abstract for nearly any original paper for all except the earliest Medline entries and I can view the entire text and any figures for some journals.

Patients are clearly taking advantage of the scientific literature search resources on the Web as well. The National Library of Medicine (NLM) first made its literature search capabilities available to the public on the Web in 1996. The number of searches performed using the NLM Web interface increased from 7 million in 1996 to 120 million in 1997.[13] It seems likely that a large part of this increase in activity was due to searches by "patients" and other non-health professionals.

GENERAL WEB SEARCHING TOOLS

Web users will find information on virtually any topic. I challenge anyone to try to find a topic so obscure that they can't find it somewhere on the Web. Both of the current dominant Web browsers have "Search" as one of the most basic functions. Netscape Communicator responds to this choice by making several of the search engines available. The capabilities and response of each of these search engines seems to change rapidly and frequently. My current favorite choice is Google (*www.google.com*) because it always seems to give relevant responses to search requests. Microsoft Internet Explorer responds to its search choice with the proprietary Microsoft search engine, although the other search engines can be used if their URLs are known. My experience with the Explorer proprietary search engine has been that it provides less relevant responses to search requests and I prefer the ease of use of Netscape Communicator. Many individual physicians and health organizations have Web pages. There are Web pages dedicated to many disease entities from the common to the very uncommon. It is important for individuals and organizations that create and post such pages to "register" them so that the search engines are more likely to find them.

PROFESSIONAL SOCIETY COMMUNICATIONS AND MANAGEMENT

The activity of professional medical societies include communication with members, educational program development, meeting management, meeting registration, committee work, professional and public education, public relations, billing and collection of dues, and other society financial management services. All of these can be and have to some extent been moved to the Internet[14] in nearly all international, national, and larger regional medical societies in North America and Europe. Submission of abstracts of work to be considered for presentation at scientific meetings is now at least optional and is even mandatory for some societies like the American Association for Vascular Surgery and Society for Vascular Surgery. Review, scoring, and selection of abstracts by program committees has been nicely implemented using the Internet and can now be easily completed without any physical meeting of the Program Committee members. Larger national and international societies may spend well into 5 or even 6 figures (US dollars) per year on postage alone, not including stationery and envelopes, for routine mailings to members. These sums are not inconsequential as many societies find their balance sheets increasingly unfavorable. Such paper mailings are increasingly unnecessary and this task is very amenable to electronic e-mail. Conversion to all electronic mail is likely to be discussed in the Executive Committees of virtually all North American and European medical professional societies in the next few years. We were intrigued to learn that only about a third of the members of our regional vascular society have e-mail addresses known to our management company (and more than 20% of those appear to be incorrect!). Results of a test e-mailing to members of the Society for Vascular Surgery in spring 2002 were similar. Converting to all electronic correspondence may produce a little grumbling among the members, but if high school students can start and run successful Web page development companies, then it's fair to say that physicians can learn how to read their electronic mail.

VascularWeb (*www.VascularWeb.org*) is a pertinent example of how the Internet can be used to facilitate the activities of professional societies. VascularWeb was established under the sponsorship of the Joint Council of the American Association for Vascular Surgery and the Society for Vascular Surgery and the initial elements of the page went live in July of 2001. VascularWeb is now the World Wide Web organ of the AAVS, SVS, affiliated societies including The Canadian Society for Vascular Surgery, The Peripheral Vascular Surgery Society, Society for Clinical Vascular Surgery, The Association of Program Directors in Vascular Surgery, regional vascular societies in North America, and other member vascular specialty organizations. SVS, AAVS, and Midwestern Vascular Surgical Society are live as of the time of this writing and other member societies' pages will go live sequentially over the next several months.

VascularWeb provides a single portal for members and non-members wishing to learn more about member societies and vascular disease. Users can search for individual members of member societies with detailed information available only to other individual members of member societies with password protection. There is access to literature searches and to the Societies' official *Journal of Vascular Surgery*. Electronic submission of abstracts for consideration for presentation was required for the first time (no paper submissions were allowed) for the June 2002 meeting and VascularWeb was and will continue to be the interface used for these electronic submissions. There were a few technical problems, but these appear to have been solved and this same interface was used for the spring 2002 submissions for the Midwestern Vascular Surgical Society annual meeting in September 2002. VascularWeb has or will have sections for public education, for discussion of interesting, unusual, or difficult cases, a section for vascular fellows including educational materials and self assessment tests, and opinions of recognized leaders in the treatment of vascular disease. Committee work and electronic communication among committee members can also be facilitated using the tools available in VascularWeb.

ELECTRONIC PUBLISHING

It appears that despite interest in electronic publication, the activity of conventional printed journals has remained quite stable over the last 40 years.[15] Despite more than

20 years of time since electronic publication became technically possible, the number of articles published in conventional print journals appears highly correlated with the number of scientists. However, there has also been a proliferation of new electronic only "publication" using the Web implying an increase in total content published (print and electronic combined). PubMed Central is an electronic archive sponsored by the NIH providing full text and graphics from articles in many print and electronic only life sciences journals. This archive posts both peer-reviewed and non-reviewed materials and purports to clearly distinguish these. Print publishers are understandably concerned about their own future, but they can see that their future includes electronic publishing. Journal costs have risen faster than consumer prices, particularly the library subscription prices.[15] This has sparked considerable resentment among librarians and a strong debate in the research and publishing communities. Many if not most professional society sponsored journals, such as the *Journal of Vascular Surgery*, are now available with full text and graphics on-line to subscribers. CrossRef is a publisher initiated alternative to PubMed Central. CrossRef articles will require a subscription (fee), but publishers understandably point out that this funds the editorial and administrative functions so necessary to provide quality. CrossRef claims 142 participating publishers, more than 6,000 journals, and 5.1 million available articles, whereas PubMed Central claims more than 4,000 journals and 11 million articles as of June 2002. This conflict between "free" and "non-free" archives has spawned some rather unpleasant exchanges.[16,17]

Individuals may post "Web pages" or other text and image information on the Internet as fast as they can compose "content." The cost of space on servers is very low and in many cases, members of academic or business organizations may have free access to server space and to the Internet. Thus, we can conceive of a future where scientific publications would be found primarily on the Internet and not in printed journals. However, increased ease of publication and resultant increased volume of published information, as is clearly the potential result of the availability of the Web, may make good information more difficult to find and more expensive.[18] This may lead to a relative "information famine."

It seems likely that there will be an expanded role for information that never gets printed on paper, but we depend on the important peer review and editorial activities that have developed in the print journal world to provide the best possible papers. Abandoning these important filters as part of a move to electronic only journals would likely mean an increase in the amount of material and a decline in quality and reliability. It is too soon to tell how this will evolve, but we can only hope that critical editorial function will somehow be adapted for electronic only journals.[19]

DISCUSSION

The Internet and the various tools it provides are unquestionably destined to be critical means of information exchange. For vascular surgeons, this will likely include patient information, image files (angiograms, CT and MRI, ultrasound, etc.), financial and insurance information, academic and educational information, and professional society communications. Like it or not, if you plan to practice vascular surgery in the 21st century, you will need to learn how to make the Internet work for you and your patients. As more and more information related to vascular surgery appears on the

Web it will educate our consumers and inform our colleagues and our competition. One will be able to view the latest abstracts, obtain meeting information, abstract deadlines, and obtain registration forms. Instead of mailings from the various societies, those that wish may receive an e-mail message that the latest mailing is now at the Web site if one wants to examine it. In fact, many societies have or will soon insist that active members establish e-mail addresses and eliminate the use of "snail-mail" completely. Further directions that the Internet and Web will take are limited only by our imagination.

There are many hurdles yet to be crossed before the Internet becomes an indispensable resource for the practice of medicine. Yet, as has always been the case in medical progress during the last 100 years, clinical need drives progress and there is no question that the practice of medicine is information "hungry." Technologies that improve information exchange and can do so at lower costs will be very attractive to practicing physicians, payors, and patients.

Smithline and Christenson provide a careful review of pertinent literature on each of the questions they pose in the quote in the Introduction of this chapter.[3] The results are clearly mixed. The business solutions have made good progress and have the potential to allow great returns in terms of office staff productivity. On the other hand, the EMR remains cumbersome and has yet to be a real tool in most of the world.

There is no question that Information Technology can provide tools to improve patient care.[20] A major problem is that most institutions and organizations still see the Web primarily as a marketing tool.[21] This appears to be changing as organizations begin to provide more useful Web pages and patient use of the Internet for health information is growing at 3–4 times the general rate of Internet growth.[22] As of mid-2001, it was estimated that there were more than 70,000 health related Web sites available and more than 50 million people used the Internet seeking health information.[23] Despite this increasing activity, Health Internet companies are, like their non-health "dot com" fellows, going through a period of difficulty.[24]

The first challenge for software developers and marketers in particular is to develop tools that do improve workflow. Their products will be spurned without this. The frustrations of wasted time and effort in my practice and that of virtually every reader of this chapter, I suspect, provide ample opportunity for improvement. The second challenge for developers will be to convince users that their tools work. We have all been disappointed by promises from software manufacturers that were unfulfilled. The complexities of, for examples, electronic medical records and billing 1 of the 1,500 or so payors in the United States dwarf the task posed by past software needs. If the developers stumble trying to build an accounts receivable system for small business, can they possibly integrate all the information required for billing and collection for an enterprise that currently represents one-seventh of the Gross Domestic Product in the United States? We have learned to be skeptical about promises made by software developers. On the other hand, developers who can solve the technical problems and make a strong case that their tools provide a cost-effective solution to the present problem of information overload faced by physicians will likely succeed in their business.

The Internet brings the promise of information integration so that that information can be available to anyone in the world with an appropriate access to that information. The care of patients can only improve with better information management. This may be the area of greatest potential for improvement in quality of both patient care and resource management in the immediate future.

REFERENCES

1. Schneider JR, Lindsay TF. The Internet and vascular surgery: A brief description of the Internet, the World Wide Web, and some of the vascular surgical resources available. *Vasc Surg.* 1997;31:605–613.
2. Feied C. Telecommunications and the next generation Internet for health care. *Ann Emerg Med.* 2001;38:293–302.
3. Smithline N, Christenson E. Physicians and the internet: Understanding where we are and where we are going. *J Ambulatory Care Manage.* 2001;24:39–53.
4. McCormack J. The top 10 ways the Internet is changing health care I.T. *Health Data Manage.* 1999;7:34–39.
5. Runy LA. How the net will reshape health care. *Hosp Health Netw.* 2000;74:suppl 4–7.
6. Robinson JC. The end of managed care. *JAMA.* 2001;285:2622–2628.
7. Fischman J. A logon a day keeps the doctor away. Patients have someone to watch over them. *US News and World Report.* 1999;127(16):65
8. Rubin R. The virtual doctor will see you now. *USA Today.* June 10, 2002, page 1.
9. Goedert J. Do-it-yourself online records. *Health Data Manage.* 1999;7(7):28–29.
10. Terry K. How the device in your hand can put more money in your pocket. *Med Econ.* 2001;78:44–50.
11. Terry K. E-health gurus still expect to transform your world. *Med Econ.* 2001;78:20–22.
12. O'Reilly M. Are more online conferences on the way? *Can Med Assoc.* J 2000;163:322.
13. Sieving PC. Factors driving the increase in medical information on the web-One American perspective. *J Med Internet Res.* 1999;1:e3.
14. Allen J. Surgical Internet at a glance: Volume IX. *Amer J Surg* 1999;177:183.
15. Tenopir C, King DW. Lessons for the future of journals. *Nature.* 2001;413(6857):672–674.
16. Marshall E. Publish and perish in the Internet world. *Science.* 2000;289:288–289.
17. Macilwain C. Internet publishing camps renew hostilities. *Nature.* 2000;406:112.
18. Coiera E. Information economics and the Internet. *J Am Med Inform Assoc.* 2000;7:215–221.
19. Harris ED. Printed journals and the Internet: A functional relationship. *Pharos.* 2000;63:1.
20. Gawande AA, Bates DW. The use of information technology in improving medical performance-Part II. Physician-support tools. *Medscape Ge Med.* 2000;2. *http://www.medscape.com/viewarticle/408033*
21. Weber DO. Web sites of tomorrow. How the Internet will transform health. *Health Forum J.* 1999;May-June:40–45.
22. Bell H. Going interactive. Once the laggards of interactivity, hospitals are beginning to build Web sites consumers can use. *Healthcare Informatics.* 2000;April:85–92.
23. Cline JW, Haynes KM. Consumer health information seeking on the Internet: the state of the art. *Health Educ Res.* 2001;16(6):671–692.
24. Larkin M. Are health internet companies heading for extinction? *Lancet.* 2001;357(9253):368.

The following articles are not cited in the text, but may be of interest to those seeking a more basic historical perspective on the Internet and medicine

Cimino JJ, Socratous SA, Clayton PD. Internet as clinical information system: application development using world wide web. *J Am Med Informatics Assoc.* 1995;2:273–284.
Ellenberger B. Navigating physician resources on the Internet. *Can Med Assoc J.* 1995;152: 1303–1307.
Glowniak JV, Bushway MK. Computer networks as a medical resource. Accessing and using the Internet. *JAMA.* 1994;271:1934–1939.
Glowniak JV. Medical resources on the Internet. *Ann Intern Med.* 1995;123:123–131.
Lindberg DA, Humphreys BL. Computers in medicine. *JAMA.* 1995;273:16671668.
Millman A, Lee N, Kealy K. ABC of medical computing. The Internet. *Brit Med J.* 1995;311: 440–443.

APPENDIX

A Brief Listing of Interesting World Wide Web Pages
Selected Academic, Society, and Journal URL

http://www.VascularWeb.org
VascularWeb (includes Society for Vascular Surgery, American Association for Vascular Surgery, and several other affiliated societies)

http://www.harcourthealth.com/scripts/om.dll/serve?action=searchDB&searchDBfor= home&id=vs
Journal of Vascular Surgery (also via link from VascularWeb)

http://www.nih.gov/
NIH Home Page

http://www.esvs.org/
European Society for Vascular Surgery

http://www.harcourt-international.com/journals/ejvs
European Journal of Vascular and Endovascular Surgery

http://www.ama-assn.org/
AMA Home Page

http://www.facs.org/
American College of Surgeons

Selected Business to Consumer (B2C) URL

http://www.cbsnews.com/sections/health/main204.shtml
CBS Health Watch

http://www.drkoop.com/
(named for former Surgeon General C. Everett Koop)

http://www.webmd.com/
WebMD consumer target Web site plus practice management software

http://www.intelihealth.com/
InteliHealth sponsored by Aetna

http://www.healthfinder.gov/
HealthFinder US Dept. of Heath and Human Services

http://www.wellmed.com/wellmed/
WellMed

http://www.lifemasters.com/
LifeMasters

http://www.healthgrades.com
HealthGrades hospital ratings (and probably physicians soon)

http://www.healthweb.org/
HealthWeb (health information for both consumers and practitioners)

http://www.subimo.com/
    Subimo health information provided by subscription

Selected Business to Business (B2B) URL (many sites in the B2C section above provide both B2C and B2B content)

http://www.medunite.com/
    MedUnite, a consortium of several health insurance companies

http://www.ePocrates.com
    Prescription drug information for Personal Digital Assistants
    Electronic Publishing Archives and Electronic Search URL

http://www.pubmedcentral.nih.gov/
    PubMed Central NIH archive of life sciences journals

http://www.crossref.org/
    CrossRef a publisher initiated journal archive

http://www.nlm.nih.gov/
    National Library of Medicine

VII

Aorta and Its Major Branches

23

Endovascular Management of Renovascular Disease

Thomas T. Terramani, MD and
Elliot L. Chaikof, MD, PhD

Renovascular disease is a progressive process that, while often silent in its initial clinical presentation, can result in 2 clinical syndromes—hypertension with all its associated sequelae and renal ischemia with parenchymal loss and a decrease in excretory renal function. The most common cause of renovascular disease is renal artery stenosis (RAS) of which 80–90% of cases are due to atherosclerosis and 10–15% attributed to fibromuscular dysplasia. Significantly, renovascular hypertension may affect up to 2 million people in the United States, and, as many as 40% of patients with a hemodynamically significant stenosis will progress to complete renal artery occlusion.[1] In this regard, abundant evidence suggests that untreated disease will progress to chronic renal failure, which has been substantiated by a 12% incidence of renal artery atherosclerosis observed among patients receiving dialysis.[2]

Despite numerous clinical reports, 5 randomized clinical trial,[3–7] and 2 recent meta-analyses[8,9] the optimal role of catheter based interventions for symptomatic renovascular disease associated with uncontrolled hypertension or ischemic nephropathy remains incompletely defined. Characteristically, medical therapy for atherosclerotic RAS results in persistent renal ischemia with eventual loss of renal mass and a risk of dialysis dependency.[10,11] Over the past 3 decades, surgical reconstruction, including endarterectomy and bypass grafting, has been the mainstay of treatment for renal artery disease with excellent long-term results and an acceptable morbidity and mortality. Nonetheless, encouraging outcomes reported during the past 10 years for percutaneous transluminal renal angioplasty and percutaneous transluminal renal artery stenting has lead to their adoption as preferred modalities with increasing frequency.

In 1978 Grüntzig et al.[12] introduced the technique of percutaneous transluminal angioplasty for the treatment of RAS and within a decade balloon-expandable stents were introduced by Palmaz et al.[13] to reduce restenosis due to elastic recoil and as a "bailout" for suboptimal or complicated angioplasty. Shorter hospital stay, reduced complication rates, and the avoidance of major surgery have all driven the adoption of angioplasty and stenting despite the absence of conclusive randomized clinical trials.

In this chapter, we review current available data regarding endovascular treatment options for the management of symptomatic RAS.

DIAGNOSIS

The diagnosis of renovascular disease should be entertained in any patient that exhibits acute worsening of previously well-controlled hypertension, malignant hypertension, or new onset hypertension after the age of 55 years. Likewise, significant asymmetry in kidney size, unexplained renal dysfunction, or a deterioration of renal function that is precipitated by angiotensin-converting-enzyme inhibitors should also initiate an evaluation for renovascular disease. Unfortunately, a single reliable test to determine whether a RAS is responsible for hypertension or excretory renal dysfunction does not exist. With that said, noninvasive evaluations remain a critical initial step for identifying those patients that have significant anatomic disease of the renal artery. Moreover, since conventional angiography may be associated with renal artery atheroembolism, contrast associated nephropathy, and puncture site complications, it should not be utilized in the initial evaluation of RAS. The principle role of contrast angiography is to confirm the diagnosis made by the noninvasive studies and to evaluate lesion extent and distribution.

Renal artery duplex ultrasonography has been advocated as a useful, inexpensive, and noninvasive screening tool for RAS. For example, 2 recent reports have demonstrated that a renal artery peak systolic velocity that exceeded 180–200 cm/sec is a reliable indicator of a stenosis that exceeds 60% with a sensitivity of 91–94%.[14,15] In an effort to identify patients with significant intraparenchymal renal artery disease, Radermacher and associates[16] have proposed the use of a renal artery resistance index defined as:

$$\text{Resistance Index} = (1 - [\text{end-diastolic velocity/maximal systolic velocity}]) \times 100$$

In their analysis of 138 patients who underwent renal artery angioplasty or surgery, a renal resistance-index value of greater than 80 reliably identified patients with a RAS in whom angioplasty or surgery did not lead to improved renal function, blood pressure, or kidney survival. Among institutions that do not have sufficient expertise in ultrasonography, magnetic resonance angiography (MRA) has become the preferred initial diagnostic study. In contrast to computed tomography angiography, gadolinium may be administered to patients with renal insufficiency. However, while MRA is associated with very few false negatives, differentiating between a moderate and severe stenosis may be difficult. Additional functional studies, such as captopril renal scintigraphy and renal vein renins, may occasionally be helpful in assessing the functional significance of a lesion. However, these studies are generally unreliable in the presence of bilateral renal artery disease.

TECHNIQUE

Appropriate pre-interventional therapy is a prerequisite for optimizing the likelihood of a successful treatment outcome. Patients are hydrated overnight and no oral intake permitted 8 hours prior to the procedure. Aspirin (81 mg) is initiated 24 hours prior to intervention and all antihypertensive medications are held the morning of the procedure in order to avoid a precipitous decrease in blood pressure that may occur following angioplasty.

Technological advancements in guidewires, catheters, and stents have lead to more reliable, safer and less traumatic renal artery interventions. Improvements in guidewire design include the addition of hydrophilic coatings, atraumatic tips, and high torque control; and have all been implemented on wires of increasingly smaller diameter (e.g., 0.018 and 0.014 mm). Many of these same features have been incorporated into the development of preshaped diagnostic catheters and guiding sheaths of increasingly smaller caliber and improved torque control. Likewise, angioplasty balloon catheters are now produced with lower profiles, greater trackability, and improved inflation/deflation properties.

Percutaneous access is best obtained from the ipsilateral femoral artery approach. If there is a marked downward angulation of the renal artery a left brachial artery approach may be helpful. A preshaped diagnostic catheter (Motarjame, Cobra, or RDC) is used to engage the renal artery, which is confirmed with a small hand injection of contrast dye. Patients are systemically heparinized prior to crossing the stenosis with a 0.035 mm Bentson guidewire. The catheter is then advanced across the lesion and a pressure gradient can be measured. We typically administer 100–200 μg of nitroglycerin intra-arterially to reduce the risk of vessel spasm. Once the renal artery has been selected, a guiding sheath is advanced to the ostium of the renal artery. At this stage, the Bentson wire is exchanged for a 0.018 or 0.014 mm guidewire. The size of the adjacent normal renal artery will dictate the selection of the balloon catheter, which should be slight oversized. Once the angioplasty is completed, a selective angiogram is performed to assess the result and to exclude dissection, rupture, or occlusion. Pressure measurements can also be performed at this time.

The role of stent placement has evolved from an adjunct initially applied primarily for suboptimal angioplasty due to restenosis, dissection, or residual stenosis to a primary treatment option for atherosclerotic ostial lesions of the renal artery.[3,17,18] The technique of percutaneous stent placement is similar to angioplasty. We generally favor predilating the stenosis, often with a 4 mm balloon, prior to advancing a catheter-mounted stent. We prefer balloon expandable stents for renal artery lesions since they undergo minimal foreshortening and have greater hoop strength than most self-expanding stents. Once the stent is in position, contrast injection through the guiding sheath will facilitate final positioning and optimal deployment.

After peripheral interventions, blood pressure should be closely monitored after the procedure and medications adjusted accordingly. Our current practice is to place all patients on aspirin and clopidogrel (Plavix) with an initial 300 mg loading dose followed by 75 mg per day for 3 to 6 months. Most studies involving the use of thienopyridines, such as clopidogrel or ticlopidine, and arterial stents have focused on their application in coronary artery disease. In the STARS trial 1965 patients undergoing coronary stenting were randomized to aspirin alone, aspirin and warfarin, and aspirin and ticlopidine.[19] Patients who received aspirin and ticlopidine had a significantly lower rate of stent thrombosis compared to the other 2 groups. The clinical benefit was noticed up to 12 months although no reduction in restenosis was observed.

COMPLICATIONS OF PERCUTANEOUS RENAL ARTERY INTERVENTIONS

The complication rate of percutaneous renal artery interventions has been reported to be as high as 14%[20,21] and may include cholesterol emobolization, dissection, thrombosis, contrast induced nephrotoxicity, vasospasm, guidewire perforation, and arterial rupture. While surgical intervention may be required for renal salvage, endovascular approaches may be appropriate in selected patients.[22,23] For example, Salam et al.[22] reported our experience with the treatment of 10 patients with acute renal artery occlusion, most often associated with angioplasty, by local infusion of a thrombolytic agent. Revascularization was achieved in 7 of 10 patients without major bleeding or death. Likewise, Morris et al.[23] described the treatment of 13 patients with acute iatrogenic renal artery complications after percutaneous renal artery interventions, all of who were managed without surgery. Five patients with acute rupture of the renal artery were treated immediately with balloon tamponade or with placement of an additional stent or stent-graft. Six patients suffered acute thrombotic occlusion; 5 were successfully treated with thrombolysis, and 1 was successfully treated without thrombolysis by the placement of an additional stent. Presumed distal guidewire perforation caused subcapsular hematoma in 1 patient and a perirenal and pararenal hematoma in another. Both events were successfully treated with conservative management. During a mean clinical follow-up period of 19 months, 1 patient required long-term hemodialysis, but no other patient required additional treatment.

The most significant recent innovation designed to reduce iatrogenic renal artery injury has been the reduction in guidewire and catheter dimensions to accommodate 0.014 mm systems. In addition, use of intravascular protection devices has also been proposed as an adjunctive technique to eliminate embolic events to the renal parenchyma during a percutaneous intervention. Characteristically, microembolization is associated with catheter and guidewire manipulations, but the true incidence of this problem during percutaneous procedures of the renal arteries remains unknown. Despite some uncertainty of the magnitude of this problem, Henry et al.[24] used a distal protection device (PercuSurge) in 28 patients during renal artery stenting. The technical success rate was 100% with debris retrieved in all instances. After a mean follow-up period of 6 months, improvement in renal function was observed in 5 patients and was otherwise stable in the remainder.

RANDOMIZED CLINICAL TRIALS

To date, the utility of percutaneous renal artery interventions has been addressed in 5 randomized trails. Three reports have compared angioplasty with antihypertensive medical therapy,[4,5,7] one study compared angioplasty and stenting,[3] and an additional review evaluated angioplasty with surgical management.[6] van Jaarsveld and associates[4] enrolled 106 patients from 26 centers in a prospective randomized trial of medical therapy versus angioplasty for the management of renovascular hypertension. No significant difference in mean blood pressure or serum creatinine levels was observed between the 2 treatment groups at 12 months. However, angioplasty was associated with a greater reduction in the number of antihypertensive medications than the drug treatment group (2.1 vs. 3.2). Moreover, within 3 months nearly half of all patients in the medical arm of this trial crossed over to angioplasty because of poorly controlled hypertension while on 3 of more antihypertensive agents. Notably, renal artery occlusion occurred in 9% of patients on drug therapy group, while no occlusions were observed among those patients treated by angioplasty. Nonetheless, a 42% incidence of restenosis was noted after angioplasty leading the authors to recommend that this intervention should be restricted to patients with poorly controlled hypertension (>3 medications) or those demonstrating a progressive decrease in renal function.

In a similar effort, Plouin and associates[7] randomly assigned 49 patients with renovascular hypertension to drug therapy or angioplasty. Despite a 13% restenosis rate at 6 months, anti-hypertensive medications were discontinued in 26% of patients treated with angioplasty and many of the remaining patients were well controlled on fewer medications. As anticipated, drug requirements persisted in the medical group. The short-term benefit of angioplasty has also been confirmed by Webster and associates.[5] While all of these results are promising, a paucity of clinical follow-up data beyond 12 months remains a significant limitation of these investigations. In addition, it is also noteworthy that while primary technical success rates as high as 93% have been reported with angioplasty alone, these results are substantially better than those noted by others. For example, Isles[8] and Leertouwer[9] have reported technical success rates of 42% and 77%, respectively.

In an effort to reduce the risk of restenosis that is all too often associated with ostial lesions, a randomized prospective trial was designed to compare the efficacy of stenting or angioplasty among 85 patients with ostial renal artery disease.[3] Among patients treated with angioplasty alone, the technical success rate was a sobering 57% and within 6 months primary patency was reduced to a mere 29% with a 48% incidence of restenosis. Stent placements lead to significantly improved outcomes with a technical success rate of 88%, a 6-month patency of 75%, and a 14% incidence of restenosis. Surprisingly, improved patency rates were not associated with a commensurate benefit in clinical outcome. Improvement or cure of hypertension was observed in roughly half of all patients with little difference in serum creatinine levels between the 2 groups. Limitations of this report include the absence of follow-up beyond 6 months and the failure or inability to confirm the clinical significance of the target lesion.

META-ANALYSIS

Leertouwer et al.[9] has recently published a meta-analysis of 14 studies in which patients were treated by angioplasty and stent placement (678 patients) and an additional 10 reports in which the mode of therapy was angioplasty alone (644 patients). The technical success rate of stenting was 98% with an 11% incidence of in-hospital morbidity and restenosis in 17% of treated vessels over a mean follow-up period of 17 months. Hypertension was cured in 20% and improved in 49% of patients. Among patients with renal insufficiency, function was improved in 30% and stabilized in an additional 38% of patients. In contrast, the technical success rate of angioplasty was 77%, with restenosis occurring in 1 of every 4 treated lesions.

In a review of our own experience at Emory, we recently assessed our results in 73 patients that underwent angioplasty and stenting of 85 renal arteries for predominately ostial disease.[25] Stents were selectively deployed for sub-optimal angioplasty (52%) or dissection (24%). Our overall primary technical success was 89% with an assisted technical success rate of 94%, and a 30-day mortality of 1.4%. Major complications occurred in 9.1% of patients including access artery thrombosis (n = 4), renal artery extravasation (n = 1), renal artery thrombosis (n = 1), and hematoma requiring operation (n = 2). Long-term clinical data were available on 69 (95%) patients at 20 ± 17 months. Sixty-one patients (84%) had a systolic blood pressure less than or equal to 160 mm Hg, and 65 (89%) had a diastolic blood pressure less than or equal to 90 mm Hg. Four patients

(5.5%) were off all anti-hypertensive medications. In 16 patients (22%) serum creatinine decreased by more than 20% and was stable in an additional 35 patients (48%). Deterioration of renal function (increase of >20%) was observed in 18 patients (25%) and of these 9 patients (12%) required dialysis at an interval of 17.4 ± 13.0 months (range, 0.8–39.1 months) after angioplasty. Five of these patients had preoperative serum creatinine levels greater than 4.0 mg/dL and has served to identify for our group a population that, more often than not, shows little benefit to intervention.

Routine follow-up imaging was not routinely performed in our population. However, angiography was performed for worsening hypertension or recurring renal insufficiency in 15 patients (20.5%) who had initially responded favorably to renal artery stenting. There were 14 in-stent restenoses (15%) in 14 renal arteries of 10 patients occurring at 11.3 ± 10.3 months. Eleven (79%) of the restenotic lesions were ostial. Intervention was not advocated for 5 patients in which a moderate restenosis was noted. Of the remaining lesions, 50% were successfully treated by angioplasty alone (n=4), stent implantation (n=3), or surgical revascularization (n=2).

As in our series, most series lack long-term clinical outcome and patency data. However, Rodriquez et al.[26] reported encouraging primary and secondary patency rates of 74% and 85%, respectively, at 36 months in a retrospective analysis of 108 patients with 125 renal artery lesions that were all treated with angioplasty and stenting. Given the ongoing risk of restenosis, we recommend continued duplex ultrasonography surveillance following intervention.[27] Notably, ferromagnetic artifacts caused by the stent material limits the use of magnetic resonance angiography.

STENTING OR ANGIOPLASTY ALONE FOR ATHEROSCLEROTIC RAS?

Angioplasty alone has been shown to be very effective in the treatment of most types of renal artery fibromuscular dysplasia lesions. The procedure is successful in 82 to 100% of patients with an associated restenosis rate of 10 to 11%.[28,29] Branch vessel disease, however, is less amenable to angioplasty. Overall, angioplasty alone is also less effective in the treatment of atherosclerotic RAS because of increased vessel rigidity, elastic recoil, and inherent risk of vessel dissection. In particular, failure rates for ostial lesions have been relatively high with associated restenosis rates of 10 to 45%. Since ostial lesions are a continuation of aortic plaque that encroaches and protrudes within the renal artery, these lesions are more resistant to dilatation and have an increase risk of dissection, acute thrombosis, and elastic recoil as compared with non-ostial atherosclerosis. Undoubtedly, the introduction of stents has significantly improved the clinical success of angioplasty. While the initial motivation of this adjunct was as a means to improve suboptimal outcomes of angioplasty, there is a growing consensus that stent placement should be a component of the routine management of renovascular occlusive disease with the exception of fibromuscular dysplasia.

CONCLUSIONS

Renovascular disease is often subtle in presentation and progressive in nature and a high clinical suspicion is required to identify patients with a treatable lesion. The clinical progression to renal failure and the sequelae of hypertension is often irreversible in the absence of intervention and the objectives of treatment remain cure or improvement of hypertension along with preservation of excretory renal function. Surgical revascularization yields excellent long-term results, but is associated with a significant risk of major morbidity and a prolonged period of convalescence. Outcomes following endovascular management of RAS have improved since its inception and gains will likely be achieved with newer devices and technologies. As such, the recent introduction of drug eluting stents, that have dramatically reduced the risk of restenosis after coronary artery angioplasty, holds much promise for improving the efficacy of renal artery interventions. Nonetheless, major morbidity, and even death, can occur even in the hands of a skilled interventionalist and it is often difficult to discern those patients that will achieve maximum benefit. Thus, in the absence of carefully analyzed long-term outcomes, it will remain difficult to determine whether angioplasty and stenting is the preferred intervention for all patients or best reserved for those at high risk for surgical treatment with poorly controlled hypertension and/or deteriorating renal function.

REFERENCES

1. Schreiber MJ, Pohl MA, Novick AC. The natural history of atherosclerotic and fibrous renal artery disease. *Urol Clin North Am.* 1984;11(3):383–392.
2. Mailloux LU, Napolitano B, Bellucci AG, et al. Renal vascular disease causing end-stage renal disease, incidence, clinical correlates, and outcomes: A 20-year clinical experience. *Am J Kidney Dis.* 1994;24(4):622–629.
3. van de Ven PJ, Kaatee R, Beutler JJ, et al. Arterial stenting and balloon angioplasty in ostial atherosclerotic renovascular disease: A randomized trial. *Lancet.* 1999;353(9149):282–286.
4. van Jaarsveld BC, Krijnen P, Pieterman H, et al. The effect of balloon angioplasty on hypertension in atherosclerotic renal-artery stenosis. Dutch Renal Artery Stenosis Intervention Cooperative Study Group. *N Engl J Med.* 2000;342(14):1007–1014.
5. Webster J, Marshall F, Abdalla M, et al. Randomized comparison of percutaneous angioplasty vs. continued medical therapy for hypertensive patients with atheromatous renal artery stenosis. Scottish and Newcastle Renal Artery Stenosis Collaborative Group. *J Hum Hypertens.* 1998;12(5):329–335.
6. Weibull H, Bergqvist D, Bergentz SE, et al. Percutaneous transluminal renal angioplasty versus surgical reconstruction of atherosclerotic renal artery stenosis: A prospective randomized study. *J Vasc Surg.* 1993;18(5):841–852.
7. Plouin PF, Chatellier G, Darne B, et al. Blood pressure outcome of angioplasty in atherosclerotic renal artery stenosis: A randomized trial. Essai Multicentrique Medicaments vs Angioplastie (EMMA) Study Group. *Hypertension* 1998;31(3):823–829.
8. Isles CG, Robertson S, Hill D. Management of renovascular disease: A review of renal artery stenting in ten studies. *QJM.* 1999;92(3):159–167.
9. Leertouwer TC, Gussenhoven EJ, Bosch JL, et al. Stent placement for renal arterial stenosis: Where do we stand? A meta-analysis. *Radiology.* 2000;216(1):78–85.
10. Scoble JE, Maher ER, Hamilton G, et al. Atherosclerotic renovascular disease causing renal impairment-A case for treatment. *Clin Nephrol.* 1989;31(3):119–122.
11. Zierler RE, Bergelin RO, Davidson RC, et al. A prospective study of disease progression in patients with atherosclerotic renal artery stenosis. *Am J Hypertens.* 1996;9(11):1055–1061.
12. Gruntzig A, Kuhlmann U, Vetter W, et al. Treatment of renovascular hypertension with percutaneous transluminal dilatation of a renal-artery stenosis. *Lancet.* 1978;1(8068):801–802.
13. Palmaz JC, Kopp DT, Hayashi H, et al. Normal and stenotic renal arteries: experimental balloon-expandable intraluminal stenting. *Radiology.* 1987;164(3):705–708.
14. Hua HT, Hood DB, Jensen CC, et al. The use of colorflow duplex scanning to detect significant renal artery stenosis. *Ann Vasc Surg.* 2000;14(2):118–124.
15. Motew SJ, Cherr GS, Craven TE, et al. Renal duplex sonography: Main renal artery versus hilar analysis. *J Vasc Surg.* 2000;32(3):462–471.

16. Radermacher J, Chavan A, Bleck J, et al. Use of Doppler ultrasonography to predict the outcome of therapy for renal-artery stenosis. *N Engl J Med.* 2001;344(6):410–417.
17. Blum U, Krumme B, Flugel P, et al. Treatment of ostial renal-artery stenoses with vascular endoprostheses after unsuccessful balloon angioplasty. *N Engl J Med.* 1997;336(7):459–465.
18. Bakker J, Goffette PP, Henry M, et al. The Erasme study: A multicenter study on the safety and technical results of the Palmaz stent used for the treatment of atherosclerotic ostial renal artery stenosis. *Cardiovasc Intervent Radiol* 1999;22(6):468–474.
19. Leon M, Baim DS, Popma JJ, et al: A clinical trial comparing three antithrombotic-drug regimens after coronary-artery stenting. *N Eng J Med.* 1998;339(23):1665–1671.
20. Mahler F, Triller J, Weidmann P. Complications in percutaneous transluminal dilatation of renal arteries. *Nephron.* 1986;44 Suppl 1:60–63.
21. Martin LG, Casarella WJ, Alspaugh JP. Renal artery angioplasty: Increased technical success and decreased complications in the second 100 patients. *Radiology.* 1986;159(3):631–634.
22. Salam TA, Lumsden AB, Martin LG. Local infusion of fibrinolytic agents for acute renal artery thromboembolism: Report of ten cases. *Ann Vasc Surg.* 1993;7(1):21–26.
23. Morris CS, Bonnevie GJ, Najarian KE. Nonsurgical treatment of acute iatrogenic renal artery injuries occurring after renal artery angioplasty and stenting. *AJR Am J Roentgenol.* 2001;177(6):1353–1357.
24. Henry M, Klonaris C, Henry I, et al. Protected renal stenting with the PercuSurge GuardWire device: A pilot study. *J Endovasc Ther.* 2001;8(3):227–237.
25. Bush RL, Najibi S, MacDonald MJ, et al. Endovascular revascularization of renal artery stenosis: Technical and clinical results. *J Vasc Surg.* 2001;33(5):1041–1049.
26. Rodriguez-Lopez JA, Werner A, Ray LI, et al. Renal artery stenosis treated with stent deployment: Indications, technique, and outcome for 108 patients. *J Vasc Surg.* 1999;29(4):617–624.
27. Sharafuddin MJ, Raboi CA, Abu-Yousef M, et al. Renal artery stenosis: Duplex US after angioplasty and stent placement. *Radiology.* 2001;220(1):168–173.
28. Tegtmeyer CJ, Selby JB, Hartwell GD, et al. Results and complications of angioplasty in fibromuscular disease. *Circulation.* 1991;83(2 Suppl):I155–61.
29. Kidney DD, Deutsch LS. The indications and results of percutaneous transluminal angioplasty and stenting in renal artery stenosis. *Semin Vasc Surg.* 1996;9(3):188–197.

24

Endovascular Interventions for Chronic Mesenteric Ischemia

*Jeffrey V. Behar, MD, Alan H. Matsumoto, MD,
J. Fritz Angle, MD, David J. Spinosa, MD,
Klaus D. Hagspiel, MD, Dorothy L. Cage, MSN, ACNP,
and Daniel A. Leung, MD*

Chronic mesenteric ischemia develops when visceral blood flow is unable to support the physiologic demands of the gastrointestinal tract. Although the abdominal aorta and mesenteric arteries are frequently affected by atherosclerosis, the clinical manifestations of mesenteric ischemia are uncommon. Bowel viability is usually preserved due to the abundant collateral circulation that exists among the mesenteric vessels. Mesenteric hypoperfusion usually results from compromised blood flow in at least 2 of the mesenteric arteries, but may occur due to significant disease in a single mesenteric artery. Once intestinal angina develops, patients will exhibit symptoms of postprandial abdominal pain, "fear of food," and progressive weight loss. Nausea, vomiting, and diarrhea are less common symptoms, and are nonspecific for mesenteric ischemia. Patients may also present with acute ischemic symptoms due to progression of chronic disease.

DIAGNOSTIC EVALUATION

Patients with symptoms of chronic mesenteric ischemia traditionally have been evaluated with biplane abdominal aortography to thoroughly define the origins of the celiac, superior mesenteric, and inferior mesenteric arteries. Patients with hemodynamically significant stenosis in 1 or more mesenteric arteries are candidates for endovascular revascularization. Lesions are considered significant when narrowing of the cross sectional area is equal to or greater than 70% or a diameter stenosis of greater than 50%. Stenoses are also considered significant when the cross sectional area narrowing is 50 to 70%, with a translesion peak to peak systolic pressure gradient of greater than 20 mmHg.[1]

Noninvasive imaging may be useful to screen patients in whom there is concern for chronic mesenteric ischemia, reserving the use of catheter angiography as the "gold standard" prior to surgical or percutaneous intervention or in cases in which the noninvasive study is not definitive in excluding significant mesenteric vascular disease. Duplex sonography has been used to measure arterial velocity, however, evaluation is limited due to patient habitus, shadowing from bowel gas, aorta pulsatility and operator inexperience.[2,3] Lack of uniform criteria for the diagnosis of hemodynamically significant stenoses limits the reproducibility of songraphic evaluation. Blebea et al. recently compared the use of contrast-enhanced duplex ultrasound to duplex ultrasound alone in the evaluation of mesenteric arteries in 17 patients with symptoms of chronic mesenteric ischemia. Including the aorta, the study consisted of 68 vessels. Duplex ultrasound alone identified 38 of 48 normal vessels (79% accuracy). Contrast-enhanced duplex ultrasound identified 44 of 48 normal vessels (90% accuracy). Duplex ultrasound alone identified 5 of 11 stenoses ≥50% and 6 of 9 occlusions (45% and 67% accuracy, respectively), whereas the use of contrast-enhanced ultrasound improved the diagnosis of stenoses ≥50% to 7 of 11 (78% accuracy) without altering the accuracy of detecting occluded vessels. Despite the use of experienced sonographers, 12 of 68 vessels were not visualized with duplex ultrasound alone, and 3 of 68 vessels were not visualized with contrast-enhanced ultrasound. Despite the small sample size of this report, contrast-enhanced ultrasound appears to improve the visualization of mesenteric arteries and may improve the diagnosis of mesenteric arterial stenosis. However, the routine use of duplex sonography for the detection of clinically significant mesenteric arterial stenoses remains very challenging at most institutions.

CT has been utilized for the evaluation of the abdominal aorta, renal arteries, and mesenteric arteries. With the advent of multi-detector CT, routine studies can be performed much faster and with thinner collimation than with single detector CT, allowing CT angiography to become a more useful and reproducible technique for vascular imaging. Direct comparisons of CT angiography and catheter angiography for the evaluation of the mesenteric arteries have not been reported, however, several studies suggest that CT angiography compares favorably with catheter angiography for the evaluation of renal artery stenosis.[4–7] Rapid scanning eliminates respiratory motion artifact and allows imaging during both the arterial and venous phases. Narrow beam collimation (0.5–1 mm) reduces volume averaging artifacts, improves vessel edge conspicuity, and allows visualization of small vessel branches. Additionally, CT potentially allows for the evaluation of some of the secondary signs of bowel ischemia, such as bowel wall thickening, submucosal hemorrhage, abnormal bowel wall enhancement, stranding within the mesenteric fat due to edema, and/or pneumatosis. Ingestion of water may also be utilized as a low-attenuation oral contrast without limiting the evaluation of mesenteric arteries.[8]

Gadolinium-enhanced 3-D MR angiography (MRA) allows for noninvasive imaging of the aorta, and the proximal portions of the mesenteric and renal arteries without the administration of nephrotoxic contrast agents or exposure to radiation. Carlos et al. have reported on the interobserver variability in the evaluation of chronic mesenteric ischemia with gadolinium-enhanced 3-D MRA as compared to catheter angiography. Two readers, blinded to the catheter angiography results, reviewed the gadolinium-enhanced MRA in 26 patients. The relative sensitivity and specificity of 3-D gadolinium-enhanced MRA compared well to catheter angiography, with a cumulative accuracy of 0.98 with a 95% confidence interval of 0.91–1.0 for lesions equal to or greater than 75%, and 0.94 with a 95% confidence interval of 0.84–0.98 for lesions ranging from 50%–75%. Image resolution is the greatest disadvantage of gadolinium-enhanced 3-D MRA. Current MR imaging abilities have a maximum spatial resolution of 1 mm,[3] while catheter angiography has submillimeter resolution (Figure 24–1). Currently, 3-D gadolinium-enhanced MRA does not provide sufficient resolution to image distal emboli, nonocclusive low flow states, small vessel occlusion, or vasculitis, and, therefore, is not a good screening tool to exclude acute mesenteric ischemia, unless mesenteric venous thrombosis is the primary concern. Additionally, an insignificant mild proximal stenosis may limit detection of distal disease.[9]

TREATMENT

Revascularization of the mesenteric circulation in patients with symptoms of mesenteric ischemia greatly improves the patient's prognosis. Surgical revascularization of occlusive mesenteric ischemia consists of transaortic endaterectomy and/or end-to-end aortomesenteric grafting. The technical success rate of surgical procedures approaches 95%,[10–12] with long-term clinical success rates ranging from 61% to 100%.[13–18] Operative morbidity ranges from 20% to 54%, with a 30-day mortality rate of 0% to 8%. The 5-year survival rate following surgery is about 61%–64%.[2,17]

Direct comparison of endovascular and surgical techniques have not been reported. However, a review of the literature indicates that endovascular therapy is an effective alternative to surgery in patients with chronic mesenteric ischemia.[1]

Percutaneous transluminal angioplasty (PTA) in the treatment of atherosclerotic stenosis of the mesenteric arteries was first described in 1980.[18] Since then, the literature has predominately consisted of small series and case reports.[19–21] In the largest

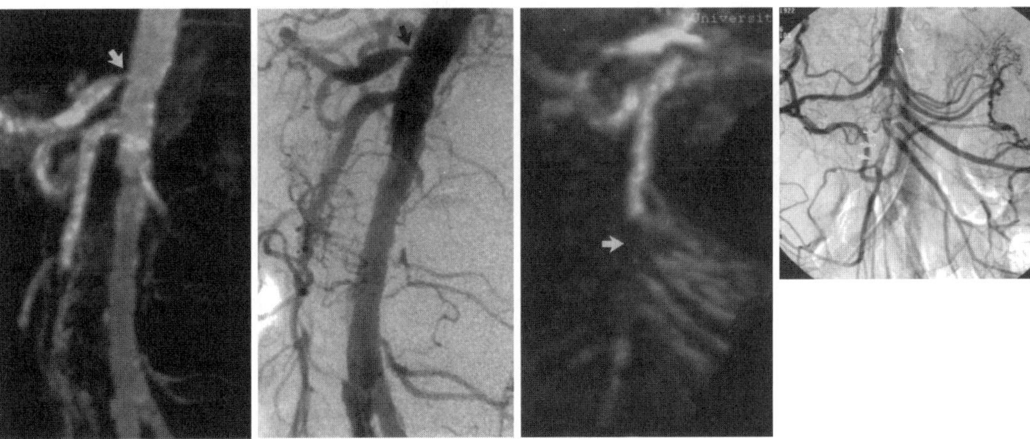

Figure 24–1. (A) The sagital gadolinium-enhanced MRA demonstrates a high grade stenosis at the origin of the celiac artery (white arrow). The SMA origin is widely patent. **(B)** The angiographic correlate demonstrates similar findings of both the SMA and celiac arteries (black arrow). **(C)** A coronal reformation of the gadolinium-enhanced MRA demonstrates a lack of contrast in the mid-SMA (white arrow) with enhancement of the jejunal branches suggesting a segmental occlusion. **(D)** The angiographic correlate demonstrates mid-SMA thrombus (white arrows) with perfusion of the jejunal branches. This patient underwent successful catheter directed thrombolysis of the SMA and subsequent stenting of the celiac artery.

published series, Matsumoto et al. reported on the treatment of 47 vessels in 33 patients over an 18-year period.[20,21] The patient population consisted of 12 men and 21 women whose ages ranged from 40 to 89 years (mean age of 63 years). Risk factors for atherosclerosis included tobacco use (52%), hypertension (58%), coronary artery disease (52%), and diabetes (9%). Eighty-eight percent of the patients presented with the classic symptoms of postprandial abdominal pain. Seventy percent of patients presented with weight loss, ranging from 6 to 80 pounds (median 28 pounds). "Fear of food" was elicited in 49% of the patients. Sixteen of the 33 (49%) patients had endoscopic, CT, or biopsy results consistent with intestinal ischemia. Twenty-one patients underwent PTA alone in 32 vessels and 12 patients underwent PTA and stenting in 15 vessels. Etiologies of the stenosis were atheroscleroses in 22 (67%), fibromuscular dysplasia in 1 (3%), intimal hyperplasia in a surgical bypass graft in 3 (9%), and median arcuate ligament in combination with atherosclerosis or fibromuscular dysplasia in 7 patients (21%). No attempts were made to treat total arterial occlusions.

PTA and stenting were performed as previously described[1] (Figures 24–2 and 24–3). Most procedures were performed via a high left brachial artery approach, although the right femoral, left femoral, and right brachial artery approaches were also used. Balloon diameters and stent lengths were determined based on measurements from either a biplane cut-film abdominal aortogram or digital subtraction aortogram using intrinsic measurement software (Polytron, Siemens Medical Systems, Erlangen Germany). A bolus of heparin (2,000 to 4,000 IU) was used during the procedure and

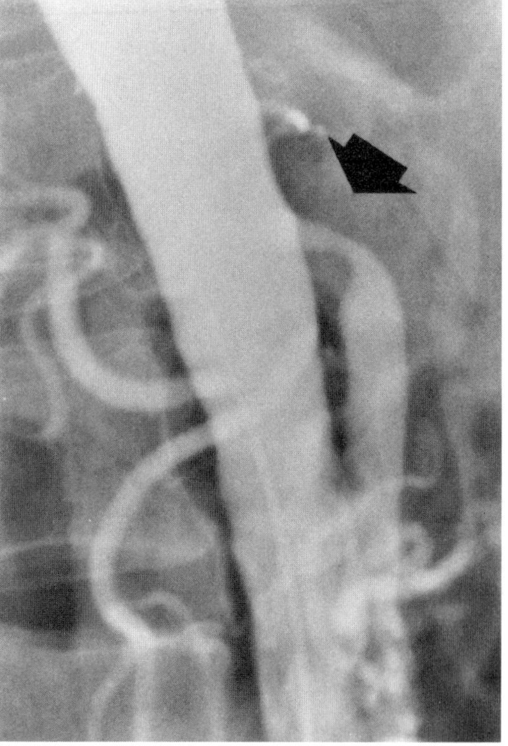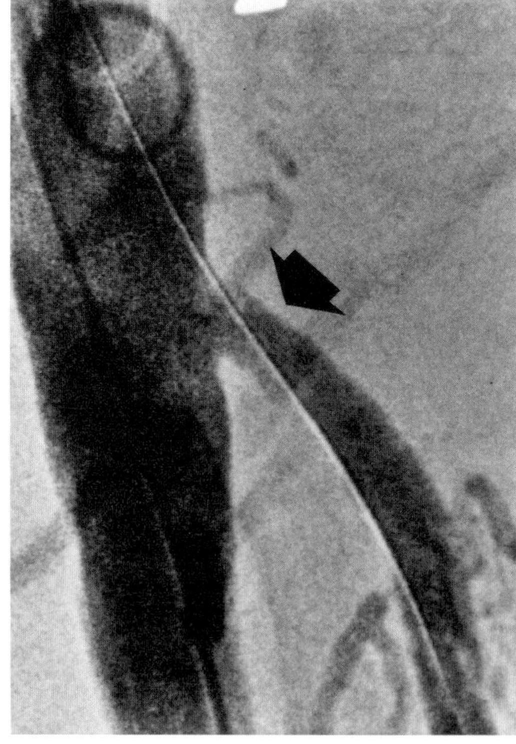

Figure 24–2. (A) A high-grade stenosis is present at the origin of the SMA (black arrow) on the lateral aortic angiogram. **(B)** Successful PTA (black arrow) of the proximal SMA lesion.

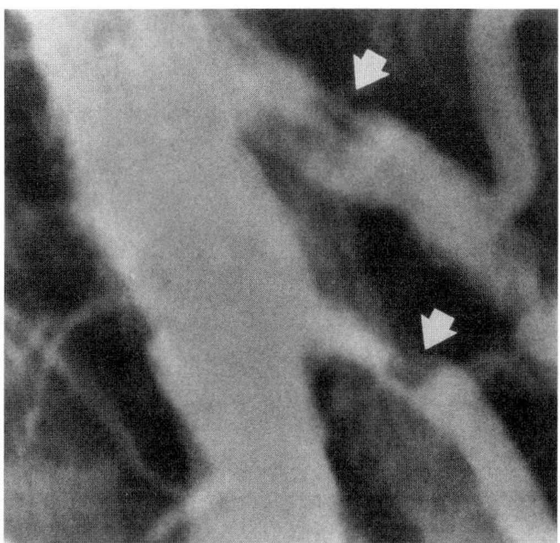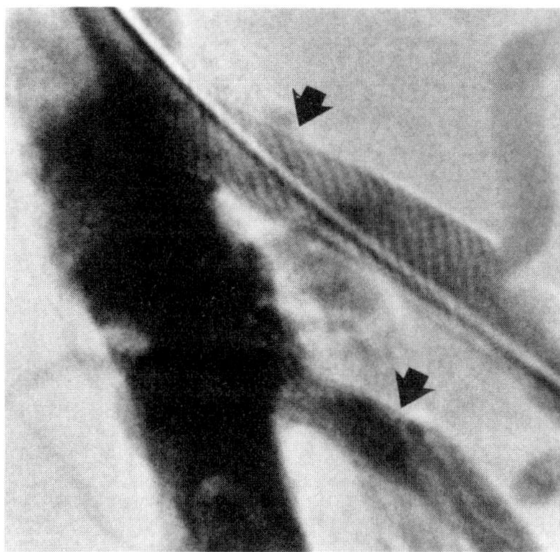

Figure 24–3. **(A)** An eccentric stenosis is identified at the origin of the proximal celiac artery and SMA on the lateral aortic angiogram (white arrows). **(B)** The patient underwent successful PTA and stenting (black arrows) of both lesions.

intraarterial vasodilators were not routinely used. No intraprocedural thrombolytic agents were given. Whenever possible, patients were given a dose of 325 mg acetylsalicylic acid once a day for life, and up until 1996, 75 mg dipyridamole, twice a day, for 6 months after the procedure.

The initial technical success rate for PTA was 81% (per vessel) and 100% for PTA and stenting (per vessel). The primary clinical success rate per patient was 82% (27 of 33 patients) for complete resolution of symptoms and 6% (2 of 33 patients) for partial, but significant improvement in symptoms. Four immediate clinical failures were encountered (12%). Two of these patients were subsequently found to have malignancies (pancreatic carcinoma and adenocarcinoma with metastasis to the porta hepatis) that were believed to be responsible for their symptoms of abdominal pain and weight loss. Both patients were treated prior to 1986, when CT scans were not routinely obtained as part of the initial evaluation. A third patient underwent a technically successful PTA of the celiac artery, with untreated total occlusions of the SMA and IMA. The patient experienced incomplete resolution of symptoms and subsequently underwent aortobifemoral bypass grafting for distal aortic and iliac disease. At that time, IMA endarterectomy was also performed and the patient's symptoms completely resolved. The fourth immediate clinical failure occurred in a patient with complete occlusion of the celiac and inferior mesenteric arteries. An SMA stenosis with the characteristic appearance of median arcuate ligament compression was treated with PTA without significant improvement in the stenosis. The PTA was done as much for diagnostic reasons to demonstrate the rapid recoil of the vessel following balloon deflation. The patient underwent surgical release of the MAL with complete resolution of symptoms.

Follow-up data were available in all 29 patients who experienced an initial clinical benefit for the procedure. The mean duration of clinical follow-up was 38 months, with a range of 1 to 123 months. The median duration of follow-up was 25 months. Angiographic follow-up was obtained in 15 of the 29 patients (52%), at a mean of 20 months (1 to 99 months). Three patients were eventually lost to follow-up, but had a minimum follow-up of at least 20 months (range 20 to 35 months). All 3 of these patients were asymptomatic at the time of being lost to follow-up. Eight of the 29 patients died 2 to 117 months (mean 46 months) after their procedure.

Of the 29 patients who experienced an initial clinical benefit from the procedure, 5 developed recurrent symptoms between 5 and 19 months. Four of these patients underwent repeat PTA with clinical improvement for a primary assisted success rate of 97% (28 of 29 patients). The fifth patient was initially treated with PTA of a 90% atherosclerotic stenosis of the celiac artery with superimposed MAL compression of the celiac artery. The procedure was a technical failure with a 50% residual stenosis due to persistent MAL compression of the celiac artery. However, the patient's clinical symptoms resolved until 19 months post procedure. At that time, the patient presented with recurrent symptoms and underwent surgical repair.

Including the patient encounters for the treatment of recurrent stenoses, there were 39 procedures performed. Five (13%) major complications occurred; 3 were access site thromboses and 2 were hematomas that required further treatment. No episodes of acute mesenteric ischemia developed secondary to any of the procedures. The 30-day mortality rate was 0% (0 in 39 patient encounters).

In the 39 patient procedures, there were 34 brachial and 24 femoral accesses used. Only 1 of the femoral access sites (4.2%) was associated with a major complication, and 4 of the 34 brachial punctures (11.8%) were associated with a major complication. In the 24 procedures in which PTA alone was used, 4 access site complications (19%) occurred. Three of these complications occurred during the era in which large balloon catheters (7-to 8-F catheters shafts) were used. In the 15 procedures in which PTA and stenting were performed, only 1 major access site complication (6.7%) occurred.

A total of 58 vessels were treated in the 39 patient encounters. With the initial 33 procedures, the celiac artery was treated 14 times, SMA 21 times, IMA 9 times, and bypass grafts 3 times. For recurrent stenoses, a total of 11 vessels were retreated in 6 patients (2 patients were retreated once and 2 patients were retreated twice). The celiac artery, SMA, and IMA were retreated 5, 5, and 1 time(s), respectively. When evaluating the primary clinical success rate by the number of vessels initially treated, there was no statistical difference between patients who had more than 1 vessel treated. When evaluating the primary success rate by whether or not the SMA was treated, there was no statistically significant difference. Four patients had the IMA treated alone and have done well.

In the 12 patients in whom stents were used during the initial procedure, 16 stents were placed in 15 vessels. The primary technical success rate was 100%, and the primary clinical success rate was 100% (Figure 24–2). The mean follow-up period for patients who had a stent placed was 15 months (range 1 to 48 months). Recurrent symptoms occurred in 1 patient secondary to in-stent restenosis at 14 months. The restenosis was successfully treated with PTA.

When comparing the primary clinical success rate of those patients who underwent PTA alone versus those patients who underwent PTA plus stenting, there was no statistical difference in the primary long-term clinical success.

The 5-year survival rate for the 29 patients was 76.1%. In the 21 patients who underwent PTA alone, 5-year survival was 70.6%. In the patients who underwent PTA and stenting, the longest follow-up was 48 months. Based on Life Table Analysis, the 5-year survival was 87.5%. The difference in survival between patients who underwent PTA alone versus PTA and stenting was not statistically significant (Figure 24–4). When evaluating survival based on whether 1 vessel or more than 1 vessel was

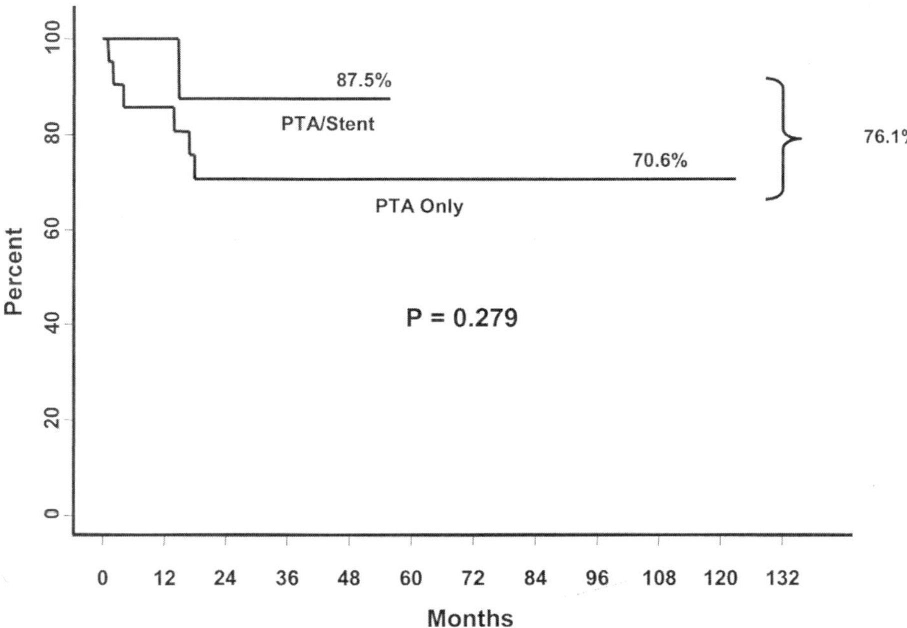

Figure 24–4. Survival by procedure type. PTA, percutaneous transluminal angioplasty. Reprinted with permission *JACS*.

treated, there was no statistical difference (Figure 24–5). When comparing whether or not survival was affect by intervention on the SMA, there was also no statistical difference (p = 0.654).

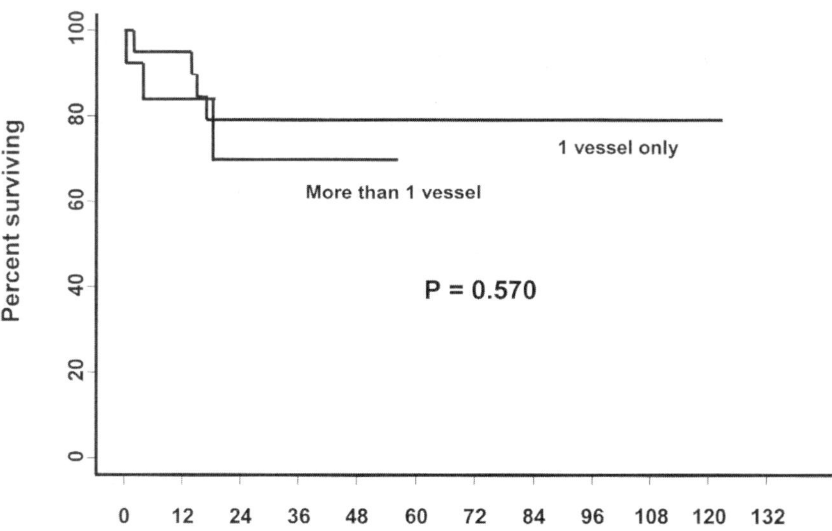

Figure 24–5. Survival by number of vessels initially treated. Reprinted with permission *JACS*.

Sheeran et al. have reported on the treatment of 12 patients with 10 focal atherosclerotic stenoses and 3 chronic occlusions with stent placment. Vessels treated included 9 SMA, 3 celiac, and 1 aorto-SMA bypass graft. The initial technical success was 92% (12 of 13 vessels). The 1 technical failure occurred due to rupture of the angioplasty balloon while deploying a balloon expandable stent. The stent was recaptured and deployed in the iliac artery. Despite a residual pressure gradient after PTA, the patient reported improved symptoms at 6-month follow-up. Primary stent placement was utilized for calcified ostial stenoses, chronic occlusions, and high-grade eccentric stenoses in 8 of 13 stent placements. Patients underwent secondary stent placement for residual stenoses of more than 30%, significant residual pressure gradients, and flow limiting dissections after PTA. Of the 12 patients, short-term mortality (<30 days) was reported in 1 patient secondary to bowel ischemia. This patient presented with acute worsening of chronic abdominal symptoms, but was deemed a nonsurgical candidate and underwent a technically successful stent placement procedure of the SMA. There were no complications associated with the puncture site, acute vessel occlusion, or distal embolization occurred.[19]

At this time, surgical revascularization remains the mainstay in the treatment of complete mesenteric arterial occlusions. However, Sheeran et al. have reported on the treatment of 3 patients (2 SMA and 1 aorto-SMA bypass graft) with chronic occlusions using PTA and stent placement. All 3 patients remained asymptomatic at 13 to 38 months of follow up.[19]

DISSCUSSION

Recent improvements in balloon catheters, guidewire, and stent technology have allowed for endovascular therapy to have an increased role in the treatment of patients with chronic mesenteric ischemia. Recent data suggests that the initial complication and mortality rates associated with PTA and stent placement can be minimized, while survival and clinical success rates comparable to surgical revascularization can be achieved. Treatment of chronic mesenteric occlusions may be technically more challenging with endovascular techniques, however, with the ability of stent technology, it now appears more feasible.

Prophylactic PTA of asymptomatic visceral artery stenosis remains controversial due to the adequacy of mesenteric arterial collateral flow. However, the development of mesenteric ischemia following reconstructive abdominal aorta surgery is known to be associated with a high peri-operative mortality rate.[22,23] In addition, Thomas et al. did a respective analysis of 980 consecutive aortograms to try to determine the natural history of patients who were found to have asymptomatic mesenteric arterial stenoses.[24] In this study, a total of 60 patients were found to have a 50% stenosis of at least 1 mesenteric artery and were monitored for 1–6 years. Fifteen of the 60 (25%) patients were found to have 3 vessel mesenteric arterial disease. Thirteen of these 15 (86%) patients developed mesenteric ischemia, 4 (27%) had other vague abdominal symptoms or died. The over-all mortality rate in the 60 patients was 40% during the follow-up period, reflecting the generalized nature of atherosclerotic disease. The authors concluded that patients with significant 3-vessel mesenteric arterial occlusive disease should be considered for prophylactic vascular reconstruction, even in the absence of symptoms. Therefore, prophylactic treatment of compromised visceral arterial circulation may be indicated in patients with 3 vessel mesenteric arterial disease or prior to performing a complex surgical repair of the abdominal aorta and iliac vessels. In the series reported by Matsumoto et al., 4 patients were treated with mesenteric PTA for this indication.[20] Two of these patients had significant disease of the SMA, IMA, abdominal aorta, and both common and internal iliac arteries. The SMA was balloon dilated in both patients due to concern for the development of mesenteric ischemia following an aortobifemoral bypass graft. The third patient had 100% occlusion of the SMA, 90% stenosis of the celiac, and 10% stenosis of the IMA, as well as a large abdominal aortic aneurysm. The patient underwent prophylactic PTA of the celiac artery. The abdominal aortic aneurysm was surgically repaired without sequelae. The fourth patient developed complete occlusion at the site of an ostial IMA stenosis following PTA of the abdominal aorta. Balloon dilatation of the IMA was performed to reestablish flow in the IMA distribution. None of these 4 patients have developed signs or symptoms of mesenteric ischemia during a follow-up period ranging from 7 to 73 months.

Mesenteric PTA in patients with atypical symptoms for chronic mesenteric ischemia or with nonostial stenosis of the celiac artery appears to be less effective. Extrinsic compression of the celiac artery due to median arcuate ligament does not respond favorably to PTA. The placement of a balloon expandable stent, such as the Palmaz stent, may lead to collapse or distortion of the stent due to extrinsic compression, and possibly abrupt occlusion of the artery. In addition, symptoms secondary to MAL compression may be related to pressure on the celiac ganglion. Surgical therapy remains the treatment of choice for patients with median arcuate ligament syndrome.

Occult abdominal or retroperitoneal malignancies may mimic the symptoms of chronic mesenteric ischemia. Therefore, an immediate technical or clinical failure of endovascular treatment of the mesenteric arteries should raise the suspicion of extrinsic compression or an occult malignancy, respectively.

Recent advances in CT angiography and gadolinium-enhanced 3-D MRA have allowed these modalities to assume a much greater role in the noninvasive screening of patients with suspected chronic mesenteric ischemia. However, catheter angiography with hemodynamic evaluation still remains the gold standard for evaluating the mesenteric arterial circulation prior to either surgical or percutaneous intervention, especially when the noninvasive studies do not clearly define the anatomy in question. It is also important to emphasize those patients who present with abdominal pain and weight loss should undergo CT evaluation prior to intervention in order to exclude other diagnoses such as malignancy.

REFERENCES

1. Matsumoto AH, Tegtmeyer CJ, Angle JF. Endovascular interventions for chronic mesenteric ischemia. In: Baum S, Pentecost MJ eds. *Abram's angiography: Interventional radiology.* Vol III. New York: Little, Brown & Co; 1997:326–338.
2. Miralles M, Cairols M, Cotillas J, et al. Value of Doppler parameters in the diagnosis of renal artery stenosis. *J Vasc Surg.* 1996;23:428–435.
3. Blebea J, Volteas N, Neumyer M, et al. Contrast enhanced duplex ultrasound imaging of the mesenteric arteries. *Ann Vasc Surg.* 2002;16:77–83.
4. Kim TS, Chung JW, Park JH, et al. Renal aretery evaluation: comparison of spiral CT angiography to intra-arterial DSA. *J Vasc Interv Radiol.* 1998;9:553–559.
5. Bergi JP, Elkohen M, Deklunder G, et al. Helical CT angiography compared with arteriography in the detection of renal artery stenosis. *AJR.* 1996;167:495–501.

6. Galanski M, Prokop M, Chaven A, et al. Renal arterial stenoses: spiral CT angiography. *Radiology.* 1993;189:185–192.
7. Rubin GD, Dake MD, Napel S, et al. Spiral CT of renal artery stenosis: comparison of three-dimensional rendering techniques. *Radiology.* 1994;190:181–189.
8. Horton KM, Fishman EK. Multi-detector row CT of mesenteric ischemia: can it be done? *Radiographics.* 2001;21:1463–1473.
9. Carlos RC, Stanley JC, Stafford-Johnson D, et al. Interobserver variability in the evaluation of chronic mesenteric ischemia with gadolinium-enhanced MR angiography. *Acad Radiol.* 2001;8:879–887.
10. Foley MI, Moneta GI, Abou-Zamzam AM, et al. Revascularization of the superior mesenteric artery alone for treatment of intestinal ischemia. *J Vasc Surg.* 2000;32:37–47.
11. Mateo RB, O'Hara PJ, Hertzter NR, et al. Elective surgical treatment of symptomatic chronic mesenteric occlusive disease: early results and late outcomes. *J Vasc Surg.* 1999;29:821–832.
12. Baxter BT, Pearce WH. Diagnosis and surgical management of chronic mesenteric ischemia. In: Strandness DE, van Breda A, eds. *Vascular diseases: surgical and interventional therapy.* New York: Churchill-Livingstone, 1994:795–802.
13. McMillian WD, McCarthy WJ, Bresticker MR, et al. Mesenteric artery bypass: objective patency determination. *J Vasc Surg.* 1995;21:729–741.
14. Calderon M, Reul GH, Gregoric ID, et al. Long-term results of the surgical management of symptomatic chronic intestinal ischemia. *J Cardiovasc Surg.*1992;33:723–728.
15. Rheudasil JM, Stewart MT, Schellack JV, et al. Surgical treatment of chronic mesenteric arterial insufficiency. *J Vasc Surg.*1988;8:495–500.
16. Rapp JH, Reilly LM, Qvarfordt PG, et al. Durablity of endarterectomy and antegrade grafts in the treatment of chronic visceral ischemia. *J Vasc Surg.* 1986;3:799–806.
17. Reul GJ Jr, Wukasch DC, Sandiford FM, et al. Surgical treatment of abdominal angina: review of 25 patients. *Surgery.* 1974;75:682–689.
18. Furrer J, Gruntzig A, Kugelmeier J, et al. Treatment of abdominal angina with percutaneous dilatation of an arteria mesenterica superior stenosis. *Cardovasc Intervent Radio.* 1980;3:43–44.
19. Sheeran SR, Murphy TP, Khwaja A, et al. Stent placement for treatment of mesenteric artery stenosis or occlusions. *JVIR.* 1999;10:861–867.
20. Matsumoto AH, Tegtmeyer CJ, Fitzcharles EK, et al. Percutaneous transluminal angioplasty of visceral arterial stenoses: results and long-term clinical follow-up. *JVIR.* 1995;6:165–174.
21. Matsumoto AH, Angle JF, Spinosa DJ, et al. Percutaneous transluminal angioplasty and stenting in the treatment of chronic mesenteric ischemia: Results and long-term follow-up. *J AM Coll Surg.* 2002;194:S22–31.
22. Gonzalez LL, Jaffe MS. Mesenteric arterial insufficiency following abdominal aortic resection. *Arch Surg.* 1966;93:10–20.
23. Rogers DM, Thompson JE, Garrett WV, et al. Mesenteric vascular problems: a 26-year experience. *Ann Surg.* 1982;195:554–565.
24. Thomas JH, Blake K, Pierce GE, et al. The clinical course of aymptomatic mesenteric arterial stenosis. *J Vasc Surg.* 1998: 27: 840–844.

VIII

Lower
Extremity
Ischemia

25

Popliteal Entrapment Syndromes: Different Causes, Different Treatments

William D. Turnipseed, MD

The term "popliteal entrapment" was coined by Love and Whelan in 1965 to describe the unique constellation of neuromuscular and ischemic symptoms in the lower extremity resulting from pathologic impingement behind the knee.[1] Numerous congenital musculotendinous variations in the development and insertion of the gastrocnemius and popliteus muscles have been associated with this condition (Table 25–1).[2] These anatomic variations are associated with an increased risk of threatening lower limb ischemia. More recent clinical observations suggest that popliteal impingement can occur without any evidence of anatomic abnormality and that symptoms associated with this condition rarely occur. Functional popliteal impingement appears to be a normal physiologic variant which may become symptomatic and cause neuromuscular claudication and paresthesias when repetitive overuse or orthopedic injury occur.[3,4]

TABLE 25–1. ANATOMIC ENTRAPMENT CLASSIFICATION

TYPE I	Medial deviation of popliteal artery around medial insertion of gastrocnemius muscle. (One patient: 17-year-old male {claudication})
TYPE II	Minimal medial deviation of popliteal artery with entrapment by aberrant medial attachments of gastrocnemius muscle. (Two patients: 42-year-old male {digital ischemia}; 69-year-old female {claudication})
TYPE III	Normally positioned popliteal artery with entrapment by aberrant lateral attachments of medial gastrocnemius muscle. (Three patients: 46-year-old male {claudication}; 42-year-old male {digital ischemia}; 53-year-old male {digital ischemia})
TYPE IV	Normally positioned popliteal artery entrapped by popliteus muscle.
TYPE V	Above abnormalities entrap popliteal artery and/or vein. (One patient: 33 year-old-female {calf swelling})

Clinical similarities and differences between anatomic and functional forms of popliteal entrapment will be discussed in this chapter. The clinical syndromes resulting from anatomic and functional entrapment differ considerably as do the indications and surgical procedures required for their treatment.

PATIENTS AND METHODS

Between 1990 and 2001, 276 patients (84 males, 192 females) were referred from our sports medicine clinic because of atypical symptoms of lower extremity claudication and a failure to detect an orthopedic cause for the extremity complaints. Most had long-standing symptoms (mean duration >24 months) classically manifest by swelling and cramping of isolated muscle groups with occasional plantar paresthesias. Symptoms were usually aggravated by vigorous athletic activity, would abate with rest, and rarely limited day-to-day activity. Although the age range varied widely (12–71 years), the median age for patients in this group was 29 years. These patients were routinely evaluated in our clinic with stress positional plethysmography to screen for popliteal entrapment. Compartment pressures were selectively performed when symptoms were referable to the anterolateral or posterior superficial muscle compartments. Compartment pressures were measured using the Stryker Computer System (Stryker Surgical, Kalamazoo, MI). Normal resting compartment pressures were considered to be <15 mmHg. Resting pressures between 16 and 24 mmHg were considered highly suggestive of chronic compartment syndrome and pressures exceeding 25 mmHg were considered diagnostic of this condition. Pressure measurements were not routinely performed in patients with deep posterior muscle compartment symptoms because of the increased chance of neurovascular injury and because of the difficulty in determining which compartments were actually being measured. Those individuals with absent or weak distal pulses on physical examination had pulse volume recordings performed at rest and after exercise (1.5 mph/10-degree elevation for 5 min). Symptomatic patients with abnormal pulse volume recordings (PVRs) suggesting intrinsic arterial disease because of abnormal resting or post-exercise studies and those with abnormal stress positional noninvasive tests suggesting popliteal entrapment had lower extremity Magnetic Resonance Angiography (MRA) or Digital Subtraction Arteriograms (DSA) performed. Those individuals suspected of having popliteal entrapment had static and stress positional arteriograms performed with the knee extended and the foot in neutral and dorsi/plantar flexion positions.

RESULTS

The large majority of patients in this clinical series (238 = 86%) were found to have chronic compartment syndrome. The diagnosis was based on presenting clinical symptoms and the documentation of abnormally elevated compartment pressures. Only 7 patients (3%) in this series had physical findings or noninvasive tests suggesting the presence of intrinsic vascular occlusive disease. A larger number of the patients had positive noninvasive entrapment screening tests (82 = 30%). However only 21 patients (<8%) actually had symptoms referable to these findings. Closer attention will be focused on this subgroup of young claudicators with abnormal noninvasive screening tests. The 7 patients with evidence of peripheral vascular disease were older (mean age 43.6) than the cohort of patients with chronic compartment syndrome (28.4 years). Five of the 7 were males (71%) whereas patients with chronic compartment syndrome were more commonly female (192 = 70%). The most common symptoms for patients with evidence of intrinsic occlusive vascular disease included claudication (43%), ischemic skin change (43%), or paresthesia (14%), whereas symptoms of chronic compartment syndrome were most commonly manifested by isolated muscle cramping or claudication (100%), and occasional plantar paresthesia (20%). Of the 7 patients with abnormal vascular screening tests, 2 had abnormal resting ankle brachial indices; 4 had normal resting pressures, but abnormal post-exercise pulse volume recordings and 1 patient with positional calf swelling had stress positional duplex venography suggesting the presence of extrinsic popliteal vein compression. All 7 patients with clinical symptoms and abnormal noninvasive tests had vascular studies performed using Digital Subtraction or Magnetic Resonance Imaging techniques. Only 2 of these had the diagnosis of popliteal entrapment made preoperatively. One patient with calf swelling and a positive venous duplex stress test had anatomic entrapment confirmed with contrast Digital Subtraction Venography. The other, a 17-year-old male, had the presumptive diagnosis of popliteal entrapment made on the basis of initial angiographic findings which included displacement of the proximal popliteal artery medial to the medial head of the gastrocnemius muscle and the presence of a minimally stenotic plaque in the mid-portion of the popliteal artery. Confirmation of the diagnosis was made by performing stress positional arteriography. The diagnosis of popliteal entrapment was initially missed in the 5 remaining patients with clinical evidence of peripheral ischemia. One patient had digital embolic infarcts and a palpable popliteal aneurysm; 2 had calf claudication with mid-popliteal artery stenosis documented on arteriography; and 2 had digital ischemia with normal appearing peripheral arteriograms and negative cardiac and hematology workups. The 2 patients with isolated popliteal artery stenoses were treated with balloon angioplasty and anticoagulation and the 2 patients with peripheral embolization and no documented pathology were started on Coumadin prophylaxis. All 4 of these patients, as well as the one individual with popliteal artery aneurysm, subsequently had noninvasive popliteal entrapment stress tests which were strongly positive. All 7 patients were ultimately operated on for popliteal entrapment using the posterior geniculate approach. The 17-year-old male was treated with arterial transection, popliteal endarterectomy, and end-to-end re-anastomosis placing the vessel in the normal midline position. The patient with venous impingement symptoms had an unclassified form of entrapment caused by compression of the plantaris muscle and tendon and torquing of the popliteal vein by geniculate branches that originated medially traversing the posterior surface of the vein to drain the lateral thigh muscles. This patient was treated with resection of the plantaris muscle, transection of the aberrant veins, and venolysis. The patient with popliteal aneurysm and digital ischemia had resection of the aneurysm, primary end-to-end popliteal anastomosis, and resection of aberrant muscle fibers. The 2 patients treated initially with balloon angioplasty for focal popliteal artery stenoses had resection of aberrant muscle fibers. The 2 patients with digital ischemia and no evidence of intrinsic disease were treated by partial musculotendinous resection of the medial gastrocnemius muscle. The posterior surgical approach used in these patients provided better exposure of the proximal and mid-portions of the popliteal artery and/or vein and enabled the surgeon to directly repair vascular lesions and resect abnormal musculotendinous structures in the popliteal fossa. Autogenous artery repair without bypass were performed in all 7 patients. Although the medial approach is appropriate when distal bypass is required, none of these direct vascular repairs would have been easy to perform through a medial approach.

Over the same 10-year period, 30 patients have been treated for "functional entrapment syndrome." In contrast to patients with anatomic entrapment syndrome these patients were younger (mean age 24.5 years), more commonly female (20 = 66%) and for the most part were well-conditioned athletic individuals. Unlike patients with chronic compartment syndrome where bilateral symmetry of symptoms was common, bilateral complaints referable to functional entrapment were present in only 7 of the 30 patients (23%). The most common symptoms of functional entrapment included soleus muscle cramping (100%), plantar paresthesia (43%), and calf swelling (7%). Fourteen of the 30 patients with symptomatic functional entrapment (47%) had coexisting complaints of chronic compartment syndrome or had previous surgery for this condition. Confirmation of popliteal impingement was established by using stress positional duplex or plethysmography with the knee extended and the foot in neutral and forced plantar and dorsiflexion positions. Confirmatory vascular imaging using DSA or MRA demonstrated normally positioned popliteal vessels with lateral compression of the neurovascular bundle against the soleal band of fascia traversing the distal outlet of the popliteal fossa. The mechanism of compression appeared to be contraction of the medial gastrocnemius and plantaris muscles. All of these patients were treated by: excision of the fascia investing the medial head of the gastrocnemius muscle, resection of the soleal band, and resection of the plantaris muscle. Of the 30 patients in this series, 27 were athletically active and returned to full activity. Three retired from active lifestyles because of other injuries including Achilles tendinitis, stress fracture, or the development of compartment syndromes in other muscle groups. Daily activity levels in these 3 patients normalized. All patients have been followed with noninvasive tests which have demonstrated complete resolution of the popliteal impingement. There have been no recurrent symptoms in this treatment group. Follow-up has ranged from 1 month to 11 years (mean 65 months).

DISCUSSION

For surgeons it's important to understand that clinical syndromes resulting from anatomic and functional impingement, their prognosis, and procedures required for their treatment are considerably different. Patients with anatomic entrapment usually have abnormal compressive bands of tendon or fascia which are associated with the development of intrinsic arterial disease and subsequent ischemic symptoms.[5] Individuals with functional entrapment develop neurovascular symptoms that result from lateral compression of the popliteal neurovascular bundle against the band of soleal fascia that at the lower border of the popliteal fossa. Patient demographics for anatomic and functional syndromes differ as well (Table 25–2). Those with anatomic entrapment are more commonly male, older, more sedentary, have more restrictive claudication symptoms, and more frequently have noninvasive test evidence of peripheral occlusive or aneurysmal disease. In contrast, patients with functional entrapment are younger, more commonly female, well-conditioned athletes with active lifestyles, and have normal vascular screening tests. The functional entrapment syndromes appear to result from overuse injury and are much more likely to occur in the same population that are effected with chronic compartment syndromes. Entrapment screening tests routinely performed in patients with chronic compartment syndrome are positive in over 30% of the patients; however less than 10% ever developed clinical symptoms referable to these findings. For comparison, positive entrapment screening tests were detected in about 15% of asymptomatic age group controls.[4,6]

TABLE 25–2. POPLITEAL ENTRAPMENT DEMOGRAPHICS

	FUNCTIONAL		ANATOMIC	
	30 PATIENTS (22 FEMALES, 8 MALES) MEAN AGE 24.5 YEARS (RANGE 15–47)		7 PATIENTS (5 MALES, 2 FEMALES) MEAN AGE 43.6 (RANGE 17–69)	
SYMPTOMS	#	%	#	%
CLAUDICATION	30	100	3	43
PARESTHESIA	13	43	1	14
CALF SWELLING	2	7	1	14
DIGITAL ISCHEMIA	0	0	3	43
POSITIVE STRESS TEST				
PVR/ABI	30	100	7	100
DUPLEX	30	100	7	100

Although plethysmography and/or duplex are useful screening methods for detecting popliteal impingement, they are not capable of distinguishing anatomic from functional mechanisms of entrapment.[7] Although arteriography has been used as the "Gold Standard" for establishing the diagnosis and basing treatment of patients suspected of having popliteal entrapment, we feel that stress positional Magnetic Resonance Arteriography and T-weighted soft tissue imaging are the best tests for diagnosing popliteal entrapment and distinguishing the anatomic from functional form of the disease. T-weighted musculoskeletal studies provide detailed information regarding the relationship between vascular and musculotendinous structures within and around the popliteal fossa. Intrinsic vascular disease can be distinguished from extrinsic compression and the mechanics of impingement can be characterized with dynamic MR imaging.[8,9]

The decision to use the posterior or medial calf approach for release of popliteal entrapment should be decided on the basis of planned surgical treatment. The posterior exposure seems more appropriate when local repair of the popliteal artery and/or resection of musculotendinous anomalies associated with anatomic impingement in the popliteal fossa is intended. When vein bypass to infra-geniculate popliteal or tibial vessels is necessary because of occlusive or aneurysmal changes or when resection of the soleal band and plantaris muscle is required for functional entrapment, the medial calf approach provides excellent exposure of these structures with minimal dissection (Table 25–3).

Our experience in younger patients that have calf claudication suggests that noninvasive testing such as stress plethysmography, duplex imaging, and pulse volume recordings are important. Those individuals with noninvasive tests who have appropriate claudication symptoms and positive popliteal impingement screening tests should have peripheral arteriography with dynamic plantar and dorsiflexion of the foot. We prefer to use Magnetic Resonance Arteriography because it affords the risk free opportunity to evaluate musculoskeletal and vascular structures in the popliteal fossa at the same time. Surgical treatment for symptomatic forms of anatomic entrapment make sense as does prophylactic treatment of asymptomatic contralateral disease when anatomic impingement is detected because of the association with popliteal artery injury. However, surgical correction of functional impingement without associ-

TABLE 25-3. DIAGNOSTIC AND TREATMENT ALGORITHM

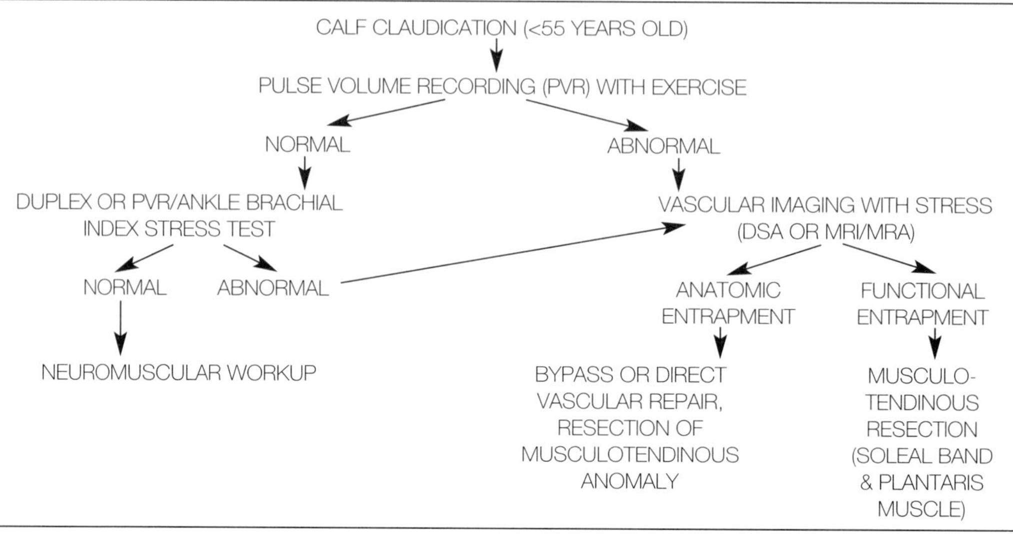

ated symptoms in our opinion does not seem appropriate. There is no indication that patients with functional entrapment are increased risk for later vascular complications and until this association can clearly be established, therapeutic intervention is only indicated when symptoms develop.

REFERENCES

1. Love JW, Whelan TJ. Popliteal artery entrapment syndrome. *Am J Surg.* 1965;109:620.
2. Insua JA, Young JR, Humphries AW. Popliteal artery entrapment syndrome. *Arch Surg.* 1970;101:771–775.
3. Rignault DP, Pailler JL, Lunel F. The "functional" popliteal entrapment syndrome. *Int Angiol.* 1985;4:341–343.
4. Turnipseed WD, Posniak M. Popliteal entrapment as a result of neurovascular compression by the soleus and plantaris muscles. *J Vasc Surg.* 1992;15:285–294.
5. Hamming JJ. Intermittent claudication at an early age, due to an anomalous course of the popliteal artery. *Angiology.* 1959;10:369–370.
6. Erdoes, LS, Devine JJ, Bernhard, et al. Popliteal vascular compression in a normal popluation. *J Vasc Surg.* 1994;20:978–986.
7. di Marzo L, Cavallaro A, Sciacca V, et al. Diagnosis of popliteal artery entrapment syndrome: The role of duplex scanning. *J Vasc Surg.* 1991;13:434–438.
8. McGuinness G, Durham JD, Rutherford RB, et al. Popliteal artery entrapment: Findings at MR imaging. *JVIR.* 1991;2:241–245.
9. Fujiwara H, Sugano T, Fujii N. Popliteal artery entrapment syndrome: accurate morphological diagnosis utilizing MRI. *J Cardiovasc Surg.* 1992;33:160–162.

26

Update on Thrombolytic Therapy 2002

Kenneth Ouriel, MD

Acute limb ischemia develops when a peripheral arterial occlusion occurs abruptly and in the absence of preexisting collateral channels. The underlying etiology is usually thrombosis of a native artery or bypass graft, but embolic events continue to account for 10 to 20% of cases.[1] Irrespective of etiology, the acute occlusive event may be catastrophic for the patient; with great risk to the patient's limb and life (Table 26–1). A now classic study by Blaisdell, published over 20 years ago, documented amputation and mortality rates in excess of 25% each following open surgical repair for acute leg ischemia.[2] Despite improvements in operative technique and postoperative patient care, more recent series continue to verify unacceptably high rates of morbidity. Jivegård and colleagues observed a 20% mortality rate in patients treated operatively.[3] Even the more recent prospective studies of operatively treated patients documented rates of limb loss and death that exceeded desired targets.[4–7]

Thus, the risk of morbidity and mortality following open surgical intervention remains at an unacceptably high level. What factors explain this finding? Clearly, the baseline medical status of the patients that present with acute peripheral arterial occlusion underlie the observation. Patients are frequently elderly, with a high rate of cardiac and other comorbidities. They are ill equipped to tolerate the insult of ischemia of

TABLE 26–1. EARLY (IN HOSPITAL OR 30-DAY) RATES OF AMPUTATION AND DEATH IN SELECTED SERIES OF PATIENTS WITH RECENT PERIPHERAL ARTERIAL OCCLUSION, TREATED WITH PRIMARY OPEN SURGICAL INTERVENTION.

Study	Year	Amputation Rate	Mortality Rate
Blaisdell	1978	25%	30%
Jivegård	1988	–	20%
Rochester	1994	14%	18%
STILE	1994	5%	6%
TOPAS	1998	2%	5%

an extremity, let alone an invasive surgical intervention to relieve the obstruction. A multivariable analysis of the data from the Rochester series uncovered several variables that were predictive of poor outcome, irrespective of the type of treatment instituted.[8] A summary of available literature would appear to confirm that individuals who present with acute, limb threatening ischemia comprise one of the sickest subgroup of patients that the peripheral vascular practitioner is asked to treat.[1]

There is some evidence to confirm the impression that a less invasive intervention is better tolerated in this very ill group of patients who develop acute limb ischemia. Poor technique, inadequate devices, and inferior agents colored the initial experiences with catheter-directed thrombolytic therapy. For instance, the now well-accepted principle of ensuring infusion of the thrombolytic agent directly into the substance of the occluding thrombus was not always ardently adhered to. End-hole catheters were employed; it was not until the late 1980s that multisided-hole catheters were available. Lastly, streptokinase was the most frequently used agent until the landmark article of McNamara in 1985 documented improved results with locally administered high-dose urokinase.[9]

PHARMACOLOGY OF THROMBOLYTIC AGENTS

In 1933, Tillett and Garner at the Johns Hopkins Medical School discovered that filtrates of broth cultures of certain strains of hemolytic streptococcus bacteria had fibrinolytic properties.[10] This streptococcal byproduct was originally termed *streptococcal fibrinolysin*. The purity of this agent was poor, however. Clinical use, of necessity, awaited adequate purification. Tillett and Sherry administered streptokinase intrapleurally to dissolve loculated hemothoraces in the late 1940s,[11] but intravascular administration was not attempted until the following decade. Tillett first reported intravascular administration of a thrombolytic agent in an article published in 1955.[12] A concentrated and partially purified SK (Varidase®, Lederle Laboratories) was injected into 11 patients. This investigation was performed with the intent to gain data on the safety of the agent in volunteers; in no case was the SK administered to dissolve pathologic thrombi. Fever and hypotension developed as the amount of SK approached therapeutic levels. Whereas fever was generally mild and controllable with antipyretics, hypotension was sometimes prominent. The mean fall in systolic pressure was 31 mm Hg and 3 of the patients manifested systolic pressures below 80 mm Hg. These untoward reactions were more likely a result of contaminants in the preparation rather than the SK itself. Despite these reactions, systemic proteolysis was observed, with a decrease in fibrinogen and plasminogen, concurrent with a mild increase in the prothrombin time.

These early studies were followed by reports on the use of SK in patients with occluding vascular thrombi. In 1956, E. E. Cliffton, at the Cornell University Medical College in New York, was responsible for the first brief description of the clinical effectiveness of intravascular thrombolytic administration.[13] The following year, Cliffton published his results in 40 patients with occlusive thrombi treated with a SK-plasminogen in combination.[14] The location of the thrombi was diverse, and included peripheral arterial thrombi, venous thrombi, pulmonary emboli, retinal occlusions, and, in 2 patients, occlusive carotid thrombi. Cliffton's clinical results were far from exemplary, recanalization was not uniform and bleeding complications were frequent. Nevertheless, he must be credited with the first use of thrombolytic agents for the treatment of pathologic thrombi, as well as with the first use of catheter-directed administration of a thrombolytic agent.

Several schemes may be used to classify thrombolytic agents. The agents may be grouped by their mechanism of action, those that directly convert plasminogen to plasmin verus those that are inactive zymogens and require transformation to an active form before they can cleave plasminogen. Thrombolytic agents can be grouped by their mode of production, those that are manufactured via recombinant techniques and those that are of bacterial origin. Of interest, recombinant agents harvested from a bacterial expression system such as *Escherichia coli* do not contain carbohydrates, while products of mammalian hybridoma (e.g. recombinant prourokinase from mouse hybridoma SP2/0 cells) are fully glycosylated. Thrombolytic agents can be classified by their pharmacologic actions, those that are "fibrin-specific" (bind to fibrin but not fibrinogen) versus non-specific and those that have a great degree of "fibrin-affinity" (bind avidly to fibrin) versus those that do not. We have found it most useful to classify thrombolytic agents into groups based on the origin of the parent compound. It is most efficient to divide the agents into 4 groups, the streptokinase compounds, the urokinase compounds, the tissue plasminogen activators, and an additional, miscellaneous group consisting of novel agents are distinct from agents in the 3 other groups.

Streptokinase Compounds

Streptokinase (SK), originating from the streptococcus bacteria, was the first thrombolytic agent to be described.[4] SK is a 50 kDa molecule with a biphasic half-life comprising a rapid $t^{1/2}$ of 16 minutes and a second, slower $t^{1/2}$ of 90 minutes.[15] Whereas the initial half-life is accounted for by complexing of the molecule with SK antibodies, the second half-life represents the actual biologic elimination of the protein. SK differs from other thrombolytic agents with respect to the stoichiometry of plasminogen binding. Whereas other agents directly convert plasminogen to plasmin, SK must form an equimolar stoichiometric complex with a plasmin or plasminogen molecule to gain activity. Only then can this SK-plasmin(ogen) complex activate a second plasminogen molecule to form active plasmin; thus, 2 plasminogen molecules are utilized in SK-mediated plasmin generation. Unfortunately, SK suffers from the limitation of antigenic potential. Preformed antibodies exist to a certain extent in all patients who have been infected with the Streptococcus bacterium. Similarly, patients with exposure to Streptokinase may have high antibody titers on repeat exposure. These neutralizing antibodies inactivate exogenously administered streptokinase. SK antibodies may be overwhelmed through the use of a large initial bolus of drug, and a large initial SK loading dose may be employed in this regard. Some investigators have recommended measurement of antibody titers prior to beginning SK therapy, gauging the loading dose on the basis of this titer.[16] SK administration is complicated by allergic reactions in approximately 2% of patients treated, with the development of urticaria, periorbital edema and bronchospasm. Pyrexia may also occur, but is usually adequately treated with acetaminophen. The major untoward effect associated with SK is hemorrhage. SK-associated hemorrhage may be no different that bleeding associated with any thrombolytic agent. The primary cause is likely the actions of systemic agent on the thrombi sealing the sites of vascular disintegrity. The generation of free plasmin, however, can contribute to the problem, with degradation of fibrinogen and other serum clotting proteins, as well as the release of fibrin(ogen)-degradation products that are potent anticoagulants themselves and exacerbate the coagulopathy.

Recognizing potential limitations with SK, anisoylated plasminogen-streptokinase activator complex (APSAC) was developed by pharmacologists at Beecham Laboratories.[17, 18] APSAC has a longer half-life than SK, since acylation rendered the complex less susceptible to degradation. Because of this property, it was anticipated that APSAC would be associated with a reduced risk of rethrombosis. Contrary to expectations, APSAC offered little clinical benefit over other agents, and, at present, is not used to treat thrombi in the peripheral vasculature.

Urokinase Compounds

Macfarlane first described the fibrinolytic potential of human urine in 1947.[19] The active molecule was extracted, isolated and named "urokinase" (UK) in 1952.[20] This urokinase-type plasminogen activator is a serine protease composed of 2 polypeptide chains, occurring in a low molecular weight (32 kDa) and high molecular weight (54 kDa) form. The high molecular weight form predominates in UK isolated from urine, while the low molecular weight form is found in UK obtained from tissue culture of kidney cells. Unlike SK, UK directly activates plasminogen to form plasmin; prior binding to plasminogen or plasmin is not necessary for activity. Also in contrast to SK, preformed antibodies to UK are not observed. The agent is nonantigenic and untoward reactions of fever or hypotension are rare. Presently, the most commonly employed UK in the United States is of tissue-culture origin, manufactured from human neonatal kidney cells (Abbokinase®, Abbott Laboratories, North Chicago, IL). UK has been fully sequenced, and a recombinant form of UK (r-UK) was tested in a single trial of patients with acute myocardial infarction and in 2 multicenter trials of patients with peripheral arterial occlusion.15 r-UK is fully glycosylated, since it is derived from a murine hybridoma cell line. r-UK differs from Abbokinase® in several respects. First, r-UK has a higher molecular weight than Abbokinase. Second, r-UK has a shorter half-life than its low-molecular weight counterpart. Despite these differences, however, the clinical effects of the 2 agents have been quite similar.

A precursor of UK was discovered in urine in 1979.[21] Prourokinase was characterized and subsequently manufactured by recombinant technology using *Escherichia coli* (nonglycosylated) or mammalian cells (fully glycosylated).[22] This single-chain form is an inactive zymogen, inert in plasma, but can be activated by kallikrein or plasmin to form active 2-chain UK. This property accounts for amplification of the fibrinolytic process—as plasmin is generated, more prourokinase is converted to active urokinase, and the process is repeated. Prourokinase is relatively fibrin specific, that is, its fibrin degrading (*fibrinolytic*) activity greatly outweighs its fibrinogen degrading (*fibrinogenolytic*) activity. This feature is explained by the preferential activation of fibrin-bound plasminogen found in a thrombus over free plasminogen found in flowing blood. Nonselective activators such as SK and UK activate free and bound plasminogen equally and induce systemic plasminemia with resultant fibrinogenolysis and degradation of factors V and VII. Given the potential advantages of prourokinase over urokinase, Abbott Laboratories produced a recombinant form of prourokinase (r-ProUK) from a murine hybridoma cell line. This recombinant agent was named Prolyse® (Abbott Laboratories) is converted to active 2-chain urokinase by plasmin and kallikrein. Prolyse® and has been studied in the settings of myocardial infarction, stroke and peripheral arterial occlusion. To date, it appears that r-ProUK offers the advantages associated with an agent that does not originate from a human cell source. Fibrin specificity, however, may be lost at the higher dose levels necessary to effect more rapid thrombolysis than Abbokinase®.

Tissue Plasminogen Activators

Tissue plasminogen activator, or "t-PA," is a naturally occurring fibrinolytic agent produced by endothelial cells and intimately involved in the balance between intravascular thrombogenesis and thrombolysis. Wild-type t-PA is a single-chain (527 amino acid) serine protease with a molecular weight of approximately 65 kDa. Plasmin hydrolyses the Arg275-Ile276 peptide bond, converting the single-chain molecule into a 2-chain moiety. In contrast to most serine proteases (e.g. urokinase), the single-chain form of t-PA has significant activity. t-PA has potential benefits over other thrombolytic agents. The agent exhibits significant *fibrin specificity*.[23] In plasma, the agent is associated with little plasminogen activation. At the site of the thrombus, however, the binding of t-PA and plasminogen to the fibrin surface induces a conformational change in both molecules, greatly facilitating the conversion of plasminogen to plasmin and dissolution of the clot. t-PA also manifests the property of fibrin affinity, that is, it binds strongly to fibrin. Other fibrinolytic agents such as prourokinase do not share this property of fibrin affinity. Recombinant t-PA (rt-PA, "alteplase") was produced in the 1980s after molecular cloning techniques were used to express human t-PA DNA.[24] Activase® (Genentech, South San Francisco, CA), a predominantly single-chain form of rt-PA, was eventually approved in the United States for the indications of acute myocardial infarction and massive pulmonary embolism. rt-PA has been studied extensively in the setting of coronary occlusion. In the GUSTO-I study of approximately 41,000 patients with acute myocardial infarction, rt-PA was more effective than SK in achieving vascular patency.[25] Despite a slightly greater risk of intracranial hemorrhage with rt-PA, overall mortality was significantly reduced. In an effort to lengthen the duration of bioavailability of t-PA, the molecule was systematically bioengineered. Initial investigations identified regions in kringle 1 and the protease portion of t-PA that mediated hepatic clearance, fibrin specificity and resistance to plasminogen activator inhibitor. Three sites were modified to create TNK-tPA, a novel molecule with a greater half-life and fibrin specificity.[26] The longer half-life of TNK-t-PA allowed successful administration as a single bolus, in contrast to the requirement for an infusion with rt-PA. In addition, TNK-tPA manifests greater fibrin specificity than rt-PA, resulting in less fibrinogen depletion. In studies of acute coronary occlusion, TNK-tPA performed at least as well as rt-PA, concurrent with greater ease of administration.[27]

Reteplase

Similar to TNK-tPA, the novel recombinant plasminogen activator reteplase comprises the kringle 2 and protease domains of t-PA. Reteplase was developed with the goal of avoiding the necessity of a continuous intravenous infusion, thereby simplifying ease of administration.[28] Reteplase (Retavase®, Centocor), produced in *Escherichia coli* cells, is non-glycosylated, demonstrating a lower fibrin-binding activity and a diminished affinity to hepatocytes.[29] This latter property accounts for a longer half-life than rt-PA, potentially enabling bolus injection versus prolonged infusion. The fibrin affinity of reteplase was only 30% of that exhibited with t-PA, similar to UK. The decrease in fibrin affinity was hypothesized to reduce the incidence of distant bleeding complications, in a manner similar to that of SK over rt-PA in the GUSTO trial. In fact, several properties of reteplase may account for a decreased risk of hemorrhage, including poor lysis of platelet-rich, older clots. Reteplase has demonstrated some benefit over rt-PA in the RAPID 1 and RAPID 2 studies, as well as in GUSTO III.[30] To date, peripheral arterial and venous studies remain few in number.[31]

Miscellaneous Agents

There exist a wide variety of novel thrombolytic agents, all of which have undergone extensive preclinical study but few of which have been adequately evaluated in patients. Vampire bat plasminogen activator ("bat PA") was cloned and expressed from the saliva of the vampire bat Desmodus rotundus.[32] This agent manifests extraordinary fibrin specificity, the plasminogenolytic activity is over 100,000 times greater in the presence of fibrin. The half-life of bat PA is 5 to 9 times slower than that of rt-PA, offering some potential advantages with respect to ease of administration. To date, clinical trials have been limited to Phase I study with healthy volunteers.[33] Fibrolase is a metalloproteinase originating from venom of the southern copperhead snake.[34] Fibrolase is a unique fibrinolytic agent that does not require plasminogen for its activity. Rather, the agent directly degrades fibrin without the requirement of any other blood components. Staphylokinase is a byproduct of Staphylococcus aureus bacterium, was originally mentioned in the classic streptococcal fibrinolysin paper of Tillett and Garner in 1933.[10] Staphylokinase has been produced by recombinant techniques and has been studied in the settings of myocardial infarction, peripheral arterial occlusion and deep venous thrombosis.[35] Like SK, staphylokinase is inactive and must bind to plasminogen to activate other plasminogen molecules. Unlike SK, staphylokinase is relatively fibrin-specific and spares circulating plasminogen and fibrinogen. While staphylokinase is antigenic, antigenicity has been reduced with newer recombinant mutants and the initial clinical results have been quite acceptable.[36]

COMPARISON OF THE AGENTS IN STUDIES OF PERIPHERAL VASCULAR DISEASE

To date, there have been few well-designed clinical comparisons of various thrombolytic agents in the peripheral vasculature. There exist a variety of in vitro studies and retrospective clinical trials, most pointing to improved efficacy and safety of UK and rt-PA over SK. In an analysis of data collected in a prospective, single institution registry at the Cleveland Clinic Foundation, UK demonstrated a diminished rate of bleeding complications when compared with rt-PA.[37] Efficacy was not evaluated in this trial.

There have been 2 prospective, randomized comparisons of UK and rt-PA. Neither was blinded. Meyerovitz and associates from the Brigham and Women's Hospital randomized 32 patients with peripheral arterial or bypass graft occlusions of less than 90 days duration to rt-PA (10 mg bolus, 5 mg/hr to a maximum of 24 hr) or UK (60,000 IU bolus, 4,000 IU/min for 2 hr, 2,000 IU/min for 2 hr, then 1,000 IU/min to a maximum of 24 hr total administration).[38] There was significantly greater systemic fibrinogen degradation in the rt-PA group (p = 0.01), indicating that the fibrin-specificity of rt-PA was lost at this dosing regimen. rt-PA patients achieved more rapid initial thrombolysis, but efficacy was identical in the 2 groups by 24 hr. The trade-off to more rapid thrombolysis was a trend toward a higher rate of bleeding complications in the rt-PA treated patients (p = 0.39). The second randomized comparison of and rt-PA was the STILE trial, a 3-armed multicenter comparison of UK (250,000 IU bolus, 4,000 IU/min for 4 hr, then 2000 IU/min for up to 36 hr), rt-PA (0.05 to 0.1 mg/kg/hr for up to 12 hr), and primary operation.[6] There was 1 intracranial hemorrhage in the UK group (0.9%) and 2 in the rt-PA group (1.5%, no significant difference). Although actual rates of overall bleeding complications and efficacy were not reported for the 2 thrombolytic groups, the authors remarked that there were no significant differences detected in any of the outcome variables. In a subsequent "re-analysis" of the data, reported in 1999, the frequency of complete clot lysis was similar with urokinase and rt-PA at the time of the early arteriographic study.[39] This recent data suggests that the rate of thrombolysis may be quite similar, in direct contradistinction to the popularly held view that rt-PA is a much more rapidly acting agent. A multicenter, blinded trial compared the results of thrombolysis with UK vs r-UK in 300 patients with peripheral arterial occlusion. This data was never published. There were no significant differences noted between the 2 agents. A North American multicenter trial compared 3 different doses of r-ProUK to UK in 241 patients with lower extremity arterial occlusions of less than 14 days duration.[40] While the higher r-ProUK dose was associated with slightly greater percentage of patients with complete (>95%) clot lysis at 8 hours, there was a mild increase in the rate of bleeding complications compared with either the UK or the lower dose r-ProUK groups. The fibrinogen levels fell in the higher r-ProUK group, suggesting that fibrin specificity is lost at the higher dose regimens for this compound.

THROMBOLYSIS VS SURGERY AS
THE INITIAL INTERVENTION: OBJECTIVE DATA

There have been 3 well-controlled, randomized comparisons of thrombolytic therapy versus primary operation in patients with recent peripheral arterial occlusion. The first study, the Rochester series, compared urokinase to primary operation in 114 patients presenting with what has subsequently been called "hyperacute ischemia."[4] Enrolled patients in this trial all had severely threatened limbs (Rutherford Class IIb) with mean symptom duration of approximately 2 days. This was a single-center trial that was partially funded by the Thrombolysis and Thrombosis Program Project NIH grant at the University of Rochester. After 12 months of follow-up, 84% of patients randomized to urokinase were alive, compared to only 58% of patients randomized to primary operation (Figure 26–1). By contrast, the rate of limb salvage was identical at 80%. A

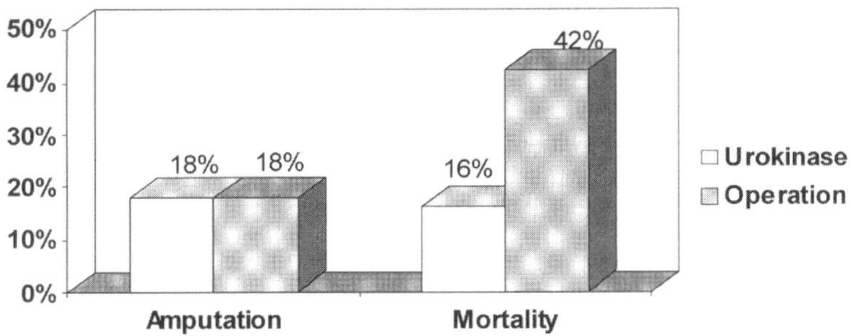

Figure 26–1. The rate of amputation was identical in the 2 treatment groups in the Rochester Trial, but the mortality rate was significantly lower in patients assigned to the thrombolytic arm.

closer inspection of the raw data revealed that the defining variable for mortality differences was the development of cardiopulmonary complications during the periprocedural period. The rate of long-term mortality was high when such periprocedural complications occurred but was relatively low when they did not occur. It was only the fact that such complications occurred more commonly in patients taken directly to the operating theatre that explained the greater long-term mortality rate in the operative group.

The second prospective, randomized analysis of thrombolysis versus surgery was the Surgery or Thrombolysis for the Ischemic Lower Extremity (STILE) trial.[6] Genentech (South San Francisco, CA), the manufacturer of the Activase brand of rt-PA, funded the study. At its termination, 393 patients were randomized to 1 of 3 treatment groups, rt-PA, urokinase or primary operation. Subsequently, the 2 thrombolytic groups were combined for purposes of data analysis when the outcome was found to be similar. While the rate of the composite endpoint of untoward events was higher in the thrombolytic patients, the rate of the more relevant and objective endpoints of amputation and death were equivalent (Figure 26–2). There appeared articles that comprised subgroup analyses of the STILE data, 1 relating to native artery occlusions[41] and 1 to bypass graft occlusions. Thrombolysis appeared more effective in patients with graft occlusions. The rate of major amputation was higher in native arterial occlusions treated with thrombolysis (10% thrombolysis vs 0% surgery at 1 year; p = 0.0024). By contrast, amputation was lower in patients with acute graft occlusions treated with thrombolysis (p = 0.026). These data suggest that thrombolysis may be of greatest benefit in patients with acute bypass graft occlusions of less than 14 days.

The third and final randomized comparison of thrombolysis and surgery was the Thrombolysis or Peripheral Arterial Surgery (TOPAS) trial, funded by Abbott Laboratories (Abbott Park, IL). Following completion of a preliminary dose-ranging trial in 213 patients,[42] 544 patients were randomized to a recombinant form of urokinase or primary operative intervention.[5] After a mean follow-up period of 1 year, the rate of amputation-free survival was identical in the 2 treatment groups, 68.2% and 68.8% in the urokinase and surgical patients, respectively (Table 26–2). While this trial failed to document improvement in survival or limb salvage with thrombolysis, fully 31.5% of the thrombolytic patients were alive without amputation with nothing more than a percuta-

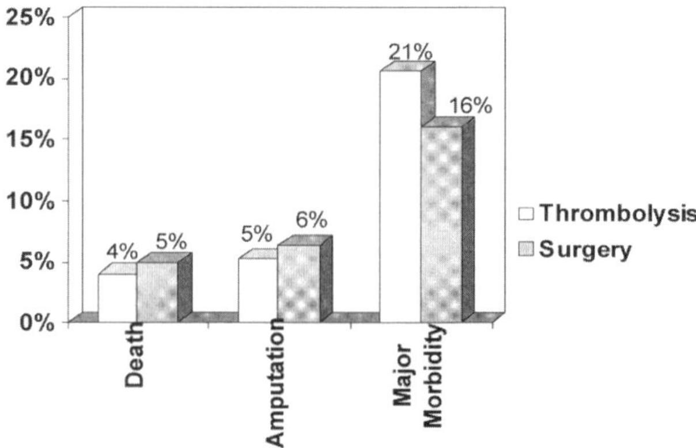

Figure 26–2. Outcome measures from the STILE data after 30 days of follow-up. Note that the rate of death and amputation are similar.

TABLE 26–2. RESULTS OF THE TOPAS TRIAL, DEMONSTRATING SIMILAR MORTALITY RATES AND AMPUTATION-FREE SURVIVAL RATES IN THE THROMBOLYTIC AND SURGERY GROUPS

Intervention	Native-Artery Occlusions (N = 242)			Bypass-Graft Occlusions (N = 302)		
	Urokinase (N = 122)	Surgery (N = 120)	P Value:	Urokinase (N = 150)	Surgery (N = 152)	P Value:
Complete dissolution of dot on final angiogram—no/total no. of patients (%)	67/112 (60)	NA	—	100/134 (75)	NA	—
Increase in ankle-brachial index	0.44±0.04	0.52±0.04	0.15†	0.48±0.03	0.50±0.03	0.76†
Mortality—%						
6 mo	20.8	15.9	0.33‡	12.1	9.4	0.45‡
1 yr	24.6	19.6	0.30‡	16.2	15.0	0.77‡
Amputation-free survival—%						
6 mo	67.6	76.1	0.15‡	76.2	73.9	0.79‡
1 yr	61.2	71.4	0.10‡	68.2	68.8	0.9‡

*Plus-minus values are means ±SE. NA denotes not applicable.
†The P value was based on one-way analysis of variance.
‡The P value was based on Kaplan-Meier analysis.

neous procedure after 6 months of follow-up (Table 26–3). After 1 year, this number had decreased only slightly, with 25.7% alive, without amputation and with only percutaneous interventions. Thus, the original goal of the TOPAS trial, to generate data on which regulatory approval of recombinant urokinase would be based, was not achieved. Nevertheless, the findings confirmed that acute limb ischemia could be managed with

TABLE 26–3. THE THROMBOLYTIC GROUP IN THE TOPAS TRIAL ACHIEVED SIMILAR RATES OF LIMB-LOSS AND MORTALITY WITHOUT THE NEED FOR OPEN SURGICAL INTERVENTION IN A SIGNIFICANT NUMBER OF PATIENTS.

Intervention or Outcome	(N=272)		(N=272)	
	6 Mo	1 Yr	6 Mo	1Yr
		no. of interventions		
Opertive Intervention				
Amputation	48	58	41	51
Above the knee	22	25	19	26
Below the knee	26	33	22	25
Open surgical procedures	315	351	551	590
Major	102	116	177	193
Moderate	89	98	136	145
Minor	124	137	238	252
Percutaneous procedures	128	135	55	70
		% of patients		
Worst outcome†				
Death	16.0	20.0	12.3	17.0
Amputation	12.2	15.0	12.9	13.1
Above the knee	5.6	6.5	6.1	7.5
Below the knee	6.6	8.5	6.8	5.6
Open surgical procedures	40.3	39.3	69.0	65.4
Major	23.6	24.3	39.3	39.3
Moderate	10.3	8.7	16.3	13.4
Minor	6.4	6.3	13.4	12.7
Endovascular procedures	16.9	15.4	2.1	1.7
Medical treatment alone	14.6	10.3	3.7	2.8

catheter-directed thrombolysis, achieving similar amputation and mortality rates but avoiding the need for open surgical procedures in a significant percentage of patients.

TREATMENT OF THE UNDERLYING LESION

Once successful recanalization of the arterial segment or bypass graft has achieved, any underlying culprit lesion must be addressed; thrombolytic therapy alone is seldom sufficient therapy for acute arterial occlusion and must be followed by definitive therapy to address the underlying lesion that caused the occlusion. In fact, when no such lesion can be found, the risk of early rethrombosis is unacceptably high.[43] As testimony to this caveat, Sullivan observed post-thrombolytic 2-year patency rates of 79% in bypass grafts with flow-limiting lesions identified and corrected by angioplasty or surgery versus only 9.8% in those without such lesions. Multiple view arteriography, duplex ultrasound and even intravascular ultrasound interrogation of a bypass graft should all be considered. Only after a wide array of diagnostic interrogations has been exhausted should one elect to merely treat the patient with long term anticoagulation.

Surgical revascularization is unquestioned as appropriate therapy for addressing an underlying arterial lesion, and there exist 3 basic choices: endarterectomy, patch angioplasty, and placement of a new bypass graft. Endarterectomy is an acceptable option when truly localized disease is present, for example, narrowing of the aorta and common iliac arteries alone.[44] Presently, however, endarterectomy is infrequently utilized after successful thrombolytic recanalization; the same lesions appropriate for endarterectomy are suitable for percutaneous procedures. Patch angioplasty continues to play an important role in the treatment of focal lesions uncovered after successful thrombolysis. This is particularly true for lesions within saphenous vein bypass conduits. While satisfactory results have been reported after balloon angioplasty of short vein graft lesions, many continue to advocate a localized operative approach. Patch angioplasty can be performed under local anesthesia with minimal morbidity. Lesions at anastomoses may be best treated with patch angioplasty as opposed to balloon dilatation,[45] and long term success can be anticipated.

A localized procedure is not appropriate when thrombolysis uncovers a diffusely diseased arterial segment or bypass graft. Fotunately, the procedure can usually be delayed until the patient is adequately prepared for this major operative intervention. The traditional operation for aortoiliac occlusive disease is an aortofemoral bypass, performed with a prosthetic graft due to the large caliber of the vessels. Infrainguinal bypass procedures are best performed with autogenous vein grafts, although the results of prosthetic bypasses are acceptable if the graft does not cross the knee joint.[46] The results of bypass procedures are correlated with the level of the disease; aortofemoral reconstructions are associated with higher patency rates than infrainguinal procedures. Nevertheless, with a nondiseased saphenous vein of adequate caliber the long-term patency rate of bypass to even the infrapopliteal (crural) vessels is quite satisfactory, approximating 70% to 80% at 5 years irrespective of whether the vein is reversed or left in situ with the valves disrupted.[47,48] Considering the quite dismal results of percutaneous angioplasty and stenting for disease in the crural arteries, autogenous vein bypass to the distal vessels should be considered as first line therapy in patients with limb-threatening ischemia and distal disease.[48]

Percutaneous catheter interventions to treat occlusive lesions of the lower extremities, first described by Dotter and Judkins in 1964,[49] are attractive alternatives to open surgical procedures such as bypass and endarterectomy. Procedural indications have been liberalized as compared to those for surgical procedures, arguing that the minimally invasive nature of percutaneous modalities warrants broadened application. Nevertheless, although devices and results have improved over time, the long-term patency of percutaneous interventions remains inferior to open surgical techniques. Moreover, the use of primary stenting versus stenting only after inadequate balloon dilation has never been proved to be advantageous when compared to the placement of a stent only after an inadequate balloon dilatation.[50,51]

Proponents of endovascular therapy site 2 contentions to justify continued use of these modalities; first, the decrement in durability is offset by the less invasive nature of endovascular interventions and resultant decreased morbidity, and second, it is infrequent for a patient to experience clinical or angiographic worsening upon failure of an endovascular intervention and the interventions can be repeatedly performed after they fail. In a meta-analysis of 2,116 patients who underwent aortoiliac percutaneous balloon angioplasty (PTA) and stent placement, the 30-day mortality rate was less than 1%.[50] The patency of PTA and stenting for aortoiliac stenoses averages 86% at 3 years, falling to 62% when aortoiliac occlusions are treated.[51] The results of infrainguinal PTA and stenting are not as good, with 3-year patency rates below 60%. Thus, available data would suggest that long-term durability is greater with surgical revascularization compared to endovascular therapy, but periprocedural complications are lower when percutaneous modalities are employed. The risk-benefit ratio associated with endovascular versus open surgical revascularization is a question that can only be answered through the performance of well-designed comparative clinical trials. In patients with anatomically appropriate lesions, however, most practitioners employ endovascular interventions preferentially; a practice based on the presumption of lower risks to the patient when open surgical procedures are avoided.

REFERENCES

1. Dormandy J, Heeck L, Vig S. Acute limb ischemia. *Semin.Vasc Surg.* 1999;12(2):148–153.
2. Blaisdell FW, Steele M, Allen RE. Management of acute lower extremity arterial ischemia due to embolism and thrombosis. *Surgery.* 84, 822–834. 1978.
3. Jivegård L, Holm J, Scherstén T. Acute limb ischemia due to arterial embolism or thrombosis: Influence of limb ischemia versus pre-existing cardiac disease on postoperative mortality rate. *J Cardiovasc Surg.* 1988;29:32–36.
4. Ouriel K, Shortell CK, DeWeese JA, et al. A comparison of thrombolytic therapy with operative revascularization in the initial treatment of acute peripheral arterial ischemia. *J Vasc Surg.* 1994;19(6):1021–1030.
5. Ouriel K, Veith FJ, Sasahara AA. A comparison of recombinant urokinase with vascular surgery as initial treatment for acute arterial occlusion of the legs. *N Engl J Med.* 1998;338: 1105–1111.
6. Anonymous. Results of a prospective randomized trial evaluating surgery versus thrombolysis for ischemia of the lower extremity. The STILE trial. *Ann Surg.* 1994;220(3):251–266.
7. Ouriel K, Kandarpa K, Schuerr DM, et al. Prourokinase versus urokinase for recanalization of peripheral occlusions, safety and efficacy: the PURPOSE trial. *J Vasc Interv Radiol.* 1999;10(8):1083–1091.
8. Ouriel K, Veith FJ. Acute lower limb ischemia: determinants of outcome. *Surgery.* 1998;124: 336–342.
9. McNamara TO, Fischer JR. Thrombolysis of peripheral arterial and graft occlusions: improved results using high-dose urokinase. *AJR American J Roentgenol.* 1985;144:769–775.
10. Tillett WS, Garner R.L. The fibrinolytic activity of hemolytic streptococci. *J Exper Med.* 1933;58:485.

11. Tillett WS, Sherry S. The effect in patients of streptococcal fibrinolysin (streptokinase) and streptococcal desoxyribonuclease on fibrinous, purulent, and snaguinous pleural exudations. *J Clin Invest.* 1949;28:173.
12. Tillett WS, Johnson AJ, McCarty WR. The intravenous infusion of the streptococcal fibrinolytic principle (streptokinase) into patients. *J Clin Invest.* 1955;34:169–185.
13. Cliffton EE, Grunnet M. Investigations of intravenous plasmin (fibrinolysin) in humans. *Circulation.* 1956;14:919.
14. Cliffton EE. The use of plasmin in humans. *Ann NY Acad Sci.* 1957;68:209–229.
15. Reddy DS. Newer thrombolytic drugs for acute myocardial infarction. [Review] [130 refs]. *Indian Exp Biol.* 1998;36(1):1–15.
16. Jostring H, Barth U, Naidu R. Changes of antistreptokinase titer following long-term streptokinase therapy. In: Martin M, Schoop W, Hirsh J, editors. *New Concepts of Streptokinase Dosimetry.* Vienna: Hans Huber; 1978. p. 110.
17. Smith RAG, Dupe RJ, English PD, et al. Fibrinolysis with acyl-enzymes: a new approach to thrombolytic therapy. *Nature.* 1981;290:505.
18. Markland FS, Friedrichs GS, Pewitt SR, et al. Thrombolytic effects of recombinant fibrolase or APSAC in a canine model of carotid artery thrombosis. *Circulation* 1994;90(5):2448–56.
19. Macfarlane RG, Pinot JJ. Fibrinolytic activity of normal urine. *Nature.*1947;159:779.
20. Sobel GW, Mohler SR, Jones, NW, et al. Urokinase: an activator of plasma fibrinolysin extracted from urine. *Am J Physiol.* 1952;171:768–769.
21. Husain SS, Lipinski B, Gurewich V. Isolation of plasminogen activators useful as therapeutic and diagnostic agents (single-chair, high-fibrin affinity urokinase).4,381,346. 1979.
22. Gurewich V. Pro-urokinase: history, mechanisms of action, and clinical development. In: Loscalzo J, Sasahara AA, editors. *New Therapeutic Agents in Thrombosis and Thrombolysis.* New York: Marcel and Dekker;1997. p.539–559.
23. Tanswell P, Tebbe U, Neuhaus KL, et al. Pharmacokinetics and fibrin specificity of alteplase during accelerated infusions in acute myocardial infarction. *J Am Coll Cardiol.* 1992;19:1071–1075.
24. Hoylaerts M, Rijken DC, Lijnen HR, et al. Kinetics of the activation of plasminogen by human tissue plasminogen activator: role of fibrin. *J Biol Chem.* 1982;257:2912.
25. The GUSTO Investigators. An angiographic study within the global randomized trial of aggressive versus standard thrombolytic strategies in patients with acute myocardial infarction. *N Engl J Med.* 1993;329:1615.
26. Cannon CP, McCabe CH, Gibson CM, et al. TNK-tissue plasminogen activator in acute myocardial infarction. Results of the Thrombolysis in Myocardial Infarction (TIMI) 10A dose-ranging trial. *Circulation.* 1997;95(2):351–356.
27. Cannon CP, Gibson CM, McCabe CH, et al. TNK-tissue plasminogen activator compared with front-loaded alteplase in acute myocardial infarction: results of the TIMI 10B trial. Thrombolysis in Myocardial Infarction (TIMI) 10B Investigators. *Circulation.* 1998;98(25):2805–2814.
28. Martin U. Clinical and preclinical profile of the novel recombinant plasmiogen activator retelplase. In: Sasahara AA, Loscalzo J, editors. *New Therapeutic Agents in Thrombosis and Thrombolysis.* New York:Marcel Dekker;1997. p.495–511.
29. Meierhenrich R, Carlsson J, Seifried E, et al. Effect of reteplase on hemostasis variables: analysis of fibrin specificity, relation to bleeding complications and coronary patency. *Int J Cardiol.* 1998;65(1):57–63.
30. Anonymous. A comparison of reteplase with alteplase for acute myocardial infarction. The Global Use of Strategies to Open Occluded Coronary Arteries (GUSTO III) Investigators [see comments]. *N Engl J Med.* 1997;337(16):1118–1123.
31. Ouriel K, Katzen B, Mewissen MW, et al. Initial Experience with Reteplase in the Treatment of Peripheral Arterial and Venous Occlusion. *J Vasc & Intervent.Radiol.* 2000. Ref Type: In Press
32. Hawkey C. Plasminogen activator in the saliva of the vampire bat Desmodus rotundus. *Nature.* 1966;211:434–435.

33. Verstraete M, Lijnen HR, Collen D. Thrombolytic agents in development. *Drugs.* 1995;50(1): 29–42.
34. Randolph A, Chamberlain SH, Chu HL, et al. Amino acid sequence of fibrolase, a direct-acting fibrinolytic enzyme from Agkistrodon contortrix contortrix venom. *Protein Science.* 1992;1(5):590–600.
35. Collen D. Staphylokinase: a potent, uniquely fibrin-selective thrombolytic agent. *Nat Med.* 1998;4(3):279–84.
36. Heymans S, Vanderschueren S, Verhaeghe R, et al. Outcome and one year follow-up of intra-arterial staphylokinase in 191 patients with peripheral arterial occlusion. *Throm Haemost.* 2000;83(5):666–671.
37. Ouriel K, Gray BH, Clair DG. Complications associated with the use of urokinase and recombinant tissue plasminogen activator for catheter-directed peripheral arterial and venous thrombolysis. *J Vasc & Intervent. Radiol.* 2000;
38. Meyerovitz M, Goldhaber SZ, Reagan K, et al. Recombinant tissue-type plasminogen activator versus urokinase in peripheral arterial and graft occlusions: A randomized trial. *Radiology.* 1990;175:75–78.
39. Comerota, AJ A re-analysis of the STILE data. Montefiore Vascular and Endovascular Symposium, Nov 17th, 1999, New York City, NY.
40. Ouriel K, Kandarpa K, Schuerr DM. Prourokinase vs. Urokinase for Recanalization of Peripheral Occlusions, Safety and Efficacy: The PURPOSE Trial. *J Vasc & Intervent Radiol.* 1999;10:1083–1091.
41. Weaver FA, Comerota AJ, Youngblood M. Surgical revascularization versus thrombolysis for nonembolic lower extremity native artery occlusions: results of a prospective randomized trial. The STILE Investigators. Surgery versus Thrombolysis for Ischemia of the Lower Extremity. *J Vasc Surg.* 1996;24(4):513–521.
42. Ouriel K, Veith FJ, Sasahara AA. Thrombolysis or peripheral arterial surgery: phase I results. TOPAS Investigators. [see comments.]. *J Vasc Surg.* 1996;23(1):64–73.
43. Sullivan KL, Gardiner GAJ, Kandarpa K, et al. Efficacy of thrombolysis in infrainguinal bypass grafts. *Circulation.* 1991;83(2:Suppl):Suppl–105.
44. Brewster DC, Darling RC. Optimal methods of aortoiliac reconstruction. *Surgery.* 1978;84: 739–748.
45. Whittemore AD, Donaldson MC, Polak JF, et al. Limitations of balloon angioplasty for vein graft stenosis. *J Vasc Surg.*1991;14(3):340–345.
46. Veith FJ, Gupta SK, Ascer E, et al. Six-year prospective multicenter randomized comparison of autologous saphenous vein and expanded polytetrafluoroethylene grafts in infrainguinal arterial reconstructions. *J Vasc Surg.* 1986;3(1):104–114.
47. Taylor LM Jr., Edwards JM, Porter JM. Present status of reversed vein bypass grafting: five-year results of modern series. *J Vasc Surg.*1990;11;193–206.
48. Belkin M, Knox J, Donaldson MC, et al. Infrainguinal arterial reconstruction with nonreversed greater saphenous vein. *J Vasc Surg.*1996;24:957–962.
49. Dotter CT, Judkins MP. Transluminal treatment of arteriosclerotic obstruction: description of a new technique and a preliminary report of its application. *Circulation.*1964;30:654–670.
50. Bosch JL, Hunink MG. Meta-analysis of the results of percutaneous transluminal angioplasty and stent placement for aortoiliac occlusive disease. *Radiology.*1997;204:87–96.
51. Vorwerk D, Günther RW, Schürmann K, et al. Primary stent placement for chronic iliac artery occlusions: follow-up results in 103 patients. *Radiology.* 1995;194:745–749.

27

Calciphylaxis in Hemodialysis Patients

R. James Valentine, MD

Calciphylaxis is a rare disorder characterized by vascular calcification and tissue necrosis in patients with end-stage renal disease (ESRD). Lesions typically begin as skin mottling (livedo reticularis) and rapidly progress to ulceration and gangrene. The natural history is one of steady deterioration, with high rates of amputation and death.[1–5] Although revascularization has little role in the treatment of calciphylaxis, ulceration and gangrene in affected patients may be misinterpreted as complications of peripheral vascular disease. The purpose of this review is to familiarize the vascular surgeon with the disorder and to outline the currently available treatment methods.

HISTORY

The term "calciphylaxis" was first introduced in 1962 by Selye to describe local tissue calcification induced in rats.[6] In the experimental model, rats were exposed to "sensitizing" agents such as vitamin D, parathyroid hormone (PTH), or a diet high in calcium and phosphorus. The animals were then "challenged" with other agents including iron salts, egg albumin, and glucocorticoids. The resulting skin ulcers contained visible deposits of calcium salts, which the investigators called "calciphylaxis."

The term was used several years later to describe similar lesions in a small group of uremic patients.[7] Since affected patients also had secondary hyperparathyroidism, it was widely theorized that hypercalcemia led to "sensitization," and that calciphylaxis was the result of myriad "challenging" agents, including local trauma. This theory was given credence by numerous reports of lesions appearing at subcutaneous injection sites. Although the Seyle model was used to explain the pathogenesis of the syndrome for many years, it has become apparent that there are important differences between the original lesions described in rats and those typically seen in humans.[8] Most importantly, vascular calcification, a uniform finding in humans with calciphylaxis, was not present in the rat model.[9] To distinguish between the lesions associated with the Seyle model from those seen in humans, Coates et al.[1] have suggested substituting the term "calcific uremic arteriolopathy" in the latter group because it is more descriptive of the histologic findings. Regardless of the term used, the etiology of the syndrome is no longer ascribed to the mechanisms used in the Seyele model (see below).

CLINICAL PRESENTATION AND RISK FACTORS

The vast majority of affected patients have chronic renal failure and secondary hyperparathyroidism, but calciphylaxis has been reported to develop in the setting of primary hyperparathyroidism in patients with normal renal function.[10] It has also been associated with alcohol-related cirrhosis[1] and with Crohn's disease.[11] The syndrome is rare, even among patients with ESRD. The overall incidence has been estimated at less than 1% of patients with ESRD, but the incidence may be increasing. In a retrospective review of 242 patients undergoing hemodialysis for ESRD, Angelis et al.[12] diagnosed calciphylaxis in 10 (4.1%). The rising incidence of calciphylaxis in patients with ESRD has been attributed to decreased use of aluminum-containing phosphate binders in favor of calcium-containing agents, with resulting increases in skin calcium content.[9]

A number of clinical risk factors for calciphylaxis have been evaluated among patients with ESRD. Race and gender appear to be determinants, as the majority of reported patients have been caucasian women.[2,3,13,14] Patient age and duration of hemodialysis may also be important factors: in the prevalence study of 242 hemodialysis patients noted above, Angelis et al. reported that patients with calciphylaxis were significantly younger and had a longer mean duration of dialysis compared to unaffected patients.[12] A number of investigators have established obesity as a risk factor, presumably because adipose tissue is associated with a reduction in local blood flow.[4,13,14] Conversely, malnutrition has also been associated with calciphylaxis. Compared to case controls, affected patients have lower serum albumin levels.[2, 13] Coates et al. have also identified weight loss >10% body weight over 6 months as another important risk factor.[1] Purported serum markers for calciphylaxis include elevated levels of serum calcium,[12] serum phosphate,[2,14] alkaline phosphatase,[12] and parathyroid hormone.[1,3,12]

DIAGNOSIS

The diagnosis of calciphylaxis is based on clinical findings. Patients typically present with mottling (livedo reticularis) and painful, indurated subcutaneous nodules. Lesions usually appear on the upper or lower extremities (Figure 27–1), but involvement of the abdominal wall, breast, and penis has also been described.[1,15,16] Proximal involvement (abdomen, thigh, and buttock) generally carries a worse prognosis compared to more distal involvement (below the knee or elbow).[4,14] Although the thighs and buttocks are the areas most commonly affected, vascular surgeons will more likely be consulted to evaluate patients with distal foot involvement. The vascular examination will usually reveal normal pulses in the affected part: acral gangrene in a hemodialysis patient with normal pedal pulses is considered to be pathognomonic of the disorder.[17,18] However, normal pulses are not always present, as involvement of medium sized arteries may lead to more proximal ischemia in some patients. Reduced or absent pulses may also be indicative of concomitant atherosclerosis. In any event, these findings may confound the diagnosis and delay treatment (see below).

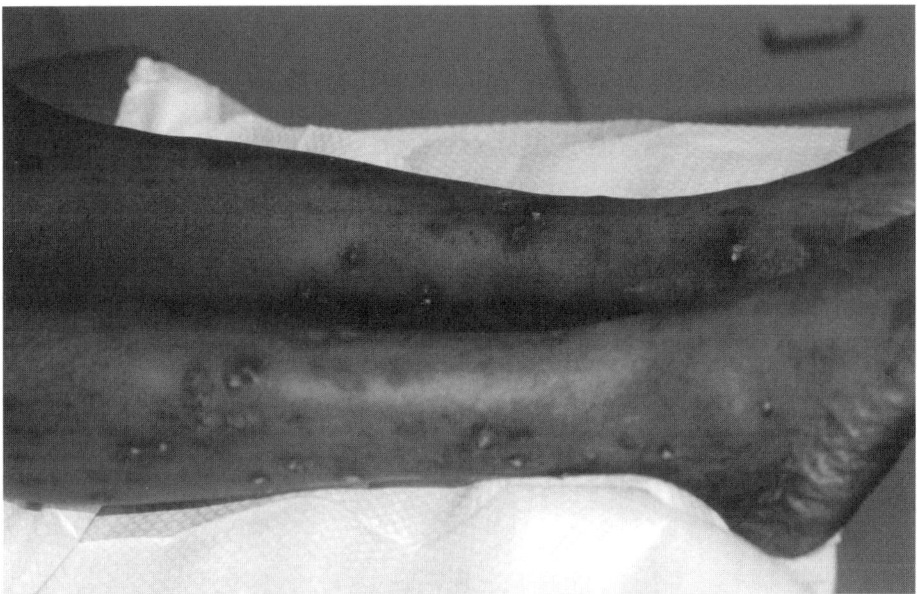

Figure 27–1. Early lesions in calciphylaxis are typically bilateral. Note indurated subcutaneous nodules and ulceration.

The natural history of calciphylaxis is characterized by progression to skin necrosis. Skin lesions are often bilateral and rapidly progress to superficial ulcerations, cutaneous necrosis, and gangrene (Figure 27–2). Plain radiographs of the affected parts typically demonstrate extensive calcification of small and medium-sized arteries (Figure 27–3). While this finding is considered to be a *sine qua non*, it is not specific for calciphylaxis. Among patients without calciphylaxis, vascular calcification is seen in up to 20% with ESRD, in up to 60% with secondary hyperparathyroidism, and up to 70% with tertiary hyperparathyroidism.[12] On the other hand, it is unusual for tissue necrosis to occur in the absence of vascular calcification in patients with ESRD.[9]

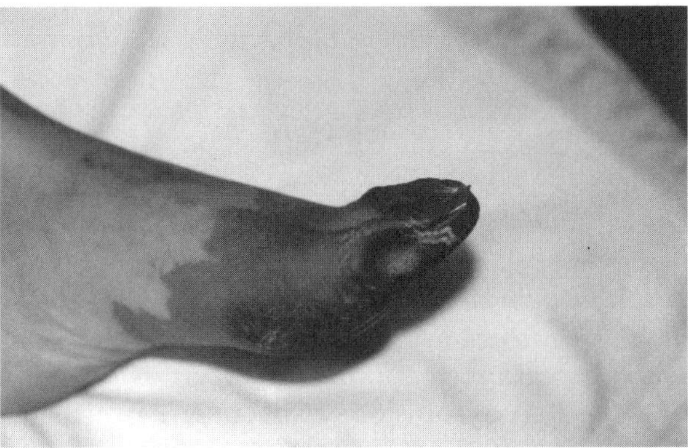

Figure 27–2. Acral gangrene in a patient with calciphylaxis.

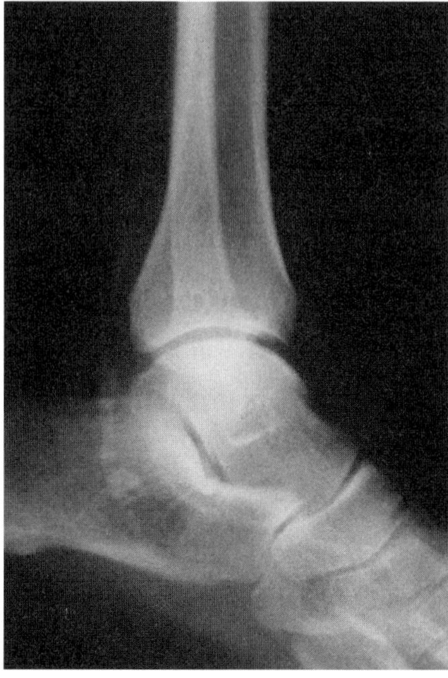

Figure 27–3. Ankle radiograph demonstrating calcification of the posterior tibial artery.

Clinical evaluation should include measurement of serum calcium, phosphorus, and parathyroid hormone levels. Secondary hyperparathyroidism is an important feature of the syndrome, and abnormal calcium deposition has been ascribed a central role in pathogenesis. While most patients have an elevated PTH level, its role is unclear because elevated levels are not universally present. Nevertheless, calcium toxicity is still considered to be an important influence in the development of calciphylaxis, and current treatment regimens are aimed at reducing serum calcium levels (see below). An elevated calcium-phosphorus product [CaXP] >70 mg^2/dl is considered to be a better marker than either serum PTH or calcium levels alone, in part because phosphorus may the critical ion.[14]

The diagnosis of calciphylaxis is confirmed by biopsy. Histologic examination reveals calcification in the tunica media of small arteries of the skin, with variable amounts of luminal narrowing, thrombosis, and acute inflammation[1,14] (Figure 27–4).

PATHOPHYSIOLOGY

Medial calcinosis is considered the hallmark of calciphylaxis, and recent investigations suggest that the process of vascular calcification is not passive. In vitro studies of isolated vascular smooth muscle cells have demonstrated that the cells can dedifferentiate into osteoblast-like precursors capable of elaborating matrix proteins that lead to calcification.[19] One such protein, osteoponin, has been used as a marker in calcified tissues. In a case-controlled study of biopsy specimens from 10 patients with calciphylaxis, Ahmed et al.[14] identified osteoponin in all calcified vessel specimens, but never in noncalcified vessels. The authors concluded that medial calcification is the

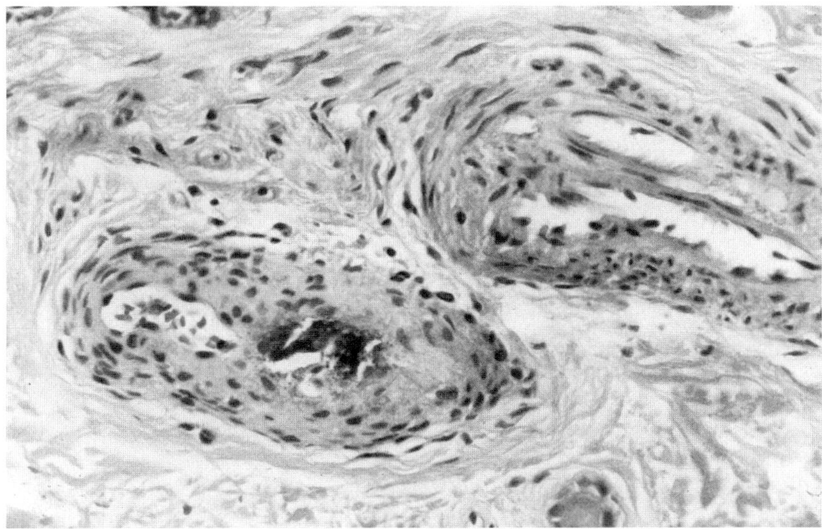

Figure 27–4. Punch biopsy from an area of acral gangrene demonstrating medial calcification and intraluminal thrombus.

associated with increased expression of osteoponin by vascular smooth muscle cells, which adds credence to the theory that the process is cell-mediated.

The common pathologic feature of calciphylaxis is widespread deposition of calcium in small and medium arteries. According to recent theory, calcium deposition leads to medial disruption, progressive luminal encroachment, and ischemia. Tissue ischemia is not limited to areas of advanced skin necrosis. Wilmer et al.[20] demonstrated low transcutaneous oxygen tension levels in patients with calciphylaxis compared to controls, even in areas without skin lesions. Since the low levels did not increase with administration of 100% FIO_2, the authors concluded that calciphylaxis is associated with a fixed insufficiency of the skin vessels.

TREATMENT

Therapy is aimed at control of sepsis and reduction of serum calcium levels. The importance of aggressive wound care cannot be overstated, since sepsis is the most common cause of death in patients with calciphylaxis. Early lesions should be treated with dry dressings, and areas of superficial necrosis should be debrided. In our experience, local wound care is not adequate to control infection in patients who have already developed gangrene.[18] Despite multiple debridements in the operating room and application of skin grafts, all of our patients with lower extremity gangrene developed superimposed infection. Since sepsis is the leading cause of death in these patients, we believe that major amputations are indicated to control rapidly evolving lesions in the extremity. For proximal lesions, wide debridement with application of skin grafts should be performed before infection develops. Judicious use of systemic antibiotics is indicated in patients with necrosis to reduce the risk of invasive infection. The use of adjuvant techniques such as hydrotherapy[18] and hyperbaric oxygen therapy[21] may have limited value in some patients.

Control of serum calcium levels appears to aid healing of superficial lesions and prevent the appearance of future lesions in some patients.[1,3,4,9] The CaXP should be normalized by controlling serum phosphate levels and by lowering serum calcium. This should include a low phosphate diet and use of phosphate binders that do not contain calcium or aluminum.[4,9] Calcium levels can be rapidly lowered by use of calcium-free dialysates.[9] Although controversial, many have advocated routine parathyroidectomy. The operation may not benefit all patients, but those undergoing parathyroidectomy tend to have a better outcome with prompt normalization of the CaXP and rapid wound healing.[3,22,23] Parathyroidectomy is most likely to benefit patients with very high levels of parathyroid hormone,[3] but it is of little value in patients who have already developed gangrene.[18] Because of the tendency for rapid progression, many surgeons advocate performing parathyroidectomy on an urgent basis.[3] Most experienced surgeons recommend total parathyroidectomy; the disease may progress in some patients after subtotal parathyroid resection or autotransplantation.[3]

OUTCOME

Despite aggressive wound therapy and control of serum calcium, the prognosis for patients with calciphylaxis is poor. Reported 1-year survival rates are less than 50%, with a median survival of 9.4 months.[2,3] Parathyroidectomy may confer some benefit in terms of months added to an individual patient's life. Kang reported that the median survival of patients undergoing parathyroidectomy was 14.8 months, which was not significantly different compared to 6.3 months for nonsurgical patients.[3] Published series indicate that sepsis is the cause of death in 60%–90% of affected patients.[1,2,4,8,9,18] Mortality is high among patients undergoing limb amputations, probably because the amputations are performed too late to control advanced sepsis. Surviving patients tend to have prolonged hospitalizations, and healing is notoriously slow.[1–5] The incidence of recurrence among survivors is not known.

VASCULAR RECONSTRUCTION IN PATIENTS WITH ESRD

Previous reports have documented a higher rate of limb loss after revascularization among patients with ESRD compared to patients with functioning kidneys.[24–26] A likely explanation for this discrepancy is that the ESRD populations included patients with calciphylaxis. In a study of 245 patients undergoing distal bypass, Edwards et al.[24] reported that 19 patients with ESRD had a similar bypass patency compared to patients without ESRD, but limb salvage rates were significantly worse. Because 5 of 7 patients with leg lesions >2 cm required amputation for progressive gangrene despite patent bypasses, the authors concluded that patients with ESRD who have large ischemic foot ulcerations proximal to the toes should undergo primary amputation.[24] Others have also reported significantly worse 1-year limb salvage rates in patients with ESRD undergoing bypass for gangrene.[25,26] The vast majority of patients who suffered limb loss had patent bypass grafts at the time of amputation. Although many ESRD patients with less advanced tissue loss may benefit from revascularization, Meyerson et al.[26] have reported that dialysis-dependent patients fare worse than patients with functioning kidneys who have the same degree of tissue loss. The degree of ischemia appears to be the critical factor when considering bypass in a patient with

ESRD: primary amputation is recommended for patients with gangrene involving more than 1 or 2 toes.

SUMMARY

Calciphylaxis is a rare disorder in patients with ESRD, but recent evidence suggests that the incidence is increasing. Affected patients usually present with livedo reticularis, followed by the appearance of subcutaneous nodules that progress rapidly to ulceration and gangrene. The diagnosis is made on clinical grounds, supported by serum markers, and confirmed by tissue biopsy results. The mainstay of treatment is aggressive wound management, with early amputation in patients who have developed extremity gangrene. Some patients with elevated PTH levels appear to have improved wound healing and increased survival after total parathyroidectomy. However, parathyroidectomy seldom improves patients who have developed advanced tissue necrosis. Revascularization procedures are of little benefit in patients with calciphylaxis due to the tendency for ongoing necrosis despite patent bypass grafts. To avoid unnecessary operations, the diagnosis of calciphylaxis should be considered in all ESRD patients presenting with ischemic tissue loss. Amputation, rather than bypass, may be the more appropriate operation in this setting.

REFERENCES

1. Coates T, Kirkland GS, Dymock RB, et al. Cutaneous necrosis from calcific uremic arteriopathy. *Am J Kidney Dis.* 1998;32:384–391.
2. Mazhar AR, Johnson RJ, Gillen DL, et al. Risk factors and mortality associated with calciphylaxis in end-stage renal disease. *Kidney Int.* 2001;60:324–332.
3. Kang AS, McCarthy JT, Rowland C, et al. Is calciphylaxis best treated surgically or medically? *Surgery.* 2000;128:967–972.
4. Mathur RV, Shortland JR, El Nahas AM. Calciphylaxis. *Postgrad Med J.* 2001;77:557–561.
5. Mureebe L, Moy M, Balfour E, et al. Calciphylaxis: A poor prognostic indicator for limb salvage. *J Vasc Surg.* 2001;33:1275–1279.
6. Seyele H. *Calciphylaxis.* Chicago:University of Chicago Press;1962.
7. Anderson DC, Stewart WK, Pierce DM. Calcifying panniculitis with fat and skin necrosis uremia with autonomous hyperparathyroidism. *Lancet.*1968;2:323–325.
8. Oh DH, Eulau D, Tokugawa DA, et al. Five cases a case of calciphylaxis and a review of the literature. *J Am Acad Dermatol.*1999;40:979–987.
9. Llach F. The evolving pattern of calciphylaxis: therapeutic considerations. *Nephrol Dial Transplant.* 2001;16:448–451.
10. Pollock B, Cunliffe , Merchant WJ. Calciphylaxis in the absence of renal failure. *Clin Exper Derm.* 2000;25:389–392.
11. Barri YM, Graves GS, Knochel JP. Calciphylaxis in a patient with Crohn's disease in the absence of end-stage renal disease. *Am J Kidney Dis.* 1997;5:773–776.
12. Angelis M, Wong LL, Myers SA, et al. Calciphylaxis in patients on hemodialysis: A prevalence study. *Surgery* 1997; 122: 1083–1090.
13. Bleyer AJ, Choi M, Igwemezie B, et al. A case control study of proximal calciphylaxis. *Am J Kidney Dis.* 1998;32:376–383.
14. Ahmed S, O'Neill KD, Hood AF, et al. Calciphylaxis is associated with hyperphosphatemia and increased osteoponin expression by vascular smooth muscle cells. *Am J Kidney Dis.* 2001;37:1267–1276.

15. Patetsios P, Bernstein M, Kim S, et al. Severe necrotizing mastopathy caused by calciphylaxis alleviated by total parathyroidectomy. *Amer Surg.* 2000;66:1056–1058.
16. Jhaveri FM, Woosley JT, Fried FA. Penile calciphylaxis: Rare necrotic lesion in chronic renal failure patients. *J Urol.* 1998;160:764–767.
17. Kasirajan K, Obermyer RJ, Lucarelli MR, et al. Calciphylaxis: Calcific angiopathy resulting in acral gangrene. Case reports. *Vasc Surg.* 1998;5:447–453.
18. Davis CA, Valentine RJ. Wet gangrene in hemodialysis patients with calciphylaxis is associated with a poor prognosis. *Cardiovasc Surg.* 2001;9:565–570.
19. Campbell GR, Campbell GH. Vascular smooth muscle and arterial calcification. *J Cardiol.* 2000;2:54–62.
20. Wilmer WA, Voroshilova O, Singh I, et al. Transcutaneous oxygen tension in patients with calciphylaxis. *Am J Kidney Dis.* 2001;37:797–806.
21. Vassa N, Twardowski ZJ, Campbell, et al. Hyperbaric oxygen therapy in calciphylaxis-induced skin necrosis in a peritoneal dialysis patient. *Am J Kidney Dis.* 1998;32:884–891.
22. Janigan DT, Hirsh DJ, Klassen GA, et al. Calcified subcutaneous arterioles with infarcts of the subcutis and skin ("calciphylaxis") in chronic renal failure. *Am J Kidney Dis.* 2000;35:588–597.
23. Kriskovich MD, Holman JM, Haller JR. Calciphylaxis: Is there a role for parathyroidectomy? *Laryngoscope.* 2000;110:603–607.
24. Edwards JM, Taylor LM Jr, Porter JM. Limb salvage in end-stage renal disease (ESRD). Comparison of modern results in patients with and without ESRD. *Arch Surg.* 1988;123:1164–1168.
25. Johnson BL, Glickman MH, Bandyk DF, et al. Failure of foot salvage in patients with end-stage renal disease after surgical revascularization. *J Vasc Surg.* 1995;22:280–286.
26. Meyerson SL, Skelly CL, Curi MA, et al. Long-term results justify autogenous infrainguinal bypass grafting in patients with end-stage renal failure. *J Vasc Surg.* 2001;34:27–33.

28

Contemporary Management of Foot Ulcers

Bauer E. Sumpio, MD, PhD and Peter A. Blume, DPM

BIOMECHANICS OF WALKING AND ULCER FORMATION

Gait is a complex set of events which require triplanar foot motion and control of multiple axes in order for complete bipedal ambulation (Figure 28–1A).[1] When the heel hits the ground, its outer edge touches first. Soft tissues (muscles, tendons, and ligaments) relax. The foot is able to flatten, adapt to uneven surfaces, and absorb the shock of touchdown. During midstance, the heel lies below the anklebone, and the front and back of the foot are aligned and the foot easily bears weight. As the heel lifts, it swings slightly to the inside. Muscles, tendons, and ligaments tighten. The foot regains its arch, allowing your toes to push your weight off the ground.

Sensory input from visual, vestibular, and proprioceptive information from the lower extremities is necessary to modify learned motor patterns and muscular output to execute the desired action. There are a variety of external and internal forces[2] that can impact on foot function. Friction and compressive forces are produced by the body weight pushing down and ground reactive forces pushing up. Shear results from the bones of the foot sliding parallel to their plane of contact during pronation and supination. Foot deformities or ill-fitting footwear will enhance pressure points since they focus the forces on a smaller area. When the foot flattens too much (overpronation), the ankle and heel do not align during midstance and some bones are forced to support too much weight. The foot strains under the body's weight. The muscles pull harder on these areas, making it more difficult for tendons and ligaments to hold bones and joints in place. Over time, swelling or pain on the bottom of the foot or near the heel may occur. Bunions may form at the toe joint. Abnormal foot biomechanics resulting from limited joint mobility, foot deformities will magnify the shearing forces and plantar pressure on the foot during ambulation and represent critical causes for tissue breakdown.

Ulcers are breaks in the dermal barrier with subsequent erosion of underlying subcutaneous tissue. In severe cases the breach may extend to muscle and bone. Although

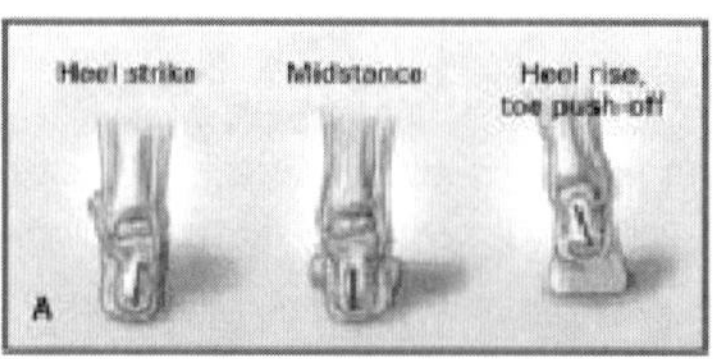

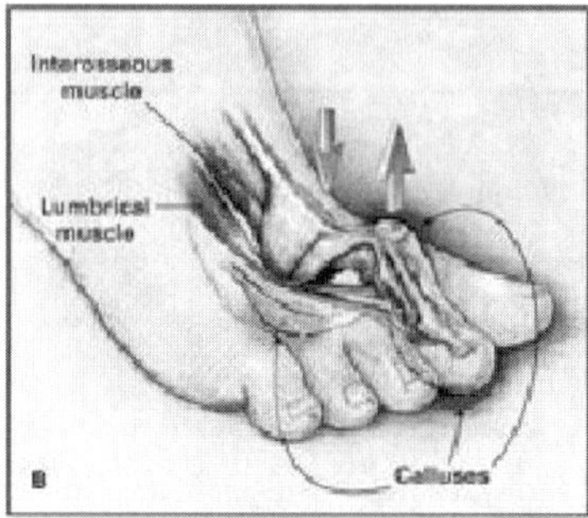

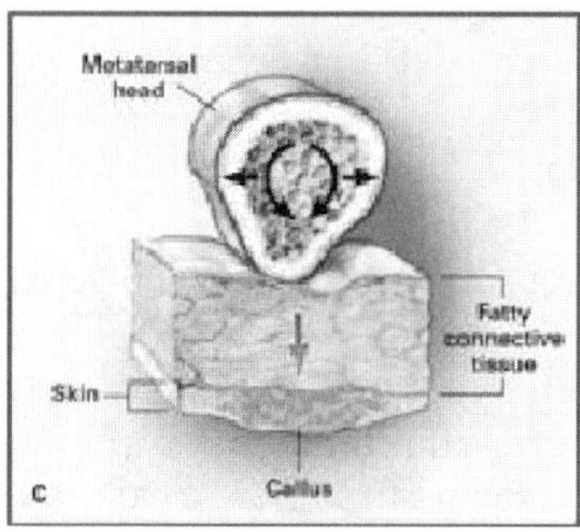

Figure 28–1. (A) Biomechanics of gait. The normal mechanics of the foot and ankle are the combined effects of muscle, tendon, ligament and bone function. Gait is classically broken into 4 distinct segments: 1) heel strike, where the lateral calcaneus makes contact with the ground and the muscles, tendons and ligaments relax providing for optimal energy absorption, 2) mid-stance, where the foot is flat and is able to adapt to uneven terrain, maintain equilibrium and absorb the shock of touchdown. The calcaneus is just below the ankle, keeping the front and back of the foot aligned for optimum weight bearing. 3) heel rise, where the calcaneus lifts off, the foot pronates and the muscles, tendons, and ligaments tighten and the foot regains its arch, 4) toe push off. **(B)** Forces on the foot. Friction and compressive forces are produced by the body weight pushing down and ground reactive forces pushing up. Friction and pressure combine as a shear force during dynamic walking as a result of the bones of the foot sliding relative to each other in a direction parallel to their plane of contact during pronation and supination. Wasting of intrinsic muscles of the foot results in an imbalance in the forces acting on the bony structures. This can lead to toe deformities, prominent metatarsal heads, equinus deformity, varus position of the hind foot and proximal malalignment. **(C)** Consequences of callus formation. Inadequate distribution of the forces of weight bearing or the presence of foot deformities can lead to abnormal movement which produces excessive stress and results in breakdown of connective tissue and muscle. (From ref 4)

simple cutaneous breakdown is not infrequent because of shearing forces or direct trauma, healing is the rule unless the wound repair mechanisms are suboptimal due to impairment of perfusion, infection or repeated, continuous traumatic insults. Lack of sensation allows the damage to cascade to ulceration. Lack of perfusion decreases tissue resilience and leads to rapid death of tissue and impedes wound healing for tissue repair. Broadly speaking, therefore, the progression to foot ulceration can be attributed to impaired arterial supply, neuropathy, musculoskeletal deformities or a combination of these factors (Table 28–1).[3] The etiology of the majority of foot ulcers can be ascertained quite accurately by a careful problem-focused history and physical

TABLE 28–1. RISK FACTORS FOR THE DEVELOPMENT AND NON-HEALING OF FOOT ULCERS

1. Arterial Insufficiency (Atherosclerosis, Vasculitis)
     - TcPO2 ≤30 mm Hg
     - Ankle pressure ≤40 mm Hg, toe pressure ≤30 mm Hg
2. Venous hypertension
3. Sensorimotor neuropathy
4. High plantar pressure
     - history of prior ulceration
     - prior surgery involving metatarsal heads
     - callus, blister or macerated skin,
5. Altered biomechanics
     - limited joint mobility,
     - limited toe dorsiflexion
6. Musculoskeletal deformity
     - severe nail pathology
     - prominent metatarsal heads, claw toes
     - Charcot foot
     - other plantar bony prominences
8. Infections
9. Trauma
10. Diabetes

examination. Early recognition of the etiology of these foot lesions and prompt management of the ulcer is essential for good functional outcome. In many cases, successful salvage of an extremity is dependent upon a multidisciplinary team of specialists and timely consultation is warranted.[4]

Vascular Insufficiency

Arterial insufficiency is suggested by a history of underlying cardiac or cerebrovascular disease, complaints of leg claudication or impotence or pain in the distal foot when supine (rest pain). Findings of diminished or absent pulses, pallor on elevation, dependent rubor, sluggish capillary toe refill, and absence of toe hair or thickened nails are consistent with impaired arterial perfusion to the foot. Ischemic ulcers are characterized by absence of bleeding, pain, and a precipitating trauma or underlying foot deformity. They often develop on the dorsum of the foot (Figure 28–2A), and over the first (Figure 28–2B) and fifth metatarsal heads (Figure 28–2C). Ischemic ulcers are uncommon on the plantar surface as the pressure is usually less sustained, and perfusion better. A heel ulcer can develop from constant pressure applied while the heel is in a dependent position or during prolonged immobilization and bed rest (Figure 28–2D). It should not be a surprise that a patient with relatively mild symptoms of arterial insufficiency develop limb-threatening extremity ulcers. This is due to the fact that once an ulcer is present, the blood supply necessary to allow healing of an ulcer is greater than that needed to maintain intact skin. This will develop into a chronic ulcer unless the blood supply is improved.

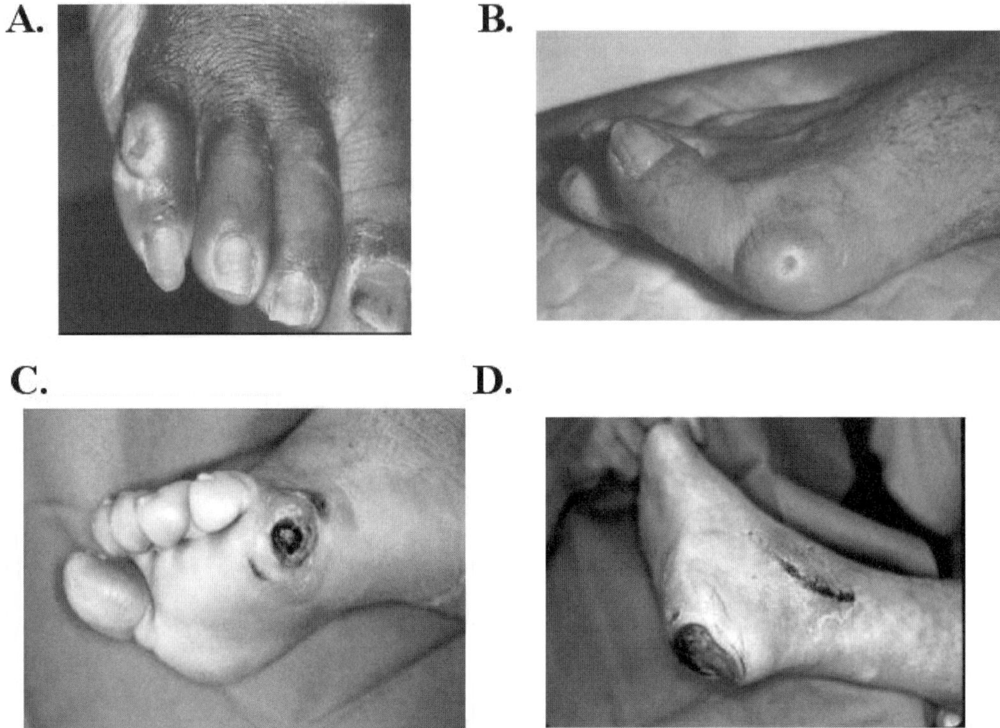

Figure 28–2. (A) 5th digit hammer toe with neurotrophic ulcer **(B)** halluxabductovalgus neurotrophic ulcer **(C)** necrotic 5th metatarsal head ulcer **(D)** heel ulcer

Elevated venous pressures due to perforator or deep vein incompetency or venous thrombosis reduce the pressure gradient for perfusion and results in inadequate tissue perfusion because the elevated venous pressures and the venous stasis hinders clearance of breakdown products. However, venous ulcers rarely present in the foot and are commonly located in the "gaiter" distribution of the leg, around the medial malleolus, where the venous pressures are highest, and are associated with a swollen leg with a distinctive skin appearance (Figure 28–3).

Four foot-related risk factors have been identified in the genesis of pedal ulceration: peripheral neuropathy, evidence of increased pressure, altered biomechanics, and limited joint mobility, bony deformity or severe nail pathology.[3]

Neuropathy

Neuropathy is the most common underlying etiology of foot ulceration and frequently involves the somatic and autonomic fibers. Loss of protective sensation due to peripheral neuropathy is the most common cause of ulceration. Neurotrophic ulcers typically form on the plantar aspect of the foot at areas of excessive focal pressures, which are most commonly encountered over bony prominences of the metatarsal heads and the forefoot region due to the requirements of midstance and heel off during the gait cycle (Figure 28–4). Sensory dysfunction affects mainly the proprioreception, light touch and pain fibers and therefore, results in increased shearing forces and repeated trauma to the foot. Autonomic nerve involvement results in tissues that are anhydrotic, warm, and at greater risk of cracking and fissuring.[5]

A.   **B.**

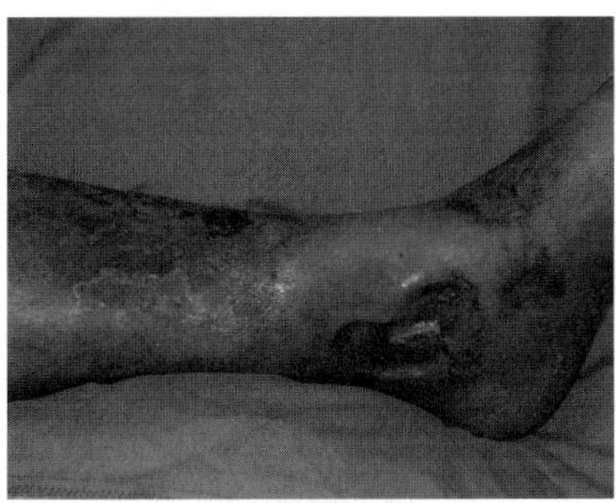
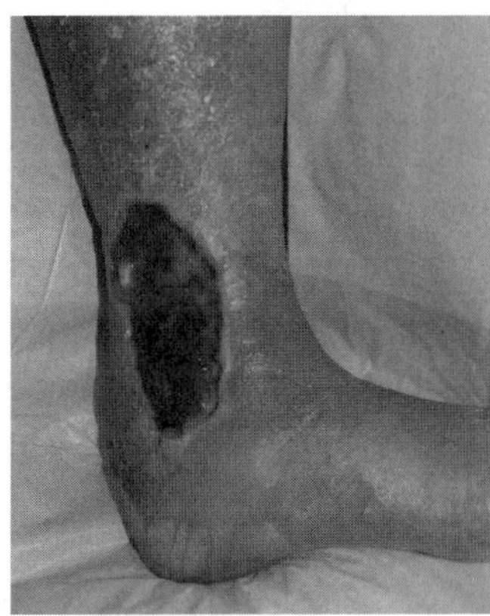

Figure 28–3. Examples of venous stasis ulcers. Note the typical location in the "gaiter" region of the leg.

Neuropathic patients have inadequate protective sensation during all phases of gait, therefore high loads are undetected due to loss of pain threshold. This results in prolonged and increased forces.[6,7] These problems manifest as abnormal pressure points, increased shearing, and greater friction to the foot.

Musculoskeletal Deformities

Atrophy of the small muscles within the foot results in nonfunctioning intrinsic foot muscles or an "intrinsic minus foot" (Figure 28–1B).[8] An intrinsic minus foot causes loss of stability as these muscles help stabilize the metatarsal-phalangeal joints during midstance of gait. For example, atrophy of the lumbrical and interosseous muscles of the foot resulting in collapse of the arch, overpowering by extrinsic muscles leads to digital contractures and cocked up toes, equinuus deformity at the ankle and a varus hind foot (Figure 28–4). These extrinisic weakesses allow for the development of hammer toes, toes with increased retrograde pressure on the metatarsal heads with anterior displacement of the protective plantar fibro-fatty padding.[9] A cavovarus foot type leads to decreased range of motion of the pedal joints, an inability to adapt to terrain, and low tolerance to shock (Figure 28–5). In essence a mobile adapter is converted to a rigid lever. Pressure is equal to body weight divided by surface area, thus decreasing surface area below a metatarsal head with concomitant rigid deformities leads to increased forces or pressure to the sole of the foot. When neuropathic foot disease is associated with congenital foot deformities, such as long or short metatarsals, a plantar-flexed metatarsal, abnormalities in the metatarsal parabola or a Charcot foot (Figure 28–6), there is a higher propensity towards breakdown as a result of increased abnormal plantar foot pressures.

Increasing body weight and decreasing the surface area of contact of the foot components with the ground will increase pressure. A low pressure but constant insult over an extended period can have the same ulcerogenic effect as high pressure over a

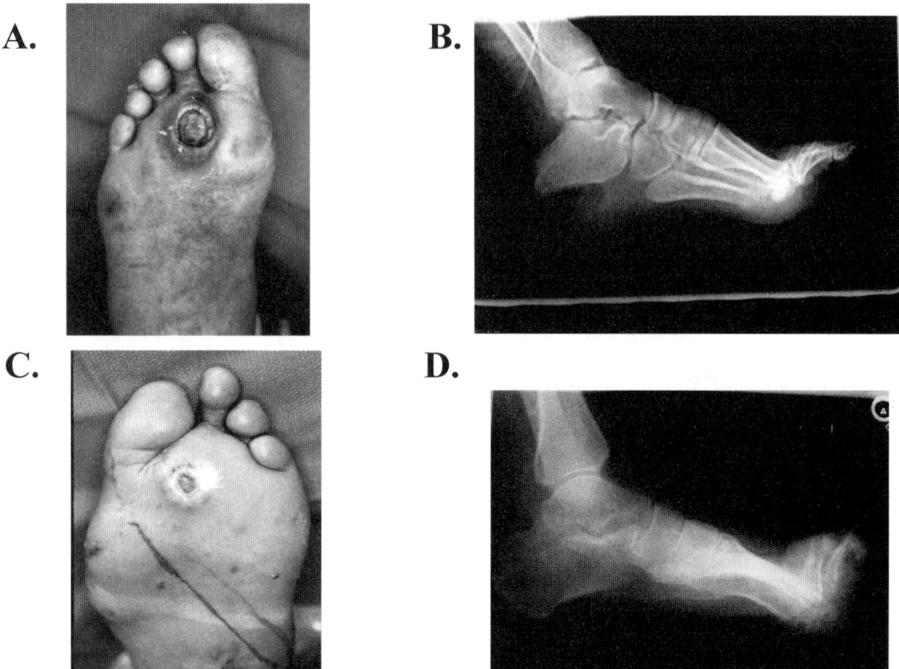

Figure 28–4. (A) 2nd metarsal head ulcer ,well perfused, but neurotrophic **(B)** corresponding foot x-ray of patient in Figure A. Note the foot deformity and hammer toes. **(C)** 2nd submetatarsal ulcer **(D)** corresponding foot x-ray or patient in Figure C. Note the cavus foot deformity, retrograde buckling and global hammer toe deformities

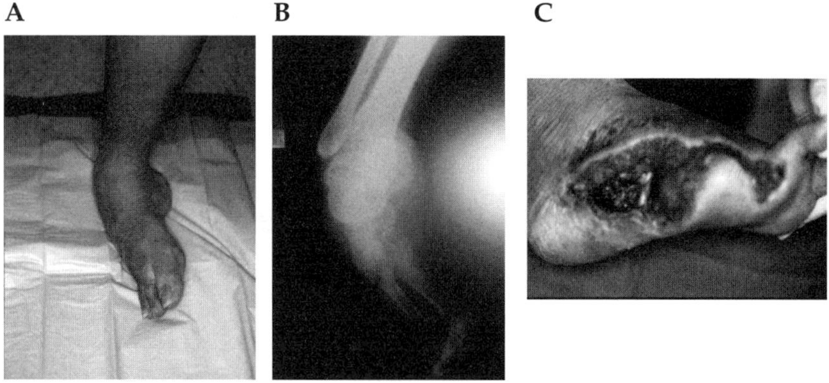

Figure 28–5. Patient with an equinovarus deformity of foot, secondary to resection of the peroneal complex **(A)** Picture of the leg **(B)** x-ray of the leg, **(C)** foot wound along the lateral edge due to equinovarus

shorter period. This is typical of the effect of tight fitting shoes. If the magnitude of these forces in a given area is large enough either skin loss or hypertrophy of the stratum corneum (callus) occurs (Figure 28–1C). The presence of callus in patients with neuropathy should raise a red flag since the risk of ulceration in a callused area is increased by 2 orders of magnitude. Clinical findings predicitive of high plantar pressure are summarized in Table 28–1.

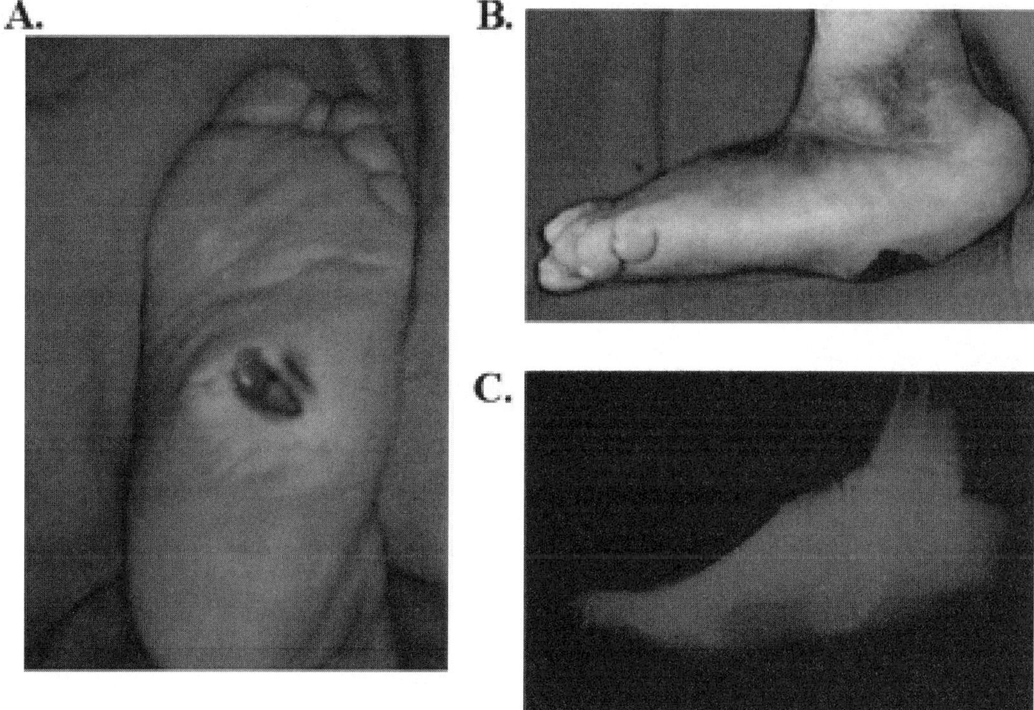

Figure 28–6. Example of an ulcer occurring in a patient with a Charcot foot. **(A)** Plantar view of the ulcer. **(B)** lateral view of the ulcer. Note the severe equinous deformity and the rockerbottom foot **(C)** x-ray of the foot demonstrating the subluxed cuboid bone.

Diabetes

Diabetic patients are particularly prone to foot ulcers. Approximately 16 million people, comprising 6% of the U.S. population is estimated to have diabetes.[10] In 1996 alone, there were 798,000 new cases of diabetes diagnosed. This becomes even more significant with increasing age as the prevalence of diabetes increases to 18% in the population over age 65.[10] Of the U.S. diabetic population, it is estimated that 15% will develop manifestations of diabetic foot disease in their lifetime.[11] In addition, diabetics have an annual incidence of 2–3% for developing a foot ulceration.[11] Although representing only 6% of the population, diabetics account for 46% of the 162,000 hospital admissions for foot ulcers annually.[11] This prevalence of foot disease in the diabetic population results in significant clinical and economic impact. Data from the National Hospital Discharge Survey demonstrates that approximately 51% of non-traumatic lower extremity amputations are performed on diabetics.[12] The age adjusted amputation rate is between 15–40% higher in diabetics than non-diabetics.[12]

The American Diabetes Association consensus group identified increased risk in patients with diabetes for >10 years, are males, have poor glucose control or have cardiovascular, retinal or renal complications.[3] Diabetics are prone to atherosclerotic disease and neuropathy. As the disease process of diabetes progresses, patients can experience alterations in distal perfusion and a neuropathic component may become apparent which can be adversely affected as a result of these complications. Neuropathy is shown to be present in 42% of diabetics after 20 years[13] and is usually a distal symmetric sensorimotor polyneuropathy affecting both myelinated type A fibers and un-myelinated type C fibers. Type A fibers are associated mainly with proprioception, light touch, pressure sensation, vibratory perception, and motor nerves to the muscle spindles. Type C fibers are associated with free nerve endings which appear to help detect noxious, painful, and thermal stimuli. Diabetic neuropathy manifests reduced or absent reflexes, sensory loss in stocking and glove distribution, and intrinsic muscle wasting. Furthermore, the ability of diabetic people to ward off even superficial infections is impaired. Purely ischemic diabetic foot ulcers are uncommon, representing between 10–15% of ulcers.[14] More commonly, ulcers have a mixed ischemic and neuropathic origin representing 33%.[14]

WOUND ASSESSMENT AND MANAGEMENT

Management of foot ulcers can be categorized into 2 parts: the initial local wound care and recognition and correction of the underlying etiology of the ulcer.

Assessment of the ulcer consists of a determination of the size and depth of the wound and inspection of the surrounding area for local signs of infection or gangrene. A number of classification systems have been devised.[15]

The absence of systemic manifestations such as fever, chills or leukocytosis is an unreliable indicator and the use of plain films of the foot, to rule out osteomyelitis, or culture of the base of an ulcer are frequently needed. Aggressive mechanical debridement, systemic antibiotic therapy and strict non-weight bearing are the cornerstones for effective wound care. Sharp debridement in the operating room or at the bedside, when applicable, allows for thorough removal of all necrotic material and optimizes the wound environment. Foot soaks, whirlpool therapy, or enzymatic debridement are rarely effective and may lead to further skin maceration or wound breakdown. There are no prospective randomized studies which demonstrate the superiority of dressing products compared to standard saline wet to dry sterile gauze in establishing a granulation bed. Use of moist dressings in clean, granulating wounds has been recommended to enhance the wound environment. In cases of gross wound infections and rampant cellulitis, use of a silver containing medication such as Silvadene may be necessary in the intitial setting to reduce the bacterial load. Oral antimicrobial therapy should be instituted based on the suspected pathogen and clinical findings. Intravenous antimicrobials should be administered for severe infections. Future advances such as use of bioactive drugs (e.g. Recombinant PDGF, Regranex) or skin substitutes (e.g. Apligraf, Dermagraft) are currently being evaluated and may be useful under specific circumstances.

VASCULAR ASSESSMENT AND MANGEMENT

Once the wound has been evaluated and initially managed as above, the emphasis is on early accurate assesment of impairment of perfusion. Adequacy of perfusion and healing potential of the wound is assessed by non-invasive physiological studies.[16]

These include measurement of segmental limb pressures, pulse volume waveform assessment and transcutanous oxygen measurements. It must be emphasized that any given patient may require only selected tests.

Segmental limb pressures are an extension of the bedside ankle-brachial index. This non-invasive test is indicated in any patient for whom history and physical examination suggests peripheral vascular disease. By obtaining pressures at successive levels of the extremity, the level of disease can be localized in most cases. Measurement of an ankle pressure <40 mm Hg suggests a low likelihood of healing. Diabetics with medial sclerosis and patients with chronic renal insufficiency often have non-occlusive pressures with ABIs greater than 1.3 limiting the utility of segmental pressures in the evaluation of peripheral vascular disease in these populations. In patients with calcified vessels, such as diabetics or patients with long standing renal failure, use of toe pressure measurements, transcutaneous oximetry, or waveform analysis may be necessary.

The toe-brachial index is a more reliable indicator of foot perfusion in diabetics because the small vessels of the toes are often spared of medial calcification. The absolute toe pressures are of value in the estimation of the healing potential ulcer with a pressure greater than 30 mm Hg favorable for ulcer healing.[17]

An adjunctive method to establish the disease level is through waveform analysis with pulse volume recordings. Pulse volume recordings are obtained through the application of sequential blood pressure cuffs with an air pleythysmographic technique. The normal PVR waveform has a sharp upstroke and peak with a reflected wave present before returning to baseline. With mild obstruction, the reflected wave is lost, the upstroke delayed and the peak blunted. Moderate to severe obstruction produces a bowing of the downstroke away from the baseline. A flat PVR is irregular with low amplitude and indicates severe obstruction.

Segmental blood pressure testing, toe brachial index measurements, and waveform analysis can be performed before and after exercise to unmask occlusive disease not apparent on resting studies. With exercise, blood flow normally increases 3- to 5-fold to meet the increased demand and resistance in the muscular bed falls. The presense of a significant stenosis limits this compensatory response and magnifies the pressure gradient across the lesion. A normal response to exercise is a slight increase or no change in the ankle systolic pressure compared to baseline and rules out vascular insufficiency as the cause of symptoms. A fall in ankle pressure by more than 20% of baseline or below an absolute pressure of 60 mmHg which requires more than 3 minutes to recover is considered abnormal.[18] Single level disease is inferred with a recovery time less than 6 minutes with greater than a 6 minute recovery time associated with multilevel disease. The administration of pharmacologic agents such as priscoline or the induction of reactive hyperemia can be performed in place of exercise testing in patients with limited exercise ability due to cardiopulmonary disease of musculoskeletal problems.

Transcutaneous oxygen measurement may provide supplemental information regarding local tissue perfusion. Platinum oxygen electrodes are placed on the chest wall and legs or feet. Either the absolute value at the oxygen tension at the foot or leg or a ratio of this value to that of the chest wall may be evaluated. A normal value at the foot is 60 mmHg and a normal chest/foot ratio is .9.[19] Controversy exists regarding the optimal level for tissue healing. It is generally accepted that wounds are likely to heal if oxygen tension is greater than 40 mmHg (foot/chest ratio >.5) and that healing is not likely to with a value less than 20 mmHg. Transcutaneous oxygen measurements can also be obtained in conjunction with exercise testing. Normally the value will not diminish, however, in the patient with arterial occlusive disease, the value will fall

In summary the assessment of the patient with peripheral vascular disease encompasses a thorough history and physical examination with the adjunctive use of the non-invasive vascular laboratory to confirm, localize, and grade lesions. While multiple non-invasive and invasive methods are available to assess the peripheral vasculature, it should be obvious that not every patient requires a exhaustive battery of tests in order to evaluate their vascular status. In general, only those tests which are likely to provide information which will alter the course of action should be performed. Differing clinical syndromes mandate the extent of peripheral vascular testing. It is imperative that flow-limiting arterial lesions are evaluated and reconstructed or bypassed.

NEUROPATHY AND MUSCULOSKELTAL ASSESSMENT AND MANGEMENT

Cutaneous pressure perception measured by Semmes-Weinstein monofilaments has been widely considered to be an ideal screening instrument for neuropathy and potential for ulceration because of its simplicity, sensitivity, and low cost.[20–22] People with normal foot sensation can usually feel the 4.17 filament (equivalent to 1g of linear pressure). Patients who cannot feel the 5.07 monofilament (equivalent to 10 g of linear pressure) when it buckles are considered to have lost protective sensation.[23] Several cross-sectional studies indicated that foot ulceration and elevated cutaneous pressure perception thresholds were strongly associated and more predictive than biothesiometry. Magnitudes of association, however, were provided in a case-control study by McNeely et al.,[24] who reported an unadjusted sevenfold risk of ulceration in those patients (97% male) with insensitivity to the 5.07 monofilament. Abnormal mechanical forces that can result in ulcerations should be addressed with the use of offloading devices in order to assist in wound healing.

The presence of neuropathy mandates attention to the biomechanics of the foot. The role of the podiatrist or foot surgeons in the evaluation of these patients cannot be underscored enough. Use of F scan to assess potential sites of breakdown has led to greater use of orthotic devices in the prevention of skin breakdown. This computerized gait analysis system uses an ultra-thin Tekscan sensor consisting of 960 sensor cells (5 mm^2 each). The sensor is used in a floor mat system designed to measure barefoot or stocking-foot dynamic plantar pressures indicating those subjects with pressures ≥ 6 kg/cm^2. Off-loading strategies such as use of total contact cast or a removable walker, has resulted in significant decrease in healing times. The stresses placed upon the foot can be intrinsic in nature as was previously described with respect to digital contractures, or stresses may be extrinsic in nature. These external forces can result from inappropriate footwear, traumatic injury, and/or foreign bodies. Shoes that are too tight or too shallow are a frequent, yet preventable component to the development of neuropathic ulcers. Boulton et. al.[6] and Veves et. al.[7] have demonstrated that there is an increase in both static and dynamic foot pressures when evaluating the neuropathic foot. To date, high pressures alone have not been shown to cause foot ulceration. Masson et. al.[25] evaluated high plantar foot pressures in rheumatoid patients with no sensitivity deficit and there was no evidence of foot ulceration noted. A variety of shoe modifications such as rocker sole design and different types of insoles, have shown that it is possible to reduce plantar foot pressures thus decreasing risks of ulceration.[26–28]

Reconstructive foot surgery may often become the conservative treatment in order to avoid major amputations in these chronic neuropathic wounds. The endpoint for chronic diabetic foot wounds should include reduction in the number of major amputations, prevention of infection, decrease probability of ulceration, maintaining skin integrity, and improvement of function. Successful outcomes for diabetic foot reconstruction should result in less intrinsic pressures via minor amputations, arthroplasties, osteotomies, chondylectomies, exostectomies, tendon procedures, and joint arthrodeisis. Open wounds can be treated in 1 stage and are primarily closed with premorbid tissue using local flap reconstruction and soft tissue repair.[29] Plastic surgical repair of these wounds can help avoid the production of inelastic scar tissue over weight bearing surfaces. Extrinsic pressures and intrinsic pressures can be further neutralized with post-op accommodative shoe gear. Prophylactic diabetic foot surgery may prevent recurrent ulceration and decrease the risk of major amputations.[30,31] Surgical biomechanics, plastic and soft tissue reconstruction, as well as appropriate off loading are all essential to creating a stable platform from which

SUMMARY

It was estimated that in 1986, "chronic skin ulcers" accounted for $150 million of cost.[12] The average cost of a lower extremity amputation in the nineties was calculated to be between $24,000 and $40,000.[32] In 1990, $600 million was spent on the 54,000 lower extremity amputations performed that year.[12] The role of the vascular surgeon in the evaluation, diagnosis, and management of foot ulcers is critica.[33] Foot disease is a common complication of diabetes that can have tragic consequences. For the majority of patients with foot ulcers, adherence to the principles outlined above will suffice for optimum treatment of these wounds (Figure 28–7).

Tight glucose control can reduce microvascular diabetic complications, including peripheral sensory neuropathy and thus development of foot ulcers. Patient education is essential for risk-factor reduction and early recognition of foot complications (Table 28–2). Awareness and training of healthcare providers in diagnosing and treating diabetic foot disease are paramount and may begin with such simple measures as adding a wall poster or chart reminder to conduct foot examinations in all diabetic patients at every office visit.

The population affected by disease represents a significant portion of the elderly and diabetic community. The major areas of influence include neuropathy, arterial vascular disease and infection. These patients require special attention directed towards these issues in attempt to limit morbidity and extend limb life in the diabetic patient. These include patient education and frequent inspection of the neuropathic foot. Careful assessment of vascular disease leading to bypass surgery when indicated, evaluation and management of biomechanical abnormalities, and aggressive treatment of any infections is also required to affect the natural history of this disease.[34] The multidisciplinary approach to limb salvage will enable us to provide a comprehensive treatment protocol which yields greater long term viability of the lower extremity.

Advances in telemedicine will allow both the patient and care-provider greater opportunity for interaction and, hopefully, improve patient management. The Internet will allow for both real-time evaluation of wounds from the home setting and decrease transportation needs and costs. Other initiatives include photographic tools, especially digital photography; e.g., it is probable that soon diabetic patients and their physicians will be able to access ulcer history and progression from a diskette that forms part of the medical record. Such systems require a way for the care-providers to categorize and share critical data, which is simple to use, yet powerful enough to communicate management options.

ACKNOWLEDGEMENT

The authors wish to acknowledge the assistance of Christopher Moore, D.P.M. in collating the clinical figures. This work supported in part by the North American Foundation for Limb Preservation.

Assessment and Management of Foot Ulcers

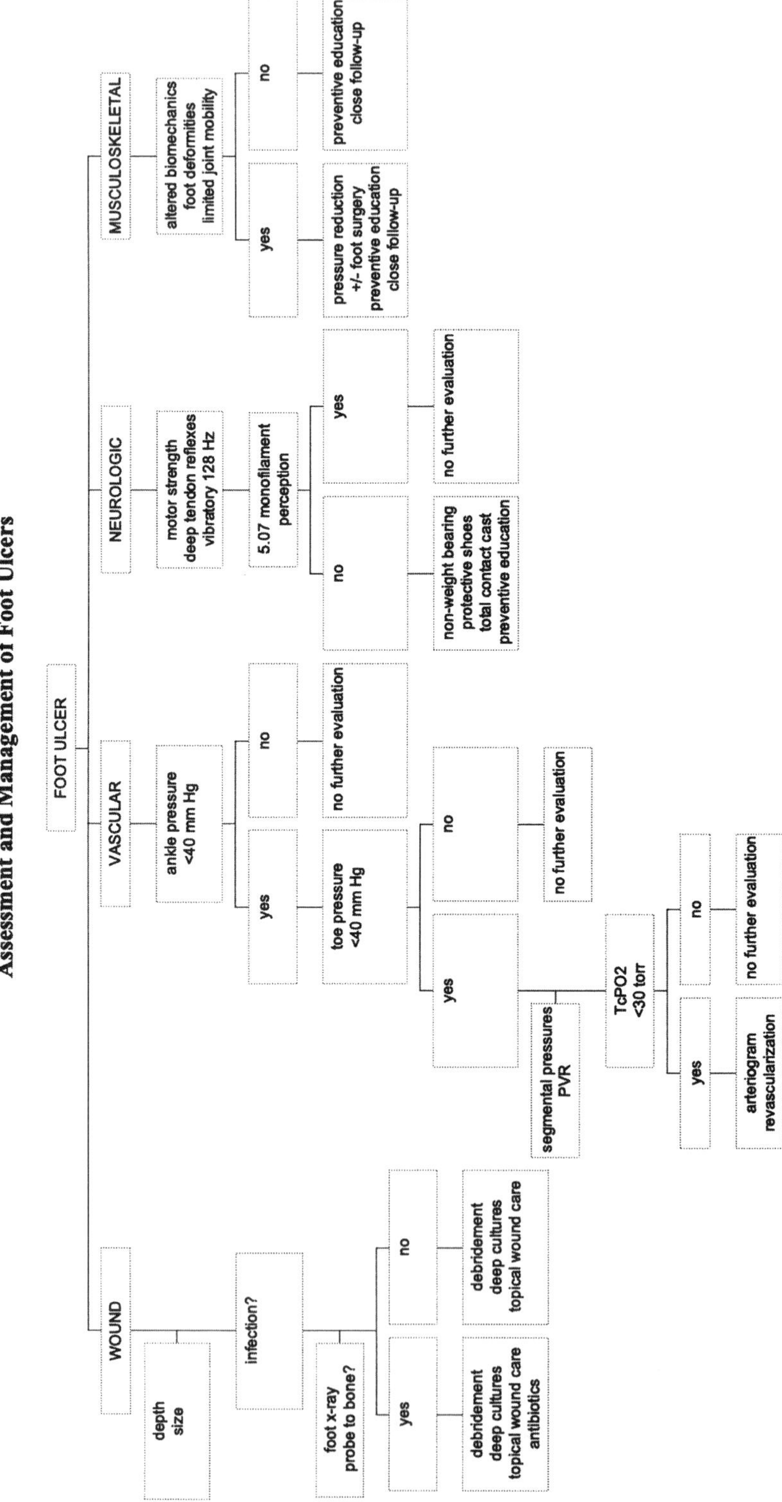

Figure 28–7. Alogrithm for the assessment and management of foot ulcers.

TABLE 28–2. THE SIX PS OF PREVENTION

PODIATRIC CARE

- Regular visits, examinations and foot care
- Risk assessment
- Early detection and aggressive treatment of new lesions

PULSE EXAMINATION

- Evaluation for claudication and rest pain
- Assessment of foot pulses; non-invasive vascular testing when indicated

PROTECTIVE SHOES

- Adequate room to protect from injury; well cushioned
- Walking sneakers, extra depth, custom-molded shoes
- Special modifications as necessary

PRESSURE REDUCTION

- Pressure measurements
- Cushioned insoles, custom orthoses, padded hosiery

PROPHYLACTIC SURGERY

- Correct structural deformities-hammertoes, bunions, Charcot
- Prevent recurrent ulcers over deformities
- Intervene at opportune time

PREVENTIVE EDUCATION

- Patient education-need for daily inspection and necessity for early intervention
- Physician education-significance of foot lesions, importance of regular foot examination and current concepts of diabetic foot management

REFERENCES

1. Hutton W, Stokes I. The mechanics of the foot. In: Klenerman L, editor. *The foot and its disorders*. Oxford: Blackwell Scientific Publications; 1991. p. 11–25.
2. Murray H, Boulton A. The Pathophysiology of Diabetic Foot Ulceration. *Clin Podiat Med Surg*. 1995;12(1):1–17.
3. AmericanDiabetesAssociation. Preventive foot care in people with diabetes [position statement]. *Diabetes Care*. 1999;22(Suppl 1).
4. Sumpio B. Foot ulcers. *N Engl J Med*. 2000;343(11):787–793.
5. Boulton A. Peripheral neuropathy and the diabetic foot. *Foot*. 1992;2:67–72.
6. Boulton A, Hardisty C, Betts R, et al. Dynamic foot pressure and other studies as diagnostic and management aids in diabetic neuropathy. *Diabetes Care*. 1983;6:26–33.
7. Veves A, Fernando D, Walewski P, et al. A study of plantar pressures in a diabetic clinic population. *Foot*. 1991;2:89–92.
8. Habershaw G, Chzran J. Biomechanical considerations of the diabetic foot. *Management of Diabetic Foot Problems*. 2nd Edition. ed. Philadelphia, Pennsylvania: W.B. Saunders Co.; 1995. p. 53–65.
9. Cavanagh P, Young M, Adams J, et al. Correlates of structure and function in the diabetic foot. *Diabetologia*. 1991;34(Suppl 2):A39.
10. U.S. Department of Health and Human Services National Diabetes Fact Sheet; 1998.
11. Reiber G, Lipsky B, Gibbons G. The burden of diabetic foot ulcers. *Am J. Surg*. 1998;176:5S–10S.
12. Reiber G, EJ B, Smith D. Lower Extremity Foot Ulcers and Amputations in Diabetes. In: Harris, editor. *Diabetes in America*. 2nd ed. Bethesda, MD:National Institutes of Health Publication;1995. p. 409–427.

13. O'Brien I, Corrall R. Epidemiology of diabetes and its complications. *N Eng J Med.* 1988;318(24): 1619–1623.
14. Laing P. The development and complications of diabetic foot ulcers. *Am J Surg.* 1998;176:11S–19S.
15. Frangos S, Kilaru S, Blume P et al. Classification of Diabetic Foot Ulcers: Improving Communication. *Int. J. Angiol.* 2002;11.:1–7.
16. Collins K, Sumpio B. Vascular Assessment. In: Blume P, editor. *Clinics in Podiatric Medicine and Surgery.* Philadelphia: W. B. Saunders; 2000.
17. Orchard T, Strandness DJ. Assessment of peripheral vascular disease in diabetes: report and recommendation of an international workshop sponsored by the American Diabetes Association and the American Heart Association, September 18–20, 1992 New Orleans, Louisiana. *Circulation.* 1993;88:819–832.
18. Weitz J, Bynre J, Clagett P. Diagnosis and treatment of chronic arterial insufficiency of the lower extremitites: A critical review. *Circulation.* 1996;94:3026–3033.
19. Byrne P, Provan J, Ameli F, et al. The use of transcutaneous oxygen tension measurements in the diagnosis of peripheral vascular insufficiency. *Ann Surg.* 1984;200:159–167.
20. Lavery L, Armstrong D, Vela S. Practical criteria for screening patients at high risk for diabetic foot ulceration. *Arch Intern Med.* 1998;158(2):157–162.
21. Kumar S, Fernando D, Veves A, et al. Semmes-Weinstein monofilaments: a simple, effective and inexpensive screening device for identifying diabetic patients at risk of foot ulceration. *Diabetes Res Clin Pract.* 1991;13:63–68.
22. Simeone L, Veves A. Screening techniques to identify the diabetic patient at risk of ulceration. *J Am Podiatr Med Assoc.* 1997;87:313–317.
23. Birke J, Sims D. Plantar sensory threshold in the ulcerative foot. *Leprosy Review.* 1986;57:261–267.
24. McNeely M, Boyko E, Ahroni J, et al. The independent contributions of diabetic neuropathy and vasculopathy in foot ulceration: how great are the risks? *Diabetes Care.* 1995;18:216–219.
25. Masson E, Hay E, Stockley I, Veves A, Betts R, Boulton A. Abnormal foot pressures alone may not cause ulceration. *Diabetic Med.* 1989;6:426–428.
26. Barrow J, Hughes J, Clark P, et al. A study of the effect of wear on the pressure-relieving properties of foot orthosis. *Foot.* 1992;1:195–199.
27. Boulton A, Franks C, Betts R, et al. Reduction of abnormal foot pressures in diabetic neuropathy using new polymer insole material. *Diabetes Care.* 1984;7:42–46.
28. Nawoczenski D, Birke J, Coleman W. Effect of rocker sole design on plantar forefoot pressures. J Am Podiatr Med Assoc. 1988;78:455–460.
29. Blume P, Partagas L, Sumpio B, et al. Single stage surgical treatment of noninfected diabetic foot ulcers. *J Plastic Reconst Surg.* 2002;109:601–609.
30. Armstrong D, Lavery L, Stern S, et al. Is prophylactic diabetic foot surgery dangerous? *J Foot Ankle Surg.* 1996;35(6):585–589.
31. Catanzariti A, Blitch E, Karlock L. Elective foot and ankle surgery in the diabetic patient. *J Foot Ankle Surg.* 1995;34(1):23–41.
32. Ollendorf D, Kotsanos J, Wishner W, et al. Potential economic benefits of lower extremity amputation prevention strategies in diabetes. *Diabetes Care.*1998;21:240–245.
33. Knox R, Dutch W, Blume P, Sumpio B. Diabetic Foot Disease. *Int J Angiol.* 2000;1(1):1–6.
34. Yeager R, Moneta G, Edwards J, et al. Predictors of outcome of forefoot surgery for ulceration and gangrene. *Am J Surg.* 1998;175(5):388–390.

IX

Infrainguinal Revascularization

29

Long-Term Follow-Up of Endoscopic Harvested Vein Graft

Francisco Alcocer, MD and William D. Jordan, Jr., MD

Since its emergence on the vascular surgery field, the endoscopic harvesting of the greater saphenous vein (EVH) has slowly gained supporters among vascular and cardiac surgeons. The noticeable cosmetic result and improvements in wound morbidity[1] were initially confronted with the increased operative time and the potential harm of the vein as a result of increased manipulation. There has been concern that this greater need for manipulation of the vein during the dissection may cause more vein trauma that may, in turn, lead to a higher rate of graft failure secondary to an injury-response phenomenon. However, as experience has been gained with this technique and better instruments have become available, the operative time and the vein manipulation have been reduced. Some reports have addressed the results of this technique with regards to graft patency in addition to the better cosmetic and functional results[2,3] (Figure 29–1). However, a feared consequence of increased vein manipulation during harvesting leading to increased intimal hyperplasia may likely to be reflected in the long-term follow-up, when hyperplasia plays a more important role in the pathogenesis of vein graft stenosis. Our experience on the long-term impact of EVH shows minimal effect on mid- and long-term graft patency.

MECHANISMS OF INJURY IN VEIN GRAFTS

It has been shown that vein injury elicits a biological response that may promote the development of intimal hyperplasia and that there is a linear relationship between the magnitude of the original insult and the intensity of the vascular response. This response to injury represents an attempt to limit the injury and repair the lesion; however, the reaction can become uncontrolled and lead to an abnormal cell proliferation and extracelular matrix deposits that can cause graft failure. Several factors have been correlated with the development of the intimal hyperplastic lesion and most of those factors are a direct response to the surgical trauma.

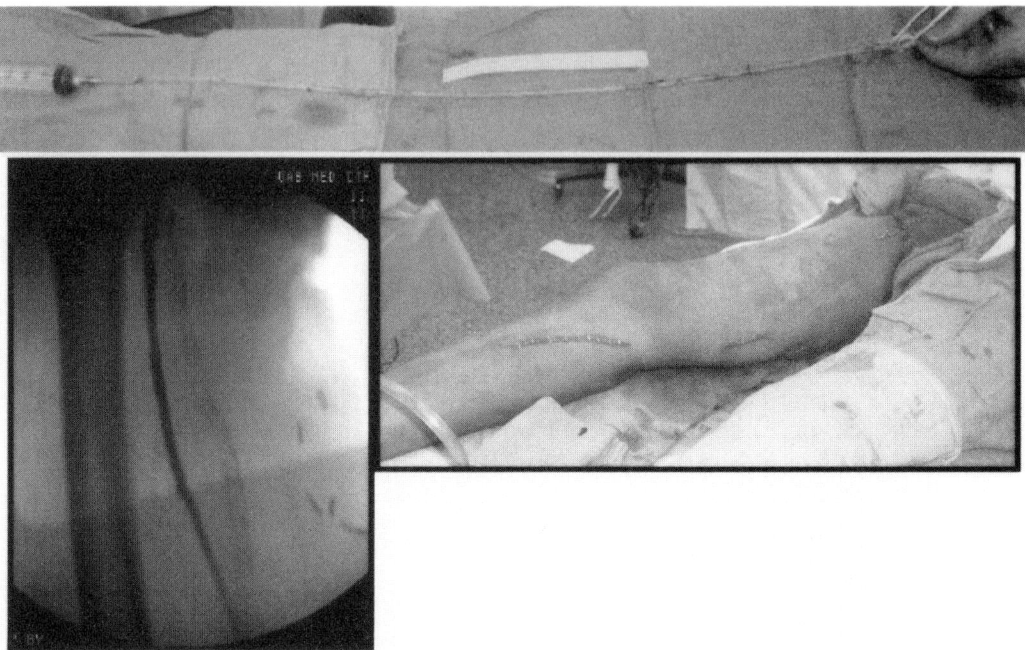

Figure 29–1. A full-length vein obtained with EVH for a below-knee femoro-popliteal bypass. The incisions for arterial exposure are used for introduction of the videoscope. Only a small incision was added to complete dissection safely. Intraoperative arteriogram shows a patent bypass.

Regardless of the harvesting technique employed, vein graft injury begins with disruption of the endothelium. Three different degrees of injury have been described:[4]

    Type I: minimal endothelial injury (no denuding).

    Type II: complete loss of the endothelium.

    Type III: transmural disruption of the vein wall

Even with the most careful technique, most of the current vein dissection techniques result in Type III injuries. Vein wall ischemia due to disruption of the vasa vasorum (a more prominent feature with translocated grafts) may result in generation of toxic free radicals. This injury, in turn, causes endothelial damage, which can result in a proliferative response of the smooth muscle cell (SMC) and subsequent hyperplasia. Moreover, after grafting, a reperfusion period occurs, which can even worsen the insult.[5] Immediately after the blood starts flowing through a vein graft, leukocyte and platelets adhere to the denuded surface. Within 96 hours after graft placement, circulating monocytes, macrophages and neutrophils migrate into the intima.[6] After endothelial loss, smooth muscle cells migrate from the media toward the intima and at least half of these cells are dividing while migrating.[7]

While vein injury uniformly occurs, different techniques may lead to varying degrees of injury. Histological studies of reversed saphenous vein grafts have shown that harvesting, preparation and implantation cause significant ischemic damage to the endothelium, while the in situ technique leads to mechanical endothelial and media damage due to the passage of the valvulotome.[8] During the course of EVH, the vein is typically exposed to more manipulation than in the traditional open harvest. Injury to the vein may occur during three different phases of the vein harvest: 1) when instrumentation is first placed into the subcutaneous cavity along the tract of the vein, 2) during the dissection of the vein with the videoscopic equipment, and 3) during retraction of the vein for dissection and removal (Figure 29–2). The vein stress can be severe with blunt dissection but mechanical manipulation seems to be most evident where the side branches are found and not as severe at the tubular portions of the vein[9] (Figure 29–3). There are concerns that excess vein traction and manipulation may increase the incidence of injury; however, studies of vein

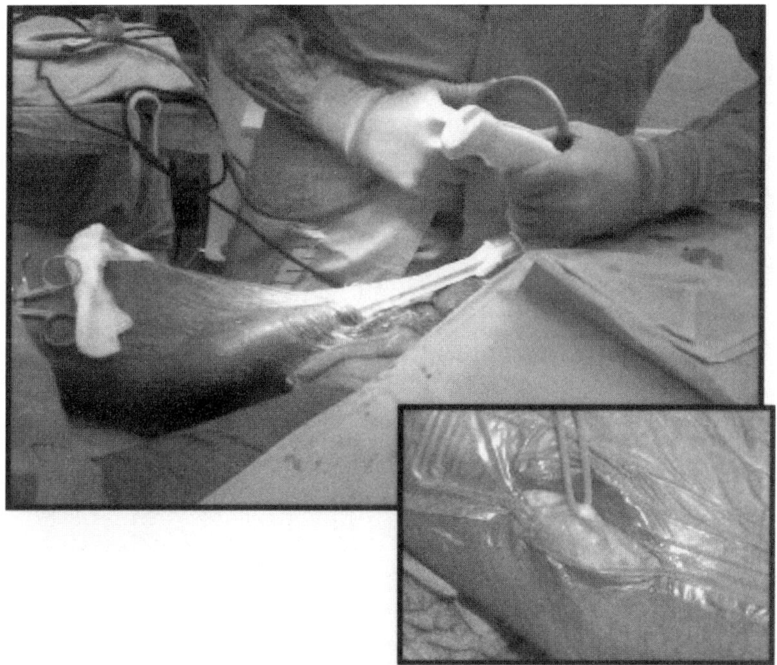

Figure 29–2. The dissector has been introduced from the right groin and is pushed forward through the perivascular tissue to create a subcutaneous space along the anterior aspect of the vein. Insert shows vein traction with vessel-loops as other possible injury mechanism.

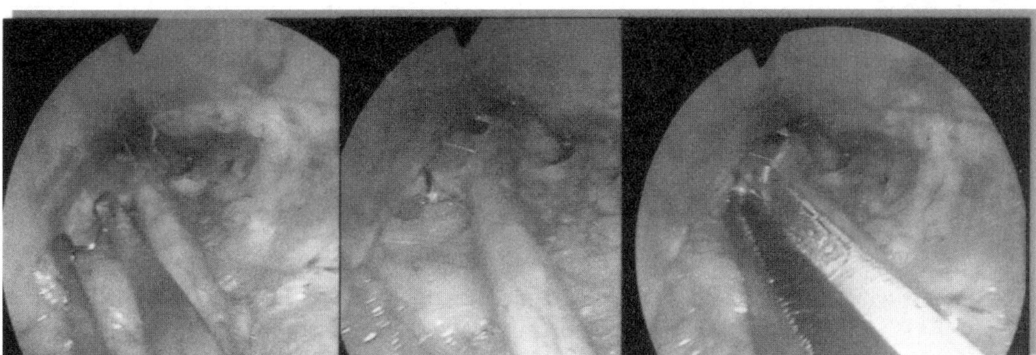

Figure 29–3. The subsequent steps for clipping and division of a side branch are shown. The blunt dissection required to expose the branches is regarded as a potential mechanism of vein injury. Intentionally, we applied clips only on the distal stump to avoid "catching" a clipped branch on the vein with the retractor. These side branches are subsequently ligated on the back table.

segments obtained with this technique have shown no morphological differences when compared with the conventional technique.[10,11] Moreover, the endothelial reactivity of vein segments harvested with endoscopic techniques is not impaired when evaluated in vein cultures in vitro suggesting endothelial preservation at least in the segments studied.[12] To date, no study has shown that a particular surgical technique or vein preparation causes less injury or improves long-term patency although gentle handling of tissue and careful technique is commonly used in hopes of reducing complications other than intimal hyperplasia, such as early thrombosis, infection, and pseudoaneurysm formation. Interestingly, despite the concern about excessive vein traction and manipulation that might occur during EVH, there is little evidence that such complications occur more frequently with this more cosmetic technique.

FIVE-YEAR RESULTS

We have been using EVH for the last eight years and recently reported our long-term experience with its use in the treatment of peripheral vascular disease.[13] The technical details have evolved some over time[14] as the instrumentation has improved. As our experience matured, we have been less likely to use veins with less than 2.5 maximum as estimated by ultrasound vein mapping. This is justified by our initial results where more graft failures occurred when small diameter veins were used. The correlation between vein mapping and graft failure has led to an adjustment of our practice so that now we consider alternative conduits when dealing with veins less than 3 mm.[15]

Our postoperative graft surveillance follows the reporting standards of the American Association for Vascular Surgery and the Society for Vascular Surgery[16] including a duplex ultrasound examination within the first postoperative week, then, at 3-month intervals during the first postoperative year. After the first year, grafts are followed at 6- to 12-month intervals, depending on the discretion of the treating physician. Grafts judged at risk for thrombosis undergo more frequent duplex scans. Grafts identified with duplex abnormalities (typically, a peak systolic velocity >220 cm/s, a peak systolic velocity <40 cm/s, or a peak systolic velocity ratio >2.5) are evaluated with angiography. If the arteriogram shows an area of stenosis that is considered to be hemodynamically significant, then the grafts are surgically explored. Following this surveillance protocol, we identified 15 grafts with flow abnormalities that warranted surgical revision. Table 29–1 shows the different anatomic positions of the bypasses. With life-table methods (Tables 29–2, 29–3, and 29–4), the five-year primary patency, primary-assisted patency, secondary patency, and limb salvage rates were 64%, 78%, and 80%, and 89%, respectively. Figure 29–4 represents the five-year graft patency rates.

IMPROVEMENTS IN WOUND COMPLICATIONS

In our experience, postoperative wound complications have been improved with the use of EVH. In a total of 185 lower extremity arterial bypass graft operations using EVH, 16 patients (8.6%) had minor wound complications during the 30-day postoperative period ranging from drainage, erythema and mild inflammation around the arterial access sites to hematomas along the subcutaneous tunnel of the harvest site. Of the 16 wound complications, 11 led to increased length of stay or a readmission after discharge, and 5 were managed with additional outpatient visits. Importantly, we have

TABLE 29–1. ANATONIC POSITIONS OF BYPASS GRAFTS

	Inflow	Outflow
Common femoral	127	0
Profunda	2	0
Superficial	27	0
Above-knee popliteal	12	47
Below-knee popliteal	5	64
Posterior tibial	0	27
Anterior tibial	1	14
Peroneal	0	20
Dorsalis pedis	0	4
Other	11	9
Total	185	185

TABLE 29–2. PRIMARY PATENCY

Interval	# at Risk	# Failed	Withdrawn	Interval Failure	Cumulative Patency	SE
					100.0	
1	**185**	16	19	0.138	86.2	2.36
6	150	24	23	0.082	79.1	2.95
12	103	12	9	0.062	74.2	3.71
18	82	6	11	0.000	74.2	4.16
24	65	0	11	0.049	70.5	4.75
30	54	3	8	0.038	67.8	5.24
36	43	2	4	0.025	66.1	5.87
42	37	1	7	0.031	64.0	6.31
48	29	1	10	0.000	64.0	7.13
54	18	0	7	0.000	64.0	9.05
60	11	0	4	0.000	64.0	11.58

TABLE 29–3. ASSISTED PATENCY

Interval	# at Risk	# Failed	Withdrawn	Interval Failure	Cumulative Patency	SE
0				100.0		
1	**185**	14	19	0.098	90.2	2.08
6	152	17	24	0.034	87.1	2.54
12	111	5	13	0.058	82.1	3.30
18	93	6	14	0.000	82.1	3.60
24	73	0	12	0.015	80.8	4.14
30	61	1	12	0.034	78.1	4.68
36	48	2	5	0.000	78.1	5.28
42	41	0	8	0.000	78.1	5.71
48	33	0	12	0.000	78.1	6.36
54	21	0	8	0.000	78.1	7.98
60	13	0	4	0.000	78.1	10.14

TABLE 29–4. SECONDARY PATENCY

Interval	# at Risk	# Failed	Withdrawn	Interval Failure	Cumulative Patency	SE
0					100.0	
1	**185**	10	19	0.099	90.1	2.08
6	156	17	225	0.027	87.7	2.46
12	114	4	15	0.019	86.1	3.01
18	95	2	15	0.000	86.1	3.30
24	78	0	12	0.014	84.9	3.74
30	66	1	13	0.032	82.2	4.27
36	52	2	6	0.021	80.4	4.93
42	44	1	9	0.000	80.4	5.36
48	34	0	12	0.000	80.4	6.10
54	22	0	8	0.000	80.4	7.58
60	14	0	4	0.000	80.4	9.51

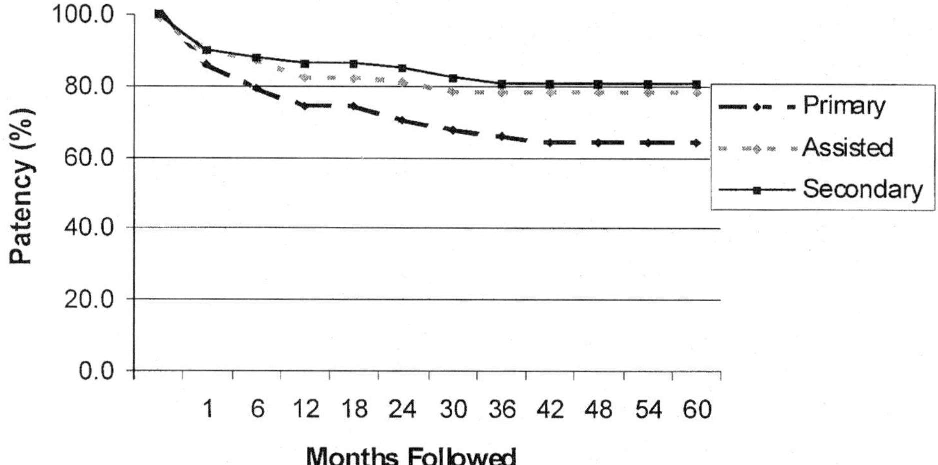

Figure 29–4. Endoscopically harvested saphenous vein grafts used as lower extremity arterial grafts: primary patency, assisted patency, and secondary patency.

not seen thigh wound breakdowns, a complication that frequently leads to protracted wound healing in these difficult vascular patients. All wound complications responded favorably to treatment and none lead to graft failure or limb loss. Although wound infection after open vein harvesting may cause a prolonged postoperative recovery, this annoying complication only rarely threatens graft patency and leads to limb loss.[17] It is difficult, therefore, to assume that the use of EVH will improve graft patency and limb salvage because of its impact on wound morbidity. However, less pain and less wound complications will be reflected in the speed of patient rehabilitation that may in turn prevent other activity-related complications.

While the improved cosmetic result and patient satisfaction with limited leg incisions are important, one must always consider the potential harmful effects that vein harvest trauma may have on intimal hyperplasia and graft failure. If this vein harvest technique does injure the vein, then the clinical benefit of reduced pain and lower infection rates must be considered in light of this potential for late failure. Carefully designed clinical studies may determine the contribution of "vein harvest trauma" to delayed graft failure.

SUMMARY

The frequent wound complications associated with conventional saphenous vein harvest are reduced with the use of EVH, a technique that has gained more acceptance among vascular and cardiac surgeons. Despite increased vein manipulation, histological and functional studies have found no significant alterations in vein injury response. Moreover, the increased vein manipulation does not seem to affect the long-term patency rates of these grafts when compared to other harvesting techniques.

REFERENCES

1. Patel AN, Hebeler RF, Hamman BL, et al. Prospective analysis of endoscopic vein harvesting. *American Journal of Surgery.* 2001;182(6):716–719.
2. Gawenda M. Minimal invasive video-assisted vein preparation (Endoscopic vein harvesting-EVH) in peripheral bypass surgery. *Chirurg.* 1999;70(12):1484–1488.
3. Jordan WD, Voellinger DC, Schroeder PT, et al. Video-assisted saphenous vein harvest: the evolution of a new technique. *J Vasc Surg.* 1997;26:405–414.
4. Kraiss LW, Clowes AN. Response of the Arterial Wall to Injury and Intimal Hyperplasia. In: Sidawy AN, Sumpio BE, et al., eds. *The Basic Science of Vascular Disease.* Armonk: Futura Publishing Company, Inc.; 1997:289–317.
5. Hagen PO, Davies MG, et al. Reduction of vein graft intimal hyperplasia by ex vivo treatment with desferrioxamine manganese. *J Vasc Res.* 1992;29:405.
6. Amano J, Suzuki A, et al. Cytokinetic study of aortocoronary bypass vein grafts in place for less than six months. *Am J Cardio.* 1991;67;1234–1236.
7. Clowes AW, Reidy MA. Prevention of stenosis after vascular reconstruction: pharmacologic control of intimal hyperplasia-a review. *J Vasc Surg.* 1991;13:885–891.
8. Sayers R, Watt P, et al. Structural and functional smooth muscle injury after surgical preparation of reversed and non-reversed (in situ) saphenous vein bypass grafts. *Br J Surg.* 1991;78:1256–1258.
9. Fabricius AM, Diegeler A, Doll N, et al. Minimally invasive saphenous vein harvesting techniques: morphology and postoperative outcome. *Ann Thorac Surg.* 2000;70(2):473–478.
10. Cable DG, Dearani JA, Pfeifer EA, et al. Minimally invasive saphenous vein harvesting: endothelial integrity and early clinical results. *Ann Thorac Surg.* 1998;66(1): 139–143.
11. Meyer DM, Rogers TE, Jessen ME, et al. Histologic evidence of the safety of endoscopic saphenous vein graft preparation. *Ann Thorac Surg.* 2000;70(2):487–491.
12. Black EA, Guzik TJ, West NE, et al. Minimally invasive saphenous vein harvesting: effects on endothelial and smooth muscle function. *Ann Thorac Surg.* 2001;71(5):1503–1507.
13. Jordan WD Jr, Alcocer F, Voellinger DC, et al. The durability of endoscopic saphenous vein grafts: a 5-year observational study. *J Vasc Surg.* 2001;34(3):434–439.
14. Jordan WD, Voellinger DC, Schroeder PT, et al. Video-assisted saphenous vein harvest: the evolution of a new technique. *J Vasc Surg.* 1997;26:405–414.
15. Patterson MA, Jordan WD, Whitley WD, et al. Pre-operative vein mapping predicts lower extremity arterial graft patency. Southern Association of Vascular Surgery, 1999.
16. Rutherford RB, Baker JD, Ernst C, et al. Recommended standards for reports dealing with lower extremity ischemia: revised version. *J Vasc Surg.* 1997;26:517–538.
17. Treiman GS, Copland S, Yellin AE, et al. Wound infections involving infrainguinal autogenous vein grafts: a current evaluation of factors determining successful graft preservation. *J Vasc Surg.* 2001;33(5):948–54.

30

Lower Extremity Bypass in Patients with Renal Failure

John C. Lantis II, MD and Michael S. Conte, MD

End stage renal disease (ESRD), defined as a lack of native renal function that requires renal replacement therapy (hemodialysis, peritoneal dialysis, or renal transplantation) is undergoing a dramatic increase in prevalence that is international in scope. Concomitant with the increase in this population at risk, critical limb ischemia secondary to ESRD arteriopathy has become a growing problem for the vascular surgeon. As evidence of this trend, the proportion of ESRD patients among all infrainguinal bypass grafts (IBG) performed at one tertiary care institution rose dramatically from 2% (1978–1992) to 14% (1993–1997) during the last decade.[1] Historically, this patient group has been characterized by increased peri-operative mortality, reduced long-term survival, diminished graft patency and poor limb salvage. Each of these issues must be carefully assessed when approaching the ESRD patient with critical limb ischemia.

EPIDEMIOLOGY

In 1999 the number of ESRD patients in the United States was 344,094, of which 114,478 had diabetes mellitus (DM).[2] The ESRD population is expected to double by 2010,[3] representing a growth rate of 7% per year.[4] In part, this reflects both the increasing prevalence of type II DM and improved medical treatment of its other end-organ complications. In 1999 there were 89,252 patients requiring renal replacement therapy for the first time, of these 38,160 were diabetic.[2] With ongoing improvements in the treatment of hypertension and coronary artery disease, more diabetic patients are developing ESRD as a late complication.[5] Furthermore, since the atherosclerotic burden in patients with type II DM is high at the outset, it may be expected that this growing fraction of the ESRD population will have a high incidence of peripheral vascular complications.

The population of patients with type II DM and ESRD continues to exhibit a limited life expectancy, with a reported 5-year survival rate of 25% in all age categories as of 1999. The 5-year survival rate ranges from 51% for the group that begins renal replacement therapy secondary to diabetes at ages 40–49 and drops to 8% for those beginning renal replacement therapy after 80 years of age.[2]

ETIOLOGY

There is a consensus among vascular specialists that lower extremity atherosclerosis associated with chronic renal failure is unique in its pattern and poor response to standard therapy. While some of the distribution of this disease mimics the lower leg arterial pathology seen in DM, the occlusive disease in ESRD appears to involve the pedal vasculature more extensively and does not respond to revascularization as successfully. The arteriopathy of ESRD is accompanied by calcification of the media of arteries of all sizes,[6] with a marked predilection for the infrageniculate vessels.

This incredibly problematic form of arteriosclerosis may exist for several interrelated reasons. These include diabetes mellitus, uremia, hyperlipidemia, hypertension, and elevated homocystine levels among others. The well defined arterioslerotic risk factors of DM and hypertension are present in nearly 100% of the patients with ESRD requiring IBG.[7] These atherogenic factors are augmented by the expression of uremic dyslipidemia; elevated cholesterol, lipoprotein A, and triglycerides, with lowered HDL levels. The increased oxidation of LDL in uremia further adds to this process,[8,9] In addition to this profile homocysteine, an independent risk factor for atherosclerosis, is consistently elevated in patients with ESRD, especially while on hemodialysis.[10,11] The medial calcinosis may be accelerated by secondary hyperparathyroidism, and chronic endothelial activation and dysfunction have been described in ESRD.[12]

OUTCOMES OF LOWER EXTREMITY REVASCULARIZATION

Perioperative Outcome and Patient Survival

This combination of atherosclerotic pathology not only affects the distal arterial tree but the coronary vasculature as well. Approximately half of all deaths in patients with ESRD are cardiac related.[2,13] This high incidence of cardiac morbidity weighs heavily in clinical decision making in ESRD patients with critical limb ischemia, elevating the surgical risk and reducing the potential long term benefits of limb salvage. Historically, operative mortality and 2-year survival rates reported in the literature ranged from 0 to 27% (mean 9 %) and 32 % to 62% (mean 49 %) respectively for ESRD patients undergoing IBG.[13] ESRD has been identified as an independent predictor of long-term mortality following IBG in patients with tissue loss.[14] While these statistics have led some authors to propose primary amputation as a safer alternative to arterial reconstruction in the ESRD patient, others have shown similar operative mortality figures for major amputation in this cohort.[15]

In our most recent experience (1993–1999), the peri-operative mortality for ESRD patients (N=60) who underwent IBG was 1.3%, not significantly different from that observed in patients without renal failure.[7] In addition, the 2- and 4-year survival rates in the ESRD group were 65% and 51% respectively, consistent with the best outcomes reported by others.[13] These results represents a significant improvement over our own previously published data,[16] and suggest that the risk/benefit ratio for performing arterial reconstruction in the ESRD patient may be somewhat more favorable than it has been generally portrayed.

Graft Patency and Limb Salvage

Modern techniques of arterial reconstruction have resulted in improved outcomes for patients with critical limb ischemia. However, the subset of patients with dialysis-dependent ESRD continues to represent one of the more difficult vascular surgical challenges. A recent review of published reports noted an early graft thrombosis rate of 14% and a greater than 14% amputation rate with a functioning graft.[13] It has long been recognized that ESRD patients undergoing IBG experience a lower rate of limb salvage as compared with graft patency.[17,18] Since 1998 there have been 5 reports, including our own, regarding the use of IBG for limb salvage in patients with ESRD[7,19, 20–22] (Table 30–1). A recent meta-analysis reviewing 16 studies of IBG in patients with ESRD from 1987 to 2000 showed promising if not ideal outcomes. The pooled results demonstrated an average graft patency rate of 74%, limb salvage rate of 73% and patient survival of 42% at 2 years.[23]

We recently reported on a series of 60 patients with ESRD undergoing IBG (N=78 procedures) for limb salvage.[7] These revascularizations were performed for rest pain (15%), ulceration (54%) or gangrene (31%), and the majority (94%) were primary bypasses. All reconstructions were performed exclusively with autogenous vein, including non-reversed greater saphenous vein (NRGSV; 51%), in-situ GSV (18%), reversed GSV (16%), spliced vein (9%), arm (4%), and lesser saphenous vein (2%) conduits. Distal inflow sites including the proximal superficial femoral artery (26% vs. 12%) and the above knee popliteal artery (23% vs. 13%) were used more frequently in patients with ESRD, as compared to a contemporaneous control group with normal renal function. Distal anastomoses were to tibial or pedal arteries in 90%, with the anterior tibial (27% vs. 15%) and the dorsalis pedis (24% vs. 9%) arteries more commonly employed in ESRD patients versus controls. This pattern of graft configurations has been observed by other authors.[21]

Primary (60%) and secondary (86%) graft patency in the ESRD cohort at 4 years was not significantly different from controls (Figures 30–1 and 30–2). Unfortunately 13% of patients with patent grafts still went on to undergo a major (transtibial or above) amputation, resulting in a 77% limb salvage rate at 4 years which, while quite encouraging, was significantly less than that observed in the control population (92%; Figure 30–3).[7]

TABLE 30–1. RESULTS FROM SELECTED SERIES OF IBG IN ESRD PATIENTS.

Author & Year	Limbs/ Patients	Periop. Mortality	Follow-Up Duration	Patency	Limb Salvage	Patient Survival
Hakaim 1998	83/76	1.2%	1 year	53% primary	63%	52%
Lantis 2001	78/60	1.3%	4 year	86% secondary	77%	51%
Cox 2001	78/63	NA	3 year	48% secondary	62%	55% (5 year)
Myerson 2001	82/64	4.9%	3 year	67% secondary	59%	60%
Biancari 2002	25/21	NA	2 year	74%	85%	23%

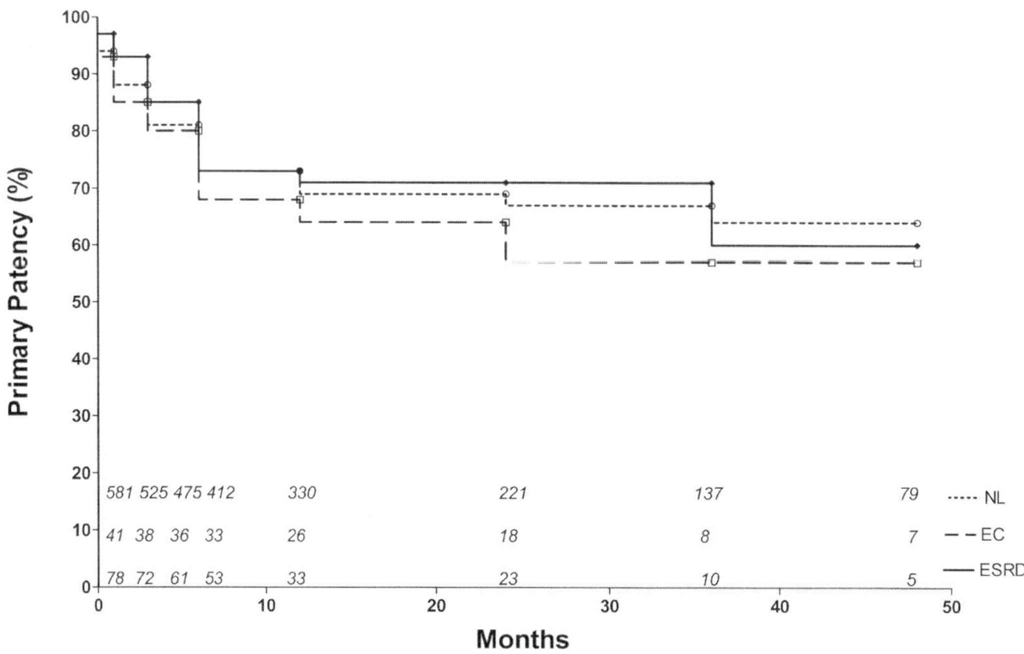

Figure 30–1. Primary graft patency for autogenous IBG performed at a single institution (1993-1999) by life table method. Patency of 3 contemporaneous groups are illustrated: normal renal function (NL; serum creatinine ≤1.2 mg/dl; N=581), elevated creatinine (EC; serum creatinine >1.2 mg/dl; N=41), and end-stage renal disease (ESRD; N=78). (by permission, *Journal of Vascular Surgery*)

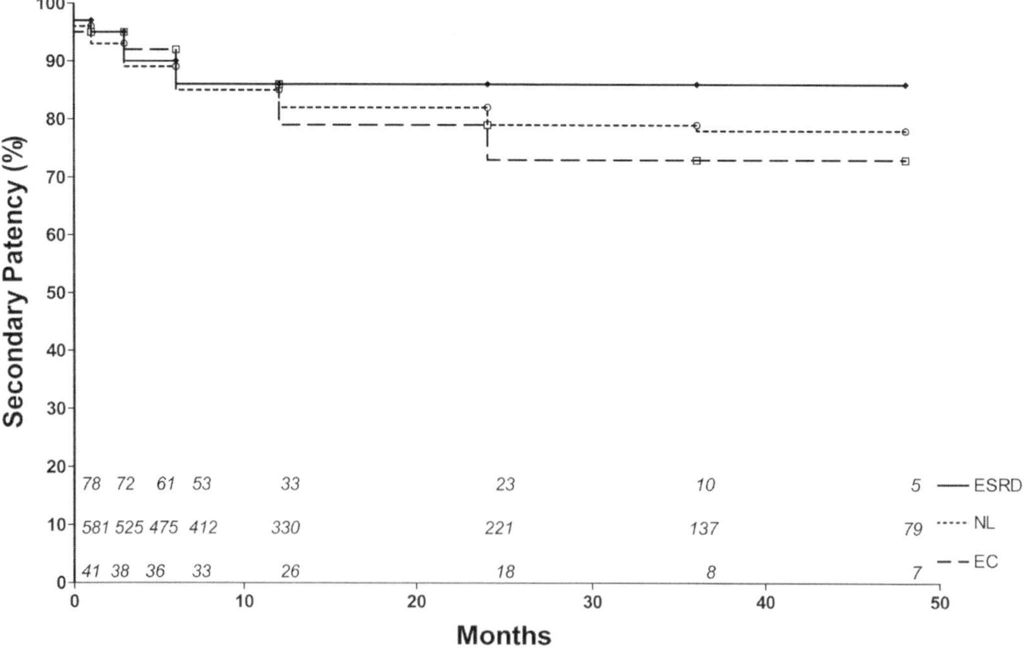

Figure 30–2. Cumulative secondary patency for autogenous IBG performed at a single institution (1993–1999), grouped by renal functional status. Groups are identical to Figure 30–1. (by permission, *Journal of Vascular Surgery*)

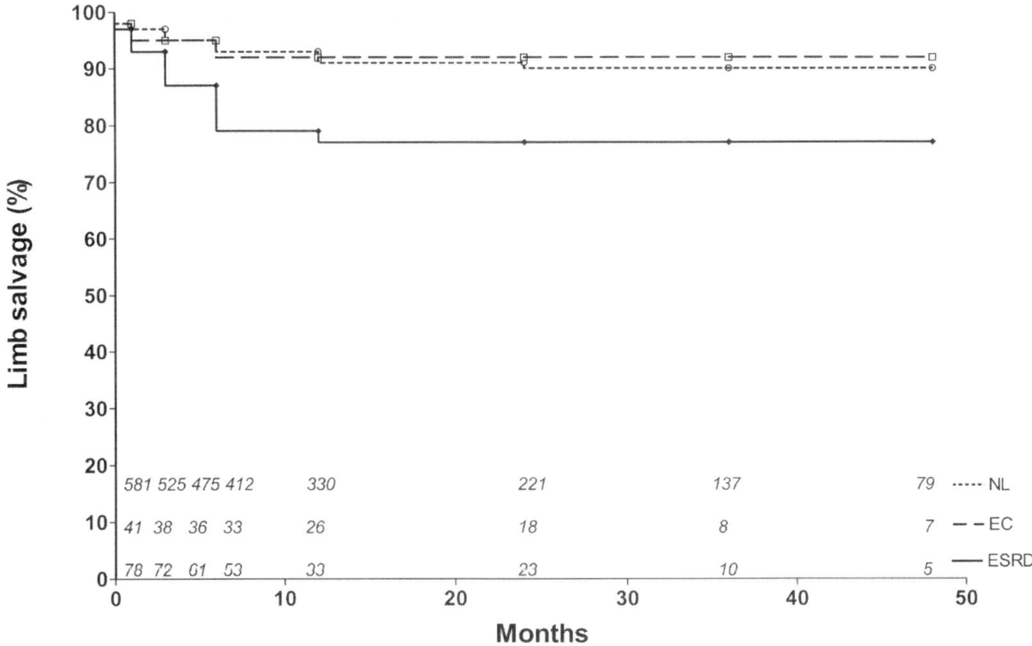

Figure 30–3. Cumulative limb salvage for a consecutive series of autogenous IBG at a single institution (1993–1999), grouped by renal functional status. Groups identical to Figures 30–1 and 30–2. (by permission, *Journal of Vascular Surgery*)

Predictors of Poor Outcome

As noted, diminished graft patency and a disturbing incidence of limb loss despite a functioning graft (hemodynamic failure) have been repeatedly observed in ESRD patients.[17] Other investigators have identified several negative predictors in this population, including pre-operative foot infection,[24] poor functional status,[25] tobacco abuse,[24] greater than 2 cm ischemic ulceration,[26] heel necrosis greater than 4 cm,[24] forefoot gangrene,[25] pre-operative toe pressures less than 20 torr, pedal angiographic resistance score of >2.5 (3.0 representing no named pedal arteries)[13] and distal vessels with only collateral outflow (SVS/ISCVS runoff score=10).[22]

In reviewing our recent experience we analyzed a number of clinical variables as predictors of poor outcome following IBG in ESRD patients.[7] Although other investigators have found that amputation despite a patent bypass was more common in patients with poor runoff scores,[27] runoff scores were not predictive of adverse outcomes in our series. ESRD patients who retained their limb had a mean runoff score of 6.0 (median 6.5). The respective mean and median runoff scores for the group who underwent amputation with an open graft and with a failed graft were 6.2/5.5 and 8.0/8.0. Furthermore age, tobacco use, type of conduit used, or use of an isolated anterior tibial target vessel were also not found to be predictive of graft or hemodynamic failure

In our analysis the only significant predictor of limb loss despite a patent graft in ESRD patients was the presence of extensive heel necrosis (>4 cm diameter). Notably, the majority of patients with smaller heel lesions went on to complete healing following IBG, even those with grafts that did not provide direct outflow to the posterior circulation. This observation is supported by previous studies demonstrating that non-direct flow bypasses in patients without ESRD will heal tissue loss.[28]

Quality of Life

The likelihood of preserving independent function and quality of life with successful limb salvage surgery is a critical aspect of the pre-operative clinical assessment. A recent report assessing Quality of Life-Class ranking in 57 patients with ESRD undergo IBG noted that these patients had significantly lower scores at both 30 days and 1 year than NL patients undergoing IBG.[29] Other recently published series have indicated that only 31% to 21% of patients with ESRD who underwent IBG were ambulating at 1 year.[29,30] One study has seen this number decrease to 6% walking independently at 2 years.[29] However, using Markov decision analysis one investigator has shown a measurable increase in the expected quality-adjusted life years for ESRD patients with tissue loss that undergo IBG.[20] This must be compared to the limited rehabilitation potential for those undergoing amputation in this severely debilitated population.

CURRENT APPROACH

Patient Evaluation

Based on our most recent experience, we have taken a fairly aggressive approach to offering IBG for limb salvage in patients with ESRD. Clearly these patients require a careful, individualized evaluation of the potential risks and benefits, and knowledge of their current quality of life and expectations weighs heavily into the treatment decisions. For those who are more debilitated and inactive, or when tissue necrosis is extensive, primary amputation is recommended. Conversely, motivated functional patients on chronic dialysis therapy should be offered attempts at limb salvage if they are otherwise stable medically and there are good options for revascularization.

Our pre-operative evaluation includes a cardiac risk assessment focusing on careful clinical review, with selective application of stress testing or cardiac catheterization. Pharmacotherapy with beta-adrenergic blocking agents for control of heart rate in the peri-operative period is the cornerstone of medical management. Antiplatelet therapy, generally using aspirin, is also standard. In order to minimize hemodynamic or electrolyte derangement we attempt to coordinate hemodialysis treatments so that pre- and post-operative dialysis sessions are both within 24 hours of surgery.

Perhaps more than any other subgroup of patients with peripheral vascular disease, diabetics with ESRD tolerate infection poorly and are prone to rapid acceleration of local sepsis in the foot. Even seemingly minor ulcerations or skin infections require aggressive treatment with surgical debridement, antibiotics, and close surveillance of wounds. When extensive debridement or multiple toe amputations are required to control infection, an assessment of the viability of remaining tissue, and the likelihood of salvage of a functional foot, is critical before proceeding with further attempts at vascular reconstruction.

For imaging of the vascular anatomy in these patients we continue to prefer digital subtraction angiography which facilitates our ability to choose the best distal outflow tract. If more than 1 infrageniculate vessel is visualized then we try to determine the vessel that appears to fill the pedal arch. If presented with 2 equal appearing target vessels, the one with the better runoff to the foot should be chosen.

When no adequate vessel is visualized on angiography, other imaging techniques may be of value. We have used MRA with gadolinium or time-of-flight techniques, as well as duplex ultrasound to help visualize target vessels in the distal calf or foot. On occasion, surgical exploration of the distal vessel is undertaken in the absence of a definable target on imaging, especially when a pedal Doppler signal is present. It is not unreasonable to take the patient with tissue loss of the foot to the operating room for exploration with an understanding that if the target vessel is unusable then a primary major amputation will be performed.

Techniques of Revascularization

Due to the anatomic pattern of disease, percutaneous interventions have a limited role in these patients. Angioplasty or stenting of inflow disease at the aortoiliac level is employed when suitable lesions with a significant pressure gradient are identified. In addition, angioplasty of focal stenoses within the superficial femoral or even popliteal segments is sometimes employed to allow for a more distal inflow site for bypass, particularly in patients who have limited autogenous conduit. Rarely, a patient with rest pain or limited tissue loss will have diseased but continuous single vessel run-off, with a series of focal lesions that are potentially amenable to angioplasty. This approach may be considered in patients with high surgical risk or lacking adequate vein, but the success rates and durability appear limited in our anecdotal experience. The extensive, circumferential calcification of the infrapopliteal arteries greatly compromises the technical success rate and increases the risk of local complications. By and large, these approaches should be reserved for patients who are not surgical candidates.

In performing infrainguinal bypass grafts in patients with ESRD, conduit usage, vessel handling, and wound management are issues requiring particular attention. For all IBG, standard surgical techniques, including loupe magnification and completion arteriography are employed. We employ Duplex ultrasound intraoperatively for vein mapping and completion imaging as well. The patients undergo general or regional anesthesia. Using a 2-team approach vein harvesting and arterial exposures can be performed simultaneously, and complex operations including those requiring spliced vein grafts can be executed more expeditiously.

Our preference for all infrainguinal revascularizations, particularly in the context of limb salvage, is to complete the bypass graft entirely with autogenous vein conduit. The use of prosthetic grafts for IBG in the ESRD patient is of little or no utility due to early occlusion. Although our group has not had to resort to this technique, other surgeons report a 27% 2 year patency with prosthetic versus a 3 year 67% patency with autogenous vein in these patients.[21]

Conduit of a minimum diameter of 3.5 mm, without discernible areas of phlebosclerosis, is utilized even if this means excising segments and performing a spliced vein graft. More than any other single factor, the quality of the venous conduit is of primary import in achieving a successful outcome with distal bypass in these challenging patients. In our experience, the use of contralateral saphenous vein or spliced vein grafts in patients without adequate ipsilateral GSV has been associated with excellent outcomes.[31,32] We believe that a flexible approach is important to make optimal use of available vein sources, particularly in the absence of ipsilateral GSV. Our preference has been to optimize the size-match between the graft and the native vessels at both the proximal and distal anastomoses, and in spliced-vein bypass, to create a gradual taper of the composite graft. To prepare non-reversed segments, valves are lysed under distension using a Mills valvulotome. Venovenostomies are performed using bevelled, end-to-end anastomoses with fine polypropylene suture. Obviously the patient undergoing hemodialysis is less likely to have available arm vein. In the face of a well functioning AVF, the use of contralateral arm vein may be cautiously considered, but we have generally avoided it to preserve alternative sites for dialysis access in the future.

Proximal and distal arterial exposures are performed via standard approaches. In the diabetic population in particular, we have found great utility in distal origin grafts where the superficial femoral or popliteal artery serves as the inflow site.[33] In our experience, the long term performance is excellent when the proximal femoral segment is minimally diseased. We will often employ the proximal GSV, harvested from the groin down and oriented in a non-reversed fashion, to complete these grafts. The advantage of translocating the proximal vein down the leg for a distal graft is that it avoids a long harvest incision in the more ischemic distal calf, allowing the bypass to be tunneled under intact skin and soft tissue. This helps to avoid difficult wound complications in this high risk population. We generally prefer subcutaneous positioning of grafts to facilitate ultrasound surveillance and revisions, but deeper tunnels are not infrequently employed in this patient group to avoid areas of potential skin breakdown or infection.

In the patient with ESRD hemostatic control and suturing of the distal vessel can be difficult secondary to medial calcinosis. In addition, choosing the best site for the anastomosis can be troublesome. We correlate the digital subtraction angiogram with the vessel and try to avoid areas of extensive calcification where possible. The vessel can also be palpated with a finger or a forcep against a right angle to find the softest spot at which to create the distal anastomosis. Techniques to facilitate the clamping and suturing of calcified vessels, such as gentle crushing of circumferential calcium or limited endarterectomy are occasionally employed and usually technically successful. Fine metal spring clamps (Yasergil or Bulldog) are often employed for hemostatic control of the distal vessel. Pneumatic tourniquets may be tried with variable success depending on the extensiveness of the proximal artery calcification; often they must be supplemented by one of the other techniques to obtain a clear field. We have also used Fogarty embolectomy balloons inflated within the lumen of the vessel Proximal anastomoses are completed first, and after the graft is carefully passed through any tunnels it is allowed to fill under arterial pressure and antegrade flow is checked. At this point the conduit is cut to length on a bevel appropriate for the target vessel. The heel of the vein is then parachuted into place and in vessels less than 2 mm the toe is often parachuted into place. Prior to completion of the anastomosis the distal outflow tract is checked for patency with a fine olive tipped coronary probe. If necessary hemostasis is augmented with topical thrombin and Gel-foam.

Wound Management

When closing incisions in the diabetic ESRD patient, extreme care must be exercised due to their poor wound healing ability. Meticulous hemostasis and careful layered closures of subcutaneous tissue is performed. Incisions in the lower calf and foot, particular those overlying the graft, are generally closed using vertical mattress nylon sutures for skin. When necessary, concominant foot debridement or toe amputations should be carried out at the completion of the bypass operation, which in this population is necessary 50% of the time. Tissue should be cut back to healthy bleeding edges.

For the heel ulcer this may require partial or near complete calcanectomy, or open transmetatarsal amputation for the forefoot. For large or complex wounds that are clean but not readily closable we have recently employed the Vacuum Assisted Closure device (Kinetic Concepts Inc., San Antonio, TX) on the wound in the operating room.[34] For lesser wounds and amputations, in the absence of surrounding sepsis, primary closure should be explored as open wounds generally heal quite slowly in the ESRD patient. Attempts at local rotational and advancement flaps may be warranted to facilitate primary closure.

Follow Up

Routine follow up should consist of post-operative visits at 1 month, and then 3 month intervals until 1 year, then at yearly intervals. Duplex scanning of the graft is the primary method of detecting occult graft lesions, and should be used at each visit. Focal increase in graft velocity (ratio >3.5:1), and decreased graft velocity (<45 cm/sec) are considered significant and are followed by arteriography and revision when appropriate. Both open and minimally invasive techniques have been employed successfully in these situations.

CONCLUSION

It is clear that a growing proportion of the patients requiring IBG for limb salvage will suffer from ESRD and DM. Recent series demonstrate that good to excellent peri-operative mortality, graft patency and limb salvage can all achieved. The actual ability of these patients to use their salvaged limb is dependent upon the individual.

Novel methods to promote wound healing in the ESRD patient need to be developed to improve the chances for successful limb preservation. Such approaches may include innovative methods of antibiotic delivery, debridement, tissue coverage and modulation of growth factors. The use of antibiotic beads, pulse irrigation at the bedside, artificial skin substitutes, growth factors, and anabolic steroids are all methods being actively investigated.

We recommend that an attempt at IBG for limb salvage in the ESRD patient is warranted in most cases not complicated by one of the following: unsalvageable wet or dry gangrene of the foot, overwhelming patient comorbidity, fixed contracture of the knee, or a level of advanced debility such that the patient would be unlikely to benefit from limb preservation.

REFERENCES

1. Conte MS, Belkin M, Upchurch GR, et al. Impact of increasing comorbidity on infrainguinal reconstruction: a 20 year perspective. *Ann Surg.* 2001 Mar;233(3):445–452.
2. Renal Data System. USRDS 2001 annual data report. Bethesda, MD.: National Institute of Diabetes and Digestive and Kidney Diseases, April 2001.
3. Luke RG. Chronic renal failure-a vasculopathic state. *N Engl J Med.* 1998;339:841–843.
4. Abt Associates, Ad Hoc Committee on Nephrology Manpower Needs. Estimated workforce and training requirements for nephrologists through the year 2010. *J Am Soc Nephrol.* 1997;8:S1–32.

5. Ritz E, Stefanski A. Diabetic nephropathy in type II diabetes. *Am J Kidney Dis.* 1996;27: 167–194.
6. Rosen H, Friedman SA, Raizener AE, et al. Azotemic arteriopathy. *Am Heart J.* 1972;84: 250–255.
7. Lantis JC. Conte MS, Belkin M, et al. Infrainguinal Bypass in Patients with End Stage Renal Disease: Improving Outcomes? *J Vasc Surg.* 2001;33:1171–1178.
8. Maggi E, Bellazzi R, Falaschi F, et al. Enhanced LDL oxidation in uremic patients: An additional mechanism for accelerated atherosclerosis? *Kidney Int.* 1994;45:876–883.
9. Becker BN, Himmelfarb J, Henrich WL, et al. Reassessing the cardiac risk profile in chronic hemodialysis patients: A hypothesis on the role of oxidant stress and other non-traditional cardiac risk factors. *J Am Soc Nephrol.* 1997;8:475–486.
10. Jungers P, Chauveau P, Bandin O, et al. Hyperhomocysteinenmia in association with atherosclerotic occlusive arterial accidents in predialysis chronic renal failure patients. *Miner Electrolyte Metab.* 1997;23:170–173.
11. Bachmann J,Tepel M, Raidt H, et al. Hyperhomocysteinemia and the risk for vascular disease in hemodialysis patients. *J Am Soc Nephrol.* 1995;6:121–125.
12. Gris JC, Branger B, Vecina F, et al. Increased cardiovascular risk factors and features of endothelial activation and dysfunction in dialyzed uremic patients. *Kidney Int.* 1994;46:807–813.
13. Dovgan PS, Shepard AD, Nypaver TJ. Critical Limb Ischemia in Patients with End-Stage Renal Disease: Do Long-Term Results Justify An Aggressive Surgical Approach? *Perspectives in Vascular Surgery,* Vol 12:1 (Editor Gloviczki, P, Thieme Pub.). p.81–92.
14. Seeger JM, Pretus HA, Carlton LC, et al. Potential Predictors of Outcome in patients with tissue loss who undergo infrainguinal vein bypass grafting. *J Vasc Surg.* 1999 Sep;30(3): 427–435.
15. Dossa CD, Shepard AD, Amos AM, et al. Results of lower extremity amputation in patients with end stage renal disease. *J Vasc Surg.* 1994;20:14–19.
16. Whittemore AD, Donaldson MC, Mannick JA. Infrainguinal reconstruction for patients with chronic renal insufficiency. *J Vasc Surg.* 1993;17:32–41.
17. Edwards JM, Taylor LM, Porter JM. Limb salvage in end-stage renal disease (ESRD). Arch Surg. 1988;123:1164–1168.
18. Seeger JM, Pretus HA, Carlton LC, et al. Potential Predictors of Outcome in patients with tissue loss who undergo infrainguinal vein bypass grafting. *J Vasc Surg* 1999 Sep;30(3):427–35.
19. Hakaim AG, Gordon JK, Scott TE. Early outcome of in situ femorotibial reconstruction among patients with diabetes alone versus diabetes and end-stage renal failure: analysis of 83 limbs. *J Vasc Surg.* 1998 Jun; 27(6):1049–1054.
20. Cox MH, Robinson JG, Brothers TE, et al. Contemporary analysis of outcomes following lower extremity bypass in patients with end-stage renal disease. *Ann Vasc Surg.* 2001 May; 15(3):374–382.
21. Myerson SL, Skelly CL, Curi MA, et al. Long term results justify autogenous infrainguinal bypass grafting in patients with end-stage renal failure. *J Vasc Surg.* 2001 Jul;34(1):27–33.
22. Biancari F, Kantonen I, Matzke S, et al. Infrainguinal endovascular and bypass surgery for critical leg ischemiain patients on long-term dialysis. *Ann Vasc Surg.* 2002 Mar;16(2): 210–214.
23. Albers M, Romiti M, Braganca Pereira CA, et al. A meta-analysis of infrainguinal arterial reconstruction in patients with end-stage renal disease. *Eur J Vasc Surg.* 2001 Oct;22(4): 294–300.
24. Baele HR, Piotrowski JJ, Yuhus J, Anderson C, Alexander JJ. Infrainguinal bypass in patients with end-stage renal disease. *Surgery.* 1995;117:319–324.
25. Simsir SA, Cabellon A, Kohlman-Trigoboff D, et al. Factors influencing limb salvage and survival after amputation and revascularization in patients with end-stage renal disease. *Am J Surg.* 1995;170:113–117.
26. Leers SA, Reifsnyder T, Delmonte R, et al. Realistic expectations for pedal bypass grafts in patients with end stage renal disease. *J Vasc Surg.* 1998;28:976–983.

27. Desai TR, Meyerson SL, Skelly CL, et al. Patency and limb salvage after infrainguinal bypass with severely compromised ("blind") outflow. *Arch Surg.* 2001 Jun;136(6):635–642.
28. Raferty KB, Belkin M, Mackey WC, et al. Are peroneal artery bypass grafts hemodynamically inferior to other tibial artery bypass grafts? *J Vasc Surg.* 1994;19:964–968.
29. Nicholas GG, Bozorgnia M, Nastasee SA, et al. Infrainguinal bypass in patients with end-stage renal disease: survival and ambulation. *Vasc Surg.* 2000;34:147–155.
30. Albers M, Fratezi A, DeLuccia N. Assessment of quality of life of patients with severe ischemia as a result of Infrainguinal arterial occlusive disease. *J Vasc Surg.* 1992;16:54–59.
31. Chew D, Conte MS, Donaldson MC, Whittemore AD, et al. Autogenous composite vein bypass for infrainguinal arterial reconstruction. *J Vasc Surg* 2001;33: 259–65.31.
32. Chew DKW, Owens CD, Belkin M, Donaldson MC, Conte MS, et al. Bypass in the absence of ipsilateral greater saphenous vein-safety and superiority of the contralateral greater saphenous vein. *J Vasc Surg.* 2002;35:1085–92.
33. Reed AB, Conte MS, Belkin M, Mannick JA, et al. Usefulness of autogenous bypass grafts originating distal to the groin. *J Vasc Surg.* 2002;35:48–55.33.
34. Argenta LC, Morykwas MJ. Vacuum-assisted closure: a new method for wound control and treatment-clinical experience. *Ann Plast Surg.* 1997:38:563–76.

31

Role of Duplex Scanning in Lower Extremity Bypass

Jonathan B. Towne, MD

Techniques used to evaluate infrainguinal autogenous vein bypass grafts has evolved over the last 2 decades. Initially, the goal was to improve operative results by developing better surgical techniques and improving patient selection with improved angiographic imaging. More recently, the emphasis has broadened to attempt to prevent patent grafts from failing in the follow up period by detecting graft threatening lesions with prospective ongoing graft surveillance protocols before the grafts occlude.[1–9] Up to one-third of grafts will require intervention to prevent failure in the follow-up period because of the development of lesions that threaten patency in the conduit, anastomatic sites, and inflow and out flow vessels.[10] The particular type of lesion varies with the time course in the follow up period. Problems related to the technical aspect of the procedure occur in the early perioperative period (less than 30 days), complications of fibrointimal hyperplasia (vein valve stenosis, graft stricture) occur during the 1–24 month period, and progression of the atherosclerotic disease in the inflow, outflow, and vein conduit itself occur beyond 24 months.[11] Because the autogenous vein is living tissue, secondary patency rates are better if lesions that lead to graft failure can be detected before thrombosis, preventing ischemic injury to the delicate venous endothelium, which reduces the incidence of conduit salvage.[12]

B-mode imaging has become a valuable adjunct to the vascular surgeon in evaluating bypass graft function. It combines the B-mode image which can visualize an anatomic defect, with Doppler spectral analysis for hemodynamic assessment. The further addition of color-coded imaging greatly facilitates vessel imaging, making this the ideal method for graft evaluation. The initial use of duplex scanning is in the operating room following completion of the arterial repair. Duplex scanning helps determine the function of the vein graft and also allows for detection of any technical errors with construction of the proximal or distal anastomosis and when the in situ technique is used it allows for identification of residual competent valves or persistent AV fistulae. When used intraoperatively, the sterile plastic sleeve is filled with saline before placing the transducer inside. The saline which is maintained inside the sheath by the application of rubber bands on the Doppler probe is needed to couple the transducer to the vessel. A vascular technologist is present to make necessary adjustments in Doppler angle assignment, sample volume placement, and color parameters in order to obtain the optimal image and accurate spectral display. Intraoperative assessment of bypass grafts has followed an evolution over the last several years. Initially, continuous wave Doppler analysis was used to assist in the evaluation of grafts. This was followed by pulsed Doppler spectral analysis and finally the current generation of color-flow duplex scanning machines. Color duplex scanning provides a rapid, accurate means of graft assessment. As the transducer is advanced slowly along the entire length of the reconstruction, the surgeon observes the color image. Uniformed colors during cardiac cycle and the absence of anatomic defects in the B-mode image indicate normal flow. A residual lesion is diagnosed when a turbulent color pattern which is indicated by a color mosaic of multiple colors and a spectral waveform with an increased Vp (>140 cm/sec) with severe spectral broadening. Graft threatening lesions and their identifying spectral characteristics are detailed in Table 31–1 and Table 31–2. Diagnostic criteria used for postoperative graft surveillance are also used for intraoperative assessment (Table 31–3).

Understanding the biology of the autogenous vein conduit is essential in attempting to maximize patency of these vascular reconstructions. The location and natural history of particular lesions that are likely to threaten patency of the bypass graft can be predicted. In the first 30 days, problems related to the operative procedure and patient selection were most likely to cause problems. These include technical errors in the construction of the anastomosis and when the in situ technique is used, residual competent valves and persistent or developing arteriovenous fistulas. In the interval between 1 and 24 months, the primary cause of graft failure was related to fibrointimal hyperplasia. This is identified as a stricture of either the proximal or distal anastomosis or more commonly as a stenosis of the conduit at the site of valve leaflets or trau-

Table 31–1. Potential technical errors: in situ saphenous vein grafts

Defect	Duplex Characteristic
Anastomotic stricture	↑ V_p, turbulent flow, visible narrowing
Intact valve leaflet	↑ V_p, turbulent flow, visible valve (gray scale)
Residual arteriovenous fistula	↑ V_p, ↑ V_d, turbulent flow, visible venous branch
Inadequate graft flow	↓ V_p, (<45cm/sec) in smallest diameter
Inadequate outflow	↓ V_p, ↓ V_d minimal turbulence

TABLE 31–2. LOWER EXTREMITY ARTERIAL DUPLEX ULTRASONOGRAPHY: CATEGORIES OF ARTERIAL STENOSIS AND VELOCITY SPECTRA CHARACTERISTICS

Diameter Reduction (%)	Peak Velocity (cm/sec)	Velocity Increase Relative to Proximal Segment (%)	Spectral Broadening
<20	<125	<30	Slight
20–49	<125	>30	Throughout pulse cycle
50–75	<125	>100	Severe
>75	>125 Diastolic >100	>100	Severe

TABLE 31–3. CATEGORIES OF DUPLEX SCAN-IDENTIFIED RESIDUAL LESIONS

Stenosis Category	PSV (cm/sec)	Vr	Interpretation & intraoperative management
Normal / Minimal	<125	1–2	Normal flow pattern; no further evaluation required
Moderate	125–180	2–3	Residual flow abnormality; rescan after 5 min with papaverine flow augmentation; consider arteriographic imaging
Severe	>180 with spectral broadening	2.5–5.0	Significant abnormality; repair defect; if not repaired perform arteriography to verify normal bypass graft segment
High-grade	>300	>5	Critical lesion, typically associated with a pulse pressure deficit and low graft flow; assess for platelet thrombus

(From: Johnson, Bandyk, Back, Avino, Roth. Intraoperative duplex monitoring of infrainguinal vein bypass procedures. *J Vasc Surg.* 2000;31(4):678–90.)

matic injury to the vein from intraluminal instrumentation required for valve disruption. Long strictures related to damage during vein harvest or abnormal veins in which fibrotic processes which may have been initiated before the bypass by previous episodes of superficial phlebitis, can also develop. After 24 months the vein graft was most likely to be placed at risk as a result of progression of atherosclerotic disease in the inflow and outflow vessels, as well as the development of atherosclerosis in the autogenous vein graft itself. In a study conducted by the authors, inflow obstruction occurred at a median of 15 months after bypass construction, and outflow obstruction developed 29 months into the life of the bypass.[11] Lesions in the native arterial system developed later than lesions in the conduit, which occurred at a median of 8.5 months.

To achieve optimal secondary patency rates, lower extremity vein grafts performed for limb salvage require considerable maintenance. Thirty percent of the grafts required at least 1 revision in the follow-up period. Even grafts that have exhibited good hemodynamics for up to 24 months are at risk subsequently for developing abnormalities that could lead to graft failure. In our study 18% of initial graft revisions occurred after 24 months. Because of the increasing incidence of progression of atherosclerosis in the inflow and outflow with long-term follow-up, a greater percentage of revisions involve inflow and outflow vessels as opposed to the conduit itself. Of the revisions performed after 24 months, 68% were to the conduit compared with 85% in the earlier time period.[11]

As the follow-up period becomes longer, degenerative changes can develop in the conduit itself. Previous work from our institution demonstrated that more than 50% of vein bypass conduits followed up for at least 5 years demonstrated evidence of atherosclerotic degeneration.[10] Often these changes represent areas of intimal thickening, but in a significant portion, the disease had progressed to form focal points of stenosis caused by atherosclerosis. As noted in this series, patients who require lower extremity bypass for limb salvage have a high long-term mortality rate, with 68% of the patients alive after 5 years and only 37% surviving 10 years. These patient deaths preclude the opportunity to monitor this group of vein grafts long enough to study the ultimate course of the degenerative process in the conduit. However, as patient longevity increases, atherosclerosis formation in the lower extremity vein graft is likely to become an increasing threat to long-term graft patency. Our studies have demonstrated that degenerative changes will develop in conduits that have been absolutely normal for several years of follow-up. The likelihood of developing graft-threatening lesions is even greater in conduits that have been previously revised or have hemodynamic abnormalities, but some conduits that have been free of abnormality for 2 years will go on to require revision.[11] Recognizing that conduits that previously have required revision are more prone to develop secondary degenerative processes allows surveillance of these conduits to be more focused.

Other authors have suggested that if the conduit has normal hemodynamics in the early perioperative period, the chance of problems are such that further surveillance may not be warranted.[12] Our study revealed that of the 67 graft revisions performed after 24 months, 37 were to previously revised conduits, but 30 were to vein grafts that required no previous revisions.[11] Conduits that are hemodynamically normal beyond 2 years evolve lesions at a significant rate to warrant on going surveillance. The average incidence of primary graft failure was 10% of the number of grafts remaining patent at each yearly time interval beyond 24 months[11] (Figure 31–1, Figure 31–2, and Figure 31–3). If vascular surgeons want to optimize long-term graft patency, surveillance must be done for the life of the conduit.

TECHNIQUE FOR SURVEILLANCE

In the past evaluation of lower extremity arterial reconstruction was limited to physical examination, which has many inherent problems as a surveillance technique. A pulse can be felt in a vein graft and a distal pulse palpated, but impending graft failure can rarely be detected by physical examination alone. Detection of distal pulses and the examination of the foot for evidence of capillary refill times are gross measures that have little predictive value in assessing potential graft problems. A noninvasive vascular laboratory is essential for the surveillance program since with duplex scan-

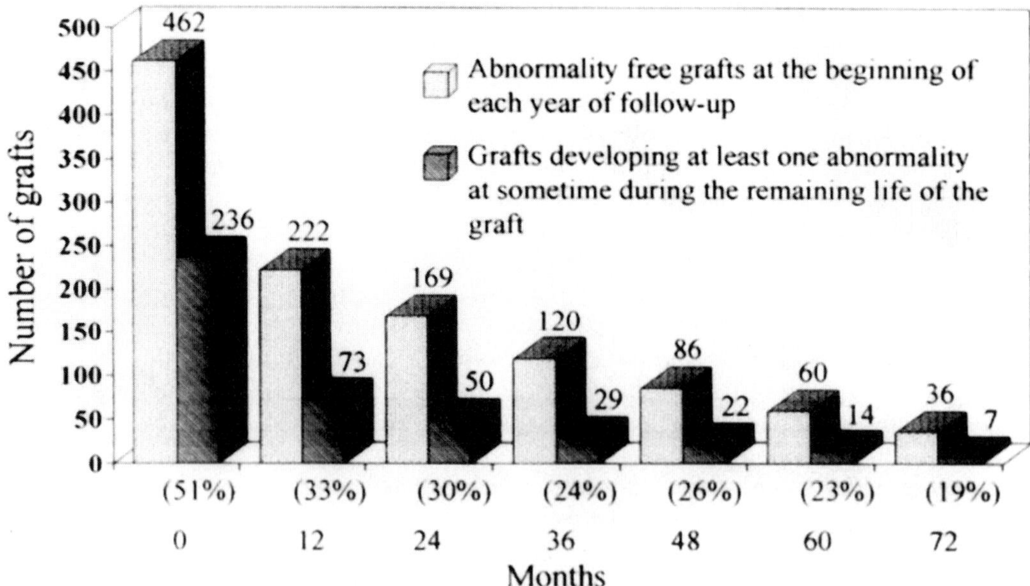

Figure 31–1. Percentage of saphenous vein in situ bypass grafts free of abnormality at beginning of each year of follow-up that subsequently develop at least 1 significant abnormality during postoperative surveillance at sometime during remaining life of graft. Reproduced with permission from Erickson LA, Towne JB, Seabrook CR. *J Vasc Surg.* 1996;23;18–27.

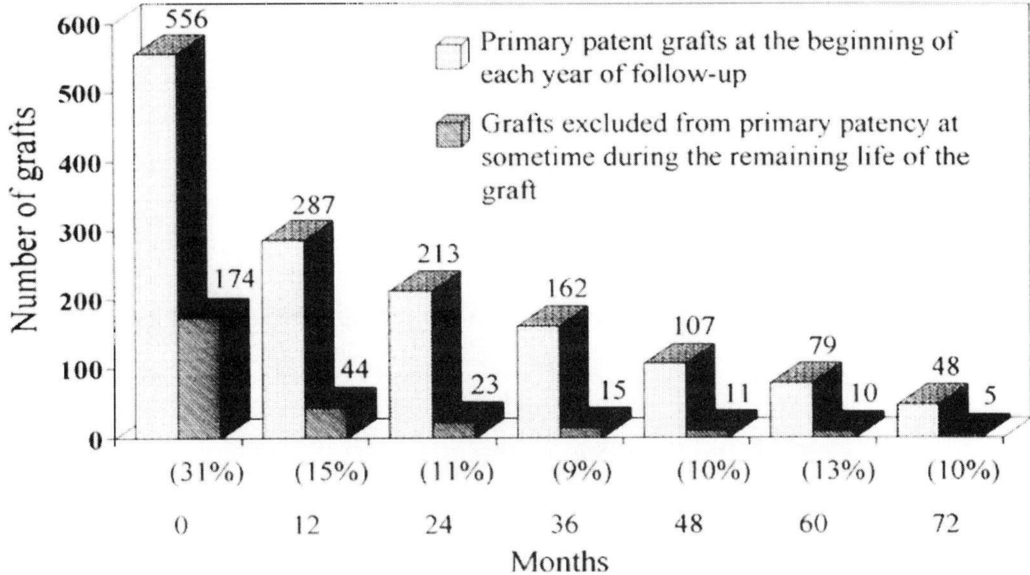

Figure 31–2. Percentage of primary patent saphenous vein in situ bypass grafts at beginning of each year of follow-up that subsequently fail at sometime during remaining life of graft. Reproduced with permission from Erickson LA, Towne JB, Seabrook CR. *J Vasc Surg.* 1996;23;18–27.

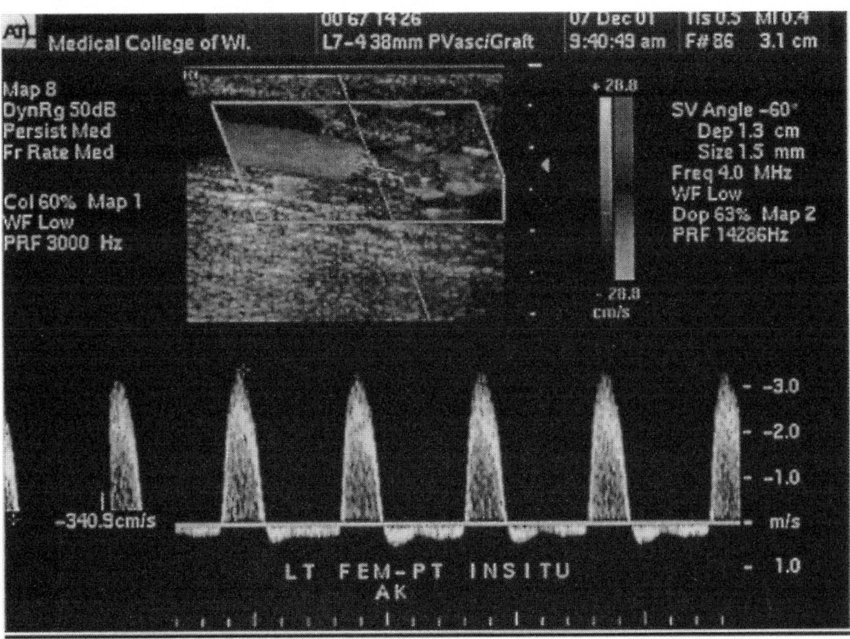

Figure 31–3. Area of graft stenosis occurring 28 months following femoral to posterior tibial in situ bypass. Peak systolic velocity was 340.9 cm/sec.

ning and measuring of ankle brachial indices precise physiologic function of the conduit can be determined. In a previous study conducted by the authors, only 1 out of 3 patients who had a lesion that was threatening to prolong graft function was identified by patient symptoms.[1] The use of ankle brachial indices alone has limitations when used for postoperative surveillance. In patients with diabetes mellitus, roughly one-third have calcification of the tibial vessels resulting in the inability to measure ankle pressures. In our practice, diabetics compose 50% of the patients, which result in a significant proportion of patients in whom ankle brachial indices are not useful. Likewise in patients in whom Doppler or ankle pressures are found to have decreased, locating the precise segment of the vascular tree that has caused this decrease is impossible.

Duplex scanning provides simultaneous color-coding of Doppler flow information based on direction of velocity within a real time B-mode image. Principle component of this instrument is the ability to assess tissue anatomy and blood flow physiology in a simultaneous or sequential manner, so the location and extent of the disease can be accurately evaluated. Most of our studies are performed with a 10 MHz linear ray transducer which permits visualization of superficially placed grafts such as the in situ saphenous vein graft. Graft assessment begins with the imaging system set for evaluation with a normal graft, and adjustments are made as necessary for imaging and Doppler assessment of stenotic lesions. The velocity range and pulse repetition frequency can be increased to prevent aliasing when a stenotic graft is found. A 3 MHz linear ray transducer is used when evaluating deeply placed grafts or when visualizing the distal anastomosis. Time gain compensation controls are often adjusted to compensate for attenuation of the ultrasound as it passes through the soft tissue.

The duplex examination of the infrainguinal bypass graft is performed with the patient in the supine position. The limb to be examined is externally rotated and slightly bent with the knee resting on a small pillow. A tape measure is positioned along the limb and held in place with tape to facilitate documentation of recording sites. It is important to have the operative report and details of any previous study available for comparison.

Duplex mapping of the graft begins in the proximal thigh where the graft is easily identified. The transducer is then advanced cephalad to the proximal anastomosis.

The graft is first imaged and assessed with the transducer in the longitudinal orientation. This orientation produces an image of a long segment of the graft for observation and for obtaining velocity spectra waveforms. Doppler spectral analysis is performed with the Doppler angle aligned to the long axis of the vessel, with the angle maintained at less than 65 degrees to obtain accurate velocity data. The transducer is then rotated so the graft diameter measurements may be obtained. These measurements are particularly important when there has been a gradual sequential decrease in graft flow velocity. Obviously, if no other technical defect is found and graft diameter has been noted to increase this will explain the decreasing velocity in the conduit.

Graft anastomosis to the below knee popliteal artery are best imaged using a posterior approach with the patient in a prone position. The hemodynamics of graft blood flow and limb arterial circulation are characterized with Doppler derived blood flow velocity analysis and limb blood pressure measurements. The blood flow velocity peak in systole is determined. Potential problems are indicated by graft flow velocities of less than 45 cm/sec in the smallest diameter segment, a decrease in graft flow velocity of 30 cm/sec, a decrease in the ankle brachial index of 0.15 on subsequent visits, or focal increases in velocity greater than 150 cc/sec.

Bandyk et al. developed the concept of velocity ratio in evaluating vein graft stenosis. The peak systolic ratio of the peak systolic velocity was divided by the peak systolic velocity proximal to the lesion (*Vr = PSV at lesion / PSV Proximal*).[13] These authors then classified the lesions into 4 categories. We use a threshold of Vr of 3 to determine the need for intervention to restore normal graft hemodynamics. Mills also used *Vr* in determining the timing of intervention to correct graft stenosis and demonstrated serial surveillance is effective for grafts with intermediate stenosis.[14]

HIGH RISK GRAFTS

Long-term studies have identified groups of grafts more likely to develop problems in the follow-up period. In a previous study of 361 saphenous vein conduits, 23% were modified to successfully complete the procedure. The modification was performed to correct an inadequate vein in 10% of the bypasses, and a technical failure occurred using inadequate vein in 13%. Technical failures were caused by vein injury, anastomotic stenosis, retained valve, bypass torsion, recurrent of platelet aggregates, and a low flow state. Primary patency at 4 years for bypasses requiring modification was 50%, significantly less than a non-modified bypass conduit 70%. The secondary patency for bypasses requiring modification 72% was significantly less than the non-modified bypass conduit (84%). In situ saphenous vein bypasses using modified conduits underwent revision 40% more frequently during the postoperative period compared to bypasses with a non-modified conduit (22%).[11]

The intraoperative modification of the vein conduit was associated with a significant increase in the incidence of late appearing lesions that require revision. The occurrence and progression of fibrointimal hyperplasia was associated with the injurious affects of bypass modification to correct the poor quality vein or technical error. As the number of technical errors decreased in our series with increasing surgical experience the quality of vein has become the most important factor determining the need for modification of the bypass conduit. We define a good quality vein as a thin walled vein greater than 2 mm in diameter with or without a bifurcated segment that has a glistening endothelial flow surface. If a technical error occurs or a poor quality segment of vein is identified, the short segment of abnormal vein can be modified with maintenance of the in situ technique. Intraoperative modification of the in situ conduit can restore normal hemodynamics and result in early bypass patency. Long-term patency is dependent on careful postoperative hemodynamic surveillance to identify and correct the bypass threatening stenosis before the thrombosis. In a subsequent study, 46% of grafts with stenosis found more than 5 years after implantation were found at sites that had previously been revised. This emphasizes the importance of noting that graft modification at the initial procedure may have implications far beyond the perioperative period. These patients should be identified and these areas of revised grafts carefully interrogated throughout the follow-up period to identify when these stenoses develop. Nineteen percent of 72 conduits were modified at the original operation to repair a venous injury or to replace a portion of unsuitable vein. Seventy-one percent of these grafts required subsequent revisons, and one-half revisions were performed at the same site that was modified at the original operation.

IMPORTANCE OF IDENTIFYING GRAFTS PRIOR TO THROMBOSIS

There is a distinct difference in long-term patency between those bypasses revised prior to thrombosis and those who were thrombosed. We noted the 3-year patency for thrombosed grafts was 47% compared to 93% for grafts that were patent at the time of revision.[9] The poor results with revising the thrombosed conduit coupled with the excellent patency of patent bypass revisions underscores the importance of monitoring graft hemodynamics with a surveillance protocol to detect a failing bypass before thrombosis.

TIMING INTERVAL

Since patients can develop graft threatening lesions throughout the life of the conduit, we feel the surveillance needs to be extended for the duration of the patient's life. The first year following the operative procedure we recommend surveillance every 3 months. After the first postoperative year well functioning grafts are then followed up with surveillance every 6 months.

REFERENCES

1. Bandyk DF, Schmitt DO, Seabrook GR, et al. Maintaining functional patency of in situ saphenous vein bypasses: the impact of a surveillance protocol and elective revision. *J Vasc Surg.* 1989;9:286–296.
2. Nehler MR, Moneta GL, Yeager RA, et al. Surgical treatment of threatened reversed infrainguinal vein grafts. *J Vasc Surg.* 1994;20:558–565.
3. Grigg MJ, Nicolaides AN, Wolfe JHN. Detection and grading of femorodistal vein graft stenoses: duplex velocity measurements compared with angiography. *J Vasc Surg.* 1988;8: 661–666.
4. Lundell A, Lindblad B, Bergquist D, et al. Femoro-popliteal-crural graft patency is improved with an intensive graft surveillance program: a prospective randomized study. *J Vasc Surg.* 1995:21:26–34.
5. Green RM, McNamara J, Ouriel K, et al. Comparison of infrainguinal graft surveillance techniques. *J Vasc Surg.* 1990;11:207–215.
6. Sladen JG, Reid JDS, Copperberg PL, et al. Color flow duplex screening of infrainguinal grafts combining low-and high-velocity criteria. *Am J Surg.* 1989;158:107–112.
7. Londrey GL, Hodgson KJ, Spadone DP, et al. Initial experience with color-flow duplex scanning of infrainguinal bypass grafts. *J Vasc Surg.* 1990;12:284–290.
8. Belkin M, Raffery KB, Mackey WC, et al. A prospective study of the determination of vein graft flow velocity: implications for graft surveillance. *J Vasc Surg.* 1995;19:259–267.
9. Bergamini TM, Towne JB, Bandyk DF, et al. Experience with in situ saphenous vein bypasses during 1981–1989: determining factors of long-term patency. *J Vasc Surg.* 1991;13: 137–149.
10. Reifsnyder TM, Towne JB, Seabrook GR, et al. Biologic characteristics of long-term autogenous vein grafts: a dynamic evolution. *J Vasc Surg.* 1993;17:207–217.
11. Erickson CA, Towne JB, Seabrook GR, et la. Ongoing vascular laboratory surveillance is essential to maximize long-term in situ saphenous vein bypass patency. *J Vasc Surg.* 1996;23: 18–27.
12. Taylor LM, Edwards JM, Porter JM. Present status of reversed vein in situ bypass grafting: Five-year results of a modern series. *J Vasc Surg.* 1990;11:193–206.
13. Johnson BL, Bandyk DF, Back MR, et al. Intraoperative duplex monitoring of infrainguinal vein bypass procedures. *J Vasc Surg.* 2000;31(4):678–690.
14. Mills JL Sr, Wixon CL, James DC, et al. The natural history of intermediate and critical vein graft stenosis: recommendations for continued surveillance or repair. *J Vasc Surg.* 2001;33(2):273–280.

32

Infrainguinal Revascularization in the Pediatric Patient

James C. Stanley, MD

Lower extremity arterial reconstructions in children are very uncommon but are a necessity in the treatment of certain vascular injuries. The most frequent vascular injury in this age group is iatrogenic, especially from femoral artery catheterization.[1–7] Such an injury if untreated in the younger child has the potential to lead to extremity growth retardation and a limb length discrepancy (LLD).[2,8–12] When LLDs are marked, gait disturbances evolve and the compensatory scoliosis that occurs leads to disabling arthritic problems in later adulthood. Early extremity revascularization to prevent these complications is quite justified.

Reversed autogenous saphenous vein bypass grafts are the most common conduit for reconstructing arteries in the lower extremities of pediatric patients (Figure 32–1). However, these vein grafts have been a matter of concern to many in the past because of documented aneurysmal changes when used for childhood vascular reconstructions in other arterial beds.[13–15] Recent experience suggests that this concern is not warranted.[1] Use of synthetic prostheses in young patients are less favored because of their inherent thrombogenicity and the fact that they need to be durable for many years longer than might be the case in the elderly patient undergoing a vascular reconstruction.

CAUSE OF LOWER EXTREMITY ISCHEMIA IN THE PEDIATRIC PATIENT

Most pediatric lower extremity vascular insufficiency, in contrast to that in adults, is due to iatrogenic causes, the majority of these vascular injuries occurring after arterial cannulation or catheterization.[16–17] Noniatrogenic causes, including penetrating trauma, knee-dislocation with popliteal disruption, and obstructive disease due to rubella, are much less common.

The incidence of catheterization-related injuries in children is not well defined. One reason may be the difficulty in accurately determining the denominator to calculate the true frequency of these events. A review of the literature supports this, with

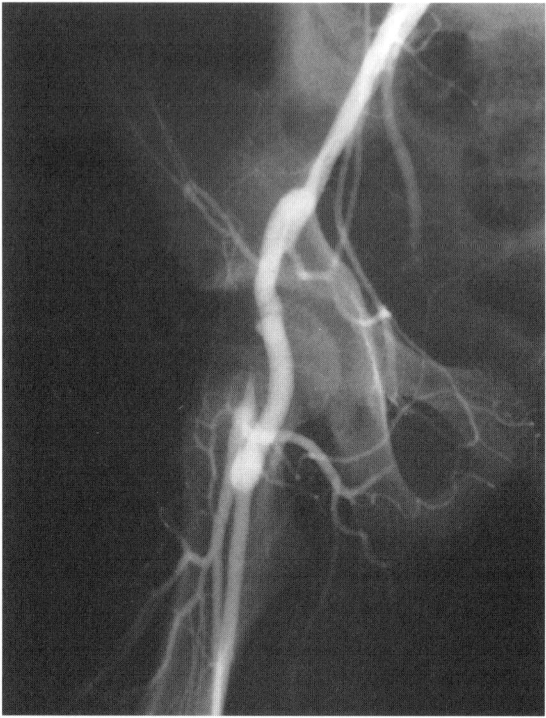

Figure 32–1. Postoperative arteriogram of a child having undergone right iliofemoral bypass graft with saphenous vein 1 week earlier. Immediate postoperative expansion of saphenous vein grafts causes them to be approximately 20% larger than the external iliac artery on the ipsilateral side, and this fact should be taken into account when determining later dilatation of vein grafts. (Reprinted with permission from Cardneau JD, Henke PK, Upchurch GR Jr, et al. Efficacy and durability of autologous saphenous vein conduits for lower extremity arterial reconstructions in preadolescent children. *J Vasc Surg.* 2001;34:34–40.)

catheterization-related vascular injuries in children reported to range from 0.2 to 37% of such procedures.[5,9,18] Nevertheless, occurrences of these injuries are likely to be toward the higher of the reported frequencies. In a recent study of 58 randomly selected children undergoing femoral artery catheterization, femoral artery occlusion was documented in 33%.[19] In the University of Michigan series, 12 (86%) of 14 patients sustained iatrogenic injuries, and all but 1 were due to femoral catheterizations during evaluation and treatment of congenital heart disease.[1]

CLINICAL MANIFESTATIONS OF LOWER EXTREMITY ISCHEMIA IN CHILDREN

Recognition of arterial insufficiency affecting a child's lower extremity may be more difficult than in an adult. Many, if not most acute injuries do not cause immediate limb-threatening symptoms, and they may go undiagnosed until years later when the consequences of chronic arterial insufficiency become apparent. Children develop extensive collaterals rapidly, and pulses in the affected extremity may even be comparable to the uninvolved side despite iliac or common femoral arterial occlusions. Physical examination of pulses is certainly not sensitive enough to predict eventual limb length changes.[8,20]

Often it is not until a LLD develops and the child complains of exercise-related symptoms or develops an abnormal gait that the diagnosis of extremity ischemia is considered. Bloom's review noted that discovery of vascular insufficiency occurred from 6 months to more than 4 years after the initial injury, when children experienced claudication or LLD.[9] It is perhaps relevant to note that some authors have not been able to correlate the degree of apparent vascular insufficiency with the manifestations of LLD severity,[2] whereas others have found a statistically significant inverse relationship between the ankle-brachial index (ABI) and LLD.[19]

DIAGNOSIS OF LOWER EXTREMITY ARTERIAL INSUFFICIENCY

Simple Doppler-derived ABI determinations may establish a diagnosis of limb ischemia. However, detection of some lesions may require performance of exercise ABIs. Postexercise reductions in the ABI and abnormal biphasic waveforms, rather than normal triphasic arterial waveforms may be evident in these circumstances. Confirmatory imaging studies to define the exact location and extent of the arterial occlusion are necessary to plan optimal treatment. Performance of conventional arteriographic studies in the very young carries the risk of a second arterial injury, and the resulting concern of pediatricians and parents over further catheterizations is justified. Newer diagnostic modalities may obviate the need for conventional arteriographic studies in many of these children. Magnetic resonance angiography often overstates a stenosis' severity and may not be precise enough to establish an exact diagnosis. However, reintroduction of intravenous digital subtraction arteriography accompanied by newer computer enhanced imaging, appears capable of defining these lesions, while avoiding further catheter-related complications (Figure 32–2). If a LLD is sus-

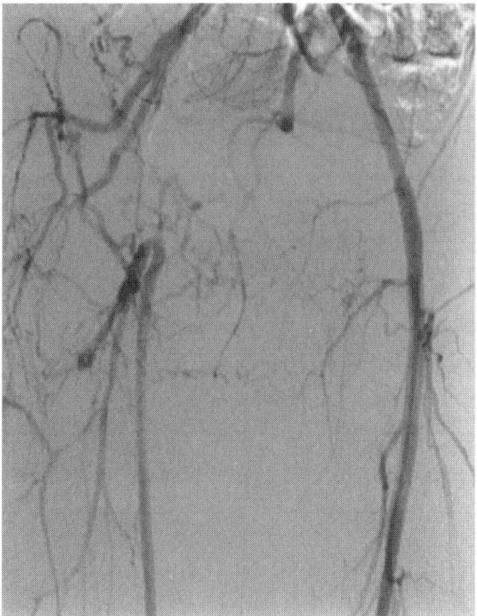

Figure 32–2. Intravenous digital subtraction arteriogram in child with occluded external iliac and common femoral arteries after diagnostic catheterization. Iodinated contrast was injected centrally through a catheter advanced through right brachial vein under fluoroscopic guidance to junction of vena cava and right atrium. (Reprinted with permission from Cardneau JD, Henke PK, Upchurch GR Jr, et al. Efficacy and durability of autologous saphenous vein conduits for lower extremity arterial reconstructions in preadolescent children. *J Vasc Surg.* 2001;34:34–40).

pected scanograms (orthoroentgenograms) should be obtained using a long ruler having radiopaque gradations placed next to the extremities, with subsequent measurements of bone length being possible to the nearest millimeter.

TREATMENT OF ACUTE LOWER EXTREMITY VASCULAR INJURIES

Definitive algorithms for the early management of children with catheterization injuries do not exist, in part because of the lack of long-term postoperative follow-up.[7] This subject becomes controversial because some believe that LLD occurs in only 0.8% of all femoral catheterizations,[10] or is even rarer, suggesting little need to treat any asymptomatic arterial obstructions in the lower extremities of children.[12] In contrast, a contemporary study on the late complications of extremity ischemia reported LLD rates of 8% after percutaneous femoral catheterizations.[19]

Treatment of acute ischemia often depends on the size of the injured vessel and, therefore, the age of the patient. Once an acute ischemic state is recognized intravenous heparin anticoagulation should be instituted. If the Doppler examination does not document that the arterial circulation has returned to near-normal by 48 hours, then a thrombectomy or reconstruction should be considered in an otherwise stable child. Unfortunately, the very young who are most prone to catheter-related vascular injuries are the most technically difficult to treat operatively. Although some advocate early revascularization of otherwise viable lower extremities because of the future risk of LLD, Smith and Green[5] asserted that good operative outcomes were in the minority when undertaken in children younger than 2 years. Klein and colleagues also argued that early operation for catheter-related injury led to poorer outcomes than nonoperative management, with an average patient age in this study of 30 months.[3] However, Flanigan and associates, in one of the largest reviews of iatrogenic pediatric vascular injuries, reported that nonoperative management led to a 23% incidence of LLD, compared with 9% for those managed operatively.[2] The mean age of children at the time of diagnosis of injury in Flanigan's study was 31 months, with 84% of the children being younger than 4 years. Furthermore, 93% of those patients treated nonoperatively with heparin had their resting ABI return to normal, supporting the tenet that a normal ABI does not necessarily eliminate the risk for the late development of LLD. Based on this latter study it seems logical that most acute injuries be addressed operatively after an early period of observation not exceeding 48 hours. Continued vigilance for the development of vascular insufficiency of the lower extremity, especially in children treated nonoperatively, is exceedingly important if one is to prevent the complication of LLD.

TREATMENT OF CHRONIC LOWER EXTREMITY ISCHEMIA

Strict guidelines are nonexistent regarding the management of children presenting with late complications of their extremity ischemia. It has been generally accepted in the past that a late operation would not reverse an existing LLD. It was thought that once a loss of limb growth had occurred that it could not be reversed, and revascularization procedures at that juncture were only preventative for additional retarded limb growth. This may have been an inaccurate perception. Various views on the subject have existed in the literature. For instance, Whitehouse and colleagues described 4 children who underwent saphenous vein bypass grafts an average of 62 months after injury for LLD.[7] Three were available for follow-up, and none of them exhibited improvement in their LLD. However, others suggest that late operations can improve, and even correct, LLDs.[9,19] Klein and his associates reported on 3 late operations for LLD with equalization of leg lengths noted approximately 2 years later in the 2 children available for follow-up.[3] Both had undergone saphenous vein revascularizations. In a similar situation, Walter and Hoffmann described a young girl with an LLD of 4 cm after catheterization that completely resolved 2.5 years after an iliofemoral bypass graft with autogenous saphenous vein.[21] Similar, but lesser degrees of LLD resolution occurred in 70% of the children in the University of Michigan series.[1]

Treatment delays for chronic ischemia may also be related to the perception that the consequences of lower extremity arterial insufficiency are not always severe enough to warrant operative intervention. After all, it may be difficult to determine what degree of LLD will become important at a later time. An LLD of 0.5 cm has been considered abnormal by some,[2,7] whereas others consider a 1.5-cm difference clinically significant.[19]

Reservations continue to exist about the stability of saphenous vein used for arterial reconstructions in the pediatric population. Bloom and associates did not use saphenous vein in any of their patients "because of its small size and poor quality in children."[9] In contradistinction to this view, the primary patency of vein grafts used in the Michigan series involving young, preadolescent children was 93% (14 of 15) at an average of 10.7 years postoperatively.[1] As a simple conduit to carry blood, these grafts appear to function well. However, the morphologic character of the vein graft in these young patients is less well defined.

Late aneurysmal degeneration of vein grafts placed in other vascular beds is known to occur in children. Nonaneurysmal saphenous vein expansion, averaging 18%, occurred in 45% of grafts used for aortorenal bypass graft in all age groups at the author's institution.[15] Greater degrees of expansion affected younger patients. An additional 8% of grafts actually became aneurysmal, with an average diameter increase of 114% (range, 62%–150%). These changes occurred at an average follow-up of only 14 months. Four of the 6 aneurysmal vein grafts occurred in patients younger than 18 years. This experience resulted in the abandonment of vein graft reconstructions of the renal arteries in children at the University of Michigan.[23] In a similar setting, Berkowitz and O'Neill cited a 33% incidence of aneurysms in unsupported saphenous veins used as aortorenal bypass grafts in children.[23]

That venous conduits in the young are more prone to aneurysmal expansion may have biologic explantations, with differences in the arborization of the vasa vasorum resulting in a greater ischemic insult to the graft during its harvest and implantation.[24] It is likely that the mild dilatation observed in most of these grafts in the lower extremity will be stable and nonprogressive.[1] Nevertheless, it may be prudent to reinforce the vein grafts with Dacron mesh in regions in which soft tissue support may not be as substantial as in the lower extremity. This would be the case in patients with deep abdominal and pelvic origins of their grafts. Proper vein harvesting techniques, including normothermic graft storage in heparinized blood without distention, may be important in maintaining the integrity of the grafts.

A recent review of the University of Michigan experience provides insight into the subject of infrainguinal revascularizations in children.[1] Fourteen children (10 boys, 4 girls), mean age of 7.3 years (range, 2–11 years), underwent 16 lower extremity revascularizations with greater saphenous vein grafts. A mean of 5.7 years elapsed between the onset of ischemia and operation. Arterial occlusions resulted from: cardiac catheterizations (11), arteritis (1), dialysis cannulation (1), and penetrating trauma (1). Indications for operation included LLD (6), claudication (4), both LLD and claudication (3), markedly diminished ABIs with a potential for LLD (2), and a traumatic transection with hemorrhage (1). The reconstructions with 15 reversed and one in situ vein grafts included iliofemoral (11), femorofemoral (1), aortofemoral (1), femoropopliteal (1), popliteal-popliteal (1), and popliteal-posterior tibial (1) arterial bypass grafts.

Among patent grafts available for follow-up in the University of Michigan experience, 36% (5 of 14) remained unchanged, 50% (7 of 14) developed nonaneurysmal dilatation, and 14% (2 of 14) exhibited nonprogressive aneurysmal expansion. One graft became occluded, and 1 graft was lost to follow-up. Collectively, the grafts manifest an 11.2% expansion at an average of 10.7 years postoperatively. ABIs increased from 0.65 preoperatively to 0.97, at an average of 11.0 years postoperatively. LLDs were reduced from 1.66 to 1.24 cm, at an average of 11.4 years postoperatively. Perhaps most surprising was the fact that preexisting LLDs were reduced in 70% of those operated upon.

It may be concluded that lower extremity ischemia in children is seldom immediately limb threatening. The ability of collaterals to evolve in children is truly noteworthy. The question of when to operate on these young patients for fear of the development or the progression of limb length inequality remains an ill-defined subject. Recent experiences suggest that documented LLDs may, in fact, improve with late operations.

REFERENCES

1. Cardneau JD, Henke PK, Upchurch GR Jr, et al. Efficacy and durability of autogenous saphenous vein conduits for lower extremity arterial reconstructions in preadolescent children. *J Vasc Surg.* 2001;34:34–40.
2. Flanigan DP, Keifer TJ, Schuler JJ, et al. Experience with iatrogenic pediatric vascular injuries. *Ann Surg.* 1983;198:430–442.
3. Klein MD, Coran AG, Whitehouse WM, et al. Management of iatrogenic arterial injuries in infants and children. *J Pediatr Surg.* 1982;17:933–939.
4. Shaker IJ, White JJ, Signer RD, et al. Special problems of vascular injuries in children. *J Trauma.* 1976;16:863–867.
5. Smith C, Green RM. Pediatric vascular injuries. *Surgery.* 1981;90:20–31.
6. White JJ, Talbert JL, Haller JA. Peripheral arterial injuries in infants and children. *Ann Surg.* 1968;167:757–766.
7. Whitehouse WM, Coran AG, Stanley JC, et al. Pediatric vascular trauma. *Arch Surg.* 1976;111:1269–1275.
8. Bassett FHI, Lincoln CR, King TD, et al. Inequality in the size of the lower extremity following cardiac catheterization. *South Med J.* 1968;61:1013–1017.
9. Bloom JD, Mozersky DJ, Buckley CJ, et al. Defective limb growth as a complication of catheterization of the femoral artery. *Surg Gynecol Obstet.* 1974;138:524–526.
10. Jacobsson B, Carlgren LE. A review of children after arterial catherterization of the leg. *Pediatr Radiol.* 1973;1:96–99.
11. Richardson JD, Fallat M, Nagaraj HS, et al. Arterial injuries in children. *Arch Surg.* 1981;116:685–690.
12. Rosenthal A, Anderson M, Thompson SJ, et al. Superficial femoral artery catheterization: effect on extremity length. *Am J Dis Child.* 1972;124:240–242.
13. Fry WJ, Ernst CB, Stanley JC, et al. Renovascular hypertension in the pediatric patient. *Arch Surg.* 1973;107:692–698.
14. O'Neill JA, Jr. Long-term outcome with surgical treatment of renovascular hypertension. *J Pediatr Surg.* 1998;33:106–111.received

15. Stanley JC, Ernst CB, Fry WJ. Fate of 100 aortorenal vein grafts: Characteristics of late graft expansion, aneurysmal dilatation, and stenosis. *Surgery.* 1973;74:931–944.
16. Villavicencio JL, Gonzalez-Cerna JL. Acute vascular problems of children. *Curr Probl Surg.* 1985;22:1–85.
17. Leblanc J, Wood AE, O'Shea MA, et al. Peripheral arterial trauma in children: A fifteen year review. *J Cardiovasc Surg.* 1985;26:325–331.
18. Mortensson W. Angiography of the femoral artery following percutaneous catheterization in infants and children. *Acta Radiol Diag.* 1976;17:581–593.
19. Taylor LM, Troutman R, Feliciano P, et al. Late complications after femoral artery catheterization in children less than five years of age. *J Vasc Surg.* 1990;11:297–306.
20. Mozersky DJ, Sumner DS, Strandness DE. Long-term results of reconstructive aorto-iliac surgery. *Am J Surg.* 1972;123:503–509.
21. Walter PK, Hoffman W. Diminished epiphyseal growth following iatrogenic vascular trauma. *Eur J Vasc Endovasc Surg.* 2000;20:214–216.
22. Stanley JC, Zelenock GB, Messina LM, et al. Pediatric renovascular hypertension: A thirty-year experience of operative treatment. *J Vasc Surg.* 1995;21:212–227.
23. Berkowitz HD, O'Neill JA, Jr. Renovascular hypertension in children. Surgical repair with special reference to the use of reinforced vein grafts. *J Vasc Surg.* 1989;9:46–55.
24. Short RHD. The Vasa Vasorum of the Femoral Vein. *J Pathol Bact.* 1940;50:419–430.

X

Endovascular Therapy

33

Transcatheter Embolization in Arteriovenous Malformation

Thomas S. Riles, MD and Glenn R. Jacobowitz, MD

The management of arteriovenous malformations (AVM) has been a challenging problem for many years. Surgical treatment alone has historically been inadequate or even disastrous, often leading to extensive damage to adjacent structures with high recurrence rates or major amputation.[1–3] As Szilagyi noted as early as 1965, "the most impressive lesson taught . . . was the realization of the futility of any attempt to cure by surgical means any but the simplest and most sharply localized of these lesions.[4] Proximal ligation of feeding vessels has been particularly troublesome, often resulting in continued enlargement of the AVM and increased recruitment of smaller feeding and draining vessels.[5] Of specific concern, such proximal ligation may in fact be contraindicated as it will make subsequent transcatheter therapy impossible by obstructing access.[2,3,5–8] The techniques of superselective catheterization of feeding vessels and the transcatheter administration of embolic agents have revolutionized the possibilities in treating these lesions. Catheter based embolization has been shown to be effective in treating vascular malformations in several anatomic areas.[9–12] The development of currently available embolization materials, particularly the rapidly polymerizing agents, has greatly improved the ability to control or eradicate complex arteriovenous connections.[13,14]

Although multiple treatments are often necessary, recently published results have shown good long-term outcomes.[8,14,15] The transcatheter therapy is usually administered by a skilled interventional radiologist with occasional subsequent surgical resection. Frequently, these patients are first seen by vascular surgeons, therefore it is imperative for the vascular surgeon to be able to recognize vascular malformations and be familiar with the best forms of treatment. At our institution, the departments of vascular surgery and interventional radiology have been part of a multidisciplinary center (the New York University Medical Center Trunk and Extremity Vascular Anomaly Center) that has treated a large volume of patients with vascular malformations. Others have also shown excellent results with the multidisciplinary structure.[15]

ETIOLOGY OF ARTERIOVENOUS MALFORMATIONS

Arteriovenous malformations are usually congenital. They may also be acquired via trauma or vessel punctures.[5] Congenital AVMs arise from improper development of the arterial, venous, and capillary systems during embryonic development. They are presumed to represent a focal persistence of primitive vascular elements. AVMs are not true neoplasms, and do not have endothelial proliferation or cellular stroma.[16,17] These lesions most commonly occur as isolated anomalies in otherwise healthy patients, and can occur anywhere in the body. The most common anatomic locations are the pelvis, extremities, and the intracranial circulation. Fortunately, they are often stable lesions requiring no specific treatment, and many of these malformations probably go undetected throughout life.

NATURAL HISTORY

The clinical behavior of AVMs is not well defined, but is likely extremely variable.[14] Several authors have shown that asymptomatic lesions may be safely observed with no intervention.[11,14,18] Evaluation of the size of the malformation and the location with respect to adjacent structures can be followed with CT scans and magnetic resonance imaging (MRI). Recent advances in MR technology have made this modality the non-invasive test of choice for imaging vascular malformations.[19,20] Treatment is usually reserved for symptomatic lesions.

PRESENTATION OF SYMPTOMS

Symptoms may include pain, hemorrhage, mass effects such as invasion or compression of adjacent structures, end-organ ischemia, impotence, or high-output heart failure. Depending on the location, a patient may initially recognize an AVM from the detection of skin discoloration or a soft tissue mass. Audible bruits may be present with hyperemic overlying skin, palpable pulses, or thrills. Rapid venous filling and venous hypertension may also be noted. Lower arterial pressure may be present distal to an AVM, and this may elevate when the AVM is compressed.

Some lesions become apparent or increase in size following trauma or during periods of hormonal stimulation such as pregnancy. Although measured cardiac output may often be increased in patients with AVMs, clinically significant cardiovascular consequences have been relatively rare in our experience.[5,14]

TREATMENT

The optimal treatment is complete surgical resection for superficial, limited lesions in the rare cases where this is possible. However, transcatheter embolization currently plays a major role in the treatment of vascular malformation in all parts of the body.[12,21] This can be performed as the sole method of therapy, or as a preoperative treatment to decrease vascularity prior to a planned surgical resection.

TRANSCATHETER EMBOLIZATION

If symptoms are present that warrant therapy, an arteriogram is performed to define the vascular anatomy and means of possible access to the nidus of the AVM. The nidus is considered to be the most central area of the arteriovenous connections within a malformation. As noted above, a CT or MRI has usually been performed prior to intravascular imaging.

The development of flexible, small-caliber catheters has allowed superselective branch vessel cannulation and angiographic delineation of the vascular malformation. Specific feeding vessels are identified and transcatheter emoblization can be performed with the goal of obliterating the nidus of the lesion

Embolization of the nidus requires material that will provide permanent occlusion of vessels at a microscopic level. Therefore, larger or non-permanent materials such as coils, detachable balloons, or absorbable gelatin sponges (gelfoam) are often ineffective. Agents used with more success have been polyvinyl alcohol foam particles (Ivalon), absolute alcohol, and the rapidly polymerizing cyanoacrylate adhesives IBCA and NBCA. Although others have had success with absolute alcohol,[15] in our experience, NBCA and IBCA have been the most effective agents in recent years.[5,14] This material polymerizes on contact with ionic material such as blood. It can be delivered by means of transarterial catheters directly into an AVM and form a cast of the multiple small vessels near the nidus of the lesion. This has been particularly effective in arteriovenous malformations, where the cyanoacrylate rapidly polymerizes in the high-flow system, acting as a glue. The cyanoacrylate adhesives must be diluted appropriately to allow for dispersion into a nidus before polymerization.[14,22] Absolute alcohol has been used more commonly for direct injection into the venous lakes of venous malformations. The low flow in these lesions allows the alcohol to remain at the injection site and effectively sclerose the area. It has been used less frequently in intra-arterial injection with AVMs because of its extreme tissue toxicity. Although several authors have reported success with the use of absolute alcohol in arteriovenous connections, it has been associated with skin or mucosal sloughing or permanent nerve damage.[15,23]

There are few large studies of transcatheter embolization used in the treatment of AVMs. The existing reports can largely be divided into those involving pelvic AVMs and those involving the extremities. Regarding pelvic AVMs, most published reports have been small case series' with emphasis on adjunctive surgical therapy with somewhat short follow-up.[13,18,24] The largest series to date is from our institution.[14] This involved 35 patients. There was a mean age of 37 years and 51% were male. Previous, unsuccessful attempted surgical resection had been attempted in 32% of patients. A mean of 2.4 embolization procedures (range 1–11) were performed over a mean period of 23 months. More than 1 embolization procedure was required in 57% of patients. These additional procedures were performed either as planned, stage embolizations (20%) or due to residual or recurrent symptoms (37%). Adjunctive surgical procedures were performed in 5 patients (15%). The rapidly polymerizing cyanoacrylate adhesives were most commonly used, and the vessels most commonly embolized were branches of the internal iliac arteries (82%) and branches of the inferior mesenteric artery (11%). At a mean follow-up of 84 months, 83% of patients were asymptomatic or significantly improved.

There does seem to be a difference between male and female patterns of congenital pelvice AVMs. In females, they tend to be more complex, with multiple feeding arteries (Figure 33–1). Although primary supply is usually from 1 or both internal iliac arteries, additional supply is often from the inferior mesenteric, middle sacral, common or deep femoral artery branches. In the male patients a distinctive pattern of malformation has been noted. It is characterized by supply from 1 internal iliac artery with massively dilated draining veins (Figure 33–2). The venous component tends to be the

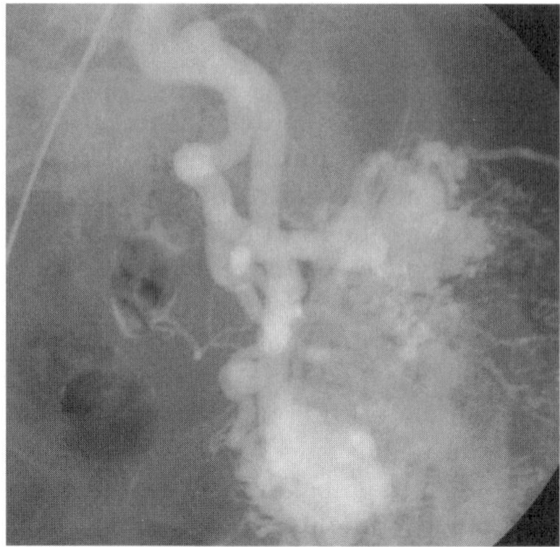

Figure 33–1. Female pattern of pelvic AVM with multiple feeding arteries

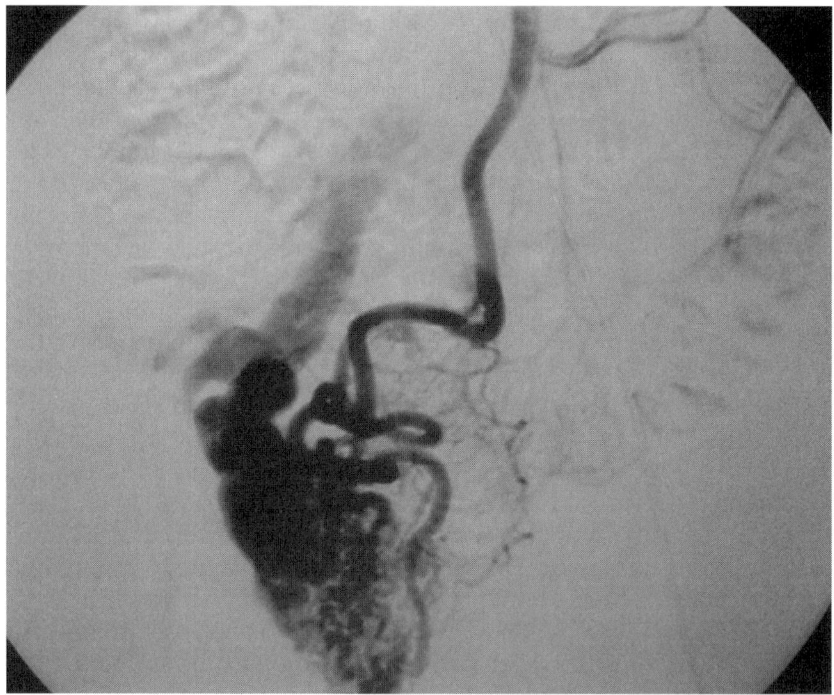

Figure 33–2. Male pattern of pelvic AVM with single large feeding artery and large draining vein

cause of symptoms, which are related to compression of surrounding structures causing pelvic pain, urinary outlet obstruction, and rectal pain. The simpler arterial supply in males most likely accounts for the tendency of these lesions to respond to embolization more favorably than females. Recurrences are more common in females. In the series from NYU, the mean number of embolizations was 3.2 for females compared with 1.7 for males. Alleviation or elimination of symptoms can be obtained equally in females with transcatheter therapy, but more frequent embolizations may be necessary.

The etiology of the more complex pelvic malformations occurring in females is unclear. It may be related to hormonal factors that affect local angiogenic mechanisms.

Several more recent studies on extremity AVMs have revealed disappointing long-term outcomes. Dickey et al. reported on 4 patients with large AVMs of the shoulder and upper extremity treated with transcatheter embolotherapy, and found these lesions refractory to intravascular treatment.[25] Mendel at al reported on 17 cases of major vascular malformations of the upper extremity, but only 3 embolizations were performed; recurrence after surgery occurred in 12 patients, and there were 4 amputations.[6] Carr et al. reported on 12 cases of extremity malformations; 8 recurred after treatment which was either surgery or embolization.[7] Most recently, however, an analysis of 20 patients with high-flow extremity AVMs treated with embolotherapy has been reported by White et al.[8] Excellent long-term results (mean, 7.4 years) were demonstrated in upper extremity cases, while 5 of 9 patients with lower extremity malformations required major amputation.

At New York University Medical Center, transcatheter embolization therapy has been performed in 50 patients with extremity vascular malformations, of which 95% were AVMs. These were evenly divided among upper and lower extremity lesions. The mean age was 22 years and 34% were male. The most commonly embolized vessels were branches of the profunda femorus and tibial arteries (83% of lower extremity lesions) and branches of the brachial and radial arteries (82% of upper extremity lesions. Patients required a mean of 1.6 embolization procedures (range 1–5) over a mean period of 57 months. Sixteen patients (32%) underwent more than 1 embolization procedure. Of these, 1 was a planned, staged procedure and 15 were for residual or recurrent symptoms. Adjunctive surgery was performed subsequent to embolization in 3 cases (6%). Ninety-two percent of patients were asymptomatic or improved at a mena follow-up of 56 months. There was 1 case of limb loss (2%). The most common agents used for embolization were the cyanoacrylate adhesives (Figures 33–3, 33–4, and 33–5).

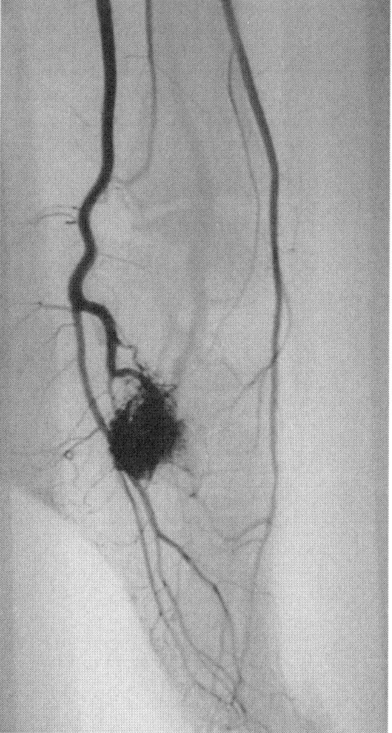

Figure 33–3. Angiogram demonstrating AVM originating in branch of lateral plantar artery

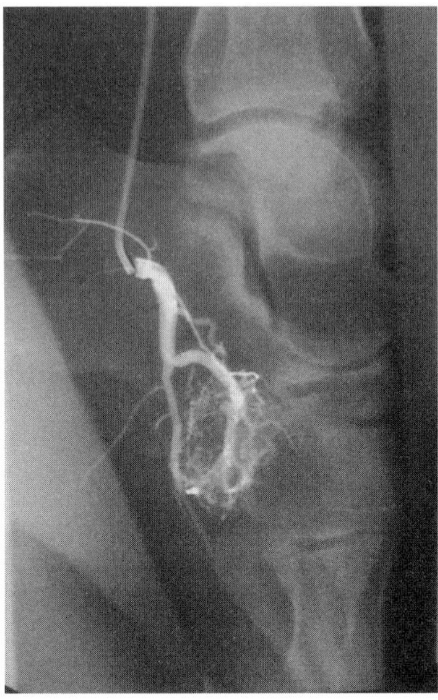

Figure 33–4. Selective catheterization of feeding artery near nidus of AVM

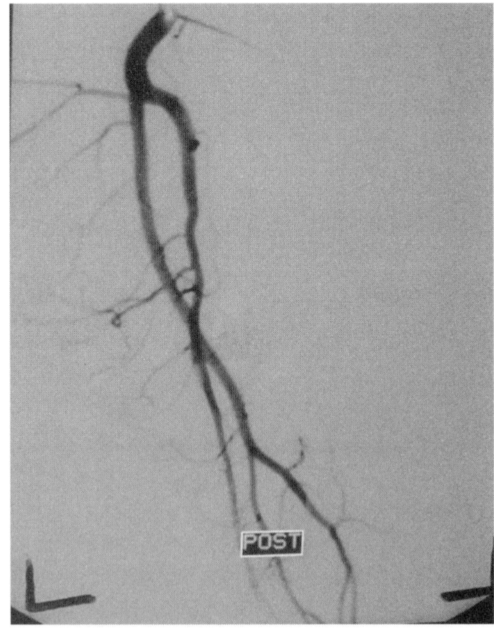

Figure 33–5. Angiogram post embolization with cyanoacrylate adhesive demonstrating obliteration of AVM

An additional type of arteriovenous malformation which deserves mention is the pulmonary AVM, which consists of a fistula-like connection between a branch of the pulmonary artery and the pulmonary vein. These lesions can be single or multiple, and may be sporadic or found in patients with Rendu-Osler-Weber syndrome. They pose the potential risk of paradoxical embolization associated with the right to left shunting. The shunting can also cause arterial desaturation, often manifested by decreased exercise tolerance. Treatment of these particular lesions is usually recommended even for those found incidentally because of the risk of embolization. They can be treated by surgical resection of an involved segment or lobe, or embolotherapy with stainless steel coils or detachable balloons via the pulmonary artery. These lesions have simpler arteriovenous connections than AVMs elsewhere in the body, making them particularly amenable to embolization with larger agents which can occlude the feeding vessels.[5]

CONCLUSION

Trancatheter embolization should be considered the current mainstay of therapy for symptomatic arteriovenous malformations. Until the last 5 to 10 years, emphasis on treating these lesions has centered largely around surgical extirpation. If a lesion is clearly resectable with respect to involvement of adjacent structures, surgical resection for cure should certainly be considered. However, after appropriate evaluation with CT scans, MR imaging, and angiography, this is usually not the case. This holds true for AVMs in the pelvis, extremities, and the lungs. For these more complex lesions, transcatheter embolization alone, although often necessary multiple times, is sufficient to eliminate or improve symptoms in a high percentage of patients. At present, the cyanoacrylate adhesives appear to the the most effective agents for embolization, administered through the technique of superselective catheterization of arterial branches allowing access to the nidus of the AVM. If a lesion is symptomatically improved with embolization, no further therapy is needed, because return of symptoms is variable.

As Szilagyi noted in 1976, it would be inaccurate to claim a "cure" for most vascular malformations and treatment with transcatheter therapy must be considered largely palliative. However, even with a high rate of recurrence, these lesions can be well controlled with additional transcatheter therapy over many years.

REFERENCES

1. Szilagyi DE, Smith RF, Elliott JP, et al. Congenital arteriovenous anomalies of the limbs. *Arch Surg.* 1976;111:423–429.
2. Coursely G, Ivins JC, Barker NW. Congenital arteriovenous fistulas in the extremities: An analysis of 69 cases. *Angiology.* 1956;7:201–217.
3. Gomes MM, Bernatz PE. Arteriovenous fistulas: a review and ten-year experience at the Mayo Clinic. Mayo Clinic Proc. 1970;45:81–102.
4. Szilagyi DE, Elliot JP, DeRusso FJ, et al. Peripheral congenital arteriovenous fistulas. *Surgery.* 1965;57:61–81.
5. Rosen RJ, Riles TS. Congenital vascular malformations. In: Rutherford RB, editor. *Vascular Surgery. 5th edition.* Philadelphia: W.B. Saunders Co; 2000. pp. 1451–1465.
6. Mendel T, Louis DS. Major vascular malformations of the upper extremity; long-term observation. *J Hand Surg.* 1997;22A:302–306.
7. Carr MM, Mahoney JL, Bowen CV. Extremity arteriovenous malformations: review of a series. *Can J. Surg.* 1994;37:394–9.
8. White RI Jr., Pollak J, Persin J, et al. Long-term outcome of embolotherapy and surgery for high-flow arteriovenous malformations. *J Vasc Int Radiol.* 2000;11:1285–1295.

9. Palmaz JC, Newton TH, Reuter SR, et al. Particulate intraarterial embolization in pelvic arteriovenous malformations. *AJR*. 1981;137:117–122.
10. Flye MW, Jordan BP, Schwartz MZ. Management of congenital arteriovenous malformations. *Surgery*. 1983;94:740–774.
11. Natali J, Merland JJ. Superselective arteriography and therapeutic embolization for vascular malformations (Angiodysplasias). *J Cardiovasc Surg*. 1976; 465–472.
12. Olcott C 4th, Newton TH, Stoney RJ, et al. Intra-arterial embolization in the management of arteriovenous malformations. *Surgery*. 1976; 79:312.
13. Widlus DM, Murray RR, White RI Jr, et al. Congenital arteriovenous malformations; tailored embolotherapy. *Radiology*. 1988;169:511–516.
14. Jacobowitz GR, Rosen RJ, Rockman CB, et al. Transcatheter embolization of complex pelvic malformations: results and long-term follow-up. *J Vasc Surg*. 2001;33:51–55.
15. Lee BB, Kim DI, Huh MD, et al. New experiences with absolute ethanol sclerotherapy in the management of a complex form of congenital venous malformation. *J Vasc Surg*. 2001;33:764–772.
16. Folkman J. Toward a new understanding of vascular proliferative disease in children. *Pediatrics*. 1984;74:850–856.
17. Mulliken JB, Zetter BR, Folkman J. In vivo characteristics of endothelium from hemangiomas and vascular malformations. *Surgery*. 1982;92:348–353.
18. Kaufman SL, Kumar AA, Roland JA, et al. Transcatheter embolization in the management of congenital arteriovenous malformations. *Radiology*. 1980;137:21–29.
19. Pearce WH, Rutherford RB, Whitehill TA, et al. Nuclear magnetic resonance imaging in patients with congenital vascular malformations of the limbs. *J Vasc Surg*. 1988;8:64–70.
20. Dobson MJ, Hartley RW, Ashleigh R, et al. MR angiography and MR imaging of symptomatic peripheral vascular malformations. *Clinical Radiology*. 1997;52: 595–602.
21. Gomes AS, Busotti RW, Baker JD, et al. Congenital arteriovenous malformations. *Arch Surg*. 1983;118:817–825.
22. Zanetti PH. Cyanoacrylate/iophenylate mixtures: modification and in vitro evaluation as embolic agents. *J Intervent Radiol*. 1987;2:65–68.
23. Yakes WF, Luethke JM, Merland JJ, et al. Ethanol embolization of arteriovenous fistulas; a primary model of therapy. *J Vasc Int Radiol*. 1990;1:89–96.
24. Laurian C, Leclef Y, Gigou F, et al. Pelvic arteriovenous fistulas: therapeutic strategy in five cases. *Ann Vasc Surg*. 1990;4:1–9.
25. Dickey KW, Pollak JS, et al. Management of large high-flow arteriovenous malformations of the shoulder and upper extremity with transcatheter embolotherapy. *J Vasc Int Radiol*. 1995;6:765–773.

34

Remote Superficial Femoral Artery Endarterectomy

David Rosenthal, MD, John H. Matsuura, MD, and Eric D. Wellons, MD

The first successful superficial femoral artery (SFA) endarterectomy was performed by the Portuguese surgeon Cid Dos Santos in 1947.[1] This "disobstruction" removed the diseased inner layer of the artery wall and was termed by Dos Santos "thromboendarterectomy." Over the years, the popularity of SFA endarterectomy waxed and waned, and the technique was gradually abandoned in the United States as published reports[2,3] demonstrated that above-knee femoral popliteal (AKFP) bypass offered superior patency rates to those of SFA endarterectomy.

With the advent of minimally invasive procedures such as percutaneous transluminal angioplasty (PTA), laser-assisted balloon angioplasty, and atherectomy, whose results have been disappointing in treatment of long segment (>10 cm) SFA occlusive disease, a reassessment of SFA endarterectomy was initiated.[4–7] Van der Heijden in 1993[8,9] reported a semiclosed endarterectomy technique using a ring stripper that achieved patency rates similar to those of AKFP bypass. Although this procedure was performed through 2 incisions, it avoided the use of prosthetic grafts and/or harvesting the saphenous vein, which could be used for subsequent cardiovascular or peripheral reconstructions. With the development of the remote endarterectomy technique reported by Ho and Moll, et al.,[10] a minimally invasive operation performed through a single incision in combination with endovascular stent or stent graft placement was devised.

This chapter describes the technique of remote superficial femoral artery endarterectomy (RSFAE) and examines medium-term results.

CLINICAL STUDY

Between March 1996 and October 2000, 60 patients underwent RSFAE as part of a retrospective multicenter study. The indications for operation were claudication in 52 cases and limb salvage in 8 patients. Forty-six patients were men, and the mean patient age was 66.2 years (range, 49–81 years). Twenty-eight patients (46.7%) had a history of cigarette smoking, 29 (48.3%) had hypertension, 26 (43.3%) had diabetes mellitus, and 21 (35.0%) had coronary artery disease.

The technique for RSFAE has been previously described by Ho and Moll, et al.[10] and is illustrated in Figure 34–1. In summary, through a small groin incision, the common, proximal profunda femoral, and proximal superficial femoral arteries are exposed. An intraoperative arteriogram is performed which documents the point of SFA occlusion and reconstitution (Figure 34–2). This image is saved and noted by a measuring tape or saved with "road mapping." By clamping the proximal SFA, flow to the profunda femoris artery is uninterrupted. After systemic heparin administration, a 3-cm arteriotomy is made from the origin of the SFA distally, and an endarterectomy is started between the inner and outer media. This intimal core is transversely cut at the SFA origin and threaded into the loop of a conventional (i.e. Vollmar) ring stripper. The ring stripper is advanced distally down the SFA beyond the occluded segment under fluoroscopic surveillance (Figure 34–3). The stripper is advanced by gentle rotating movements while holding the intimal core with a forceps. The ring stripper is exchanged for the Moll Ring cutter device (Vascular Architects, San Jose, CA), which transects the distal atheroma core (Figure 34–4). The entire core is removed through the proximal arteriotomy by pulling back the MollRing cutter, and arteriography is performed to confirm a patent distal artery (Figure 34–5).

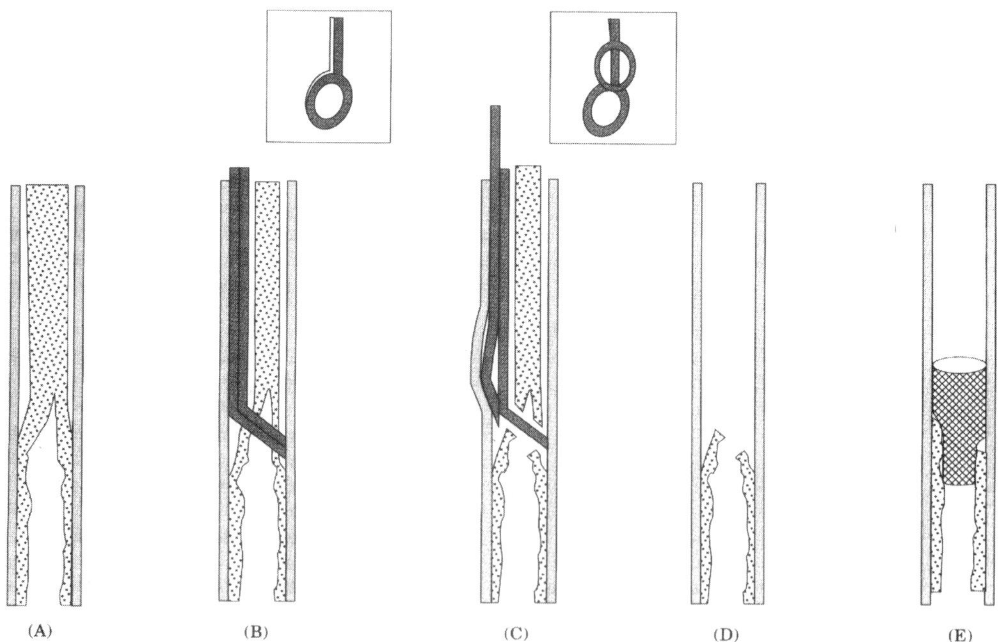

Figure 34–1. Diagram to illustrate the current technique of remote endarterectomy. **(A)** Endarterectomy has been performed by ring-stripper (not shown) just distal to end of occlusion. **(B)** MollRing cutter passed to same position in endarterectomy plane (inset shows ring cutter closed). **(C)** Ring cutter transects atheroma at chosen level (inset shows the relative movement of rings). **(D)** Atheromatous core removed proximally leaving free edge of cut atheroma. **(E)** Diagrammatic representation of Palmaz stent in position. (Reprinted from *Eur J Vasc and Endovasc Surg.* 1998;16:254–8 with permission from WB Saunders).

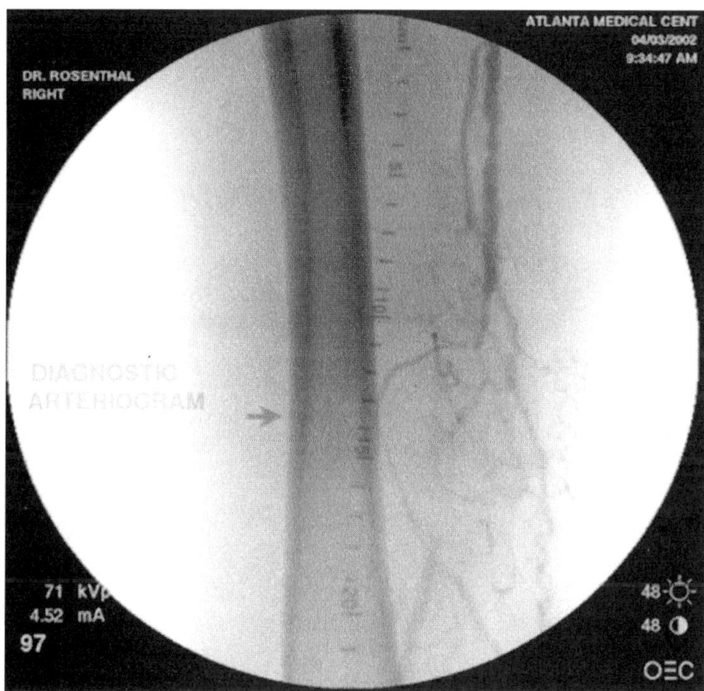

Figure 34–2. Intraoperative arteriogram documents point of SFA occlusion and reconstitution (note reference measuring tape).

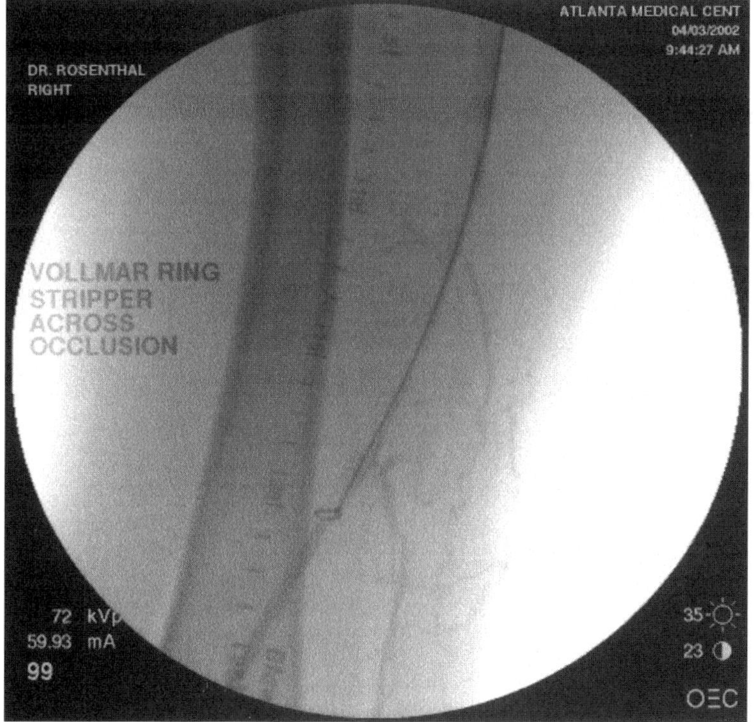

Figure 34–3. Vollmar ring stripper advanced under fluoroscopic surveillance across occlusion.

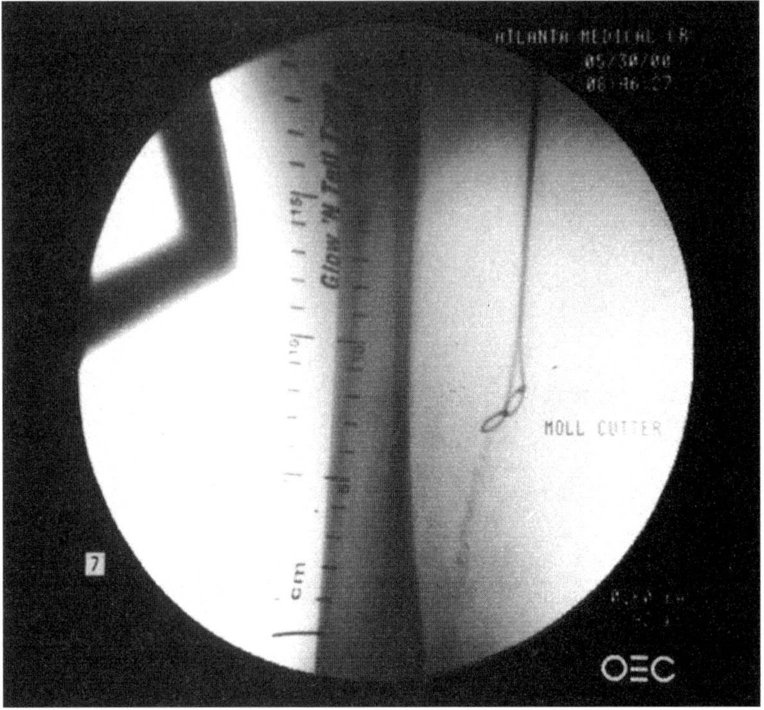

Figure 34–4. MollRing cutter transects distal atheroma core.

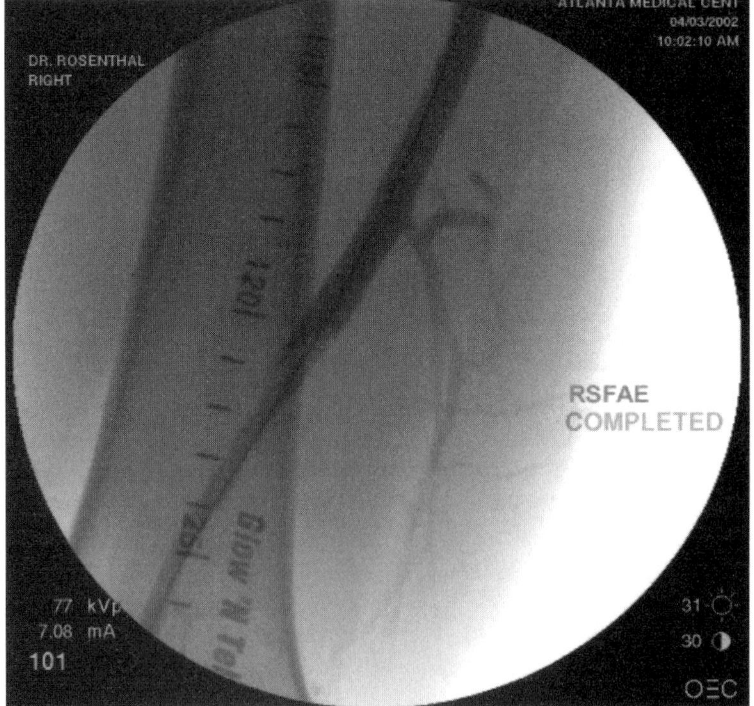

Figure 34–5. RSFAE complete. Arteriogram documents patent distal artery.

Under fluoroscopic guidance, a guidewire is passed across the distal SFA endarterectomy end point and balloon/stent angioplasty is performed, "tacking" the distal plaque to prevent further dissection (Figure 34–6). Completion arteriography verifies RSFAE patency and any outflow tract obstruction. Loose debris, visualized by arteriography, is removed with a Fogarty embolectomy or graft thrombectomy catheter (Edward Life Sciences, Vascular Division, Irvine, CA). The arteriotomy may be extended proximally to perform an open endarterectomy of the common femoral and/or profunda femoris ostia as necessary.

Technical success was defined as any recanalization of an occluded artery on completion arteriography. All patients underwent clinical evaluation during the 30-day postoperative period with duplex color-flow ultrasound scanning. The patients were followed at 3-, 6-, and 12-month intervals and at 6-month intervals thereafter with color-flow duplex ultrasound scanning. Remote superficial femoral artery endarterectomy patency was confirmed with duplex scan or arteriographic evaluation. The primary end point was any occlusion and/or radiologic or surgical intervention before occlusion. Cumulative primary and primary assisted patency rates were calculated by the actuarial life table method based on number of procedures performed.

Initial technical success was achieved in 81.4% (57/70) cases. RSFAE was successful in 3 patients, but the guidewire could not be passed across the residual popliteal plaque, and the procedure was abandoned. In 10 other patients with heavily calcified femoral arteries, RSFAE could not be performed when the ring stripper could not be passed distally and they were excluded from the study. All of the patients in whom RSFAE could not be performed underwent uneventful AKFP bypass.

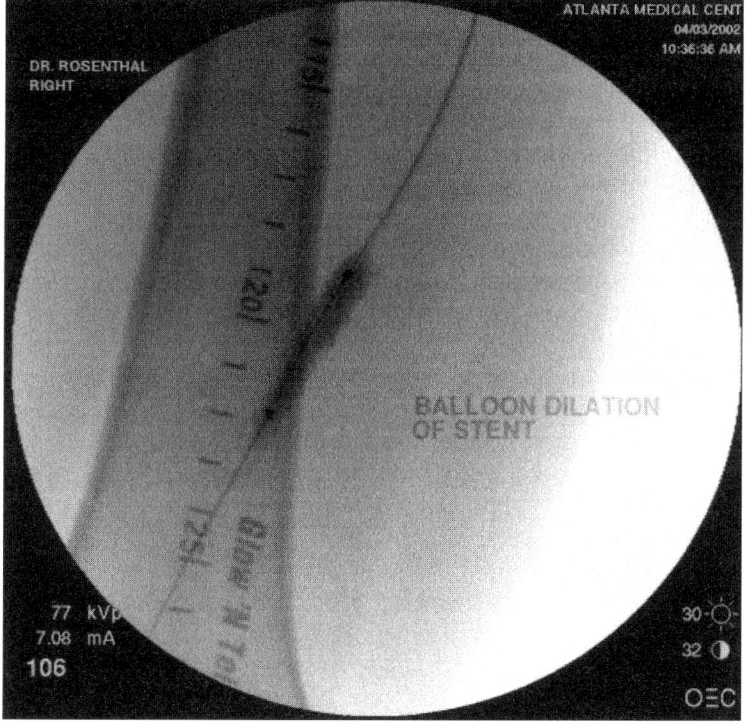

Figure 34–6. Distal balloon stent angioplasty "tacks" distal plague.

The study group, therefore, consisted of 60 patients who underwent RSFAE. The mean length of endarterectomized SFA was 22.3 cm (range 8–37 cm). In 32 patients, a common femoral and/or profunda femoris endarterectomy was performed as well. Completion arteriography demonstrated SFA thrombus in 5 cases, which was successfully removed with a Fogarty balloon catheter. In 2 other cases, arteriography showed residual fractured plaque, which was removed with a Fogarty graft thrombectomy catheter. Three patients had extravasation of contrast at completion arteriography, but this was self-limiting and required no intervention. Thirty-nine of the 60 arteriotomies were closed by patch angioplasty (16 with autogenous vein and 23 with prosthetic patch material).

The primary cumulative patency rate by life table analysis was 61.4% 9% (SE), (mean 12.9 months; range 3–36 months). Repeat radiologic intervention was necessary in 14 patients (9 PTA, 5 stent angioplasty), for a primary assisted patency rate of 82.6% 8% (Figure 34–7). The locations of the stenoses after RSFAE included 6 that were over the course of the SFA, 4 at the adductor canal in long (>20 cm) endarterectomies, 2 at the SFA origin, and 2 at the distal stent. One below-knee amputation was performed during follow-up in a patient who was diabetic and dialysis-dependent with gangrene of the forefoot. He underwent successful RSFAE, but amputation was necessary despite a patent SFA endarterectomy. There were no deaths, 1 wound complication (hematoma), and the mean hospital length of stay (LOS) was 1.4 days 0.8 days. The ankle brachial indices rose from 0.61 (0.16) preoperatively to 0.97 (0.05) postoperatively.

COMMENTS

Remote superficial femoral artery endarterectomy in combination with popliteal artery balloon/stent angioplasty offers the vascular surgeon a minimally invasive alternative to radiologic endoluminal procedures for the treatment of SFA occlusive disease. The disappointing reported results[4–7] for long segment (>10 cm) SFA occlusive disease with atherectomy, PTA, and laser-assisted balloon angioplasty, led van der Heijden and coworkers[9] to reassess semiclosed endarterectomy as a "debulking" procedure of SFA that might hopefully improve patency. They reported a technical success rate of

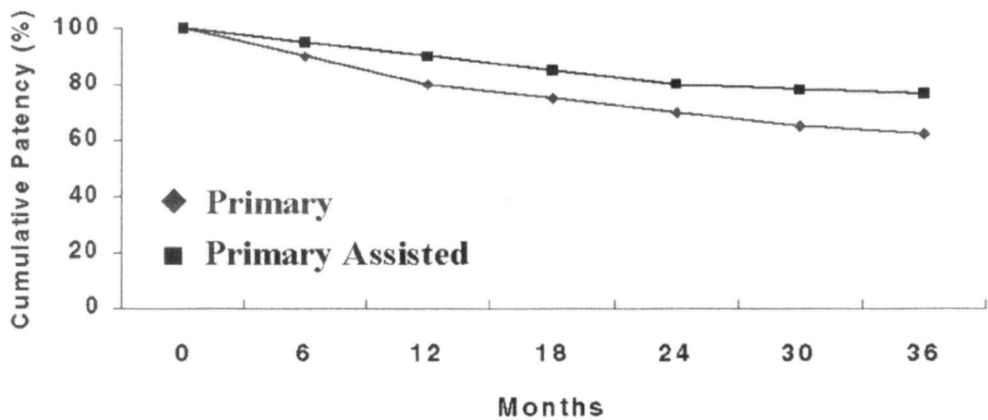

Figure 34–7. Cumulative primary and secondary patency after RSFAE.

89% and a 5-year secondary patency rate of 61% in 259 SFA endarterectomies. With this technique, a ring stripper was introduced via arteriotomies at the common femoral and above-knee popliteal arteries, and endarterectomy performed; the distal popliteal artery plaque was "tacked" with sutures. The development of the remote endarterectomy technique by Moll and colleagues,[10] performed through a single short groin incision in combination with distal plaque balloon/stent angioplasty, offered several advantages. It was minimally invasive, a second distal incision was avoided, and common femoral and profunda femoris ostial endarterectomy could be easily performed as necessary. Additionally, the technique avoided use of prosthetic material, and it could be used in the absence of saphenous vein and, alternatively, allowed preservation of the saphenous vein for subsequent reconstructions in the cardiovascular or peripheral circulation.

The 12-month (74.9%) and 36-month (61.4%) primary cumulative patency rates in this study were comparable to those reported by Ho and coworkers[11] and were similar to rates expected following AKFP bypass. Part of the "learning curve" of any new procedure is patient selection. In this study, patients with heavily calcified SFAs (i.e. diabetic, renal failure patients) fared poorly and are likely not candidates for this procedure. The incidence of stenosis formation after RSFAE was concerning in that 14 (23.3%) of 60 patients required adjunctive procedure (9 PTA, 5 stent angioplasty) to maintain SFA patency. Although the incidence (23%) of early (<2 years) stenosis in this study, likely due to intimal hyperplasia, was less than that reported by Ho, et al.[11] (46% at 1 year) and by Galland and colleagues[12] (69% at 15 months), it remains a major concern. The endarterectomized SFA, because of its long length, tortuosity, small caliber, and relatively low flow, may not be able to withstand exuberant intimal hyperplasia formation and arterial recoil. Interestingly, we observed that when a RSFAE failed, the patient's symptoms were, in general, less severe than before the procedure which may be due to "opening" of collaterals at the time of endarterectomy, or the benefit of an adjunctive profunda femoris endarterectomy in 32 patients. This remains to be proven.

"Debulking" and SFA endografting, however, may sufficiently obviate the problem of restenosis along the SFA to offer patency rates comparable to those of AKFP bypass. Information, nevertheless, on SFA endografting is limited. It is of interest to note the controversy surrounding the incidence of SFA endograft stenosis, as some authors[13-15] believe that a stent graft may limit formation of neointimal hyperplasia, while others[16] believe that the presence of an endograft accelerates neointimal hyperplasia formation.

An intriguing adjunct to RSFAE is the use of the aSpire stent (Vascular Architects, San Jose, CA). The PTFE aSpire covered stent's (Vascular Architects, San Jose, CA) unique spiral design offers flexibility and radial strength, while promoting laminar flow. The operators ability to control expansion, diameter, and length also allows preservation of arterial side branches after RSFAE (Figure 34–8).

RSFAE may also have a role in the revascularization of the ischemic lower extremity when a saphenous vein (SV) is unavailable. SV is the conduit of choice for femorodistal popliteal/tibial bypass, however, the SV has been reported to be unusable in up to 45% of cases,[17] due to anatomic inadequacy (i.e. phlebitis, sclerotic), previous stripping, harvest, or intraoperative injury. When a distal popliteal/tibial bypass is necessary and adequate SV is not available, RSFAE allows the proximal popliteal artery to serve as the "inflow site" for the distal bypass with residual SV (Figure 34–9). This procedure may prove to be a useful adjunct for limb salvage, especially in the presence of foot infection where an autogenous tissue bypass is preferred.

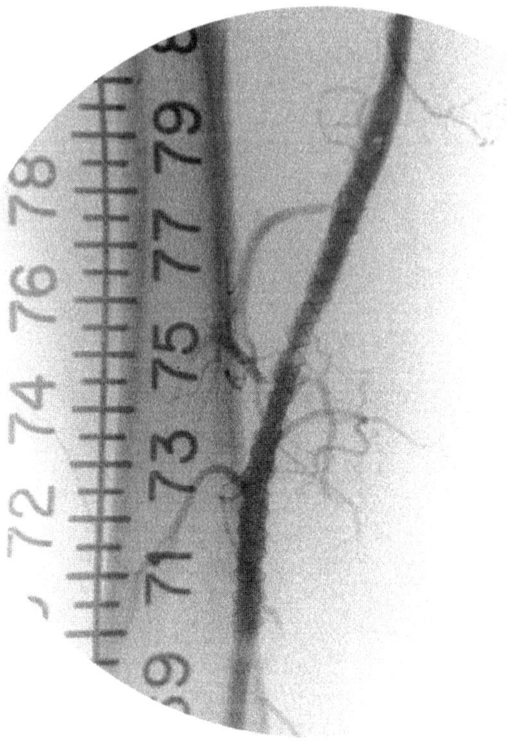

Figure34–8. aSpire covered stent deployed with preservation of arterial side branch.

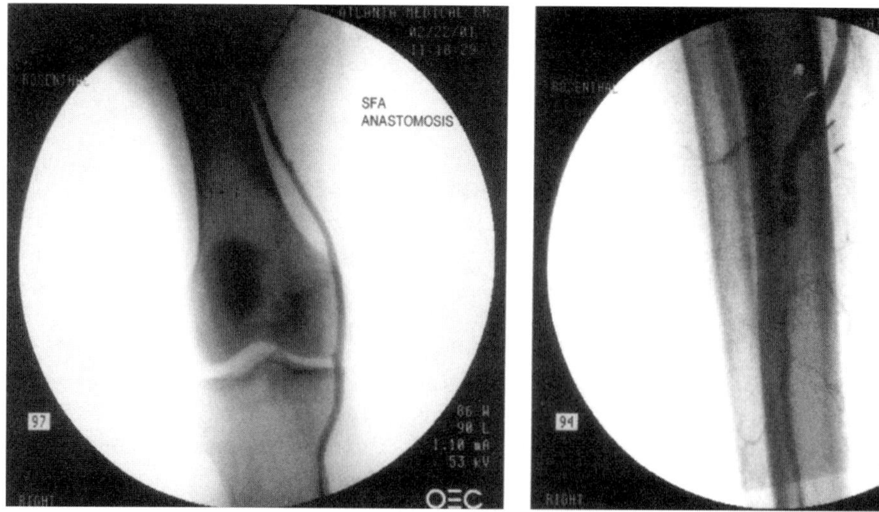

Figure34–9. Completion arteriogram after RSFAE to saphenous vein bypass anastomosis and distal peroneal anastomosis.

The treatment of femoropopliteal occlusive disease with RSFAE and popliteal stent angioplasty and/or endovascular grafts continues to evolve. Many questions, however, remain unanswered. What role does a stent at the distal endarterectomy end point play? Is it necessary to line the debulked SFA segment with an endograft? If so, what is the most appropriate graft material, and should the endograft be structurally supported? Percutaneous catheter-based radiologic SFA endografts are currently being developed by major graft companies for the treatment of SFA occlusive disease. It is incumbent upon the vascular surgeon to develop a minimally invasive alternative to these radiologic procedures that will offer patients a procedure of comparable morbidity but with patency rates similar to those of AKFP. Remote superficial femoral artery endarterectomy is a safe and moderately durable procedure that may lower operative morbidity, reduce hospital LOS, and shorten recuperation.

REFERENCES

1. Dos Santos JC. Surla desobstruction des thromboses arterieles anciennes. *Mem Acad Chir.* 1947;73:409 411.
2. DeWeese JA, Barner HB, Mahoney EB, et al. Autogenous venous bypass grafts and thromboendarterectomies for atherosclerotic lesions of the femoropopliteal arteries. *Ann Surg.* 1996; 163:205–214.
3. Darling RC, Linton RR. Durability of femoropopliteal reconstructions: endarterectomy versus vein bypass grafts. *Am J Surg.* 1972;123: 472–479.
4. Matsi PJ, Manninen HI, Vanninen RL, et al. Femoropopliteal angioplasty in patients with claudication: primary and secondary patency in 140 limbs with 1–3 year follow-up. *Radiology.* 1994;191:727–733.
5. The Collaborative Rotablator Atherectomy Group (CRAG). Peripheral arthrectomy with the rotablator: a multicenter report. *J Vasc Surg.* 1994;19:509–515.
6. Diethrich EB. Laser angioplasty: A critical review based on 1849 clinical procedures. *Angiology.* 1990;41:757–767.
7. Johnston KW, Rae M, Hogg-Johnson SA, et al. 5-year results of a prospective study of percutaneous transluminal angioplasty. *Ann Surg.* 1987; 206:403–413.
8. van der Heijden FH, Eikelboom BC, van Reedt Dortland RW, et al. Superficial femoral artery endarterectomy: a procedure worth reconsidering. *Eur J Vasc Surg.* 1993;6 651–658.
9. van der Heijden FH, Eikelboom BC, van Reedt Dortland RW, et al. Long-term results of semiclosed endarterectomy of the superficial femoral artery and the outcome of failed reconstructions. *J Vasc Surg.* 1993;8:271–279.
10. Ho GH, Moll FL, Joosten PP, van de Pavoordt ED, et al. The Mollring cutter remote endarterectomy: preliminary experience with a new endovascular technique for treatment of occlusive superficial femoral artery disease. *J Endovasc Surg.* 1995;2:278–287.
11. Ho GH, Moll FL, Hedeman Joosten PP, et al. Endovascular remote endarterectomy in femoropopliteal occlusive disease: one-year clinical experience with the ring strip cutter device. *Eur J Vasc Endovasc Surg.* 1996;12:105–112.
12. Galland RB, Whiteley MS, Gibson M, et al. Remote superficial femoral artery endarterectomy: medium-term results. *Eur J Vasc Endovasc Surg.* 2000; 19:278–282.
13. Ombrellaro MP, Stevens SL, Sciarrotta J, et al. Effect of PTFE graft placement on cell proliferation, PDGF secretion, and intimal hyperplasia. *J Surg Res.* 1996;63:110–114.
14. Ohki T, Marin ML, Veith FJ, et al. Anastomotic intimal hyperplasia: a comparison between conventional and endovascular stent graft techniques. *J Surg Res.* 1997;69:255–267.
15. Marin ML, Veith FJ, Cynamon J, et al. Effect of polytetrafluoroethylene covering of Palmez stents on the development of intimal hyperplasia in human iliac arteries. *J Vasc Interv Radiol.* 1996;7:651–656.

16. Van Sambeek MRHM, Gussenhoven EJ, Hagenaars T, et al. Vascular response in the femoropopliteal artery after implantation of an ePTFE balloon expandable endovascular graft: an intravascular ultrasound study. Submitted 2002.
17. Taylor LM, Edwards, JM, Porter JM. Present status of reversed vein bypass: five-year result of a modern series. *J Vasc Surg*. 1990:11:193–205.

35

Long-Term Outcomes of Iliac Artery Angioplasty and Stenting

Sasan Najibi, MD, Gustavo Torres, MD,
George Andros, MD, and Robert W. Oblath, MD

If long-term, complication-free durability is the yardstick by which endovascular procedures are gauged, then iliac angioplasty (PTA) is certainly to be reckoned a success; results of endoluminal treatment have become even more impressive since the introduction of stents. The promise of durable effectiveness, suggested by early reports, has been reconfirmed for 25 years by publications world wide. There is little question iliac PTA/stenting is the established "ne plus ultra" of non-coronary *interventional* therapy. But not all procedures are consistently successful; and it must be borne in mind that the results of iliac stenting must be weighed against aortofemoral bypass graft, perhaps the most successful of all *open* interventions.

Which lesions can be expected to be treatable and achieve early and late patency? What roles do stenting and re-intervention play in enhancing the results of this endoluminal procedure? The purposes of this paper are first, to review the long-term results of iliac PTA/stenting, surveying patency and complications as well; second, to evaluate the predictors of success and failure; and finally, to see whether the available evidence will provide a guide to improved patient selection and consequently enhance the outcomes of endoluminal revascularization. Isolated internal iliac artery (IIA) PTA/stent for vasculogenic impotence and discreet hip claudication are omitted because of its relative rarity and a lack of systematic studies.

TECHNIQUE

Balloon angioplasty techniques have become standardized over over the last decade. Device-related improvements, however, are ongoing. A partial list includes:

- New sheaths with thinner walls which allow smaller diameter balloon catheters and stents to be delivered

- Pre-shaped and shapable catheters and sheaths
- Improved and hydrophilically-coated guidewires in multiple sizes
- Lower profile, coated balloon catheters with increased trackability on smaller shafts
- More flexible balloon expandable (Palmaz) stents
- Self-expanding Nitinol stents with reduced foreshortening to improve precision of deployment
- Cost-reductions for many endoluminal devices

Bilateral retrograde femoral puncture and access facilitates iliac angioplasty. Access of both sides allows aortic and femoral pressures to be evaluated simultaneously or for the use of kissing balloons or stents. Bilateral access is appropriate even in cases of distal external iliac/proximal common femoral artery disease that must be treated from the contralateral artery (over the aortic bifurcation). Because of limited ipsilateral working room, the juxtafemoral lesion must be treated from the contralateral side; nevertheless, bilateral access simplifies hemodynamic assessment. The more severe the iliac lesions and, in consequence, the greater the reduction of the femoral pulse, the more problematic retrograde femoral puncture becomes. A host of easily learned techniques enable the interventionist to puncture the "pulseless" artery so that it becomes unnecessary to approach the ipsilateral lesion via contralateral femoral access across the aortic bifurcation.[1] Complete iliac artery *occlusions*, of course, can be treated "over-the-top," but these lesions are crossed much more easily from the ipsilateral side. *Stenoses*, as would be expected, can be successfully crossed from either direction with appropriate guidewires and catheters.

Our stent of choice for common iliac artery and proximal and mid-external iliac artery lesions is a second or third generation balloon expandable stent. Nitinol stents are also very useful and their applicability has been augmented by the addition of radiopaque end-markers which improve fluoroscopic visualization. We recommend pre- and post-procedural platelet inhibiting drugs and administer 40–50 units per kgm of heparin prior to angioplasty or stent deployment (the heparin is not reversed with protamine). Antibiotics are administered routinely prior to deployment and in the presence of distal ischemic or infected lesions. For large vessel angioplasty IIB/IIIA glycoprotein platelet inhibitors have no proven benefit. Sheaths are removed in the Recovery Room after 1 to 2 hours when the ACT has normalized. This approach has made the use of percutaneous closure devices unnecessary.

RESULTS

The results of balloon angioplasty of iliac stenoses have been satisfactory and durable based on objective criteria such as ankle/brachial pressure indices (ABPI) and duplex assessment. Technical success rates, based on intention to treat, exceed 95% and yield 1–3 year primary patency of approximately 80% and 65% respectively (Table 35–1).[2–6] If in the follow up of primary angioplasties, failure occurs, aggressive reintervention of the *initial lesions*, (often supplemented by stenting), will improve the secondary 3 year patency to about 75–80% (Table 35–1).[2–6] Delayed hemodynamic failure of the angioplastied limb may be the result of a new stenosis remote from the initial lesion. The frequency with which a new lesion, rather than the initial lesion, later compromises limb blood flow is not well documented, but in our experience exceeds 20% after 3 months.

TABLE 35–1. PATENCY RATES FOR PTA OF ILIAC ARTERY STENOSIS AND OCCLUSIONS

	Primary Patency (%)			Secondary Patency (%)		
	1y	3y	5y	1y	2y	3y
Balloon angioplasty of iliac stenosis[2–6]	78	66	61	92	87	77
Balloon angioplasty of iliac occlusions[2,6,15,18,19]	68	60	*	86	82	

*data not available
weighted averages

With the availability of stents after 1989, many investigators recommended primary stenting on either a selective or routine basis: both strategies increase 1 and 3 year primary patencies (Table 35–2).[7–14] At present, there are no data to support the practice of routine primary stenting for iliac artery lesions.[15] Their usefulness to control residual stenosis/recoil and dissection are, however, clearly documented.

Patency rates for PTA of iliac *occlusions* is, as expected, less than for *stenosis*, in large measure because of initial technical failure (failure to cross) of about 20% (Table 35–1).[7,16,17] Technical success and 1 and 3 year primary patency are both improved with stenting. Routine stenting appears to have become accepted practice for the treatment of chronic, complete occlusions and 1 and 3 year patencies of approximately 75% and 65% respectively can be expected with appropriate patient selection (Table 35–2).[15,18,19] Stenting of recurrent iliac artery lesions (secondary patency) will enhance patency by 5–10% at both time periods. Subintimal angioplasty, developed and championed by Bolia and Bell, has clearly carved a niche for itself for infrainguinal lesions.[20] It is too early to tell whether or not this technique will be readily applicable to iliac angioplasty. The accumulated data indicate that by combining PTA and stenting and repeat therapy when clinically indicated, very satisfactory patency of iliac artery lesions, either *stenoses* and *occlusions*, is attainable.

PREDICTORS OF SUCCESS

PTA/stenting of the iliac arteries is not uniformly successful. Not only are the results of angioplasty and stenting superior in the iliac segment than in the SFA, but other determinates of improved outcomes are well documented. These include:

- Proximal lesions[6]
    CIA > EIA

TABLE 35–2. PATENCY RATES FOR STENTING OF ILIAC ARTERY STENOSES AND OCCLUSIONS

	Primary Patency (%)		
	1y	3y	5y
Stenting of iliac stenosis[9–16]	90	74	72
Stenting of iliac occlusions[7,17,18]	72	64	*

*data not available
weighted averages

- Stenoses > occlusions[6]
- Short (<3 cm) vs long lesions[6]
- Clinical indication for intervention[6]
    Claudication > limb salvage
- Runoff [6]
    Patent vs occluded SFA (although poor runoff, e.g. SFA occlusion, is a predictor of reduced patency, there are no studies to compare patients who only undergo iliac PTA/stenting with those whose SFA occlusions are bypassed or otherwise treated).
- Gender
    Men > women

In addition to these established predictors of success, others have been addressed:

- *Calcifications:* Although the presence of focal calcium flecks in the occlusive lesion probably do not adversely affect PTA stenting, arteries with circumferential, dense calcification are poor choices for endoluminal therapy.
- *Hormone replacement therapy(HRT):*[21] Women tend to have worse outcomes than men and HRT may actually worsen women's outcomes.
- *Cigarette smoking:* As expected, long-term outcomes are worse in patients who continue to smoke.
- *Hypertension and dyslipidemia:* Based on cardiac trials, failure to control these arteriosclerotic risk factors is associated with worse outcomes. The same may be true for homocysteinemia.
- *Diabetes mellitus:*[22] Some studies suggest no deleterious effects of diabetes mellitus (DM) on outcomes. DM, however, is closely associated with infrapopliteal disease rather than with aortoiliofemoral occlusive lesions.
- *Arterial tortuosity:* No studies assess the effect of arterial tortuosity on patency.
- *Internal artery occlusive disease (IIA):* Stenosis or occlusion of the internal iliac arteries is a frequent congener of CIA + EIA lesions. There is no evidence of it being a predictor of the success or failure of iliac PTA/stenting. IIA involvement may be a marker for more extensive disease whose endoluminal treatment outcomes tend to be worse.
- *Type of stent:* Properly sized, both self-expanding and balloon expandable stents are equally effective.
- *IVUS assessed stent deployment:* IVUS has been used to determine stent-artery wall coaption and incomplete stent deployment with a residual "step-off." Hence, some workers have recommended assessment of the adequacy of stent sizing with IVUS. This modality, of course, would only be useful for balloon expandable stents. Neither cost-effectiveness nor improved patency using IVUS have been validated by appropriate randomized trials.
- *Length of the stented segment*[23] Some studies have suggested that angioplastied arteries requiring more than 2 stents (>7 cm) have a poorer prognosis. This may be the result of a) stents crossing and possibly occluding the IIA or b) longer lesions extending to the EIA with its known poorer prognosis. Whether it is necessary to cover the entire length of artery subjected to PTA with a stent(s) remains a subject of conjecture (Figure 35–1, 35–2, 35–3).

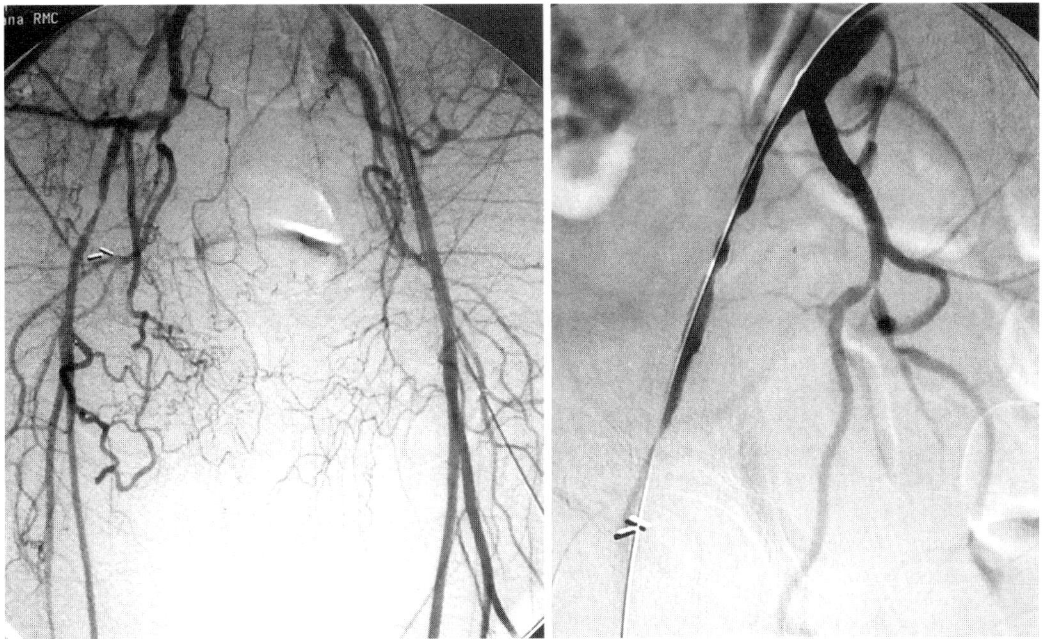

Figure 35–1. Angiogram of iliac arteries showing multisegment diffuse stenosis of right iliac artery.

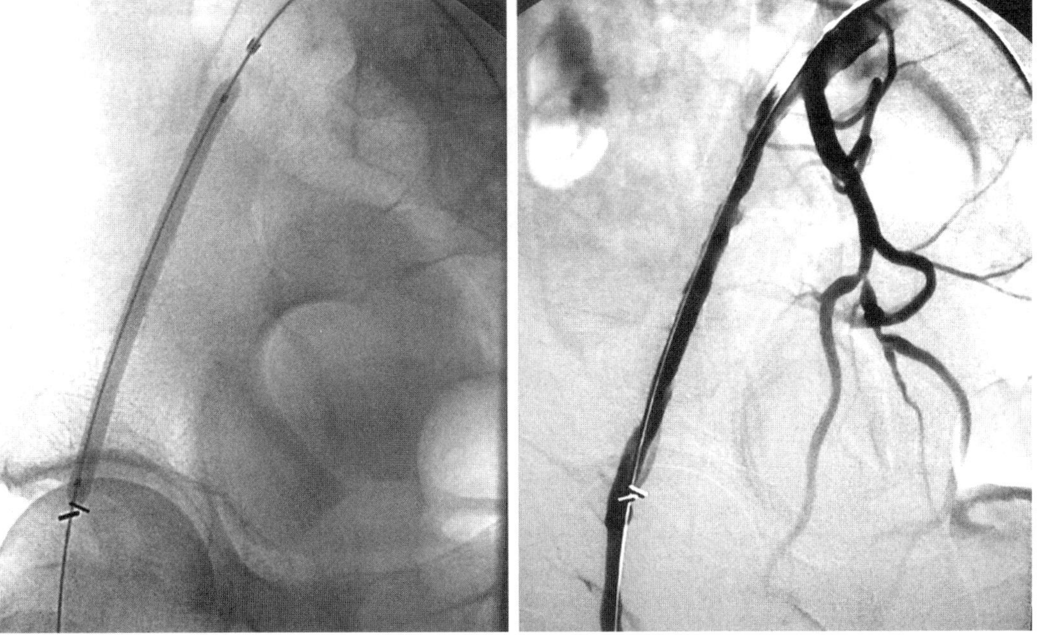

Figure 35–2. Balloon angioplasty of the right iliac artery lesion with a 6 mm x 10 cm balloon showing some improvement in the stenotic segments.

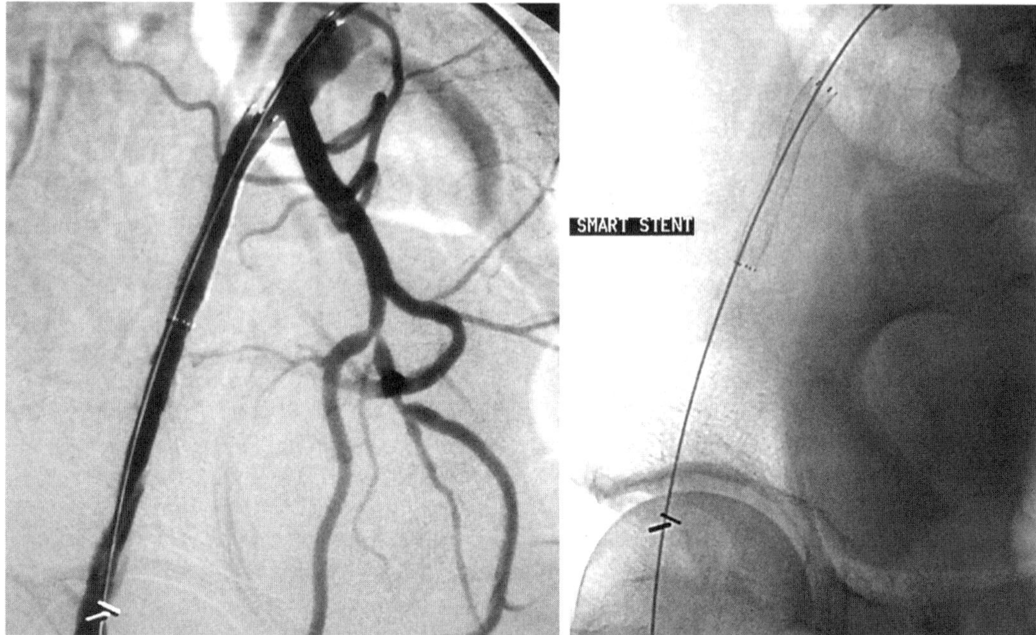

Figure 35–3. Post-stenting angiogram (smart stent 8 mm x 40 mm). Showing improved proximal stenotic segment.

DISCUSSION

The data that support the effectiveness of treating aortoiliofemoral occlusive disease with PTA/stenting are ineluctable. Underlining this success is the dramatic reduction of aortofemoral bypass grafting (ABFB) in Europe and in some centers in the USA; this both a relative and absolute decline in revascularization by open surgery. Coincident with the transformation of the treatment paradigm for occlusive disease is the substitution of endoluminal stent grafting for open repair of abdominal aortic aneurysms. Because endoluminal therapies are most effective in patients with less severe disease, those whose only therapeutic recourse is open surgery often require suprarenal cross-clamping and other technical complexities. Stratifying outcomes based solely upon the method of therapy is, therefore, inappropriate.

Moreover, until recently, therapy was further stratified with endoluminal procedures performed by interventional radiologists and open revascularizations by vascular surgeons. Now that vascular surgical fellows are being trained in endovascular techniques, their experience with open therapies can be anticipated to decline commensurately.[24] Who, then, will be left to revascularize the difficult and complex lesions not amenable to catheter-based techniques? No answer to this question is possible without comprehensive epidemiologic studies of aortoiliac disease that is left untreated and lesions treated by endoluminal or open techniques.[25] Until such data become available, it seems appropriate that therapeutic decisions should be made by doctors skilled with both methods and a vested interest in neither. It has been shown in other conditions that when the decisions are made by specialist physicians, shorter hospital lengths of stay can be achieved.[26] This sentinel outcome will doubtless gather the attention of governmental agencies and third party payers.

Because iliac PTA/stenting is applicable to less severe lesions and ABFB to the more advanced, these procedures are obviously complimentary. Viewed from the perspective of durable effectiveness, ABFB can substitute, as it did successfully for 25 years, for iliac PTA/stenting; the converse, however, is not true. By treating proximal lesions with ABFB, in patients with tandem lesions in the aortoiliac and infrainguinal segments, it has been shown that symptoms can be completely relieved in 50–75% of cases.[27] With iliac PTA stenting, essentially all patients will remain symptomatic from the more distal obstruction in the SFA. A cohort of such patients with either therapy for tandem lesions has not yet been systematically compared using objective measurements of hemodynamic and clinical outcomes. Comparison of the financial costs of ABFB and iliac PTA/stenting as primary procedures has demonstrated that there are no fiscal advantages to the less invasive approach to therapy.[28] Thus, the belief that endoluminal techniques will soon replace ABFB[29] has been likened to Mark Twain's comment on his purported imminent demise: "Report of my death greatly exaggerated."[30]

Based on the experience of the last decade, further technical advances can be anticipated. Covered stents have been recommended for ulcerated and emboligenic plaques. Combination procedures may also exploit some of the useful properties of covered stents by lining external iliac lesions that have been dilated or endarterectomized by retrograde methods from the femoral artery. Analogous to open surgical endarterectomy, simple balloon angioplasty of an extensively diseased EIA-femoral segment is quite vulnerable to restenosis. Improvements in long-term benefits in this arterial segment can only increase the applicability of endoluminal therapies.

REFERENCES

1. Andros G. Arterial Access in Endovascular Surgery. In Moore and Ahn (ed). *Endovascular Surgery, 3rd E*. Philadelphia:W.B. Saunders;2001:37–47.
2. Harris RW, Dulawa LB, Andros G, et al. Percutaneous transluminal angioplasty of lower extremities by the vascular surgeon. *Ann Vasc Surg*. 1991;5:345–353.
3. Tegtmeyer CJ, Hartwell GD, Selby JB, Robertson R, Kron IL, Tribble CG. Results and angioplasty in aortoiliac disease. *Circulation*. 1991;83(suppl I): I–53–I–60.
4. Jeans WD, Armstrong S, Cole SEA, et al. Fate of patients undergoing transluminal angioplasty for lower limb ischemia. *Radiology*. 1990;177:559–564.
5. Jorgensen B, Skovgaard N, Norgard J, et al. Percutaneous transluminal angioplasty in 226 iliac artery stenoses: role of the superficial femoral artery for clinical success. *Vasa*. 1992;21:382–386.
6. Johnston KW: Iliac arteries: reanalysis of results of balloon angioplasty. *Radiology*. 1993: 186:207–212.
7. Gupta AK, Ravimandalam K, Rao VR, et al. Total occlusion of iliac arteries: results of balloon angioplasty. Cardiovasc *Intervent Radiol*. 1993;16:165–177.
8. Bosch JL, Hunink MGM. Metaanalysis of the results of percutaneous transluminal angioplasty and stent placement of aortoiliac occlusive disease. *Radiology*. 1997;204:87–96.
9. Murphy TP, Webb MS, Lambiase RE, et al. Percutaneous revascularization of complex iliac artery stenoses and occlusions with use of wallstent: Three-year experience. *J Vasc Intervent Radiol*. 1996;7:21–27.
10. Laborde JC, Palmaz JC, Rivera FJ, et al. Influence of anatomic distribution of atherosclerosis on the outcome of revascularization withiliac stent placement. *J Vasc Intervent Radiol*.1995;6:513–521.
11. Brewster DC. Clinical and anatomical considerations for surgery in aortoiliac disease and results of surgical treatment. *Circulation*. 1991;83(suppl I):142–152.

12. Tetteroo E, van der Graaf Y, Bosch JL, et al. Randomised comparison of primary stent placement versus primary angioplasty followed by selective stent placement in patients with iliac-artery occlusive disease. Dutch Iliac Stent Trial Study Group. *Lancet.* 1998 Apr 18;351(9110):1153–1159.
13. Palmaz JC, Laborde JC, Rivera FJ, et al. Stenting of iliac arteries with Palmaz stent: experience from a multicentric trial. *Cardiovasc Intervent Radiol.* 1992; 15:291–297.
14. Strecker EP, Hagen P, Liermann D, et al. Iliac and femoropopliteal vascular occlusive disease treated with flexible tantalum stents. *Cardiovasc Interven Radiol.* 1993:16:158-164.
15. Cambria RA, Farooq MM, Mewissen MW, et al. Endovascular Therapy of iliac arteries: routine application of intraluminal stents does not improve clinical patency. *Ann Vasc Surg.* 1999;13:599–605.
16. Blum U, Gabelmann A, Redecker M, et al. Percutaneous recanalization of iliac artery occlusions: results of a prospective study. *Radiology.* 1993;189:536–540.
17. Rutherford RB, Durham J. Percutaneous balloon angioplasty for arteriosclerosis obliterans: long term results: In Yao JST, Pearce WH, ed. *Techniques in Vascular Surgery.* Philadelphia:W.B. Saunders, 1992:329–345.
18. Wolf YG, Schatz RA, Knowels HJ, et al. Initial experience with the Palmaz stent for aortoiliac stenoses. *Ann Vasc Surg.* 1993;7:254–261.
19. Hausegger KA, Lammer J, Klein GE, et al. Percutaneous recanalization of pelvic artery occlusions: fibrinolysis, PTA, stents. *ROFO.* 1991;155:550–555.
20. London NJ, Srinivasan R, Naylor AR, et al. Subintimal angioplasty of femoropopliteal artery occlusions: the long-term results. *Eur J Vasc Surg.* 1994:8(2):148–55.
21. Timaran CH, Stevens SL, Grandas OH, et al. Influence of hormone replacement therapy on the outcome of iliac angioplasty and stenting. *J Vasc Surg.* 2001;33:S85–S92.
22. Spence LD, Hartnell GG, Reinking G, et al. Diabetic versus nondiabetic limb-threatening ischemia: outcome of percutaneous iliac intervention. *AJR.* 1999;172:1335–1341.
23. Powel RJ, Fillinger M, Bettmann M, et al. The durability of endovascular treatment of multisegment iliac occlusive disease. *J Vasc Surg.* 2000;31:1178–1184.
24. Moore WS, Clagett GP, Veith FJ, et al. Guidelines for hospital privileges in vascular surgery: An update by an ad hoc committee of the American Association for Vascular Surgery and the Society for Vascular Surgery . In press (*J Vasc Surg*).
25. Management of Peripheral Arterial Disease (PAD):TransAtlantic Inter-Scociety Concensus (TASC). *J Vasc Surg.* 2000;31:S97–S112.
26. Clinical advisory board-partnering in throughput reform. August 2002.
27. Brewster DC. A surgeon's view of iliac stenting: what will be the role for aortofemoral bypass? *Prospect Vasc Surg.* 1996;9(1):67–70.
28. Ballard JL, Bergen JJ, Singh P, et al. Aortoiliac stent deployment versus surgical reconstruction: analysis of outcome and cost. *J Vasc Surg.* 1998;29;94:103.
29. Criado FJ, Wellons E, Abul-khoudoud O, et al. Endovascular intervention for iliac artery disease: indications and techniques. *Prospect Vasc Surg.* 1999;11(1):29–46.
30. Andros G. Expert commentary to "Endovascular intervention for iliac artery disease: indications and techniques." *Prospect Vasc Surg.* 1999;11(1):47–49.

36

Angioplasty and Stent for Superficial Femoral Artery Lesions

Matt M Thompson, MD, FRCS, Kevin Molloy, FRCS, Amman Bolia, FRCR, Guy Fishwick, FRCR, and Peter Bell, MD, FRCS

Percutaneous transluminal angioplasty (PTA) has become an accepted treatment for atheromatous disease of the superficial femoral artery (SFA) during the last 3 decades, during which time the number of percutaneous interventions has increased dramatically.[1] In recent years several new endovascular techniques have facilitated treatment of more severe SFA disease. Despite the apparent success of PTA in the treatment of SFA lesions, the evidence base to support the use of angioplasty, with or without stenting, is limited.

Most descriptions of the efficacy of this technique are non-randomised, observational, cohort studies, which report results from treating a diverse group of patients with both claudication and critical limb ischaemia (CLI). The majority of publications detail technical success rates, symptomatic and haemodynamic patencies for SFA interventions, but contain no control data. These limitations in the literature base make comparisons between different endovascular techniques virtually impossible.

At present, the demand for evidence-based treatments has emphasized the need for properly controlled clinical trials to compare the efficacy of angioplasty against other treatment modalities. Descriptions of trials comparing PTA against exercise therapy for claudication and PTA against surgery for CLI, have started to appear.[2] In the next 5 years, evidence from several studies worldwide, will allow the endovascular treatment of SFA disease to be rationalized.

This review will cover the historical basis of SFA angioplasty and describe the evidence for the use of newer techniques including stenting and endoluminal femoropopliteal grafting. The review concludes with a report of the approach to treating SFA lesions in our unit, with the preferential use of subintimal angioplasty.

HISTORICAL REVIEW

A general review of the historical literature suggests that the technical success rate for SFA PTA was approximately 80%.[3–5] The prime determinant of technical success was the morphological characteristic of the arterial lesion, with occlusions having a higher technical failure rate and a higher complication rate than stenotic lesions. In the long term, the patency of femoro-popliteal angioplasty was influenced by the same factors that predict the outcome of iliac and tibial PTA. Factors associated with favourable long term outcome included presentation (claudication as opposed to CLI), good run off, absence of diabetes, and lesion morphology. The presence of diffuse stenotic disease, highly eccentric plaques and arterial occlusions greater than 3 cm in length were associated with high rates of restenosis.

Life table analysis from a series of reports suggested that the 1-, 3-, and 5-year patency rates for SFA PTA were 70%, 60% and 50% respectively. However, most series of SFA angioplasties contained a high proportion of patients with claudication and stenotic disease, who would be expected to have a good outcome. The results when arterial occlusions were considered were poor. Lofberg et al.[6] reported a series of patients with limb threatening ischaemia in which the 5 year primary patency for SFA occlusions greater than 5 cm was 12%.

INDICATIONS FOR SFA PTA

In the past few years, the emphasis in treatment of intermittent claudication has changed. Previously, the mainstay of therapy for claudication revolved around endovascular or surgical revascularisation of the limb. This approach has been modified in the light of contemporary studies defining the role of medical management and exercise therapy in treating intermittent claudication.[7] Recent evidence has suggested that risk factor modification, anti-platelet and statin therapy are essential to reduce the risk of subsequent cardiovascular events. The role of PTA in treating SFA lesions responsible for claudication has been addressed in 2 small randomised clinical trials, which have compared PTA with exercise programmes. Both trials failed to show any long term benefit in the cohort undergoing PTA.[2,8] Further multi-center studies to compare exercise therapy and PTA in claudication are underway.

Whilst the role of PTA in treating stable claudication is uncertain at present, the place of PTA in limb threatening ischaemia is less controversial. Despite the absence of any controlled studies, most practitioners regard PTA as an appropriate first-line therapy in patients with CLI. Morphologically, patients with CLI often have diffuse multi-level atheromatous disease with long SFA occlusions, which have historically been associated with poor patency rates following PTA. The challenge for vascular specialists in the treatment of SFA disease will be to introduce techniques to deal with long SFA occlusions in patients presenting with CLI.

In the past few years, innovative modifications to traditional PTA techniques have evolved in an attempt to treat complex SFA occlusions with high technical success and long-term patency rates. Unfortunately, the use of laser angioplasty and percutaneous atherectomy that were popularized in the 1980s and 90s, were not associated with an improvement in short or long term patency. The technical challenge to treat patients with CLI and SFA disease include, flush lesions with no SFA stump, full-length occlusions, calcified plaques, and extension of disease into the run off. The modern approach to these problems has been to utilize different access techniques,[9] stents, remote atherectomy or sub-intimal angioplasty.

PTA AND PRIMARY STENTING

There is an assumption in the vascular community that the results of angioplasty for iliac occlusions are improved if combined with primary stent placement. There is no substantive evidence on which to base this practice, which is now widely accepted. In an attempt to improve the disappointing results following PTA of long SFA occlusions, several centers have applied experience from iliac PTA and advocated the use of primary stenting in the femoro-popliteal segment (Figure 36–1). The rationale for stent use was to minimize elastic recoil of the vessel wall, treat angioplasty induced arterial dissection and maintain a patent arterial channel.

Gordon et al.[10] reported a series of 71 limbs with atherosclerotic SFA occlusion, that underwent PTA, stent deployment and thrombolysis (27%) to manage peri-procedural thrombosis. The 1 and 3 year primary patencies were 55% and 30% respectively. On the basis of these data, the authors concluded that "PTA and stenting yielded higher patency rates than historical controls." Similar results were reported by Cheng et al.[11] in a series of limbs with 52% occlusions and 43% severe limb ischaemia. In this mixed cohort the 1 and 2 year primary patency rates were 63% and 54%.

The series described above did not contain a control group that could be used to compare clinical outcomes between PTA and PTA+stenting. This question was addressed by a clinical trial, which randomised 32 patients with femoro-popliteal occlusions to PTA alone or in combination with a Strecker stent.[12] Although underpowered, this study demonstrated no improvement in clinical or radiological patency associated with stent deployment. However, the investigation did suggest that stent placement in the SFA was associated with an increased rate of restenosis which limited the efficacy of the technique.

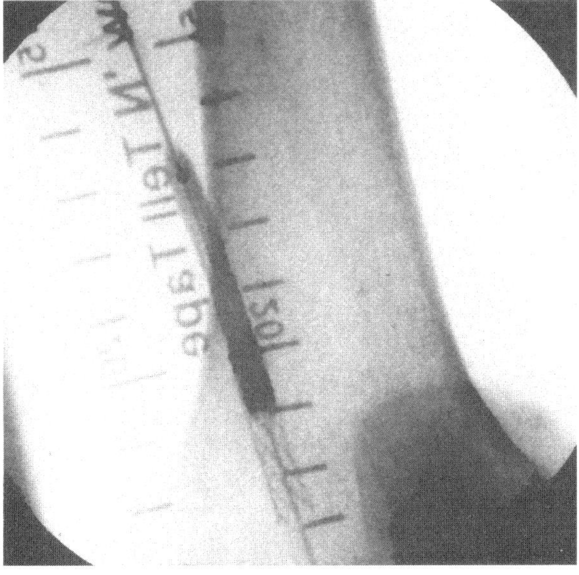

Figure 36–1. Palmaz stent being deployed in the proximal popliteal artery.

A high incidence of stent-induced restenosis was also described by Gray et al.[13] who calculated that the median time to restenosis or reocclusion following stent placement in the SFA was 6 months. At present, the major limitation to primary stent deployment following SFA PTA is the occurrence of intimal hyperplasia causing arterial restenosis and stent failure. The high incidence of stent failure in the SFA has led several authors to recommend that the use of primary stenting in the SFA be limited.[14,15] The place of stents for complications of PTA or in rescue situations has not been systematically addressed, but remains within the clinical armamentarium of most endovascular surgeons.

The development of covered stents has proved useful for the treatment of arterial rupture following balloon angioplasty of many arterial segments. In an attempt to improve stent performance in the SFA, ePTFE covered stents have been used to perform endovascular femoro-popliteal bypass after balloon dilation. Although results of several trials are still awaited, initial results have been disappointing.[16] Deutschmann et al.[17] reported a series of 18 patients, with a 6 month primary patency of only 50%. Intimal hyperplasia was observed in 39% of the grafts, and it remains likely that covered stents will suffer from a similarly high rate of restenosis as uncovered stents.

Recent developments in the treatment of intimal hyperplasia offer the possibility to reduce stent failure. Considerable progress has been made with drug eluting stents, brachytherapy, and gene therapy that offer the hope of improved stent performance in the near future.[18,19]

REMOTE SFA ENDARTERECTOMY AND ENDOLUMINAL BYPASS

Thromboendarterectomy is a standard vascular surgical technique that is still widely utilized in the treatment of carotid artery disease. Endarterectomy of the SFA became obsolete when femoro-popliteal bypass became established as the first line surgical treatment for SFA occlusions. In recent years the disappointing results obtained by endovascular techniques in the treatment of long SFA occlusions, stimulated several groups to re-assess endarterectomy, utilizing a semi-closed technique. The scientific rationale for endarterectomy was the hope that debulking the SFA would improve patency.

Remote SFA endarterectomy may be performed following exposure of the femoral bifurcation, through a small arteriotomy in the SFA. The endarterectomy is started conventionally and continued using a ring stripper. The ring stripper is advanced until the occlusion has been removed. The atheromatous core is then transected using a ring cutter device. A guide wire is then passed across the distal SFA endarterectomy end point, which is then fixed, by balloon expansion or stenting.[20] The procedure may be combined with adjunctive profunda femoris endarterectomy.

The primary patency rates of remote SFA endarterectomy have been encouraging with 1-year rates above 60%.[21] However, as with stenting, the major concern with this technique is the development of intimal hyperplasia within the SFA that may affect nearly 70% of the endarterectomised segments.[22] In an attempt to reduce this problem, several authors have suggested that the remote endarterectomy be combined with SFA endografting. The endograft utilized may incorporate a conventional proximal anastomosis (Figure 36–2) or use covered stents.

The technical feasibility of endoluminal femoro-popliteal bypass has now been established but the patency rates have been disappointing with 2 studies reporting 1 year primary patency rates of approximately 30% (16;23). Recent results of this tech-

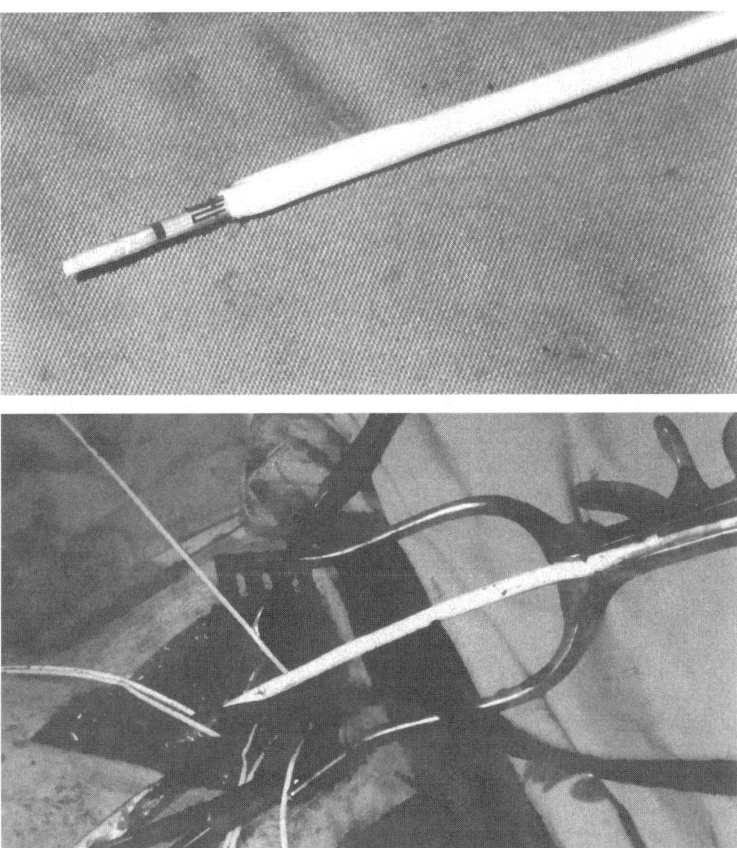

Figure 36–2. Endoluminal femoro-popliteal graft. EPTFE graft being mounted on a Palmaz stent, and subsequently on a balloon catheter. Graft is then packaged in a peel away sheath prior to being deployed in the SFA. The sheath is peeled away to uncover the ePTFE graft in the SFA. The graft is deployed by inflation of the balloon. The procedure is completed by a conventional inlay anastomosis to the femoral artery.

nique from a specialized single center have been more positive,[24] but restenosis is likely to remain a problem.

SUB-INTIMAL ANGIOPLASTY

Sub-intimal angioplasty is a technique extensively utilized in our institution. The technique was initially performed in 1987, and since that time has been utilized in over 900 femoro-popliteal occlusions. Sub-intimal PTA is now our treatment of choice in suitable patients with CLI.

Patients are selected for PTA on the basis of duplex scanning without prior arteriography. All patients with CLI and SFA occlusions are preferentially treated with sub-intimal PTA if no contra-indications are present. The main exclusion criteria for the technique are disease affecting the common femoral artery, and possibility of an acute occlusion with fresh thrombus.

TECHNIQUE OF SUB-INTIMAL PTA

The principles of sub-intimal PTA are to dissect into the sub-intimal space, cross the lesion in this plane, re-enter into the true lumen below the lesion and then to dilate the dissection channel with a balloon. This leads to spiral dissection channel in the vessel (Figure 36–3). The technique has been described in detail elsewhere but a brief review is outlined below.[25]

The procedure is performed under local anaesthesia. Assuming adequate inflow, an antegrade puncture is made in the common femoral artery. A 5F-predilating catheter is introduced into the SFA and arteriography performed to confirm lesion length and status of the run off. Following systemic heparinisation, a straight guidewire is used to enter the lesion. The guidewire is directed towards the arterial wall, and in most circumstances enters the occlusion in the subintimal plane. The catheter is then advanced with the guidewire that forms a loop within the dissection plane (Figure 36–4). Occasionally, passage into the dissection and subsequent advancement is facilitated by use of a hydrophilic wire.

An attempt is made to avoid major collateral vessels during formation of the dissection channel. Occasionally, a perforation will occur during initiation of the dissection. This is not usually serious but embolisation may be necessary. In most cases an alternative route for the dissection channel is found (Figure 36–5).

Once the lesion has been traversed, the wire loop is manipulated back into the true lumen. In most cases this occurs spontaneously as there is a discrete arterial end point where the intima is tethered to the vessel wall. Occasionally extensive catheter manipulation is required and re-entry is achieved more distally. Once the lesion has been

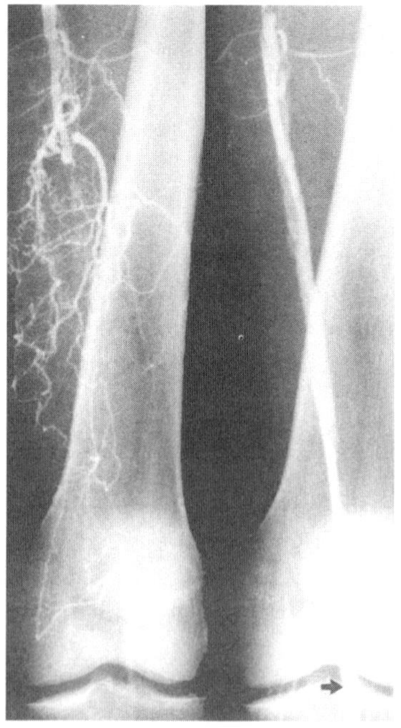

Figure 36–3. Sub-intimal PTA of a long SFA occlusion extending into the popliteal artery. Following sub-intimal PTA a spiral appearance is demonstrated which represents the spiral channel formed in the dissection plane. The distal re-entry point is illustrated with an arrow.

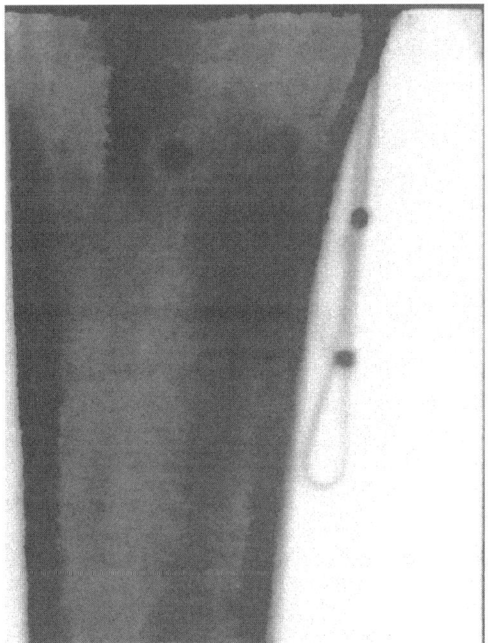

Figure 36–4. Tibial PTA. Sub-intimal passage of a wire in the dissection plane confirmed by the presence of a loop on the wire.

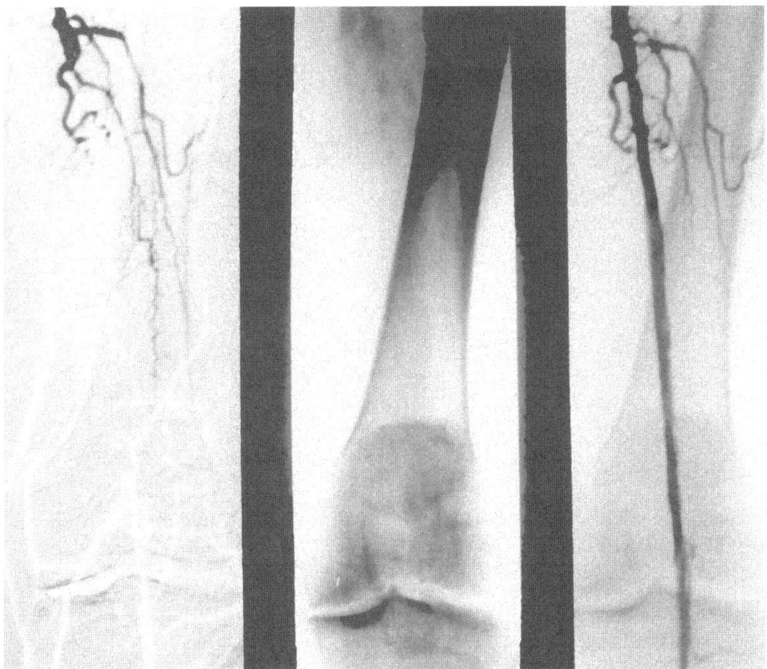

Figure 36–5. Sub-intimal PTA of an SFA lesion. A perforation occurred during the first attempt and extravasated contrast can be seen. An alternative route was found and PTA succeeded.

crossed, the entire channel is dilated with a standard balloon with particular attention being given to the proximal and distal entry points.

TECHNICAL SUCCESS AND LONG TERM PATENCY

The technical success rate for SFA sub-intimal angioplasty in our institution is approximately 90% in a series of patients with a mean occlusion length of 15 cm.[26] The majority of failures were due to an inability to re-enter the true lumen distally. The major morbidity/mortality rate was 2.5%.

The primary haemodynamic and symptomatic patencies for 200 femoro-popliteal occlusions are illustrated in Table 36–1. At present, it has not proved prospectively possible to identify the reasons for long term failure of sub-intimal PTA, but intimal hyperplasia is likely to play a significant part. In patients undergoing duplex scanning or arteriography for recurrent symptoms, restenosis has been described at all points within the dissection channel. Interestingly, in cases that remain patent for long periods, the vessel wall shows signs of remodeling (Figure 36–6).

The main advantage of sub-intimal PTA over conventional techniques is the ease in dealing with long occlusions. Once a dissection channel has been formed, it becomes relatively easy to traverse the entire length of the occlusion in the same plane. Even if the SFA occlusion extends into the popliteal or crural arteries the same technique may be applied.[27] Additionally the technique may be utilized to treat long occlusions without a SFA stump (Figure 36–7).

COMPLICATIONS OF PTA. TRANSLUMINAL VS. SUB-INTIMAL

Between 1995 and 1998, 988 patients underwent 1,377 PTAs at our institution. The majority of interventions were for the treatment of claudication (61%) or CLI (27%), and the commonest site for treatment was the femoral arteries (64%). 660 interventions (48%) were performed using a sub-intimal technique. The number of serious complications following sub-intimal and transluminal angioplasty is illustrated in Table 36–2. Despite the increased complexity of the lesions that were dealt with using the sub-intimal technique, the complication rates were similar between conventional and sub-intimal techniques.[28]

TABLE 36–1. HAEMODYNAMIC AND SYMPTOMATIC PATENCIES FOR 200 FEMORO-POPLITEAL OCCLUSIONS TREATED BY SUB-INTIMAL ANGIOPLASTY. ANALYSIS BY LIFE TABLE METHODOLOGY.[29]

	Haemodynamic Patency (%)		Symptomatic Patency (%)	
	12 Months	36 Months	12 Months	36 Months
All Procedures	56	46	58	48
Technical Success	71	58	73	61

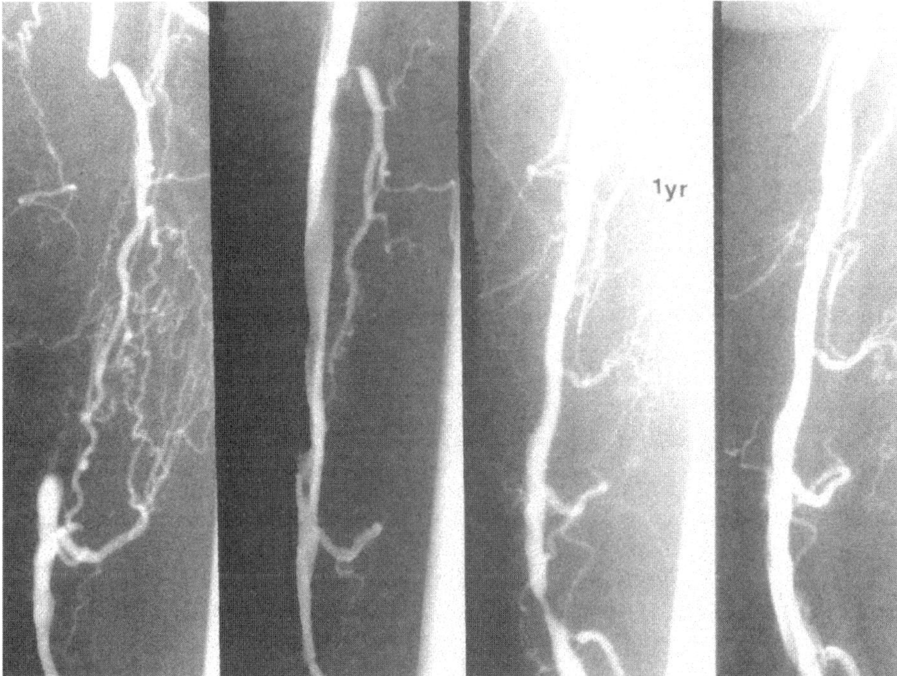

Figure 36–6. Sub-intimal PTA of a mid SFA occlusion. Following PTA, a spiral appearance is noted at the PTA site. Repeat angiography for recurrent symptoms demonstrated a stenosis distal to the PTA site, but evidence of remodeling within the dissection channel. Dilation of the stenosis was successful.

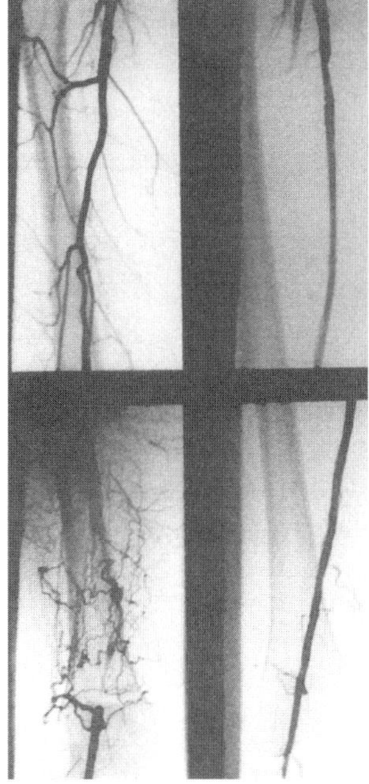

Figure 36–7. Full length occlusion of the SFA without a discernable stump. The popliteal artery refilled just above the knee. A full length SFA recanalisation was successful.

TABLE 36–2. TABLE ILLUSTRATING THE RATE OF MAJOR MEDICAL AND SURGICAL COMPLICATIONS IN A SERIES OF 1377 ANGIOPLASTIES. THE RATES OF ACUTE LIMB ISCHAEMIA AND HAEMORRHAGE INDICATE THOSE PATIENTS WHO REQUIRED EMERGENCY SURGERY.[28]

Complication	Subintimal	Transluminal
Acute limb ischaemia	1.6%	1.4%
Haemorrhage	0.6%	0.6%
Amputation	0.6%	0.5%
Death	1.1%	1.6%
Death+major morbidity	3.9%	3.1%

Role of Sub-Intimal PTA in CLI

The role of sub-intimal PTA in our practice may be illustrated by a series of prospective audits into the treatment of CLI. In 1994, 46% of the patients presenting to our unit with CLI were treated with PTA as compared to a national average for the UK of 22%.[29] In 1997, 64% of 208 critically ischaemic limbs were treated with PTA in a patient cohort with a median age of 76 years. The commonest arterial location requiring revascularisation was the SFA (42%), and 80% of the angioplasties had a sub-intimal component. The technical success rate was 78%. The cumulative mortality, amputation and symptomatic recurrence rates are illustrated in Figures 36–8 and 36–9. The 12-month limb salvage rate for the patient cohort treated with PTA was 92%.

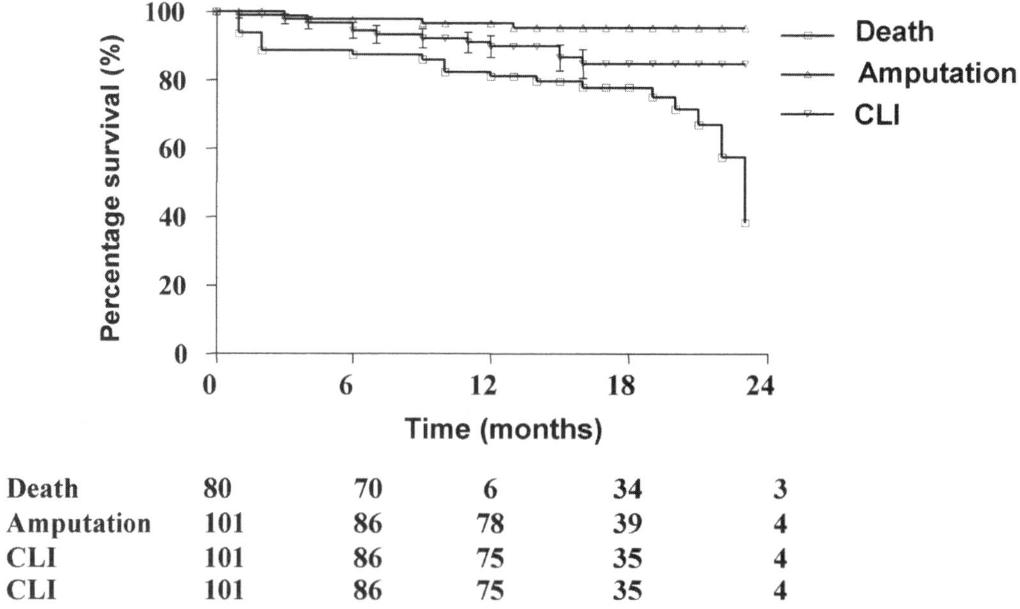

Death	80	70	6	34	3
Amputation	101	86	78	39	4
CLI	101	86	75	35	4
CLI	101	86	75	35	4

Figure 36–8. Mortality, amputation and symptom recurrence rates in patients undergoing PTA for CLI at Leicester Royal Infirmary in 1997. Graph illustrates cumulative rates in patients having a technically successful PTA. Numbers of patients at risk at each time point are tabulated.

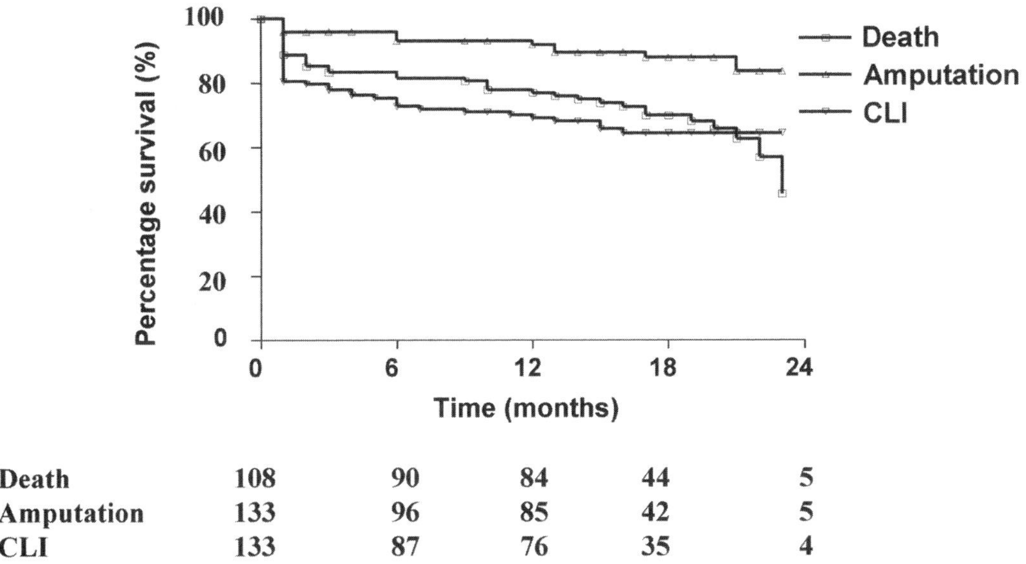

Death	108	90	84	44	5
Amputation	133	96	85	42	5
CLI	133	87	76	35	4

Figure 36–9. Mortality, amputation and symptom recurrence rates in patients undergoing PTA for CLI at Leicester Royal Infirmary in 1997. Graph illustrates cumulative rates in all patients having PTA. Numbers of patients at risk at each time point are tabulated.

CONCLUSIONS

The treatment of SFA disease remains complex and controversial. The place of PTA, surgery or conservative measures has a meager evidence base. In the future the treatment of claudicants and patients with CLI may be resolved by randomised clinical trials. Likely comparisons are exercise therapy versus PTA in claudication and PTA versus surgery in CLI. However, these trials will be difficult to design and implement and recruitment may be selective. Additionally, treatment must be compared "like with like." Comparing femoro-popliteal bypass with a graft surveillance programme against PTA and no surveillance would give a biased result.

At present, the use of PTA in the SFA remains an individual decision. PTA of isolated stenoses gives reliably durable results. Unfortunately, the treatment of long SFA occlusions remains problematic, with low rates of technical success and poor long-term patency. Several techniques have been proposed to improve these results and several approaches seem promising. Further developments in vascular biology will have application to reduce the intimal hyperplasia that affects all endovascular therapy of the SFA.

REFERENCES

1. Sayers RD, Thompson MM, Varty K, Jagger C, Bell PR. Changing trends in the management of lower-limb ischaemia: a 17-year review. *Br J Surg.* 1993;80(10):1269–1273.
2. Whyman MR, Fowkes FG, Kerracher EM, et al. Is intermittent claudication improved by percutaneous transluminal angioplasty? A randomized controlled trial. *J Vasc Surg.* 1997;26(4):551–557.
3. Capek P, McLean GK, Berkowitz HD. Femoropopliteal angioplasty. Factors influencing long-term success. *Circulation.* 1991;83(2 Suppl):I70–I80.
4. Hewes RC, White RI, Jr., Murray RR, et al. Long-term results of superficial femoral artery angioplasty. *Am J Roentgenol.* 1986;146(5):1025–1029.
5. Johnston KW, Rae M, Hogg-Johnston SA, et al. 5–year results of a prospective study of percutaneous transluminal angioplasty. *Ann Surg.* 1987;206(4):403–413.

6. Lofberg AM, Karacagil S, Ljungman C, et al. Percutaneous transluminal angioplasty of the femoropopliteal arteries in limbs with chronic critical lower limb ischemia. *J Vasc Surg.* 2001;34(1):114–121.

7. Shearman CP. Management of intermittent claudication. *Br J Surg.* 2002; 89:529–531.

8. Perkins JM, Collin J, Creasy TS, et al. Exercise training versus angioplasty for stable claudication. Long and medium term results of a prospective, randomised trial. *Eur J Vasc Endovasc Surg.* 1996;11(4):409–413.

9. Yilmaz S, Sindel T, Ceken K, et al. Subintimal recanalization of long superficial femoral artery occlusions through the retrograde popliteal approach. *Cardiovasc Intervent Radiol.* 2001;24(3):154–160.

10. Gordon IL, Conroy RM, Arefi M, et al. Three-year outcome of endovascular treatment of superficial femoral artery occlusion. *Arch Surg.* 2001;136(2):221–228.

11. Cheng SW, Ting AC, Wong J. Endovascular stenting of superficial femoral artery stenosis and occlusions: results and risk factor analysis. *Cardiovasc Surg.* 2001; 9(2):133–140.

12. Zdanowski Z, Albrechtsson U, Lundin A, et al. Percutaneous transluminal angioplasty with or without stenting for femoropopliteal occlusions? A randomized controlled study. *Int Angiol.* 1999;18(4):251–255.

13. Gray BH, Sullivan TM, Childs MB, et al. High incidence of restenosis/reocclusion of stents in the percutaneous treatment of long-segment superficial femoral artery disease after suboptimal angioplasty. *J Vasc Surg.* 1997;25(1):74–83.

14. Gray BH, Olin JW. Limitations of percutaneous transluminal angioplasty with stenting for femoropopliteal arterial occlusive disease. *Semin Vasc Surg.* 1997;10(1):8–16.

15. Lampmann LE. Stenting in the femoral superficial artery: an overview. *Eur J Radiol.* 1999;29(3):276–279.

16. Kessel DO, Wijesinghe LD, Robertson I, et al. Endovascular stent-grafts for superficial femoral artery disease: results of 1-year follow-up. *J Vasc Interv Radiol.* 1999;10(3):289–296.

17. Deutschmann HA, Schedlbauer P, Berczi V, et al. Placement of Hemobahn stent-grafts in femoropopliteal arteries: early experience and midterm results in 18 patients. *J Vasc Interv Radiol.* 2001;12(8):943–950.

18. Poon M, Badimon JJ, Fuster V. Overcoming restenosis with sirolimus: from alphabet soup to clinical reality. *Lancet.* 2002;359(9306):619–622.

19. Quarck R, Holvoet P. Restenosis and gene therapy. *Expert Opin Biol Ther.* 2001;1(1):79–91.

20. Teijink JA, van den Berg JC, Moll FL. A minimally invasive technique in occlusive disease of the superficial femoral artery: remote endarterectomy using the MollRing Cutter. *Ann Vasc Surg* 2001;15(5):594–598.

21. Rosenthal D, Schubart PJ, Kinney EV, et al. Remote superficial femoral artery endarterectomy: Multicenter medium-term results. *J Vasc Surg.* 2001;34(3):428–432.

22. Galland RB, Whiteley MS, Gibson M, et al. Remote superficial femoral artery endarterectomy: medium-term results. *Eur J Vasc Endovasc Surg.* 2000;19(3):278–282.

23. Tisi PV, Cowan AR, Morris GE. Endoluminal femoropopliteal bypass for intermittent claudication. *Eur J Vasc Endovasc Surg.* 2000;19(5):481–488.

24. Heijmen RH, Teijink JA, van den Berg JC, et al. Use of a balloon-expandable, radially reinforced ePTFE endograft after remote SFA endarterectomy: a single-center experience. *J Endovasc Ther.* 2001;8(4):408–416.

25. Reekers JA, Bolia A. Percutaneous intentional extraluminal (subintimal) recanalization: how to do it yourself. *Eur J Radiol.* 1998;28(3):192–198.

26. Bolia A, Bell PR, London N. The durability of subintimal angioplasty. In: Greenhalgh RM, editor. The durability of vascular and endovascular surgery. London: WB Saunders, 1999:3–15.

27. Bolia A, Sayers RD, Thompson MM, et al. Subintimal and intraluminal recanalisation of occluded crural arteries by percutaneous balloon angioplasty. *Eur J Vasc Surg.* 1994;8(2):214–219.

28. Axisa B, Fishwick G, Bolia A, et al. Complications following peripheral angioplasty. *Ann R Coll Surg Engl.* 2002;84(1):39–42.

29. London NJ, Srinivasan R, Naylor AR, et al. Subintimal angioplasty of femoropopliteal artery occlusions: the long-term results. *Eur J Vasc Surg.* 1994;8(2):148–155.

XI

Hemodialysis Access

37

Surveillance Program for Hemodialysis Access

Andrew N. Bowser, MD and Dennis F. Bandyk, MD

Maintenance of a functional subcutaneous arteriovenous conduit for hemodialysis remains a challenge in caring for patients with end-stage renal disease (ESRD). Both autogenous fistulas and prosthetic bridge grafts are associated with a spectrum of problems that threaten or terminate dialysis function. Thrombosis of the access conduit is the most common problem, but development of stenosis caused by myointimal hyperplasia, infection, pseudoaneurysms, upper limb venous hypertension; or hand ischemia can also lead to loss of function. Failure of dialysis access procedures is frequent with a primary patency rate, based on "intention to treat" reporting standards, of approximately 40% at 1 year for both autologous arteriovenous fistulas (AVF) and prosthetic polytetraflouroethylene (PTFE) bridge grafts.[1,2] In a significant number of patients, access function can be salvaged by secondary endovascular (thrombolysis, balloon angioplasty) or open surgical (catheter thrombectomy, patch angioplasty, graft extension or replacement) procedures. However, subsequent failure rates remain high with secondary patency rates of 46 and 60% at 1-year for salvaged AVFs and PTFE bridge grafts respectively. Based on the favorable experience of lower-limb arterial bypass grafting surveillance in improving graft patency,[3] it is logical to assume a surveillance program of dialysis access conduits would also extend functional patency if clinically important abnormalities were identified and repaired prior to thrombosis. To date, no appropriately designed clinical trials have been performed to test this hypothesis.

The utility of dialysis access surveillance is predicated on 2 assumptions. First, the surveillance technique and protocol will accurately detect lesions that increase the risk of access failure; and second, intervention to correct lesions will extend functional patency and therapeutic hemodialysis. The development of stenosis in the venous outflow vessels is most common mechanism of dialysis access failure, but occlusive lesions can also develop within the graft, arterial anastomotic site, or less commonly the inflow artery. Significant stenoses (>50% diameter-reducing, DR) are found in up to 80-90% of thrombosed access grafts following restoration of patency by thrombolysis or thrombctomy.[4-6] In the remainder of the thrombosed grafts, no anatomic lesion can be demonstrated suggesting other mechanisms, such as transient hypotension, hypovolemia, extrinsic compression, hypercoagulable states, or improper access cannulation procedures, may play a role. Hemodialysis access failure is most frequent reason for hospitalization of ESRD patients.

The National Kidney Foundation (*www.kidney.org*) in their Dialysis Outcome Quality Initiative (DOQI)[7] guidelines 9 through 11 recommends "prospective surveillance of dialysis access grafts for hemodynamically significant stenosis." Evidence-based data indicate that when combined with correction, surveillance "improves patency and decreases the incidence of thrombosis." The surveillance should include weekly physical examination; and the use of anatomic and physiologic techniques to detect stenosis or access flow reduction. Surveillance methods available to clinicians include access recirculation calculations, venous line pressures, ultrasonic dilution techniques, duplex evaluation for stenoses and volume flow measurement, and contrast fistulography.[8] The best surveillance method is one that is accurate, inexpensive, safe, and for practical considerations, reimbursed by Medicare/Medicaid or other insurance payment plans. Although duplex ultrasound appears ideally suited for dialysis access surveillance, the Center for Medicare Services (CMS) recently issued payment guidelines for CPT 93990, "duplex scan of hemodialysis access" that prevents application for routine surveillance. Reimbursement is allowed only to evaluate an access with signs and symptoms of malfunction, such as elevated dynamic venous pressure (>200 mm Hg) during dialysis at a flow of 200 ml/min, access recirculation of 12% or greater, or an otherwise unexplained urea reduction ratio of <60%. Also, CMS will not pay for a duplex scan and a fistulogram unless documentation to medical necessity for both is provided. In this chapter, each method of dialysis access surveillance will be reviewed and a protocol using duplex ultrasonography to access function after construction and during chronic hemodialysis is proposed.

METHODS OF DIALYSIS ACCESS SURVEILLANCE

Access Recirculation

Recirculation within a hemodialysis access conduit is defined as dialyzed blood returning through the venous needle that re-enters the extracorporeal dialysis circuit through the arterial needle (Figure 37–1). Measured accurately, access recirculation does not occur unless the dialysis flow rate exceeds that of the access conduit.[9] Normal levels of access recirculation are felt to be less than 10% using the 2-needle urea measurement calculation, or less than 5% when ultrasonic dilution methods are used.[7] Calculation of recirculation percentage is possible by the measurement of blood urea nitrogen (BUN) concentration in the systemic circulation (U_s), arterial blood line (U_a), and venous blood line (Uv) using the formula:

$$\text{Urea recirculation} = \frac{U_s - U_a}{U_s - U_v} \times 100\%.$$

While urea recirculation values of greater than 15% at a dialysis flow rate of 400 ml/min have acceptable accuracy for identifying access conduits with stenoses,[10,11] threshold values predictive of access failure or need for revision have not been established. A value of 12% or greater correlates with low volume flow, which is the result

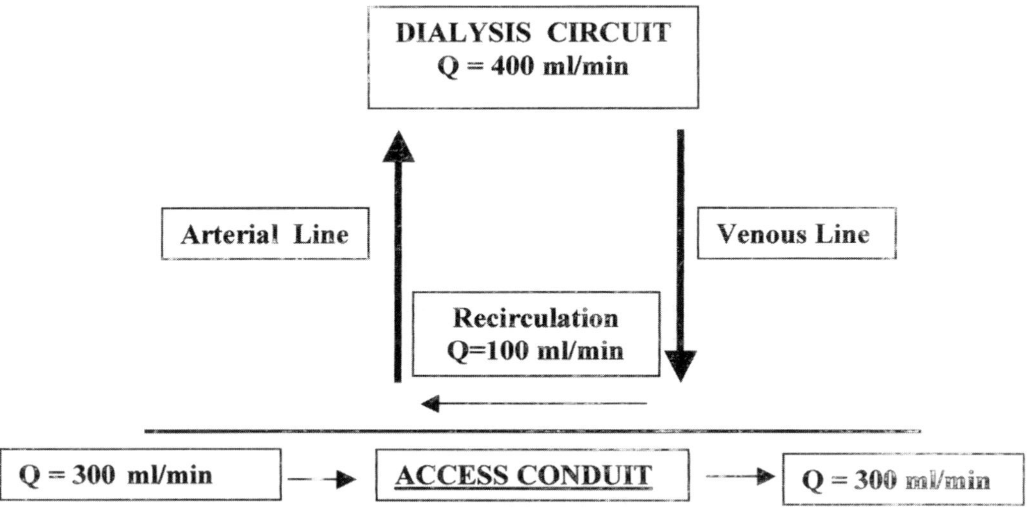

Figure 37–1. Recirculation diagram illustrating recirculation occurring when dialyzer flow exceeds fistula flow. Amount of recirculation can be calculated by measurement of blood urea nitrogen (BUN) levels from the arterial, venous lines, and systemic circulations.

of a developing stenosis. The measurement of access recirculation is not a preferred method for identifying a failing access conduit, but when used should be considered a screening test.[5,6,12–14]

Venous Line Pressure

Elevation of venous pressures measured in the drip chamber of the venous cannula downstream of the dialysis pump and membrane unit can occur with significant obstructions at the venous anastomosis or venous outflow. Since stenoses at these locations are a common cause for access conduit thrombosis, serial measurements of venous line pressures has been proposed to detect failing accesses. Accuracy of the pressure measurement is highly dependent on proper matching of the dynamic response of the catheter-transducer system, transducer zeroing relative to height differences in the system, and elimination of air bubbles or blood clots. Both static (measured with no dialyzer flow) and dynamic (with dialyzer flow) venous line pressures have been utilized. Normal values of dynamic venous pressure measurements vary with dialysis flow rate and are most reliable when flow rates are held constant at 200 ml/min for several minutes. The upper limits of normal for dynamic venous line pressure is less than 125 to 150 mmHg.[7] Static pressure measurements vary between individual patients, and the static/dynamic pressure ratio of the venous and arterial lines pressures vary between grafts and autogenous fistulae. The arterial ratios should normally be between 0.13–0.43 and 0.35–0.74 for autogenous fistulas and prosthetic bridge grafts respectively, and the venous ratios should be between 0.08 to 0.34 and 0.15 to 0.49 respectively.[7] It is important to remember that trends in the line pressures rather than absolute values are more predictive in an individual patient.

The reported diagnostic accuracy of venous line pressures to detect access stenoses or predict thrombosis vareis.[2,5,12–18] Dynamic venous pressures greater than 150 mmHg during 3 consecutive dialysis sessions achieved a 86% sensitivity and 93%

specificity for detection of >50% stenoses by fistulography within the access conduit or venous outflow.[15] The average dynamic venous pressure was significantly higher in patients with >50% DR angiographic stenosis (126 ± 35 mmHg) than in accesses without stenosis (95 ± 22 mmHg). Average static venous pressures were also significantly different between these 2 access groups (49 versus 26 mm Hg respectively).[17] However, serial[2,5,12] and single point13 measurement of dynamic venous pressures were not predictive of subsequent access stenosis or thrombosis in several prospective studies. Serial measurements of static venous pressure normalized by mean arterial pressure have identified PTFE grafts with subsequent thromboses but not with significant stenosis.[14,16] Based on these results, serial venous line pressure measurements facilitate detection of venous outlet stenoses but threshold values prompting further access evaluation are not well defined. In general, a dynamic venous line pressure >200 mm Hg at a dialysis flow rate of 200 ml/min should be considered abnormal and prompt imaging studies such as duplex ultrasound or fistulogram when high values are consistently recorded. Of note, venous line pressure measurements are not as reliable in evaluation of AVF function because of the potential development of collateral outflow veins not seen with prosthetic dialysis access grafts.[18] When venous pressure are consistently elevated the incidence of bridge graft thrombosis is 10 times great than an access with normal pressures. Dynamic pressures should be obtained weekly and are the least expensive form of access surveillance.

Contrast Fistulography

Dialysis access imaging by direct injection of iodinated contrast agents and digital subtraction angiography is considered the "gold standard" for detection of conduit stenosis. Grading of stenoses requires accurate measurement of narrowed lumens and comparison to adjacent, minimally diseased vessel or conduit segments. Stenoses of greater than 50% lumen diameter reduction are considered significant and should be considered for repair. Fistulography can also detect true and false aneurysms associated with arteriovenous hemodialysis conduits-lesions that increase thrombosis risk and should be repaired. Since contrast fistulography is invasive, expensive and has associated risks, it is not considered a surveillance method but rather should be reserved for evaluation of a documented failing access or for evaluation after thrombectomy. Its use should be avoided in patients with ESRD but not yet requiring dialysis to prevent acceleration of renal failure.

An important application of contrast fistulography is its use to monitor endovascular procedures such as catheter thrombolysis or thrombectomy, and transluminal balloon angioplasty. It is also the preferred technique for evaluation of the central (axillary, subclavian, brachiocephalic, superior vena cava) venous system for obstruction or stenotic lesions produced by prior venous catheter insertion.

Color Duplex Ultrasonography

Duplex ultrasound interrogation of dialysis accesses aims to directly identify stenotic or occluded segments within the arterial inflow, conduit, or venous outflow with precision similar to contrast fistulography. Color duplex imaging (CDI) can be done serially and is best performed by a trained vascular technologist. Recording of Doppler spectral waveforms, peak systolic and end diastolic velocities and qualitative assessment of focal disturbed flow conditions assist in identification and grading of stenoses.

Velocity waveforms within the access and venous outflow should reflect a high-flow, low outflow resistance flow condition characterized by peak systolic velocities of greater than 150–200 cm/s coupled with diastolic flow velocity values 40–60% of those during systole. Proper selection of the velocity scale set-up parameters is necessary to minimize potential aliasing artifacts and overestimation of stenosis.

Dialysis access stenosis is identified by real-time color or power Doppler imaging of >50% DR in the flow lumen, and at least doubling of the peak systolic velocity ratio compared with a normal adjacent graft segment. The presence of a tissue bruit by itself does not indicate a significant stenosis. Criteria for interpretation of duplex testing, including expected normal values and guidelines for access stenosis is listed in Table 37–1. In general, a >50% DR stenosis has duplex features of a PSV >400 cm/s, end-diastolic velocity >250 cm/sec, and residual lumen <2 mm in diameter.

The accuracy of duplex ultrasound for detection of access stenoses confirmed by contrast fistulography in the range of 80–90%, and has been documented by a number of authors.[19–24] Most studies used direct measurement of diameter reduction by B-mode and color flow imaging for identification of >50% stenoses. Tordoir et al., reporting in Doppler-derived frequency, elegantly defined different threshold values for >50% stenoses within bridge grafts, AVFs and venous outflow tract[23] that unfortunately have not been utilized elsewhere. Older et al. calculated a positive predictive value of 83% for the detection of >50% DR stenoses confirmed by fistulography were detected using a threshold PSV velocity greater than 400 cm/s or peak systolic velocity ratio greater than 3.[24] Despite an accuracy of >80% for detection of access stenoses, use of duplex surveillance to predict thrombosis is unproven. Presence of a greater than 70% reduction in cross-sectional area by duplex ultrasound has correlated with access thrombosis within 3 months. However, the detection of anatomic stenosis without concomitant measurement of access function is not helpful. In a large prospective study, Bay et al. found stenosis severity was not predictive of access failure.[13]

TABLE 37–1. INTERPRETATION GUIDELINES FOR COLOR DUPLEX ULTRASOUND TESTING (CPT 93990) OF DIALYSIS ACCESS GRAFTS AND FISTULAS.

Scan Interpretation	Recorded Velocity Spectra	Color Doppler Imaging
Normal	Arterial anastomosis >200 cm/sec Mid-graft >150 cm/sec	No conduit stenosis imaged; patent venous outflow
Moderate stenosis	Anastomosis >400 cm/sec Graft lesion >300 cm/sec Mid-graft 100–150 cm/sec	Decrease in lumen diameter; echogenic material within graft lumen; PSV ratio >2.5 at stenosis
Severe stenosis	Mid-graft velocity <100 cm/sec	Intraluminal echos; <2 mm residual lumen; >50% diameter reduction PSV ratio >3 at stenosis
Inflow stenosis	Anastomotic site: PSV >400 cm/sec	Focal lumen narrowing; <2 mm lumen at stenosis no velocity increase at venous outflow
Outflow stenosis	Arterial anastomosis: <300 cm/sec with decrease in graft velocity compared to baseline study. Focal increase in velocity >300 cm/sec	Lumen reduction in outflow veins
Occlusion	No Doppler signal	Intraluminal graft echos; occluded vein may be imaged

PSV, peak systolic velocity

Prophylactic endovascular treatment of anatomic stenoses within PTFE conduits also failed to improve access patency in a randomized, prospective study.[22] These results suggest that the presence of an access stenosis alone does not indicate impending access failure.

Duplex imaging of access grafts are useful for the diagnosis of abscess, hematoma or seroma by imaging fluid collections surrounding the prosthetic material. Aneurysms and pseudoaneurysms are readily detected by color flow imaging, and easily distinguished from hematoma by documenting the presence of flow. Small pseudoaneurysms (<5 mm diameter) caused by cannulation tend to remain stable while large pseudoaneurysms (>1 cm diameter) tend to enlarge and should be surgically repaired. Lumen thrombus can also be detected by duplex scanning and in general is a sign of access dysfunction and associated with access thrombosis.

Transit-time Ultrasonic Dilutional Access Volume Flow

Serial measurement of blood flow rates within functioning access grafts holds promise as the most accurate method for access surveillance, and newer ultrasonic dilution techniques have been used to estimate time-averaged blood flow rates. As the diameter of the vessel and time-averaged velocity can be determined ultrasonographically, volume flow can be calculated. An association between low access volume flow rates and risk of thrombosis has been demonstrated, but the relationship between presence of stensosis and conduit flow rates has not yet been fully defined. In general, a high-grade stenosis (<2 mm residual lumen, PSV >400 cm/sec, end-diastolic velocity >200 cm/sec) is required to reduce volume flow. It is felt that for therapeutic hemodialysis, access flow should exceed 600 ml/min. Changes in access flow are also important and when serial measurements, indicates reduction to <1000 ml/min over 4 months, imaging to identify a correctable lesions is appropriate.[7]

Measurement of access flow rates can be made during hemodialysis sessions using a recently described transit-time, ultrasonic dilution method.[25] Separate ultrasound transducers are placed on the arterial and venous dialysis tubing and the lines are reversed so that the arterial line is downstream of the venous line within the access conduit. The dialysis circuit flow is fixed at 200–300 mL/min and ultrafiltration turned off. Rapid injection of 5–10 ml of normal saline at body temperature into the venous line dilutes the red cell mass in blood flowing through the access and results in alteration of the Doppler-derived velocity waveform recorded by the arterial line transducer. The measured areas under the perturbed velocity versus time curve at the venous (S_v) and arterial (S_a) lines and the known dialyzer flow rate (Q_b) allow calculation of the access flow rate by the relation:

$$Q = Q_b \left(\frac{S_v}{S_a} - 1 \right).$$

Accuracy of the access flow calculation appears independent of dialyzer flow rates between 177 and 350 mL/min but requires careful positioning of the arterial needle within the centerstream of the access flow. Two or 3 access flow measurements should be made for reproducibility as the error between consecutive measurements averages 5%.[26] Clinical comparison of ultrasound dilution and Doppler-derived flow rate measurements have yielded acceptable agreement (correlation coefficients 0.79–0.83) over a wide range of access flow rates.[12,25] The ultrasound dilution technique does not tend to over- or underestimate flow rates except in accesses with stenosis; where dilution measurements are typically were lower than those obtained by duplex-derived measurements. This method is not routinely used in most dialysis centers, however it is the preferred method for dialysis access surveillance in the DOQI guidelines. As with other indirect surveillance techniques, an abnormal study identifies the access at risk for failure but indicate when and what type of intervention should be performed.

Volume Flow Measurements Using Duplex Ultrasonography

Duplex-derived conduit flow rates can be serially measured after access construction and are not subject to the measurements errors produced by the hemodynamic changes induced hemodialysis. Because of potential sources of measurement, the test is best performed in the accredited vascular laboratory by a trained technologist. Volume flow rate is calculated by the relation:

$$Q = v\,A = v\,\frac{(\pi\,d^2)}{4}$$

where v is time- and spatially-averaged velocity over the lumen cross-section, d and A are the lumen diameter and cross-sectional area at the site of velocity measurement respectively. Flow calculations are possible using software packages in most high-resolution duplex ultrasound units. Assumptions made in these calculations are that flow is minimally disturbed, axial-symmetric, and the lumen cross-section is circular.

Technical performance of duplex derived flow rates utilizes velocity measurements obtained at 3 or 4 locations along the access graft, typically 3–4 vessel diameters distal to the arterial anastomosis, mid-graft, and 3–4 diameters proximal to the venous anastomosis. The access volume flow rate is the average of the measured flow rates (Figure 37–2). Flow measurements are made at sites where no lumen narrowing or highly disturbed color Doppler flow is imaged. Accurate B-mode ultrasound cross-sectional measurement of lumen diameter must be made with the transducer oriented

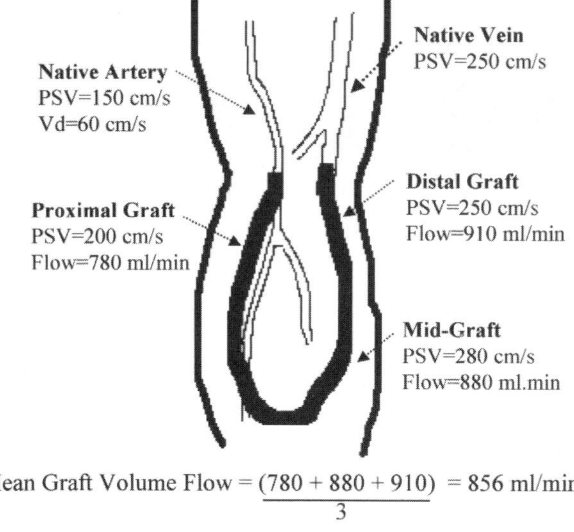

Figure 37–2. Schematic showing typical duplex values of peak systolic velocity (PSV) and volume flow recorded from a 6 mm diameter forearm loop bridge dialysis access graft. The mean access volume is the average of the 3 flow measurements recorded from proximal, middle, and distal bridge graft.

perpendicular to the long axis of the conduit. Pulsed wave Doppler insonation of the flow center-stream at an angle of 60 degrees is imperative with time averaging of the velocity waveform over 3–5 cardiac cycles (Figure 37–3). The pulsed-Doppler sample volume should be enlarged to encompass the entire flow lumen. Validation of duplex-derived volume flow measurements have been performed experimentally with good correlations at flow rates between 200–1000 ml/min.[27] The variability of the flow measurement is ± 30%.

Low access flow rates are strongly predictive of limited conduit patency in PTFE bridge grafts as shown by multiple studies.[12,13,27–31] Thrombosis risk increases greatly with falling bridge graft flows whether measured by duplex or ultrasound dilution techniques. The association between flow rate and patency of AVFs is not as strong as for prosthetic bridge grafts since lower flow rates may support autologous conduit patency. Lower access flow rates are also predictive of patent conduits with stenoses in several studies.[16,17,27] Flow rates were significantly less in conduits with stenoses than measured in functioning conduits with maintained stenosis-free patency

Controversy exists regarding the threshold access volume flow that should prompt intervention or additional imaging studies such as contrast fistulography. Based on current retrospective and uncontrolled prospective data, PTFE bridge grafts with access flow rates below 700–800 mL/min and reduced velocities in the afferent brachial artery <90 cm/sec should be imaged with contrast fistulography.[12,13] Similarly, measured flow rates less then 400 mL/min in AVFs should prompt angiographic assessment. Optimal intervals for surveillance measurement of access flow

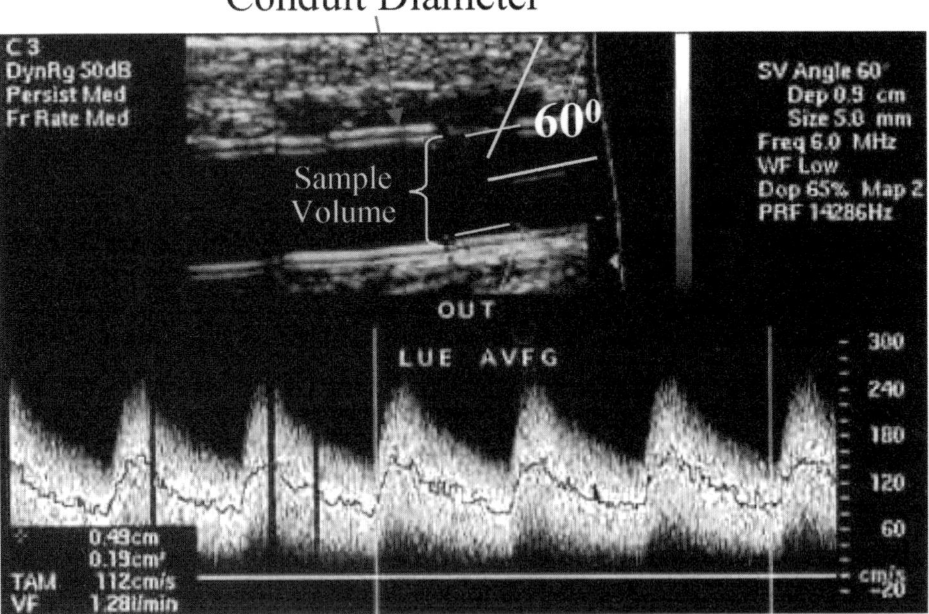

Figure 37–3. Technique of volume flow measurement using duplex ultrasonography. Conduit is imaged at a site of no stenosis and uniform diameter. Diameter is measured and the pulsed Doppler sample volume adjusted to size of the lumen. Time-averaged velocity spectra is recorded at a 60-degree Doppler beam angle and volume flow calculated based on 3 pulse cycles.

rates have not been specified and may differ with access type and graft diameters. As access failure is most common during the first postoperative year, surveillance at 2- or 3-month intervals may be required. A baseline evaluation at the time of dialysis access maturation, i.e. prior to use for hemodialysis, is recommended (Figure 37–4). This study will verify if the volume flow is adequate for hemodialysis (flow >400 ml/min) and identify if an access stenosis is present. A repeat duplex study after 4 weeks of dialysis is recommended to document any changes in volume flow, and identify any problems caused by repeated cannulation. Subsequent duplex surveillance is performed at 2–3 months intervals depending on the results of prior testing. An advantage of this approach is that duplex surveillance can detect progressive stenosis that produces reduction in volume flow, and based on CDI, focal lesions suitable for endovascular balloon angioplasty are identified.

Duplex Surveillance of Dialysis Access—The USF Experience

We have used duplex surveillance to evaluate dialysis access graft hemodynamics prior to cannulation and identify progressive high-grade stenosis that produce a reduction in access volume flow. These "hemodyanmically significant" access stenosis are repaired and changes in access hemodynamics measured. At present there is little data to guide the clinician regarding the significance of access volume flow rates. It is known that flow rates of AVFs are less than prosthetic bridge grafts, but at what level should access revision be recommended has not been defined.

Using the surveillance algorithm depicted in Figure 37–4, duplex testing of all dialysis access procedures was performed prior to initial cannulation. In a consecutive series of 100 patients with autogenous (n = 56) or prosthetic (n = 44) dialysis access fistula, volume flow was measured and the access imaged for abnormalities. Duplex mapping of the upper extremity resulted in autogenous fistula construction in 56% of patients. At the graft maturation study, access conduits were divided into 2 groups of "normal conduits" n = 73 (no abnormalities and usable conduit), and "abnormal conduits" n = 27 (abnormality of stenosis or volume flow limitation, conduit unusable for

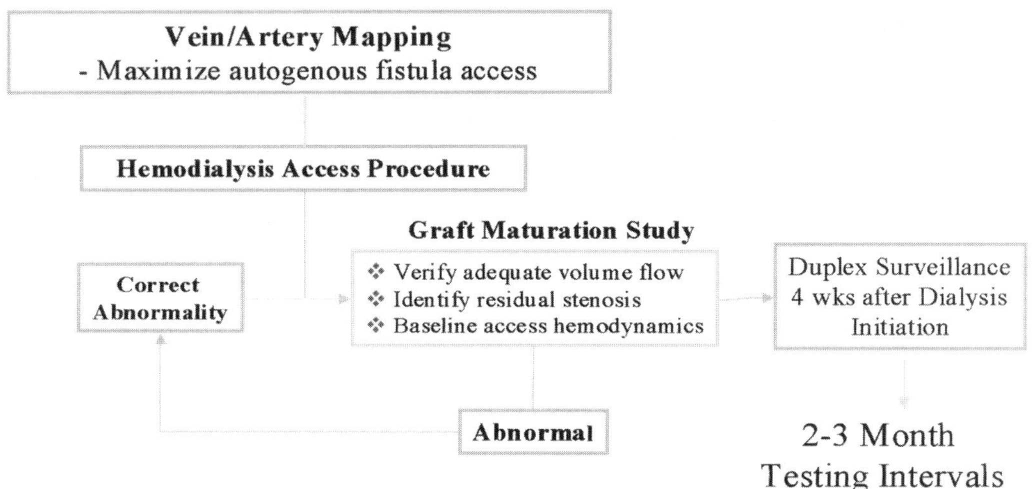

Figure 37–4. Use of duplex ultrasonography for vein-artery mapping to maximize autogenous fistula construction and access surveillance to verify adequate volume flow and development of access stenosis.

cannulation). Duplex values recorded from each group are shown in Tables 37–2 and 37–3. The mean access flow rates of "normal" in the lower arm were significantly lower than other more proximal fistulas and both forearm and arm PTFE bridge grafts. The values recorded serve as guides to expected flow rates. By comparison, volume flow rates PSV values were less (p<0.001) in "abnormal" access conduits. Based on these results, a volume flow of <500 ml/min for AVF or <800 ml/min for a PTFE bridge graft or basilic vein transposition is abnormal and the access should be imaged for a residual abnormality (inflow or outflow stenosis, anastomotic stenosis). The baseline value of volume flow is also important for comparison with subsequent serial studies, especially if an access stenosis has been detected. A PSV value of >150 cm/s is reliable indicator of adequate flow in a 6 mm prosthetic bridge graft.

Duplex surveillance has also been used to evaluate changes in access hemodynamics following revision for stenosis, inflow occlusive disease, or venous outflow abnormalities. Eleven patients with abnormal precanulation duplex scans (n = 10), or followed for decrease in volume flow in established conduits (n = 1) underwent single (n = 8) or multiple (n = 3) access revisions. The mean (± SEM) increase in volume flow

TABLE 37–2. DUPLEX-DERIVED VOLUME FLOW MEASUREMENT, ARTERIAL, AND PROXIMAL ANASTOMOSIS PEAK SYSTOLIC VELOCITY (PSV, CM/SEC) VALUES RECORDED PRIOR TO INITIAL CANNULATION FOR 73 "NORMAL" DIALYSIS ACCESS FISTULAS OR BRIDGE GRAFTS. VALUES EXPRESSED AS MEAN ± SEM.

Dialysis Access Type	No.	Flow Volume (ml/min)	Conduit PSV	Arterial Anastomosis PSV
Radiocephalic AVF	15	1093 ± 100	306 ± 76	526 ± 40
Brachiocephalic AVF	15	1589 ± 130	40 ± 77	455 ± 36
Basilic vein transposition	8	1855 ± 309	68 ± 104	435 ± 63
Forearm vein transposition	2	1046 ± 271	188 ± 42	418 ± 87
Forearm PTFE (6 mm)	16	1516 ± 120	40 ± 26	437 ± 40
Arm PTFE (6 mm)	13	1494 ± 199	216 ± 50	417 ± 53
Thigh PTFE (6 mm)	2	1040 ± 150	240 ± 31	319 ± 35

p <.001 for radiocephalic AVF volume flow rates versus other dialysis access types using Student's t-test of means
ANOVA analysis for variance between groups was significant, p = .035

TABLE 37–3. DUPLEX-DERIVED VOLUME FLOW MEASUREMENT, ARTERIAL, AND ARTERIAL ANASTOMOSIS PEAK SYSTOLIC VELOCITY (PSV, CM/SEC) VALUES RECORDED PRIOR TO INITIAL CANNULATION FROM 26 "ABNORMAL" DIALYSIS ACCESS CONDUITS WITH A DUPLEX IDENTIFIED STENOSIS.

Fistula Type	No.	Flow Volume (ml/min)	Conduit PSV(cm/s)	Arterial Anastomotic PSV (cm/s)
Radiocephalic AVF	9	458 ± 53	316 ± 73	469 ± 60
Brachiocephalic AVF	1	511	378	90
Basilic vein transposition	1	304	574	285
Forearm vein transposition	2	663 ± 318	119 ± 3	361 ± 194
Forearm PTFE graft	11	808 ± 84	119 ± 22	396 ± 58
Arm PTFE graft	1	609	133	221
Thigh PTFE	1	573	74	245

ANOVA analysis for variance between groups, p = 0.11

following 523 ± 423 ml/min (range: 400 to 1500 ml/min). The types of access revision included repair of an inflow anastomosis stenosis (n = 7), balloon angioplasty (n = 4), jump graft to more proximal outflow (n = 3), and formation new access (n = 2). All interventions except 1 produced an increase in volume flow and a usable conduit for hemodialysis.

CLINICAL APPLICATION OF DIALYSIS ACCESS SURVEILLANCE

Implementation of routine surveillance of dialysis access to facilitate identification of the "failing graft" coupled with prophylactic revision has been associated with variable efficacy. Several prospective studies have documented a significant decrease in number of thrombotic events and increased conduit patency with elective surgical or endovascular intervention of duplex- or angiographic-identified tenosis.[32-34] But, a randomized, prospective study conducted by Lumsden et al.[23] failed to demonstrate prolonged PTFE conduit patency in patients receiving prophylactic PTA of >50% DR duplex-detected stenosis compared to observation alone. These differences in surveillance outcome are due to multiple factors: difference in study design (i.e. characteristics of the control group), surveillance techniques used, and threshold criteria for intervention, and assessment of adequacy of the intervention. Benefit from elective intervention is likely to occur primarily with correction of access stenosis that is progressive and hemodynamically significant (i.e. accompanied by low access flow rate, increased venous line pressure or elevated access recirculation). Since the presence of stenoses is relatively common (prevalence of 20–30%) in adequately functioning conduits, it is not surprising that the presence of a stenosis by itself does not correlate with thrombotic failure. While the use of duplex ultrasonography without flow volume measurement can accurately detect an anatomic stenosis, interpretation of severity remains somewhat non-specific if only PSV values are used. The addition of volume flow measurement should facilitate identifying the "failing" access at increased risk for thrombosis.

Based on available data, routine surveillance of dialysis access procedure appears warranted. The "best" algorithm for access surveillance remains to be developed, including details regarding prescribed intervals of testing relative to dialysis access type, what hemodynamic parameters should be measured, and when is intervention warranted. Currently, we recommend baseline evaluation at the time of graft maturation utilizing color duplex ultrasonography with calculation of volume flow rate. Subsequent duplex evaluations at 3-month intervals are reasonable based on prior experience acquired from lower limb bypass graft surveillance. More frequent testing would be appropriate for dialysis access grafts that exhibit problems during dialysis, i.e. low flow, or have developed abnormal venous line pressures or increase urea recirculation percentages.

Access imaging combined with the calculation of volume flow by duplex ultrasound techniques should be the primary surveillance method for PTFE bridge grafts and autologous AVFs. When flow rates fall below 600 mL/min for PTFE grafts and 400 mL/min for AVFs, contrast fistulography should be considered unless duplex imaging clearly identifies a significant graft or anastomotic stenosis. Flow rates in the range of 500–800 mL/min in PTFE conduits may indicate an increased thrombosis risk and should prompt an evaluation for stenosis by duplex ultrasonography, or alternatively directly by fistulography if high quality duplex testing is not available. If measurements of access volume flow are not possible or prove to be unreliable, the vascular surgeon should intervene when a progressive duplex-identified stenosis with velocity spectra consistent with a critical stenosis (PSV>400 cm/sec, EDV >250 cm/sec, velocity ratio >3, mid graft velocity <150 cm/sec, residual lumen <2 mm diameter) is identified. These lesions typically demonstrate >60% DR on angiography and when verified elective surgical or endovascular treatment is appropriate. An important feature of a surveillance program is confirmation of improved access flow rate and hemodynamic correction of access stenosis after intervention. This assessment is best performed utilizing inter-procedural duplex ultrasonography.

The proposed surveillance algorithm of hemodialysis access requires validation by a prospective, randomized trial designed to determine if duplex surveillance and repair of identified stenoses prolongs access functional patency, and is associated with a reduction of health care costs. At present, routine duplex surveillance of access grafts or fistulas has not been approved for payment by the Center for Medicare Services and thus other health insurers.

REFERENCES

1. Hodges TC, Fillinger MF, Zwolak RM, et al. Longitudinal comparisons of dialysis access methods: risk factors for failure. *J Vasc Surg.* 1997;26:1009–1019.
2. Cinat ME, Hopkins J, Wilson SE. A prospective evaluation of PTFE graft patency and surveillance techniques in hemodialysis access. *Ann Vasc Surg.* 1999;13:191–198.
3. Mills JL, Bandyk DF, Gahtan V, et al. The origin of infrainguinal vein graft stenosis: a prospective study based on duplex surveillance. *J Vasc Surg.* 1995;21:16–22.
4. Palder SB, Kirkman RL, Wittemore AD, et al. Vascular access for hemodialysis: patency rates and results of revision. *Ann Surg.* 1985;202:235–239.
5. Strauch BS, O'Connell RS, Geoly KL, et al. Forecasting thrombosis of vascular access with Doppler color flow imaging. *Am J Kidney Dis.* 1992;19:554–557.
6. Sands JJ, Miranda CL. Prolongation of hemodialysis access survival with elective revision. *Clin Nephrol.* 1995;44:329–333.
7. National Kidney Foundation. K/DOQI Clinical practice guidelines for vascular access, 2000. *Am J Kidney Dis.* 2001 (suppl 1);37:S137–S181.
8. Beathard GA. Percutaneous transvenous angioplasty in the treatment of vascular access stenosis. *Kidney Int.* 1992;42:1390–1397.
9. Back MR, Bandyk DF. Current status of surveillance of hemodialysis access grafts. *Ann Vasc Surg.* 2001;15:491–502.
10. Besarab A, Sherman R. The relationship of recirculation to access blood flow. *Am J Kidney Dis.* 1997;29:223–229.
11. Windus DW, Audrain J, Vanderson R, et al. Optimization of high-efficiency hemodialysis by detection and correction of fistula dysfunction. *Kidney Int.* 1990;38:337–341.
12. Daniels ID, Berlyne GM, Barth RH. Blood flow rates and accesses recirculation in hemodialysis. *Int J Artif Organs.* 1992;15:470–474.
13. May RE, Himmelfarb J, Yenicesu M, et al. Predictive measures of vascular access thrombosis: A prospective study. *Kidney Int.* 1997;52:1656–1662.
14. Bay WH, Henry ML, Lazarus JM, et al. Predicting hemodialysis access failures with color flow Doppler ultrasound. *Am J Nephrol.* 1998;18:296–304.
15. Besarab A, Lubkowski T, Frinak S, et al. Detection of access strictures and outlet stenoses in vascular accesses: Which test is best? *ASAIO J.* 1997;43:543–547.
16. Schwab SJ, Raymond JR, Saeed M, et al. Prevention of hemodialysis fistula thrombosis: early detection of venous stenoses. *Kidney Int.* 1989;36:707–711.
17. Besarab A. Lubkowski T, Frinak S, Ramanathan S, Escobar F. Detecting vascular access dysfunction. *ASAIO J.* 1997;43:M539–M543.
18. Bosman PJ, Boereboom FTJ, Smits HFM, et al. Pressure or flow recordings for the surveillance of hemodialysis grafts. *Kidney Int.* 1997;52:1084–1088.

19. Besarab A, Sullivan KL, Ross RP, Moritz MJ: Utility of intra-access pressure monitoring in detecting and correcting venous outlet stenoses prior to thrombosis. *Kidney Int.* 1995;47:1364–1373.
20. Middleton WD, Picus DD, Marx MV, et al. Color Doppler sonography of hemodialysis vascular access: comparison with angiography. *AJR.* 1989;152:633–639.
21. Dousset V, Grenier N, Douws C, et al. Hemodialysis grafts: color Doppler flow imaging correlated with digital subtraction angiography and functional status. *Radiology.* 1991;181: 89–94.
22. MacDonald MJ, Martin LG, Hughes JD, et al. Distribution and severity of stenoses in functioning arteriovenous grafts: A duplex and angiographic study. *J Vasc Technol.* 1996;20: 131–136.
23. Lumsden AB, MacDonald MJ, Kikeri D, et al. Prophylactic balloon angioplasty fails to prolong the patency of PTFE arteriovenous grafts: Results of a prospective randomized study. *J Vasc Surg.* 1997;24:382–392.
24. Tordoir JHM, deBruin HG, Hoeneveld H, et al. Duplex ultrasound scanning in the assessment of arteriovenous fistulas created for hemodialysis access: comparison with digital subtraction angiography. *J Vasc Surg.* 1989;10:122–128.
25. Older RA, Gizienski TA, Wilkowski MJ, et al. Hemodialysis access stenosis: early detection with color Doppler ultrasound. *Radiology.* 1998;207:161–164.
26. Depner TA, Krivitski NM . Clinical measurement of blood flow in hemodialysis access fistulae and graft by ultrasound dilution. *ASAIO J.* 1995;41:M745–M749.
27. Zierler BK, Kirkman TR, Kraiss LW, et al. Accuracy of duplex scanning for measurement of arterial volume flow. *J Vasc Surg.* 1992;16:520–526.
28. Sands J, Glidden D. Miranda C. Hemodialysis access flow measurement: comparison of ultrasound dilution and duplex ultrasonography. *ASAIO J.* 1996;42:M899–M901.
29. Rittgers SE, Garcia-Valdez C, McCormick JT, et al. Noninvasive blood flow measurement in expanded PTFE grafts for hemodialysis access. *J Vasc Surg.* 1986;3:635–642.
30. Shackleton CR, Taylor DC, Buckley AR, et al. Predicting failure in PTFE vascular access grafts for hemodialysis: a pilot study. *Can J Surg.* 1987;30:442–444.
31. Sands J, Young S, Miranda C. The effect of Doppler flow screening studies and elective revisions on dialysis access failure. *ASAIO J.* 1992;38:M524–M527.
32. Johnson CP, Zhu Y, Matt C, et al. Prognostic value of intraoperative blood flow measurements in vascular access surgery. *Surgery.* 1998;124:729–738.
33. Brooks JL, Sigley RD, May RJ Jr, et al. Transluminal angioplasty versus surgical repair for stenosis of hemodialysis grafts: A randomized study. *Am J Surg.* 1987;153: 530–531.
34. Dapunt O, Feurstein M, Rendl KH, et al. Transluminal angioplasty versus conventional operation in the treatment of hemodialysis fistula stenosis: Results from a 5-year study. *Br J Surg.* 1987;74:1004–1005.

38

Hemodialysis Access

Britt H. Tonnessen, MD, Michael S. Conners, III, MD, and Samuel R. Money, MD, FACS, MBA

The growing population of patients with end-stage renal disease challenges the vascular surgeon to provide the most durable hemodialysis access possible. Between 1995 and 1999, there was a 7% annual increase in the total number of hemodialysis patients, with patients 65 years and older comprising 50% of the total hemodialysis population.[1] Minimizing morbidity through well-planned access procedures is important in this aging population. Techniques such as vein mapping eliminate much of the guesswork in choosing an appropriate site for access creation. Monitoring for graft dysfunction additionally benefits patients by allowing for early intervention in failing accesses. However, the ideal method for monitoring as well as the timing and type of intervention is still controversial. In the presence of appropriate anatomy, the creation of an arteriovenous fistula (AVF) for access should always be sought, given the lower risk for infection and better long-term patency results. However, achieving this goal is not always easy. We feel that achieving primary AVF placement is largely dependent on early referral to the vascular surgeon, liberal usage of duplex scan vein mapping, and the versatility of the surgeon.

PREOPERATIVE "VEIN MAPPING"

Duplex ultrasonography of upper extremity veins or "vein mapping" is a useful tool in planning access procedures. In many institutions, ultrasound mapping has replaced venography as the test of choice for evaluation of upper extremity venous anatomy. In addition to the noninvasive determination of vein size, venous duplex imaging is helpful in identifying central venous stenosis or occlusion. This information is particularly important in patients who have had central venous catheters. Passman and colleagues have reported color flow duplex imaging to be as high as 81% sensitive and 97% specific in the detection of central venous stenosis, and in most cases can replace venography as the initial test of choice in evaluating the central venous system.[2]

Clinical characteristics that are felt to be relative indications for obtaining preoperative vein mapping are the absence of a readily palpable vein, a prior history of multiple intravenous or central lines, arm edema, a previous access procedure, the presence of collateral vein development, and obesity. Some surgeons advocate routine vein mapping,[3,4] but unfortunately cost-effectiveness and reimbursement issues have limited this approach. We estimate that over 80% of our patients who undergo access procedures receive vein mapping prior to operation.

Our vascular lab utilizes a linear wide aperture 5–12 MHz probe (Advanced Technologies Lab, Bothell, Washington) to evaluate the diameter and compressibility of the superficial veins from the wrist to the axilla bilaterally. A suitable vein is felt to have a diameter be at least 2.0 mm for a wrist fistula, 2.5 mm for a forearm fistula[3] and 3 mm for an upper arm fistula.[5] The non-dominant arm is selected unless there is a substantially larger vein in the dominant arm.

Routine vein mapping aids with operative planning but may also improve outcomes. In a series of 108 patients, Silva found that 53% of AVFs were created based on vein mapping in patients who otherwise would not have received an AVF based on physical exam alone.[3] Of note, the majority were upper arm arteriovenous fistulas (UAFs) or forearm transpositions rather than the traditional distal radiocephalic (Cimino) fistulas. Robbin noticed as well that vein mapping changed the operative plan in nearly one-third of cases.[6] The selection of the "best" veins for access by preoperative vein mapping may benefit patients by reducing primary failure rates (failure of fistula maturation) and improving long-term patency. In Silva's study, the primary failure rate decreased from 36% to 8% whereas the 12-month primary patency rate increased from 48% to 83% after the institution of routine preoperative vein mapping.[3] Despite these encouraging statistics, others have been unable to demonstrate similar outcomes.[4] Nevertheless, routine vein mapping potentially increases by up to 50% the rate of AVF creation, consequently increasing the population of patients who dialyze with an AVF.[3,4,6]

PRIMARY ACCESS STRATEGIES

For first-time access the patient with end stage renal disease should receive an AVF whenever possible. The Dialysis Outcome Quality Initiative (DOQI) guidelines recommend that 50% of all new access procedures be AVFs rather than synthetic arteriovenous grafts (AVGs) and that 40% of patients in any given dialysis unit have a functional AVF.[7] AVFs offer 2 principal advantages over AVGs: durability and low infection risk. The primary patency rate of AVFs, defined as continued use without secondary intervention, ranges from 56–85% at one year and 40%–54% at 2 years. These figures exceed the primary patency rates for AVGs by up to 36%.[5,8,9] However, secondary patency rates may be similar for AVFs and AVGs.[8,9]

A distal forearm radiocephalic (Cimino) fistula is the procedure of choice in the ideal patient with a thin arm, suitable cephalic vein at the wrist, and a negative Allen's test in the non-dominant arm. However, this patient is usually the exception to the rule. More commonly, if vein mapping can demonstrate adequate cephalic vein in the upper arm, it is our preference to perform a brachiocephalic fistula in the antecubital region. For the brachiocephalic fistula, we typically make an incision several centimeters distal to the antecubital crease and perform an end-to-side anastomosis. Occasionally, the median cubital vein (Figure 38–1) or its perforating branch is used

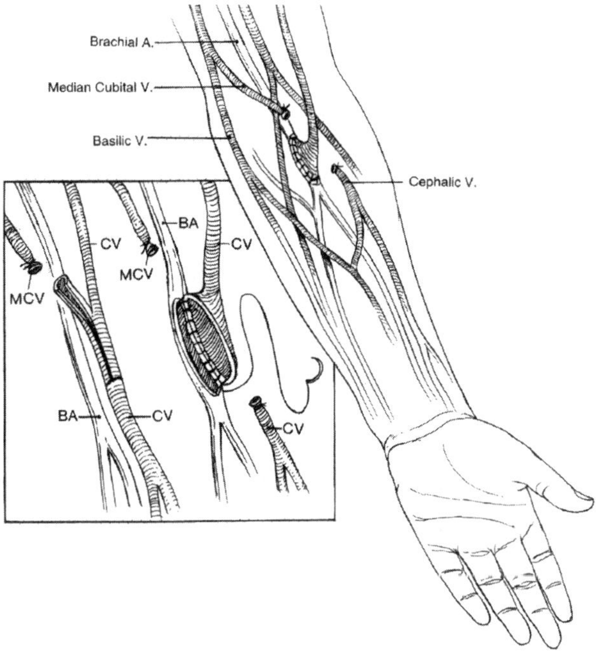

Figure 38–1 Brachiocephalic fistula, an upper arm fistula (UAF), performed distal to the antecubital crease utilizing a portion of the median cubital vein for the anastomosis.

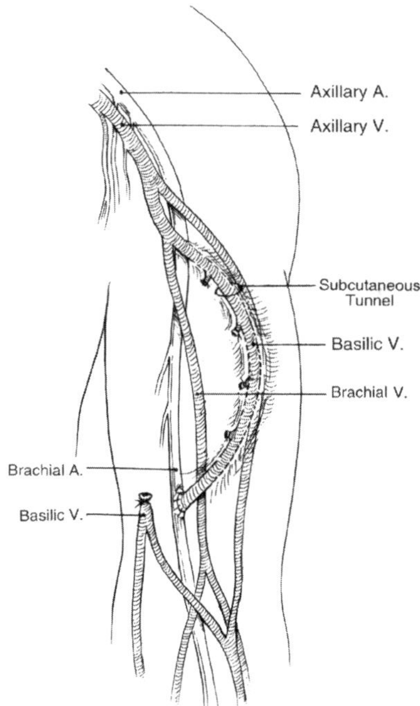

Figure 38–2. Basilic vein transposition is performed through an upper arm incision. Mobilized vein with ligated tributaries is "transposed" or tunneled through the subcutaneous tissues of the anterior arm and anastomosed to the brachial artery.

for the anastomosis. For first time accesses, these brachiocephalic fistulas may have better patency rates than wrist AVFs. In one report by Dixon and colleagues, the 1 year patency rate for upper arm fistulas (UAFs) was 71%. Their findings compared favorably to the 54% 1 year patency rates experienced by forearm AVFs which demonstrated similar patency rates to AVGs. At 5 years this advantage continued, with UAFs having 21% better patency compared with forearm AVFs (57% vs. 36%).[10]

Whereas thrombosis and infection are the main causes of AVG loss, non-maturation is the Achilles heel of AVFs. Non-maturation, also known as "primary failure," refers to failure of the vein to dilate to an appropriate diameter for cannulation within a period of 3 to 4 months after AVF creation. Primary failure may occur in 9% to 70% of fistulas, and may vary depending on gender, diabetes, and site of placement.[5,8,11,12] There appears to be no significant difference in the non-maturation rate when comparing distal forearm (Cimino) AVFs with UAFs.[5,10] The exception may be in diabetics, as Hakaim demonstrated a remarkably high 70% primary failure rate of Cimino fistulas in this population compared with a 0–27% primary failure rate for UAFs.[12] The DOQI guidelines do not dictate an acceptable percentage for primary failure in order to promote an ultimate goal: increasing the number of autogenous accesses.

Certain patient characteristics may affect the primary failure and long-term patency rates for AVFs. Women may have an increased risk for primary failure,[8,9] although this is not a consistent finding.[10,11] It is possible that average smaller vein size in women biases towards fistula failure. Diabetes may negatively affect AVF maturation and long-term patency rates, particularly for forearm fistulas.[8,11 12] The physiologic reasons for poor results in diabetics are not clear, although diseased radial arteries are thought to play a role. The effect of insulin-dependent versus non-insulin dependent diabetes on fistula outcomes is still being investigated. Upper arm fistulas, created with larger veins and less calcified arteries, may be a better choice in women and diabetics needing a first time access procedure. The effects of age, race and other co-morbid illnesses on AVF maturation and patency are less clear, although one study examining a large database of dialysis patients found that African Americans may have an increased risk of primary failure.[9]

The overall AVF creation rate increased 35% while temporary catheter insertion rate decreased 18% between 1996 and 1999.[1] In parallel with the enthusiasm for AVFs over AVGs, basilic vein transposition as a primary or secondary access procedure has increased in popularity (Figure 38–2). In contrast to the cephalic vein, the basilic vein's deeper location in the upper arm requires its "transposition" to a more superficial location in order to create an AVF. Dagher first described basilic vein transposition in 1976.[13] One year patency rates of greater than 70% compare favorably with brachiocephalic fistulas.[11,14] In examining the long-term results of basilic vein transposition, an impressive 52% patency rate at 10 years has been noted.[15] Despite concerns that creating a higher-flow AVF in the upper arm could increase the incidence of steal, an overall less than 3% incidence has been found for brachiocephalic fistulas.[10] Results vary on the incidence of steal for basilic vein transpositions, with frequencies of 2% to 15% reported.[11,14,15] The 15% incidence of steal with basilic vein transposition occurred in a "higher risk" population in which the majority of cases were not first time accesses.[14]

MONITORING ACCESS FUNCTION

Since the availability of access sites is limited, prolonged use of each site is desirable. Nephrologists have devised numerous methods for monitoring access dysfunction,

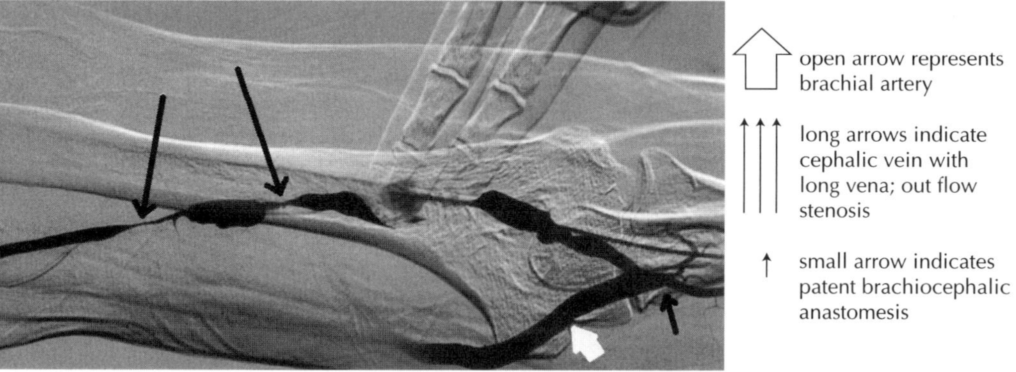

Figure 38–3A Fistulogram of a brachiocephalic fistula demonstrates a long venous outflow stenosis and patent arterial anastomosis. Fistula was revised by transposition of a sizable basilic vein.

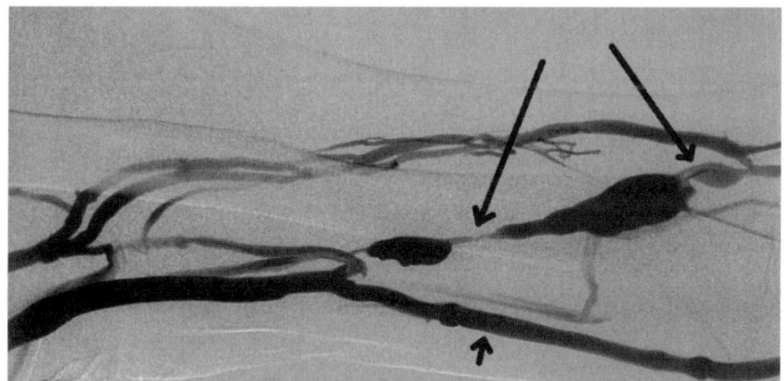

Figure 38–3B. Fistulogram of a brachiocephalic fistula demonstrates a long venous outflow stenosis and patent arterial anastomosis. Fistula was revised by transposition of a sizable basilic vein.

with the aim of intervention prior to thrombosis. Early dysfunction is more difficult to detect in AVFs than AVGs with the available technology. Furthermore, given the high rate of AVG thrombosis, a large proportion of monitoring efforts centers on AVGs. The simplest but least specific method of evaluation is the physical examination. A diminished thrill, intensified bruit, difficult cannulation, or increased pulsatility of the AVG may all be warning signs for impending thrombosis. A decrease in dialysis clearance as calculated by Kt/V (K= dialyzer clearance, t = time, V = urea distribution volume) may be a late sign of access dysfunction. During hemodialysis, the abnormal mixing of blood between the arterial and venous access sites in the presence of outflow stenosis may occur. This "recirculation" may be measured by either the urea recirculation method or the saline dilution method. A urea recirculation greater than 10–15% is usually touted as significant for evaluation, but again is usually a late sign of graft dysfunction.[7]

More sensitive methods of monitoring for access dysfunction include measuring venous pressure (Vp), either as a static value or as a dynamic part of the dialysis circuit. Rising Vp may herald graft thrombosis. Dynamic Vp is the simplest method for monitoring. On the other hand, dynamic Vp is subject to deviation related to tubing and needle size, blood pressure, and the type of dialysis machine. Dynamic Vp

>150–250 mmHg (depending on pump speed but typically 200–400 ml/min) has been used as a guideline for possible stenosis.[8,16] Static Vp, which requires specialized equipment, is measured at zero pump flow and should be divided by the mean arterial pressure to account for blood pressure differences. Static Vp is significant if the ratio exceeds 0.5.[16] An upward trend in either dynamic or static Vp is also important and measurements exceeding the baseline by threefold are significant.[7]

Access flow (Qa) is another method for monitoring access function which has been found to be equivalent in detecting hemodynamically significant stenoses when compared with Vp measurements in AVGs.[16] Qa <600–800 ml/min is considered an indicator of significant AVG dysfunction.[7,8,16] Measurements of Qa can be obtained by Doppler flow, magnetic resonance flow, or ultrasound dilution (the latter can be performed during dialysis). The prohibitive cost of routine Doppler flow measurement of Qa will likely prevent widespread use of this technique.[17] Directed intervention based upon abnormal Vp or Qa can decrease the rate of thrombosis events per patient year by over 50%.[16] The vast majority of graft stenoses occur at the venous outflow limb. However, Qa may be a more sensitive indicator of the less frequently found arterial limb or midgraft stenoses not evident by Vp or Kt/V measurements.[10,17]

ACCESS SALVAGE AND REVISION

In the failing or thrombosed access, numerous methods of salvage by a secondary procedure may be employed. With an average 18-month lifespan for AVGs, secondary procedures become an important part of "extending the life" of the graft without exhausting potential access sites. Since monitoring for access dysfunction will hopefully result in early identification of failing accesses, the question becomes "When and what type of intervention offers the most benefit for the least risk and cost?"

Endovascular interventions have been compared to surgical treatments for thrombosed AV grafts in a randomized prospective trial.[18] In this study by Marston and colleagues, one group was treated with endovascular intervention consisting mostly of mechanical thrombectomy with angioplasty, with thrombolysis and angioplasty comprising less than 20% of the procedures. In the surgical group, 70% of the patients were treated with graft revision rather than thrombectomy alone. Overall, there was no difference between the endovascular and the surgical groups in the immediate success (>70%), but surgery improved long-term patency compared with endovascular interventions at endpoints of 6 months (34% vs. 11%) and 12 months (24% vs. 9%). From these data, it is clear that the majority of thrombosed grafts do not last more than a few months, despite intervention. Unlike arterial lesions, venous stenoses are notoriously elastic and therefore may not respond as well to balloon angioplasty, which may have accounted for the better results achieved in the surgical group. The advent of liberal stent usage for venous stenoses may affect these results. The cost of endovascular interventions compared with surgical management was very similar. Regardless of whether endovascular or surgical intervention is chosen, fistulograms should be routinely performed following thrombectomy, because the majority of thrombosed grafts have an identifiable underlying cause. Although the majority of underlying graft problems are outflow venous stenoses from isolated neointimal hyperplasia at the anastomosis, long venous outflow stenoses may be the cause of thrombosis in up to 30% of cases. Surgical revision may be particularly important when long-segment venous stenosis is the problem, as these lesions are rather refractory to balloon angioplasty.[18] The methods for surgical revision are varied, but usually a jump graft or patch angioplasty is employed. Our choice is usually a short jump graft. Balloon angioplasty has been compared with patch angioplasty as adjuvant therapies to surgical thrombectomy with similar results.[19] Neither endovascular nor surgical thrombectomy for thrombosed AVFs is very effective, but occasionally with creativity, the fistula can be revised.

Clearly these salvage procedures can extend the lifespan of most grafts for a short-term, and in a minority extend function longer term. Ideally graft thrombosis would be prevented. The DOQI guidelines suggest that intervention only be pursued in the presence of a >50% stenosis which is also hemodynamically significant. Technically, it is possible to use angioplasty to improve stenoses and the hemodynamics of afflicted grafts,[20] although this technical capability does not necessarily translate to long-term patency. When patients were divided into grades of stenoses (<30%, 30–50%, >50%) as seen by Duplex ultrasound, thromboses occurred most frequently in the 30–50% stenosis group.[17] Therefore the physiologic criteria rather than the degree of measured stenosis are of the utmost significance in determining the need for intervention. A reasonable goal for angioplasty is a 50% 6 months patency rate and for surgical revision a 50% 1 year patency rate.[7]

The use of prophylactic angioplasty for the treatment of stenosis >50%, as measured by Duplex and confirmed by angiography has been evaluated in a randomized prospective trial. When compared with observation, early intervention with prophylactic angioplasty did not result in significantly improved patency at 12 months (47% vs. 51%). Only 45% of these patients had a hemodynamically significant lesion as identified by elevated venous pressure. The authors concluded that angioplasty should not be used to prophylactically to treat stenoses which are not hemodynamically significant.[21]

AVFs may require a secondary procedure to treat non-maturation as well as hemodynamically significant stenoses. In one study, secondary procedures such as vein patches, interposition vein grafts, and transpositions for these AVFs resulted in a 10% increase in cumulative fistula patency with an overall 1 year patency of 78%.[22] The authors concluded that secondary procedures, when carefully selected, are an important step in maintaining functioning fistulas. The authors advocated early angiography to identify underlying lesions in fistulas which fail to mature by 4–6 weeks.

The cause of AVF non-maturation dictates the cure. Large branching veins visualized by fistulogram may require ligation in order to facilitate maturation of the fistula. Short venous anastomotic stenosis may be treated by angioplasty, but a jump graft with vein or synthetic graft may be more durable. Occasionally patients develop long venous outflow obstruction which may be revised with either an interposition graft or with transposition of a more suitable vein (Figure 38–3A and 3B).

Central venous stenosis or occlusion is a relatively frequent problem for dialysis patients, given the frequency with which central venous lines are employed. A variety of therapies may be used. In patients with hemodialysis access on the same side as a central stenosis, there is a substantial risk for thrombosis of that graft. Thrombolysis, with or without angioplasty and with or without stenting achieves 70% patency rates of the central vein at 2 years, but there is a progressive decline in patency thereafter.[23] Stents are primarily useful in "elastic" lesions, rather than strictures or longer lesions. Percutaneous transluminal angioplasty of central veins with stent placement achieves equivalent long-term patency compared with surgical bypass in dialysis patients.[24] We routinely stent these central venous lesions. We feel the elasticity of central veins makes this a useful adjuvant therapy.

EARLY REFERRAL

Early recognition of impending hemodialysis may affect the type of access that a patient first receives. Ideally, initiating dialysis with a catheter should be avoided whenever possible given the attendant risks of central vein stenosis, infection, and procedure-related complications. However, using a tunneled catheter in the internal jugular vein as a bridge while awaiting AVF maturation is preferable to placement of an AVG. The presence of a functional arteriovenous access rather than a catheter at the initiation of dialysis is directly related to early referral to a nephrologist, as well as to the vascular surgeon. Patients who are referred to a nephrologist at least one month prior to initiation of hemodialysis are three times more likely to use an arteriovenous access than those referred within one month.[25] Among patients with arteriovenous access, 45% of those patients referred as least 4 months prior to onset of dialysis had a functional AVF, compared to only 31% when referred within four months. Young age, male gender, and the absence of diabetes all increase the likelihood of receiving an AVF for first functional access.[25]

The Healthy Start Clinic at the Ochsner Clinic Foundation is a program designed for the early education and treatment of the patient with renal insufficiency (J.S. Lindberg, M.D., unpublished data, March 2002). Specifically, patients with a creatinine >3.0 and/or expected time to dialysis of 6–12 months are included. The program focuses on patient education and initiates contact with a nephrologist, nurse educator, dietician and social worker. 49% of patients in the Healthy Start Clinic initiated dialysis with pre-existing arteriovenous accesses, compared with 23% in patients at our institution who were not enrolled. Of patients with arteriovenous access placed prior to initiation of dialysis, Healthy Start patients had a higher rate of AVF placement compared with non-Healthy Start patients (74% vs. 38%). These data exceed the 50% AVF placement recommendation by the DOQI. The Healthy Start program has increased our rate of AVF usage for dialysis initiation by nearly five times.

Hemodialysis access is a routine but often challenging part of most vascular surgeons' practices. Utilizing available techniques to increase the proportion of fistula placement and to optimize graft durability are important goals. Early intervention based on physiologically significant access dysfunction involves the cooperation and efforts of surgeons, nephrologists and interventionalists. Programs which strive for early referral of patients with renal insufficiency may play a large role in maximizing the number of patients who initiate dialysis with a functional autogenous access.

REFERENCES

1. U.S. Renal Data System, USRDS 2001 Annual Data Report: Atlas of End-Stage Renal Disease in the United States, National Institute of Health, National Institute of Diabetes and Digestive and Kidney Diseases, Bethesda, MD, 2001.
   Available at *http://www.usrds.org/atlas.htm*. Accessed May 1, 2002.
2. Passman MA, Criado E, Farber MA, et al. Efficacy of color flow duplex imaging for proximal upper extremity venous outflow obstruction in hemodialysis patients. *J Vasc Surg.* 1998;28:869–875.
3. Silva MB Jr, Hobson RW II, Pappas PJ, et al. A strategy for increasing use of autogenous hemodialysis access procedures: impact of preoperative noninvasive evaluation. *J Vasc Surg.* 1998;27:302–308.

4. Allon M, Lockhart ME, Lilly RZ, et al. Effect of preoperative sonographic mapping on vascular access outcomes in hemodialysis patients. *Kidney Int.* 2001;60:2013–2020.
5. Ascher E, Gade P, Hingorani A, et al. Changes in the practice of angioaccess surgery: impact of dialysis outcome and quality initiative recommendations. *J Vasc Surg.* 2000;31:84–92.
6. Robbin ML, Gallichio MH, Deierhoi MH, et al. US vascular mapping before hemodialysis access placement. *Radiology.* 2000;217; 83–88.
7. The Vascular Access Work Group. NKF-DOQI clinical practice guidelines for vascular access. *Am J Kidney Dis.* 1997;30(Suppl 3):S150–191.
8. Kalman PG, Pope M, Bhola C, et al. A practical approach to vascular access for hemodialysis and predictors of success. *J Vasc Surg.* 1999;30:727–733.
9. Gibson KD, Gillen DL, Caps MT, et al. Vascular access survival and incidence of revisions: a comparison of prosthetic grafts, simple autogenous fistulas, and venous transposition fistulas from the United States Renal Data System Dialysis Morbidity and Mortality Study. *J Vasc Surg.* 2001;34:694–700.
10. Dixon BS, Novak L, Fangman J. Hemodialysis vascular access survival: upper-arm native arteriovenous fistula. *Am J Kidney Dis.* 2002;39:92–101.
11. Ascher E, Hingorani A, Gunduz Y, et al. The value and limitations of the arm cephalic and basilic vein for arteriovenous access. *Ann Vasc Surg.* 2001;15(1):89–97.
12. Hakaim AG, Nalbandian M, Scott T. Superior maturation and patency of primary brachiocephalic and transposed basilic vein arteriovenous fistulae in patients with diabetes. *J Vasc Surg.* 1998;27:154–157.
13. Dagher F, Gelber R, Ramos E, et al. The use of basilic vein and brachial artery as an A-V fistula for long-term hemodialysis. *J Surg Res.* 1976;20:373–376.
14. Murphy GJ, White SA, Knight AJ, et al. Long-term results of arteriovenous fistulas using transposed autologous basilic vein. *Br J Surg.* 2000;87:819–823.
15. Humphries AL, Colborn GL, Wynn JJ. Elevated basilic vein arteriovenous fistula. *Am J Surg.* 1999;177:489–491.
16. Smits JHM, Van Der Linden J, Hagen EC, et al. Graft surveillance: venous pressure, access flow, or the combination? *Kidney Int.* 2001;59:1551–1558
17. Wang E, Schneditz D, Levin NW. Predictive value of access blood flow and stenosis in detection of graft failure. *Clin Neph.* 2000;54:393–399.
18. Marston WA, Criado E, Jaques PF, et al. Prospective randomized comparison of surgical versus endovascular management of thrombosed dialysis access grafts. *J Vasc Surg.* 1997;26:373–381.
19. Bitar G, Yang S, Badosa F. Balloon versus patch angioplasty as an adjuvant treatment to surgical thrombectomy of hemodialysis grafts. *Am J Surg.* 1997;174:140–142.
20. Bacchini G, Cappello A, La Milia V, et al. Color Doppler ultrasonography imaging to guide transluminal angioplasty of venous stenosis. *Kidney Int.* 2000;58:1810–1813.
21. Lumsden AB, MacDonald MJ, Kikeri D, et al. Prophylactic balloon angioplasty fails to prolong the patency of expanded polytetrafluoroethylene arteriovenous grafts: results of a prospective randomized study. *J Vasc Surg.* 1997;26:382–392.
22. Berman SS, Gentile AT. Impact of secondary procedures in autogenous arteriovenous fistula maturation and maintenance. *J Vasc Surg.* 2001;34:866–871.
23. Kalmen PG, Lindsay TF, Clarke K, et al. Management of upper extremity central venous obstruction using interventional radiology. *Ann Vasc Surg.* 1998;12:202–206.
24. Bhatia DS, Money SR, Ochsner JL, et al. Comparison of surgical bypass and percutaneous balloon dilatation with primary stent placement in the treatment of central venous outflow obstruction in the dialysis patient. *Ann Vasc Surg.* 1996;10:452–455.
25. Astor BC, Eustace JA, Powe NR, et al. Timing of nephrologist referral and arteriovenous access use: the CHOICE study. *Am J Kid Dis.* 2001;38(3):494–501.

XII

Vascular Trauma

39

Iatrogenic Vascular Injuries

Mark R. Nehler, MD and William C. Krupski, MD

Injuries to arteries or veins occur in approximately 3% of civilian cases of major trauma and an even higher percentage of military injuries.[1] Although civilian and military traumatic vascular injuries remain important causes of mortality and morbidity in modern society, the increasing use of arteriography, endovascular, and cardiac interventions has led to a marked increase in the number of iatrogenic vascular injuries encountered by vascular surgeons. Moreover, iatrogenic vascular complications can result from non-vascular procedures (especially orthopedic procedures), the need for indwelling monitoring devices, and new technologies (e.g., vascular injuries related to laparoscopy). The incidence of iatrogenic vascular injuries in the United States has not changed substantially in the past several decades and may be as high as 13%[2] to 15%.[3] As reported by Fingerhut and colleagues, in many European countries where accurate registries are collected, the proportion of iatrogenic injuries as a cause of vascular trauma has exceeded 40% (Table 39–1, Table 39–2).[4] Over one-half million individuals undergo percutaneous arterial catheterizations annually for diagnostic and/or therapeutic procedures, most frequently coronary arteriography,[5] and a significant number of iatrogenic arterial injuries arise from these investigations and interventions.

An iatrogenic injury is defined as an injury caused by a medical intervention or encounter. Many (but not all) iatrogenic vascular injuries are preventable. Early diag-

TABLE 39–1. EUROPE'S ESTIMATE OF THE ETIOLOGY OF VASCULAR TRAUMA

Country	No. of Years	Patients	Penetrating	Trauma Mechanism (%) Blunt	Iatrogenic
Spain	1980–1995	451	20	40	40
Sweden	1987–2000	1000	31	23	46
Finland	1991–1999	503	39	19	42
Turkey	1993–1997	190	74	25	1
Austria	1993–2001	131	32	33	35

Adapted from: reference 4

TABLE 39–2. EUROPEAN EXPERIENCE WITH CAUSES OF IATROGENIC VASCULAR INJURIES

Procedure	No.of Patients	Percentage of Patients
Orthopedic surgery	28	16
Traditional vascular surgery	27	15
Traditional general surgery	5	3
Laparoscopic surgery	21	12
Injection treatment of varicose veins	40	22
Venous surgery	30	17
Interventional radiology	27	15

nosis and repair limit litigious consequences as long as the final result is acceptable. Adar et al. classified vascular injuries as related to: a) accidental, unavoidable complications due to some unusual or rare circumstance; b) faulty technique; c) errors in judgment or management; d) incorrect recognition of anatomy; e) inappropriate interpretation of findings in the arteriograms or results of laboratory studies; f) adverse reaction to drugs including allergies, toxicity, or overdose; and g) anesthetic complications.[6] Iatrogenic vascular injuries also occur after nonvascular surgical procedures and may occur after almost any intervention on any part of the body. Even non-operative procedures, such as chiropractic manipulation of the neck, can produce serious iatrogenic arterial injuries.

FEMORAL ARTERAL PUNCTURE COMPLICATIONS

Since Gruntzig[7] performed the first percutaneous transluminal coronary angioplasty in 1977, the number of cardiac catheterizations, interventional procedures, atherectomies, stent placements, valvuloplasties, percutaneous insertion of balloon assist devices and catheters for extracorporeal bypasses, and a host of peripheral arterial endovascular` interventional procedures has increased exponentially.[8] Since the femoral artery is the preferred site for these interventions, complication rates are generally reported at this location. Complications of femoral artery access include hemorrhage (rarely fatal), thrombosis, infection, laceration, arterial dissection, embolization, arteriovenous fistula and pseudoaneurysm formation.[9–11] The risk of complications related to femoral artery punctures ranges between 1.0% and 16%.[3,12] When an intra-aortic balloon pump is placed, the incidence of vascular complications may be as high as 35%.[13]

The wide range of complication rates associated with femoral punctures is multifactorial. In part, this variation is based upon differences in definitions of complications. Some bleeding occurs after all arterial punctures. Most authorities define a hematoma as a palpable or visible accumulation of blood in the subcutaneous tissue, although this too is somewhat subjective. In general, bleeding complications and subsequent pseudoaneurysms are more frequent following therapeutic rather than purely diagnostic procedures, especially when the procedures involve insertion of intravascular devices such as arterial stents. In addition to the greater diameter of the device being inserted, patient-related factors play and important role, such as severely calcified arteries, obesity preventing adequate hemostatic compression, female gender, severe hypertension, and concurrent anticoagulation. Location of the puncture/laceration of circumflex or deep femoral branches that cannot be adequately compressed after the procedure also partially explain why hemorrhagic complications occur in some patients but not in others. The mortality rate of arteriography is 0.03% due to anaphylactic reaction to contrast and under appreciated bleeding that occurs into the retroperitoneum. Often there is minimal evidence of hemorrhage in the groin when the major blood loss is into the retroperitoneum. A high index of suspicion is required to diagnose this potentially morbid condition expediently. A falling hematocrit and the presence of a femoral nerve deficit are suggestive of significant retroperitoneal hemorrhage.

PSEUDOANEURYSM

Disruption of a portion of the injured arterial wall can lead to a pulsating hematoma—a pseudoaneurysm (also called false aneurysm) as the blood circulates from the arterial lumen through the site of penetration into the surrounding tissues, eventually forming a sac. Physical signs that a hematoma contains a pseudoaneurysm include lateral pulsations and the presence of a bruit. Hematomas are easily differentiated from pseudoaneurysms by duplex ultrasound. Surgical evacuation of post procedural hematomas have traditionally included expanding size, sufficient blood loss to require transfusion, and mass effect producing nerve compression, venous obstruction, or jeopardy to viability to overlying skin.

Traditionally, operative therapy has been recommended for almost all iatrogenic femoral artery pseudoaneurysms.[14,15] The operation was often performed under general or regional anesthesia, but the precarious condition of the patient often enhanced the danger of this approach. Moreover, the substantial cost involved with an operative approach for this relatively frequently occurring clinical problem and the potential for significant wound complications represented significant disadvantages to this approach.

This led to several natural history studies of iatrogenic false aneurysms of the femoral artery complicating femoral artery catheterizations. In 1991, Kresowik and colleagues[13] at the University of Iowa evaluated complications at the femoral puncture site in 144 patients undergoing percutaneous transluminal coronary angioplasty (PTCA) over a 14-month period. In addition to routine physical examinations, all patients had color-flow duplex scans of the involved groin. On the initial scan, 8 pseudoaneurysms, 3 arteriovenous fistulas (AVFs), and 1 combined pseudoaneurysm-arteriovenous fistula were detected for a major complication rate of 9%. Initial extravascular cavity size ranged from 1.3 to 3.5 cm. These lesions were followed with serial weekly duplex scans (even though most patients were treated with short-term anticoagulation) and only 1 of the pseudoaneurysms was repaired surgically, because the patient required long-term anticoagulation. The remaining observed pseudoaneuryms all spontaneously thrombosed within 1 to 4 weeks. Although 2 of the 3 AVFs were eventually repaired, none suffered complications despite observation for 8 weeks or more. Thus, most pseudoaneurysms underwent spontaneous thrombosis over time. When this paper was presented at the national meeting of the ISCVS in Los Angeles, several discussants arose to comment that they too had observed spontaneous resolution of this complication in their patients.

Similarly, Allen and co-workers at Washington University School of Medicine in St. Louis recommended selective non-operative management of pseudoaneurysms and arteriovenous fistulae complicating femoral artery catheterization.[16] These surgeons prospectively studied the natural history of 22 pseudoaneurysms, 8 AVFs, and 3 combined lesions identified by duplex scan in 32 patients following trans-femoral cardiac, peripheral vascular, or vascular access arterial catheterization procedures; arteriograms were performed with the use of 5–8 F introducer sheaths. Although some patients required operative intervention because long-term anticoagulation was needed and others underwent surgery for pain or enlargement of lesions, 19 arterial lesions (9 pseudoaneurysms, 8 AVFs, and 2 combined lesions) spontaneously improved over time and 17 (89%) of the lesions resolved spontaneously within 5–90 days (mean 30.7 days).

A prospective study of the clinical outcome of femoral pseudoaneurysms and arteriovenous fistulas induced by arterial puncture was performed at Beth Israel Hospital in Boston, MA, in 1993.[17] Twenty-two patients with either pseudoaneurysms (n=16) or AVFs (n=6) induced by percutaneous punctures were monitored with serial duplex scans. Nine of the 16 pseudoaneurysms and 4 of 6 AVFs closed spontaneously. Although size was not an absolute predictor of the need for repair, larger lesions (>6 cm^3) were more likely to require operative intervention. In addition, patients receiving continuous anticoagulation were more likely to undergo surgery. Neither length of the aneurysm neck, velocity in the cavity, size of the original arterial puncture, nor velocity in the AVF correlated with thrombosis. The authors concluded that many such lesions close spontaneously and repair is not required unless symptoms or signs of progressive enlargement develop.

An important contribution to the surgical literature was provided in 1997 by Toursarkissian and colleagues.[18] who studied 196 pseudoaneurysms, 81 AVFs, and 9 combined lesions that were identified by duplex scan. One hundred thirty-nine patients underwent prompt surgical repair for enlarging lesions, increasing pain, groin infection, nerve compression, limb ischemia, concomitant surgical procedures, and patient refusal or inability to comply with follow-up. However, over half of the patients (n=147) were initially managed without operation. There were no limb-threatening complications associated with nonoperative management in this subset of patients. Eighty-six percent of the lesions being observed resolved spontaneously within a mean of 23 days. By life table analysis, 90% of selected pseudoaneurysms had resolved by 2 months. The authors concluded that the natural history of stable pseudoaneurysms and AVFs is benign and frequently spontaneous resolution occurs unless the lesions are large (in this study larger than 3 cm in diameter) or other pressing indications for operation exist, properly selected patients can be managed without operation. In a comparable study of 50 clinically occult injuries of major arteries studied prospectively by serial observation, Frykberg et al.[19] reported that 89% of the followed injuries never required surgery; thus, in smaller pseudoaneurysms, AVMs, and intimal flaps, observation appears to a safe and effective management option.

ULTRASOUND-GUIDED COMPRESSION REPAIR

In an effort to avoid surgical repair of femoral artery injuries and hasten resolution, in 1991 Fellmeth first described ultrasound-guided compression repair (UGCR) of pseudoaneurysms.[20] Using this technique, duplex ultrasound is used to localize the communication between artery and pseudoaneurysm cavity, and the ultrasound probe is used to precisely compress the pseudoaneurysm, manually pressing the continuous real time B-mode ultrasound probe against the lesion to eliminate flow within the pseudoaneurysm without occluding the artery. Typically, the protocol involves compression for 20–30 minutes and the procedure is repeated if the initial UCGR is unsuccessful, which frequently occurs. However, mean compression times vary greatly, averaging 49.6 +/−33.9 minutes with a range of 300 minutes.[21]

Since Fellmeth's original report, hundreds of patients with post catheterization pseudoaneurysms and AVMs have been treated using UGCR. Initial success rates approaching 90% have been reported.[22–28,29] UCGR has even been successful in obliterating false aneurysms in as many as 70% of anticoagulated patients.[30] Ultrasound guided compression has been employed successfully for false aneurysms of varying age and size, but the best results are achieved with acute lesions less than 4 cm in diameter with well-defined "necks" of the pseudoaneurysms. Not all investigators have reported excellent initial success rates; for example Feld et al. reported a relatively low success rate of 46.7%, which could be increased to 66.7% after application of additional compressions.[31] Discomfort and pain at the treatment site are frequent complaints for the patients treated with prolonged firm compression, especially those with considerable surrounding hematomas, the procedure is very operator-dependent and requires a moderate amount of skill and judgment, patient sedation and pain control is usually required (often demanding the attendance of a physician), and many patients are simply unable to tolerate the procedure. In addition, recurrence of false aneurysms averages about 10%, so repeat scanning to confirm complete thrombosis is generally recommended. Most recurrences can be eliminated by repeat compression, although the optimal treatment strategy remains to be clarified and controversy exists regarding optimal management strategies of iatrogenic femoral artery injuries.[32] Nevertheless, many authorities remain fervent proponents of UGCR for virtually all post-catheterization femoral artery false aneurysms, recommending UGCR as the preferred treatment for all such lesions, even in patients requiring anticoagulation with pseudoaneurysms as large as 8 cm in diameter.[33]

ULTRASOUND-GUIDED THROMBIN INJECTION

Even prior to the UGCR that was introduced by the interventional radiology group at the University of California at San Diego, other investigators had considered therapeutic direct injection of pseudoaneurysms in an attempt to achieve rapid and predictable thrombosis. In 1986 Cope and Zeit described a new technique for "clotting aneurysms" by direct injection of diluted thrombin.[34] They conceived the idea based on the use of coils, cyanoacrylate glue, and balloons mixed with compression of femoral false aneurysms. In 1987 Walker et al.[35] reported the successful treatment of a large deep femoral artery pseudoaneurysm in a 33-year-old by directly injecting thrombin. Yet despite the excellent results achieved by these investigators, a decade passed before the next report of thrombin injection of pseudoaneurysms appeared. Duplex-scanning-guided thrombin injection for treatment of iatrogenic regained popularity in the late 1990s. Liau and colleagues[36] reported complete success in 5 patients with iatrogenic pseudoaneurysms of the femoral arteries within seconds of injection of a small amount of bovine-derived thrombin into the false aneurysms. Kang and colleagues at Loyola University Medical Center[37] injected thrombin in 83 pseudoaneurysms in 82 patients with excellent initial success, including success in 28 of 29 patients who were undergoing anticoagulation therapy. One distal brachial artery thrombosis resolved spontaneously. There were early recurrences in 7 patients, but in general the authors recommended widespread use as the primary treatment for this common problem. Other reports have been favorable as well.[20,38,39] Duplex-guided thrombin injection has also been successful in anticoagulated patients.[40] In one of the most recent reports of ultrasound-guided thrombin injection in the treatment of femoral pseudoaneuryms, Friedman and colleagues[41] reported 100% complete thrombosis of the femoral pseudoaneurysms treated by thrombin injection with only 1 minor complication.

Studies comparing patient satisfaction and effectiveness of thrombin injection versus duplex scanning guided compression have shown a 96% success rate in the thrombin-injected patients versus 75% in the duplex compression-treated patients. Moreover the thrombin injection required a matter of minutes compared with a mean compression time of 44 minutes.[42] However, one must balance this enthusiasm against the natural history studies that showed spontaneous resolution of most iatrogenic pseudoaneurysms (see above). In addition, serious complications of thrombin injection requiring femoral artery reconstruction or intraarterial thrombolysis for limb salvage have been reported.[20,43] Nevertheless, results of thrombin injection of femoral pseudoaneurysms have been quite good, as illustrated in Table 39–3.[34–37,40,41,44–57]

Two noteworthy comparisons of UGGR versus thrombin injection for treatment of iatrogenic femoral artery pseudoaneurysms have been recently published. Paulson and co-workers at Duke[49] compared compression therapy and thrombin injection for these disorder—both directed by continuous color Doppler US guidance. 26 patients with direct thrombin injection were compared with 281 consecutive patients who underwent US-guided compression repair. Direct thrombin injection was successful in 25 of 26 patients, for a success rate of 96%. This was significantly higher than the success rate for the patients treated with UGCR (74%). The mean thrombosis time for thrombin injection was 6 seconds compared with 41.5 minutes for compression. No compli-

TABLE 39–3. RECENT REPORTS OF THROMBIN INJECTION FOR THE TREATMENT OF PSEUDOANEURYSMS

First Author	Ref.	Year	No. Cases	Total Success	% Complications
Brophy DP	44	2000	15	100	0
Cope C	34	1986	1	100	0
Friedman SC	41	2002	40	100	5
Frusch DP	45	2000	1	100	0
Hughes MJ	46	2000	9	100	0
Kang SS	37	2000	74	100	0
La Perna L	47	2000	70	94	0
Lennox AF	40	2000	30	100	0
Liau CS	36	1997	5	100	0
Morrison SL	48	2000	39	100	0
Paulson EK	49	2000	26	96	0
Pezzullo JA	50	2000	23	96	5
Pope M	51	2000	1	100	100
Sheldon PJ	52	2000	1	100	0
Sievert H	53	2000	29	100	0
Tamin WZ	54	2000	10	100	0

cations occurred in the patients treated with thrombin injection, there were no changes in foot pulses, and none of the patients required conscious sedation. No recurrent pseudoaneurysms were seen on follow-up US at 24 hours. Thus, US-guided thrombin injection appeared to be superior to compression repair.

In the second study, similar findings were reported. Khoury et al.[42] prospectively evaluated thrombin injection versus compression therapy alone. In the 31 months of the study, 131 iatrogenic pseudoaneurysms were initially treated with injection and thrombosis was achieved in 126 of theses cases (96%). Thrombosis of the false aneurysm sac was accomplished within seconds of thrombin injection. In contrast, only 75% of the direct compression cases were cured by the technique with a mean compression time of 44 minutes. Again, direct injection of pseudoaneurysms appears to be a superior treatment modality.

PREVENTION OF ANGIOGRAPHIC COMPLICATIONS AND EARLY MOBILITY

The current goal of arteriographers is avoidance of angiographic complications in conjunction with early mobility of those undergoing both diagnostic and therapeutic femoral artery punctures. Several methods are available to achieve this end: manual compression; Perclose (Perclose Inc, Menlo Park, CA); Vasoseal (Datascope Corp, Montvale, NJ); and Angio-Seal (Sherwood Medical Co, St Louis, MO). An excellent review of these devices is provided by Heyer et al.[58] Each product provides different advantages and disadvantages; time does not permit a thorough discussion of each method. Suffice it to say, that not surprisingly, new problems have arisen from introduction of these devices. For example, we recently reported a series of 8 patients who sustained vascular complications related to percutaneous vascular suturing devices.[59] Although the products appear to be relatively safe overall, the complications that can be associated with them (albeit infrequent) can be significantly more challenging than simple acute pseudoaneurysms or hemorrhage. A thorough review is presented in our treatise. The obvious advantage of methods to achieve arteriotomy closure is earlier ambulation, decreased morbidity from prolonged recuperative bedrest, and fewer pseudoaneurysms, AVMs, etc. Yet, as with all new technology, there are prices to be paid—both literally and figuratively. Figures 39–1 through 39–4 illustrate a woman with small arteries whose femoral artery was "sewn shut" by one of these devices, requiring operative repair using an autogenous vein graft angioplasty.

As Toursarkissian et al. described, we are seeing changing patterns of access site complications with the use of percutaneous closure devices.[60] Infection, more extensive arterial injuries, entrapment of the devices within arteries, direct physical injuries to surgeons charged with removing or dealing with such devices have led to a plethora of articles in the recent past.[59, 61–64] As Dr. Nehler concluded in his recent publication, percutaneous suturing devices are gaining wide acceptance by interventional radiologists and cardiologists. With the introduction of this new technology comes a shift in patterns of arterial injuries, which are more technically demanding than straightforward iatrogenic arteriographic injuries. Whereas there appears to be an overall reduction in the number of femoral pseudoaneurysms after widespread use of percutaneous suturing devices, the resultant complications that rarely occur are more difficult to deal with. Communication with interventionalists can improve patient selection, guide the specific device used, and refine future devices.

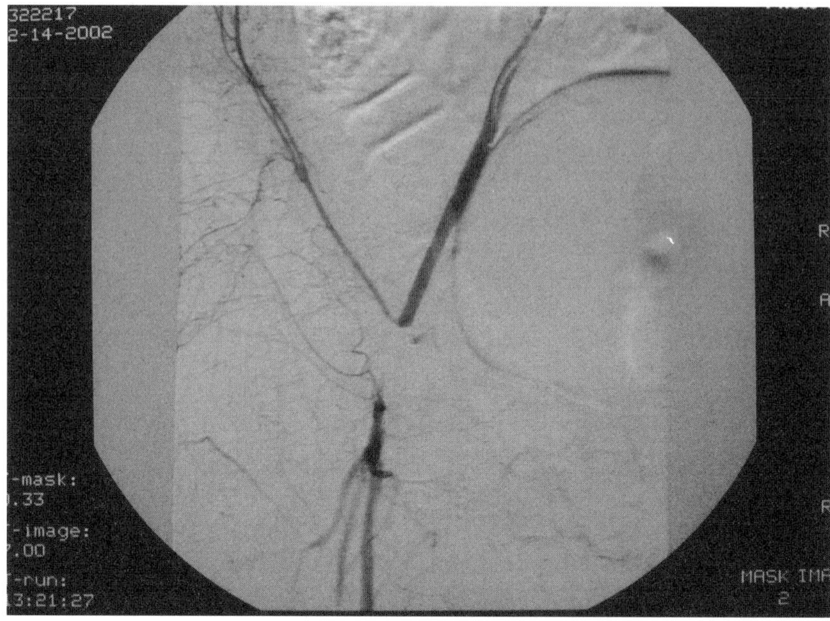

Figure 39–1 Arteriogram demonstrating occlusion of common femoral artery

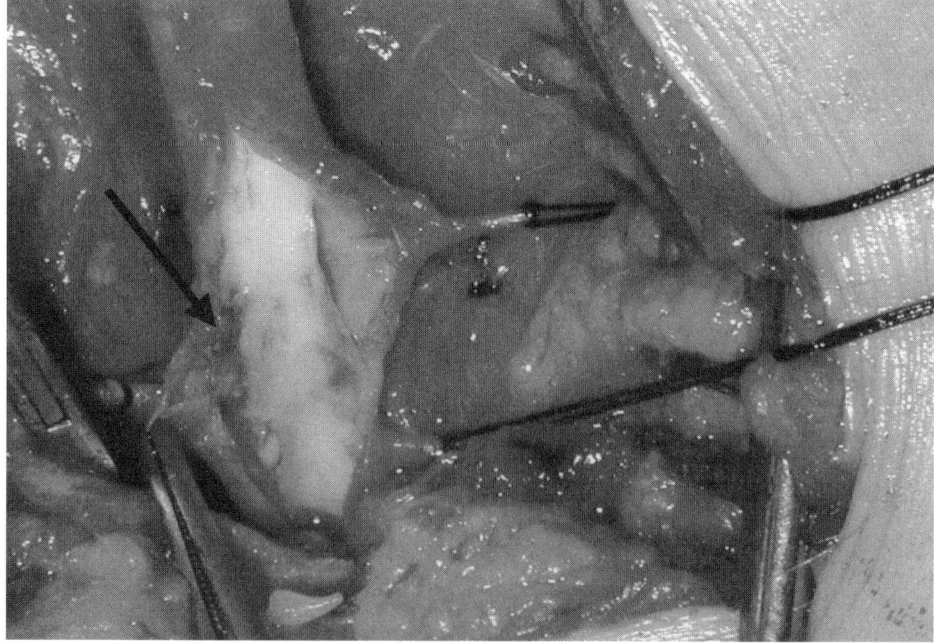

Figure 39–2 Suture through wall (arrows) and involving posterior artery plaque

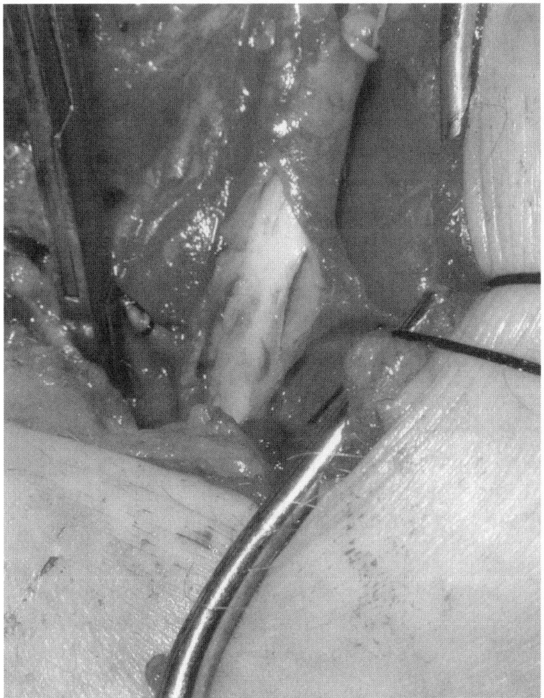

Figure 39–3 Suture released and removed

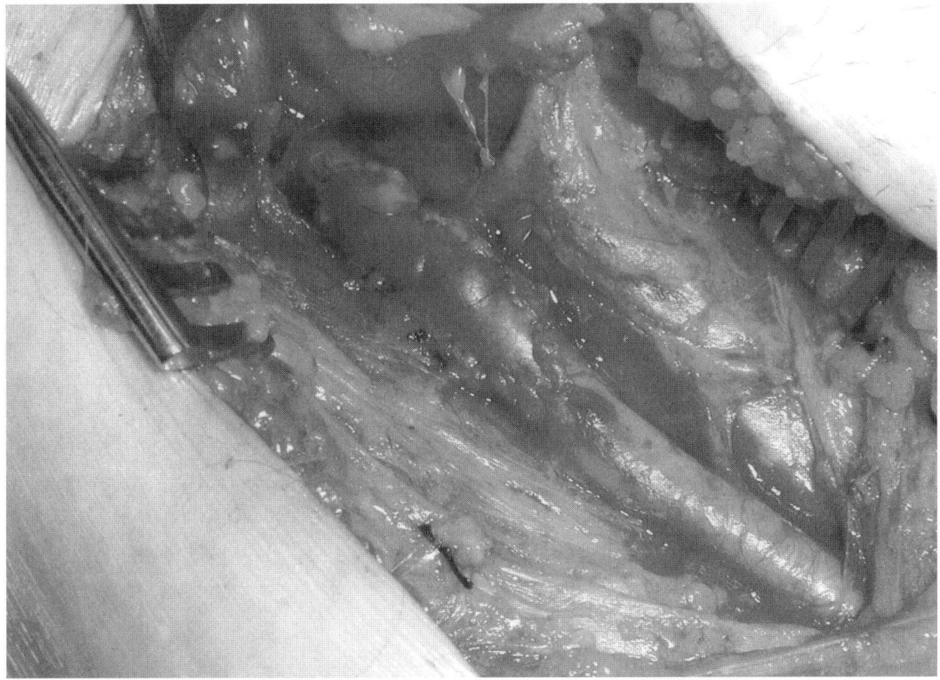

Figure 39–4 Vein patch angioplasty closure of common femoral artery

OTHER IATROGENIC TRAUMA

Use of the axillary or brachial artery when the femoral arteries are not available due to occlusive disease or previous bypass grafting creates potential for dangerous nerve compression from hematoma in the axillary sheath after arteriography. Clinical series[61,65] routinely report higher complication rates from using arterial access sites other than the femoral. Patients may develop axillary sheath hematomas and nerve compression; initially they complain of pain and sensory disturbance of the ispsilateral extremity, with motor weakness appearing later. The initial symptoms may be misinterpreted as due to local anesthetic. Symptoms usually begin within 24 hours but have been reported as late as 15 days after arteriography.[61,66] Therapy is emergency surgical decompression of the axillary sheath to reduce the occurrence of permanent major nerve impairment. Permanent nerve injury may occur even in patients whose symptoms are recognized promptly and treated appropriately.

INDWELLING INTRAVASCULAR DEVICES

As the population ages, there has been an increase in the care of critically ill patients. In addition, more patients have prolonged survival with previously fatal conditions. Most of these patients have the need for indwelling vascular monitoring or therapeutic devices.

Balloon Counterpulsation Devices

Balloon counterpulsation devices require a large bore introducer and produce constant device movement within the arterial lumen that potentiates the likelihood of intravascular injury from arterial rupture, dissection, and/or embolization. These risks are greater than for arteriography alone. The vascular complication rates with these devices are about 20 to 30% in general, but have been reported to be as high as 60%.[67,68] The most lethal complications are perforation of the iliac arteries and embolization. These are most frequently observed in patients with coexistent aortic aneurysms, both due to intra-aneurysm thrombus and associated iliac artery torturosity. Dissection and thrombosis are usually limited to the insertion site and can be locally repaired using various techniques. Ofttimes, emergency "temporary" axillobifemoral bypasses are required to preserve limb viability. There has even been a recent description of a percutaneous "bedside" femoro-femoral bypass graft for acute ischemia caused by intra-aortic balloon pumps.[69]

Arterial Pressure Monitoring Devices

The radial artery is the site of choice for intraarterial pressure monitoring. Decannulation thrombosis of this artery occurs in 15 to 20% of patients on average.[70] Because of the rich collateral supply to the hand, few patients develop frank ischemia, but this can certainly occur. In addition, infected pseudoaneurysms have been reported as an infrequent complication related to prolonged catheter duration and systemic infections.[3] If radial artery catheterizations are impossible to insert or contraindicated by a positive Allen's test, the femoral artery is a satisfactory alternative.

Pulmonary Artery Catheters

Pulmonary artery catheters have their own set of complications, including pulmonary artery rupture, pseudoaneurysm formation, hemoptysis, false readings, and a whole host of additional problems.[71,72–75] Ironically, few prospective studies have shown survival advantage in those patients with pulmonary artery catheters compared to those without them.[76]

IATROGENIC INURIES ASSOCIATED WITH OTHER SURGICAL PROCEDURES

The literature is replete with reports of iatrogenic vascular trauma from orthopedic procedures.[77–89] The range of these procedures is immense and include: lumbar disc surgery[77,80,81] hip surgery,[82–84] shoulder surgery,[85] total knee replacement,[86,87] common orthopedic and other non-vascular injuries.[78,88,89]

More and more frequently "less invasive surgery" involving trocars and laparoscopy are becoming associated with iatrogenic vascular trauma.[90–97]

It is well accepted that the association of iatrogenic vascular trauma with non-vascular operations is one of the most frequent causes of lawsuits in this country and elsewhere. It must be stressed that the occurrence of unexpected vascular trauma is multifactorial and NOT necessarily related to substandard care or malpractice. These injuries will be discussed in more detail during my presentation, but suffice it to say that a high degree of suspicion for the potential of vascular injuries from non-vascular procedures should be vigilant. Blood vessels are often in close proximity to other important structures requiring operation in the body. In addition, the positions necessary to safely carry out such procedures (e.g., the lithotomy position) lend themselves to potential adverse vascular outcomes. Unusual or abnormal anatomy of blood vessels in relation to nearby structures and the requirement for tourniquet control for safe conduct of orthopedic, neurologic, general, and gynecologic surgery place both normal and diseased blood vessels at risk for injury. In summary, we are encountering iatrogenic vascular trauma with increasing frequency as a result of the increasing frequency and magnitude of intravascular instrumentation and both new and old operative interventions. Recognition of the vascular trauma and prompt intervention are perhaps the most important lessons to be learned by these trends.

REFERENCES

1. Austin OM, Redmond HP, Burke PE, et al. Vascular trauma-a review. *J Am Coll Surg.* 1995;181:91–108.
2. Orcutt MB, Levine BA, Gaskill HV, III, et al. Iatrogenic vascular injury. A reducible problem. *Arch Surg.* 1985;120:384–385.
3. Lumsden AB, Miller JM, Kosinski AS, et al. A prospective evaluation of surgically treated groin complications following percutaneous cardiac procedures. *Am Surg.* 1994;60:132–137.
4. Fingerhut A, Leppaniemi AK, Androulakis GA, et al. The European experience with vascular injuries. *Surg Clin North Am.* 2002;82:175–188.
5. Nehler MR, Taylor LM, Jr., Porter JM. Iatrogenic vascular trauma. *Semin Vasc Surg.* 1998;11:283–293.
6. Adar R, Bass A, Walden R. Iatrogenic complications in surgery. Five years' experience in general and vascular surgery in a University Hospital. *Ann Surg.* 1982;196:725–729.
7. Gruntzig AR, Senning A, Siegenthaler WE. Nonoperative dilatation of coronary-artery stenosis: percutaneous transluminal coronary angioplasty. *N Engl J Med.* 1979;301:61–68.
8. McCleary AJ, Raptis S. Closing the loop: the role of audit in reducing groin complications associated with coronary angiography. *Clin Radiol.* 2001;56:917–921.

9. Messina LM, Brothers TE, Wakefield TW, et al. Clinical characteristics and surgical management of vascular complications in patients undergoing cardiac catheterization: interventional versus diagnostic procedures. *J Vasc Surg.* 1991;13:593–600.

10. Franco CD, Goldsmith J, Veith FJ, et al. Management of arterial injuries produced by percutaneous femoral procedures. *Surgery.* 1993; 113:419–425.

11. Davis C, VanRiper S, Longstreet J, et al. Vascular complications of coronary interventions. *Heart Lung.* 1997;26:118–127.

12. Skillman JJ, Kim D, Baim DS. Vascular complications of percutaneous femoral cardiac interventions. Incidence and operative repair. *Arch Surg.* 1988;123:1207–1212.

13. Kresowik TF, Khoury MD, Miller BV, et al. A prospective study of the incidence and natural history of femoral vascular complications after percutaneous transluminal coronary angioplasty. *J Vasc Surg.* 1991;13:328–333.

14. Waller DA, Sivananthan UM, Diament RH, et al. Iatrogenic vascular injury following arterial cannulation: the importance of early surgery. *Cardiovasc Surg.* 1993;1:251–253.

15. Perler BA. Surgical treatment of femoral pseudoaneurysm following cardiac catheterization. *Cardiovasc Surg.* 1993;1:118–121.

16. Allen BT, Munn JS, Stevens SL, et al. Selective non-operative management of pseudoaneurysms and arteriovenous fistulae complicating femoral artery catheterization. *J Cardiovasc Surg (Torino).* 1992;33:440–447.

17. Kent KC, McArdle CR, Kennedy B, et al. A prospective study of the clinical outcome of femoral pseudoaneurysms and arteriovenous fistulas induced by arterial puncture. *J Vasc Surg.* 1993;17:125–131.

18. Toursarkissian B, Allen BT, Petrinec D, et al. Spontaneous closure of selected iatrogenic pseudoaneurysms and arteriovenous fistulae. *J Vasc Surg.* 1997;25:803–808.

19. Frykberg ER, Crump JM, Dennis JW, et al. Nonoperative observation of clinically occult arterial injuries: a prospective evaluation. *Surgery.* 1991;109:85–96.

20. Fellmeth BD, Roberts AC, Bookstein JJ, et al. Postangiographic femoral artery injuries: nonsurgical repair with US-guided compression. *Radiology.* 1991;178:671–675.

21. Coley BD, Roberts AC, Fellmeth BD, et al. Postangiographic femoral artery pseudoaneurysms: further experience with US-guided compression repair. *Radiology.* 1995;194: 307–311.

22. Cox GS, Young JR, Gray BR, et al. Ultrasound-guided compression repair of postcatheterization pseudoaneurysms: results of treatment in one hundred cases. *J Vasc Surg.* 1994;19: 683–686.

23. Hajarizadeh H, LaRosa CR, Cardullo P, et al. Ultrasound-guided compression of iatrogenic femoral pseudoaneurysm failure, recurrence, and long-term results. *J Vasc Surg.* 1995;22:425–430.

24. Feng YL, Truitt RE, Coggins TR, et al. Nonsurgical repair of femoral artery pseudoaneurysm with color flow guided ultrasound transducer compression. *Echocardiography.* 1996;13:297–302.

25. Lange P, Houe T, Helgstrand UJ. The efficacy of ultrasound-guided compression of iatrogenic femoral pseudo-aneurysms. *Eur J Vasc Endovasc Surg.* 2001;21:248–250.

26. Murphy PB, Bajwa TK, Kubota J, et al. Peripheral artery pseudoaneurysm: treatment by transcutaneous compression guided by ultrasonography. *Echocardiography.* 1996;13: 483–488.

27. Langella RL, Schneider JR, Golan JF. Color duplex-guided compression therapy for postcatheterization pseudoaneurysms in a community hospital. *Ann Vasc Surg.* 1996;10:27–35.

28. Steinkamp HJ, Werk M, Felix R. Treatment of postinterventional pseudoaneurysms by ultrasound-guided compression. *Invest Radiol.* 2000;35:186–192.

29. Hye RJ. Compression therapy for acute iatrogenic femoral pseudoaneurysms. *Semin Vasc Surg.* 2000;13:58–61.

30. Dean SM, Olin JW, Piedmonte M, et al. Ultrasound-guided compression closure of postcatheterization pseudoaneurysms during concurrent anticoagulation: a review of seventy-seven patients. *J Vasc Surg.* 1996;23:28–34, discussion.

31. Feld R, Patton GM, Carabasi RA, et al. Treatment of iatrogenic femoral artery injuries with ultrasound-guided compression. *J Vasc Surg.* 1992;16:832–840.
32. Kronzon I. Diagnosis and treatment of iatrogenic femoral artery pseudoaneurysm: a review. *J Am Soc Echocardiogr.* 1997;10:236–245.
33. Kumins NH, Landau DS, Montalvo J. Expanded indications for the treatment of post-catheterization femoral pseudoaneurysms with ultrasound-guided compression. *Am J Surg.* 1998;176:131–136.
34. Cope C, Zeit R. Coagulation of aneurysms by direct percutaneous thrombin injection. *AJR Am J Roentgenol.* 1986;147:383–387.
35. Walker TG, Geller SC, Brewster DC. Transcatheter occlusion of a profunda femoral artery pseudoaneurysm using thrombin. *AJR Am J Roentgenol.* 1987; 149:185–186.
36. Liau CS, Ho FM, Chen MF, Lee YT. Treatment of iatrogenic femoral artery pseudoaneurysm with percutaneous thrombin injection. *J Vasc Surg.* 1997;26:18–23.
37. Kang SS, Labropoulos N, Mansour MA, et al. Expanded indications for ultrasound-guided thrombin injection of pseudoaneurysms. *J Vasc Surg.* 2000;31:289–298.
38. McCoy D, Scharfstein B, Walker W, et al. Ultrasound-guided percutaneous thrombin injection for femoral artery pseudoaneurysms. *Am Surg.* 2000;66:975–977.
39. Sackett WR, Taylor SM, Coffey CB, et al. Ultrasound-guided thrombin injection of iatrogenic femoral pseudoaneurysms: a prospective analysis. *Am Surg.* 2000;66:937–940.
40. Lennox AF, Delis KT, Szendro G, et al. Duplex-guided thrombin injection for iatrogenic femoral artery pseudoaneurysm is effective even in anticoagulated patients. *Br J Surg.* 2000;87:796–801.
41. Friedman SG, Pellerito JS, Scher L, et al. Ultrasound-guided thrombin injection is the treatment of choice for femoral pseudoaneurysms. *Arch Surg.* 2002;137:462–464.
42. Khoury M, Rebecca A, Greene K, Rama K, Colaiuta E, Flynn L, Berg R. Duplex scanning-guided thrombin injection for the treatment of iatrogenic pseudoaneurysms. *J Vasc Surg.* 2002;35:517–521.
43. Forbes TL, Millward SF. Femoral artery thrombosis after percutaneous thrombin injection of an external iliac artery pseudoaneurysm. *J Vasc Surg.* 2001;33:1093–1096.
44. Brophy DP, Sheiman RG, Amatulle P, et al. Iatrogenic femoral pseudoaneurysms: thrombin injection after failed US-guided compression. *Radiology.* 2000;214:278–282.
45. Frush DP, Paulson EK, O'Laughlin MP. Successful sonographically guided thrombin injection in an infant with a femoral artery pseudoaneurysm. *AJR Am J Roentgenol.* 2000;175:485–487.
46. Hughes MJ, McCall JM, Nott DM, et al. Treatment of iatrogenic femoral artery pseudoaneurysms using ultrasound-guided injection of thrombin. *Clin Radiol.* 2000;55:749–751.
47. La Perna L, Olin JW, Goines D, et al. Ultrasound-guided thrombin injection for the treatment of postcatheterization pseudoaneurysms. *Circulation.* 2000;102:2391–2395.
48. Morrison SL, Obrand DA, Steinmetz OK, Montreuil B. Treatment of femoral artery pseudoaneurysms with percutaneous thrombin injection. *Ann Vasc Surg.* 2000;14:634–639.
49. Paulson EK, Sheafor DH, Kliewer MA, et al. Sketch MH, Jr. Treatment of iatrogenic femoral arterial pseudoaneurysms: comparison of US-guided thrombin injection with compression repair. *Radiology.* 2000;215:403–408.
50. Pezzullo JA, Dupuy DE, Cronan JJ. Percutaneous injection of thrombin for the treatment of pseudoaneurysms after catheterization: an alternative to sonographically guided compression. *AJR Am J Roentgenol.* 2000;175:1035–1040.
51. Pope M, Johnston KW. Anaphylaxis after thrombin injection of a femoral pseudoaneurysm: recommendations for prevention. *J Vasc Surg.* 2000;32:190–191.
52. Sheldon PJ, Oglevie SB, Kaplan LA. Prolonged generalized urticarial reaction after percutaneous thrombin injection for treatment of a femoral artery pseudoaneurysm. *J Vasc Interv Radiol.* 2000;11:759–761.
53. Sievert H, Baser A, Pfeil W, et al. [The treatment of iatrogenic spurious aneurysm of the femoral artery by direct thrombin injection]. *Dtsch Med Wochenschr.* 2000;125:822–825.
54. Tamim WZ, Arbid EJ, Andrews LS, et al. Percutaneous induced thrombosis of iatrogenic femoral pseudoaneurysms following catheterization. *Ann Vasc Surg* 2000; 14:254–259.

55. Taylor BS, Rhee RY, Muluk S, et al. Thrombin injection versus compression of femoral artery pseudoaneurysms. *J Vasc Surg.* 1999;30:1052–1059.

56. Vermeulen EG, Umans U, Rijbroek A, et al. Percutaneous duplex-guided thrombin injection for treatment of iatrogenic femoral artery pseudoaneurysms. *Eur J Vasc Endovasc Surg.* 2000;20:302–304.

57. Wixon CL, Philpott JM, Bogey WM, Jr., et al. Duplex-directed thrombin injection as a method to treat femoral artery pseudoaneurysms. *J Am Coll Surg.* 1998;187:464–466.

58. Heyer G, Atzenhofer K, Meixl H, et al. Arterial access site closure with a novel sealing device: *Duett. Vasc Surg.* 2001;35:199–201.

59. Nehler MR, Lawrence WA, Whitehill TA, et al. Iatrogenic vascular injuries from percutaneous vascular suturing devices. *J Vasc Surg.* 2001; 33:943–947.

60. Toursarkissian B, Mejia A, Smilanich RP, et al. Changing patterns of access site complications with the use of percutaneous closure devices. *Vasc Surg.* 2001;35:203–206.

61. Eidt JF, Habibipour S, Saucedo JF, et al. Surgical complications from hemostatic puncture closure devices. *Am J Surg.* 1999;178:511–516.

62. Gonze MD, Sternbergh WC, III, Salartash K, Money SR. Complications associated with percutaneous closure devices. *Am J Surg.* 1999;178:209–211.

63. Smith TP, Cruz CP, Moursi MM, Eidt JF. Infectious complications resulting from use of hemostatic puncture closure devices. *Am J Surg.* 2001;182:658–662.

64. Sprouse LR, Botta DM, Jr., Hamilton IN, Jr. The management of peripheral vascular complications associated with the use of percutaneous suture-mediated closure devices. *J Vasc Surg.* 2001;33:688–693.

65. Kerber C, Mani RL, Bank WO, et al. Selective cerebral angiography through the axillary artery. *Neuroradiology.* 1975;10:131–135.

66. Molnar W, Paul DJ. Complications of axillary arteriotomies. An analysis of 1,762 consecutive studies. *Radiology.* 1972;104:269–276.

67. Kvilekval KH, Mason RA, Newton GB, et al. Complications of percutaneous intra-aortic balloon pump use in patients with peripheral vascular disease. *Arch Surg.* 1991;126:621–623.

68. Mackenzie DJ, Wagner WH, Kulber DA, et al. Vascular complications of the intra-aortic balloon pump. *Am J Surg.* 1992;164:517–521.

69. Lin PH, Bush RL, Conklin BS et al. Percutaneous bedside femorofemoral bypass grafting for acute limb ischemia caused by intra-aortic balloon pump. *J Vasc Surg.* 2002;35:592–594.

70. Dahl MR, Smead WL, McSweeney TD. Radial artery cannulation: a comparison of 15.2- and 4.45-cm catheters. *J Clin Monit.* 1992; 8:193–197.

71. Prentice D, Ahrens T. Controversies in the use of the pulmonary artery catheter. *J Cardiovasc Nurs.* 2001;15:1–5.

72. Becker K, Jr. Resolved: A pulmonary artery catheter should be used in the management of the critically ill patient. *Con. J Cardiothorac Vasc Anesth.* 1998;12:13–16.

73. Cruz K, Franklin C. The pulmonary artery catheter: uses and controversies. *Crit Care Clin.* 2001;17:271–291.

74. Sirivella S, Gielchinsky I, Parsonnet V. Management of catheter-induced pulmonary artery perforation: a rare complication in cardiovascular operations. *Ann Thorac Surg.* 2001;72: 2056–2059.

75. Vincent JL, Dhainaut JF, Perret C, Suter P. Is the pulmonary artery catheter misused? A European view. *Crit Care Med.* 1998;26:1283–1287.

76. Barone JE, Tucker JB, Rassias D, Corvo PR. Routine perioperative pulmonary artery catheterization has no effect on rate of complications in vascular surgery: a meta-analysis. *Am Surg.* 2001;67:674–679.

77. Quigley TM, Stoney RJ. Arteriovenous fistulas following lumbar laminectomy: the anatomy defined. *J Vasc Surg.* 1985;2:828–833.

78. Natali J. Forensic medical implications of vascular injuries in orthopedic surgery. *J Mal Vasc.* 1996; 21:206–215.

79. Freischlag JA, Sise M, Quinones-Baldrich WJ, Hye RJ, Sedwitz MM. Vascular complications associated with orthopedic procedures. *Surg Gynecol Obstet.* 1989;169:147–152.

80. Raptis S, Quigley F, Barker S. Vascular complications of elective lower lumbar disc surgery. *Aust N Z J Surg.* 1994;64(3):216–219.
81. Goodkin R, Laska LL. Vascular and visceral injuries associated with lumbar disc surgery: medicolegal implications. *Surg Neurol.* 1998; 49:358–370.
82. Karanikas I, Lazarides M, Arvanitis D, Papayanopoulos G, Exarchou E, Dayantas J. Iatrogenic arterial trauma associated with hip fracture surgery. *Acta Chir Belg.* 1993; 93:284–286.
83. Lazarides MK, Tsoupanos SS, Georgopoulos SE, et al. Incidence and patterns of iatrogenic arterial injuries. A decade's experience. *J Cardiovasc Surg (Torino).* 1998;39(3):281–285.
84. Lazarides MK, Arvanitis DP, Dayantas JN. Iatrogenic arterial trauma associated with hip joint surgery: an overview. *Eur J Vasc Surg.* 1991;5(5):549–556.
85. Weber SC, Abrams JS, Nottage WM. Complications associated with arthroscopic shoulder surgery. *Arthroscopy.* 2002;18:88–95.
86. Kumar SN, Chapman JA, Rawlinds I. Vascular injuries in total knee arthroplasty. A review of the problem with special reference to the possible effects of the tourniquet. *J Arthroplasty.* 1998;13:211–216.
87. Smith DE, McGraw RW, Taylor DC, et al. Arterial complications and total knee arthroplasty. *J Am Acad Orthop Surg.* 2001;9:253–257.
88. Jue-Denis P, Kieffer E, Le Thoai H, et al. Perioperative vascular accidents during orthopedic surgery. Apropos of 55 cases. *J Chir (Paris).* 1983;120:437–441.
89. Jue-Denis P, Kieffer E, Benhamou M, et al. Injuries to abdominal vessels after surgery of disk herniation. *Rev Chir Orthop Reparatrice Appar Mot.* 1984;70:141–145.
90. Bhoyrul S, Vierra MA, Nezhat CR, et al. Trocar injuries in laparascopic surgery. *J Am Coll Surg.* 2001;192:677–683.
91. Corson SL, Chandler JG, Way LW. Survey of laparoscopic entry injuries provoking litigation. *J Am Assoc Gynecol Laparosc.* 2001;8:341–347.
92. Fruhwirth J, Koch G, Amann W, et al. Vascular complications of lumbar disc surgery. *Acta Neurochir (Wien).* 1996;138:912–916.
93. Fruhwirth J, Koch G, Mischinger HJ, et al. Vascular complications in minimally invasive surgery. *Surg Laparosc Endosc.* 1997;7:251–254.
94. Mases A, Montes A, Ramos R, et al. Injury to the abdominal aorta during laparascopic surgery: an unusual presentation. *Anesth Analg.* 2000;91:561–562.
95. Montero M, Tellado MG, Rios J, et al. Aortic injury during diagnostic pediatric laparoscopy. *Surg Endosc.* 2001;15:519.
96. Schafer M, Lauper M, Krahenbuhl L. A nation's experience of bleeding complications during laparoscopy. *Am J Surg.* 2000;180:73–77.
97. Schafer M, Lauper M, Krahenbuhl L. Trocar and Veress needles injuries during laparoscopy. *Surg Endosc.* 2001;15;275–280.

40

Blunt Thoracic Aortic Injury

Mark H. Meissner, MD and Riyad Karmy-Jones, MD

Traumatic rupture of the aorta is responsible for 12% to 30% of blunt trauma deaths and is second only to head injury as a cause of death following blunt trauma in the United States.[1,2] This corresponds to approximately 8000 deaths per year from blunt aortic injury.[3] Motor vehicle crashes are responsible for 50% to 95% of these injuries and the incidence in fatal automobile crashes ranges from 12% to 26%.[1,4] However, a similar 12.7% incidence of thoracic aortic trauma has been reported in pedestrian fatalities.[5] The majority of such injuries, as many as 90% to 95%, occur at the aortic isthmus—that is, the descending thoracic aorta just distal to the left subclavian artery.[4,6] The isthmus is often considered to be an area of inherent weakness that is particularly vulnerable to longitudinal shearing forces. Although several mechanisms have been proposed, a combination of deceleration and chest compression appears to be responsible for injuries of the thoracic aorta.[4]

Approximately 85% of patients with traumatic aortic disruption will die before reaching the hospital.[7] However, historical autopsy series suggesting a mortality rate of 1% per hour in non-operated survivors were flawed by selection bias, diagnostic limitations in detecting minimal intimal injuries, and failure to rigorously control blood pressure.[2,5,7,8] Mortality among those surviving to hospital admission may be as low as 32%[9] and depends on the patient's early hemodynamic condition (Figure 40–1). Approximately 8% of patients with blunt aortic injury will present in extremis.[1] Mortality approaches 95% in those with massive hemothorax and cardiovascular collapse,[9] the majority of whom have complete aortic tears.[10] However, instability among patients with hypotension early after admission is related to other injuries in over 75% of cases[11] (Table 40–1). Management of other life-threatening injuries assumes priority in the absence of an expanding mediastinal hematoma or actively bleeding hemothorax. The remaining patients are hemodynamically stable, allowing thorough evaluation and staging of any intervention. Mortality in this latter group is as low as 12% to 14%.[1,12]

The management of blunt thoracic aortic injury continues to evolve with an improved understanding of the natural history and advances in diagnostic and surgical techniques. Advances in radiographic imaging, an understanding of the technical and anatomic factors that influence outcome, an appreciation of the role of delayed opera-

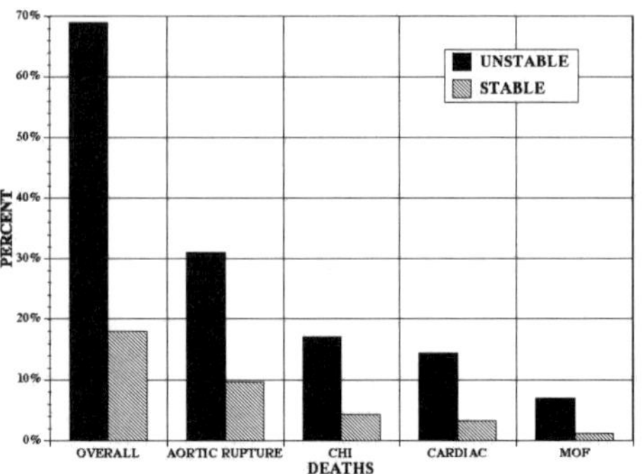

Figure 40–1. Deaths among unstable (systolic blood pressure <90 mmHg, N = 42) and stable (systolic blood pressure ≥90 mmHg, N = 78) with blunt thoracic aortic injury, stratified according to cause. Overall mortality in unstable (69%) and stable (18%) patients was significantly different (p = 0.001). CHI—closed head injury; MOF—multiple organ failure. Adapted from Karmy-Jones R, Carter YM, Nathans A, et al. Impact of presenting physiology and associated injuries on outcome following traumatic rupture of the thoracic aorta. *Am Surgeon.* 2001;67: 61–66.

TABLE 40–1. ASSOCIATED INJURIES IN BLUNT AORTIC TRAUMA (N = 122)

Associated Injuries	Number (%)
Closed Head Injury	37 (30.3%)
Pelvic Fractures	29 (23.8%)
Splenic Rupture	21 (17.2%)
Flail Chest	13 (10.7%)
Lower Extremity Fractures	16 (13.1%)
Liver Laceration	10 (8.2%)
Diaphragmatic Rupture	10 (8.2%)
Facial Injuries	7 (5.7%)
Spine Fracture	4 (3.2%)
Kidney Laceration	3 (2.5%)
Clavicular Fracture	3 (2.5%)
Upper Extremity Fractures	3 (2.5%)
Sternal Fracture	2 (1.6%)
Bladder Rupture	1 (0.8%)

From Karmy-Jones R, Carter Y, Nathens A, et al. Impact of presenting physiology and associated injuries on outcome following traumatic rupture of the thoracic aorta. *Am Surgeon.* 2001;67: 61–66. Reproduced with permission.

tive management, and the potential for endovascular repair of vascular injuries have altered the approach to the patient with aortic trauma.

DIAGNOSIS OF BLUNT AORTIC INJURY

Aortography remains the "gold standard" for the diagnosis of blunt aortic injury. The sensitivity and specificity of aortography approaches 100% and 98% respectively.[13] Small, intimal tears are responsible for most false negatives while false positives may result from atheromatous plaques, atypical ductus irregularities and other anatomic variants. However, as angiography is both invasive and expensive, some selection criteria are required to insure its cost effective use.[14]

Despite recent advances in vascular imaging, chest radiography remains the most widely used screening test for blunt aortic injury. Signs of mediastinal hematoma or significant chest wall trauma including widening of the mediastinum (>8 cm or >0.25 to 0.4 thoracic diameter), an indistinct aortic knob, opacification of the aorto-pulmonary window, an apical cap, rightward deviation of the nasogastric tube, or downward displacement of the left mainstem bronchus should prompt angiography.[3,15,16] Sternal and first rib fractures are rarely present in isolation and alone do not warrant routine angiography. [4,16,17] Approximately 85% of patients with a thoracic aortic injury will have a widened mediastinum on chest x-ray.[1,10] However, initial chest radiographs will be normal in 5% to 10% of patients with traumatic aortic rupture[1,18,19] and such findings may be absent in patients with injuries of the ascending aorta.[20] Although the sensitivity of chest radiography for aortic or great vessel injury exceeds 95%, specificity is only 10% to 45%.[16,21,22] Furthermore, the diagnostic performance of chest x-ray depends on the position in which it is performed.[14] Signs present on an upright anteroposterior film are more specific and have a higher positive predictive value than those present on supine films.[23] Unfortunately, concerns regarding spine injury may preclude upright films in many patients.

The role of computed tomography (CT) in the evaluation of blunt aortic injury is evolving. In comparison with chest radiography, CT is more sensitive (100%) and more specific (87%) in detecting mediastinal hematoma.[24] Computed tomography may be a more cost effective screening modality than the chest x-ray, potentially eliminating the need for aortography in up to 63% of patients.[14,21] However, an aortic injury is present in only approximately 20% of patients with mediastinal hemorrhage[24] and CT will unequivocally define the injury in only 74% of cases.[1] The additional time required for CT imaging and the detection of great vessel injury also remain a concern.[22] However, spiral CT appear to offer greater accuracy for the detection of blunt aortic injury and may even be sufficient to guide operative intervention without angiography.[24] Spiral CT angiography (CTA) protocols with a timed contrast bolus can precisely define most injuries, particularly when combined with three-dimensional reconstruction. Spiral CTA may be most appropriate for stable patients with an abnormal mediastinum and no high-risk signs such as massive hemothorax, differential lower extremity pulses, or supraclavicular hematoma.[25]

The cost-effectiveness of any diagnostic strategy depends upon the risk of injury.[26] Cost-effectiveness models are driven by the high false positive rate of chest radiography and the risks and costs of performing angiography on all patients with a positive chest x-ray.[14] Clinical prediction models have been developed[26] and chest CT followed by angiography for positive findings is the most cost effective strategy in patients undergoing CT for other injuries and when the risk of injury is less than 5%.[14] Aortography is the most cost-effective strategy if the prior probability of aortic injury is greater than 5%.

Other diagnostic modalities may have a role in specific circumstances. Intravascular ultrasound may be particularly useful in planning endovascular repair. Transesophageal echocardiography (TEE) may also be helpful in evaluating small injuries in atherosclerotic aortas, interrogating the aorta intra-operatively, and serially evaluating injuries that are managed non-operatively. Although their clinical relevance is unclear, TEE appears to be particularly sensitive in detecting small intimal injuries which may missed by angiography and CT.[27] However, TEE may be impossible to perform in patients with cervical spine or maxillofacial injuries and may not adequately visualize the distal ascending aorta, proximal aortic arch, and great vessels.[28]

OPERATIVE THERAPY

Operative repair remains the standard of care for the management of blunt aortic injuries. However, as delays to the operating room average 10 hours,[1] strict blood pressure control should be instituted as soon as there is a suspicion of blunt aortic injury in the stable patient.[10,19] Once the diagnosis is established, a right radial arterial line should be placed pre-operatively. If distal monitoring is desired, a right femoral line will leave the left femoral artery available for bypass. The patient's pulmonary status should permit at least transient deflation of the left lung and a double lumen endotracheal tube is usually needed to achieve adequate lung separation. Inability to deflate the left lung critically compromises exposure and is associated with prolonged cross clamp times at the very least.

A left 4th intercostal space posterolateral thoracotomy affords optimal exposure to the descending thoracic aorta.[29] Among 91 cases in which the site of an aortic injury could be retrospectively determined, 46% were <1 cm from the origin of the left subclavian artery and the remainder were >1 cm distal to origin.[30] More proximal injuries mandate control between the left common carotid and subclavian arteries, a more challenging situation than clamping distally. The dissection is deeper in the chest, may be limited by the trachea and left main bronchus, and risks injury to the vagus and recurrent nerves. There is also a tendency to dissect more distally along the lesser curve of the aorta, increasing the risk of inadvertently entering the injury. Not surprisingly, proximal injuries are associated with a significantly higher risk of death and longer cross clamp times (Figure 40–2). The risk of rupture, particularly intra-operatively, is also 5 times greater for lesions <1 cm from the subclavian artery.[30] Because of these considerations, cannulation for left heart bypass should precede dissection in stable patients. While the majority of cases require an interposition graft, primary anastamosis has been possible in 18% to 72% of patients with partial tears.[6,10–12] When feasible, primary repair has the advantages of shorter cross clamp times and avoidance of prosthetic material.[12,31]

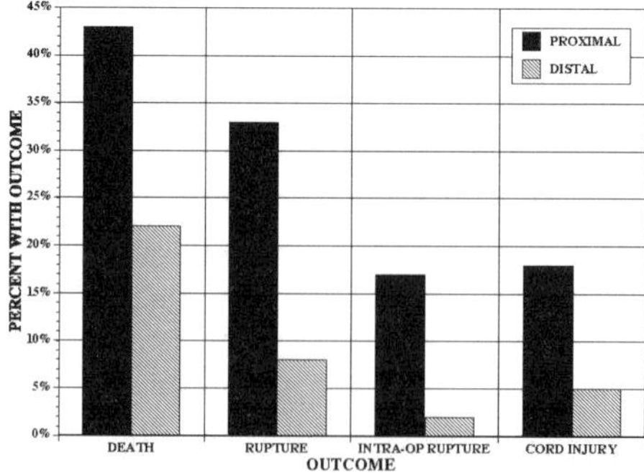

Figure 40–2. Outcome among patients with injuries ≤1 cm (proximal, N = 42) or >1 cm (distal, N = 49) from the origin of the left subclavian artery. Proximal injuries are associated with a significantly (p <0.05) greater risk of death and overall and intra-operative rupture. Differences in the incidence of ischemic spinal cord injury did not reach statistical significance (p = 0.1). Adapted from Carter Y, Meissner M, Bulger E, et al. Anatomical considerations in the surgical management of blunt thoracic aortic injury. *J Vasc Surg.* 2001; 34: 628–633.

Paraplegia complicating thoracic aortic repair has a multifactorial etiology that is influenced by anatomic and hemodynamic factors as well as associated injuries.[2] However, cross clamp times of greater than 30 minutes are associated with an increased risk of neurological deficits[1,9] and the risk of paraplegia approaches 100% at cross clamp times of 120 minutes.[9] A variety of techniques to support distal aortic perfusion have been employed including passive shunts, left heart bypass, and full cardiopulmonary bypass. In contrast to passive shunts, the use of active mechanical pumps to maintain distal aortic perfusion does appear to reduce the incidence of paraplegia. In comparison with left heart bypass and partial cardiopulmonary bypass, the "clamp and sew" technique is associated with a 3.4- to 6.4-fold increased risk of neurological deficits.[1,31] The 15% to 26% incidence of paralysis associated with the "clamp and sew" technique can be reduced to 0% to 5% with the use of left heart bypass.[1,8,9, 12,19,31,32] It has been estimated that 1 case of paraplegia is prevented for every 14 patients managed with left heart bypass.[31] In addition to maintaining spinal cord perfusion, left heart bypass may reduce left heart strain and minimize end-organ ischemia and release of inflammatory mediators.[11,12,32] Small series have reported a lower incidence of organ failure, particularly renal insufficiency, among patients repaired using left hear bypass.[32]

Left heart bypass is usually performed using a centrifugal pump (BioMedicus, Inc., Eden Prairie, MN) that, when used with heparin-bonded tubing, does not require systemic anticoagulation. Although inflow is most commonly obtained through the left atrial appendage, cannulation of the inferior pulmonary vein has several advantages.[12] This approach does not require opening the pericardium; avoids cannulating an irritable, friable appendage; and allows placement of the cannulae away from the operative field. Among 50 patients undergoing left heart bypass for traumatic aortic injuries at our institution, inflow was obtained through the left atrial appendage in 19 and via the pulmonary veins in 31. Complications, most often dysrythmias, occurred in 36.8% of patients cannulated through the atrial appendage in comparison to only 6.5% of those cannulated via the pulmonary veins.[33] Distal ischemia is minimized by maintaining perfusion pressures >60 mm Hg as monitored by a femoral arterial line. However, as pressure is difficult to manipulate with left heart bypass, increasing flow and adding volume are frequently the only useful interventions.

Unfortunately, maintenance of distal aortic perfusion is not always feasible. Approximately one-third of repairs in North America are performed without bypass.[19] These patients are frequently critically ill, hemodynamically unstable and have impending or actual aortic rupture. In addition to not being able to use left heart bypass in some of these patients, pre-operative instability is independently associated with a 5.5-fold increased risk of post-operative paralysis.[11] Other considerations to minimize cord injury include the prevention of a steal by quickly ligating any back bleeding intercostals and restoring subclavian flow as soon as the proximal anastamosis is completed.

ENDOVASCULAR REPAIR

Although the long-term benefits remain unclear, endovascular stent grafts have become an alternative to surgery for many aortic disorders, including blunt thoracic aortic injury. Several groups have reported successful repair of thoracic aortic injuries using non-commercial devices, most often constructed of modified stainless steel Z-stents fashioned into a cylindrical frame and covered with polyester or balloon dilated polytetrafluoroethylene.[34–37] Unfortunately the time required to construct (3 to 4 hours) and gas sterilize (24 to 27 hours) these devices limits their utility in the acutely injured patient.[38]

Although not currently approved for clinical use in the United States, several groups have also reported successful repairs using commercially available devices. As the mean diameter of the thoracic aorta at the site of blunt injury is 20 mm, repair using approved abdominal devices is theoretically possible. Both the Ancure (Guidant Corporation, Menlo Park, CA) tube graft and AneuRx (Medtronic AVE, Inc., Santa Rosa, CA) aortic cuffs have been successfully utilized for this purpose, although the short delivery systems require access through the iliac arteries or abdominal aorta. No approved thoracic devices are currently available in the United States. However, Orend et al.[39] repaired 8 descending thoracic aortic injuries with a variety of endografts available in Europe. Others have similarly reported 100% technical success in treating small numbers of subacute or chronic traumatic thoracic aortic injuries with MinTec or Talent stent grafts.[40,41] Both devices have an uncovered leading edge, allowing fixation across the subclavian origin. Although existing studies have included few patients and must be interpreted with caution, the risk of paraplegia has been reported to be only 0% to 3%.[34,35,38]

Although experience remains limited, some factors unique to the endovascular repair of thoracic aortic injuries are beginning to emerge. Many of the technical considerations are identical to those in the abdominal aorta-that is, the adequacy of the proximal and distal necks, the ability of the delivery device to negotiate small and tortuous arteries, and the ability to obtain an adequate seal. Most investigators have recommended a proximal neck of 10 to 15 mm and oversizing the diameter 10% to 20% larger than the proximal neck.[34,38,39] The distance from the left subclavian artery is the most important determinant of successful endovascular repair of thoracic aortic lesions.[34] In reviewing endoprostheses placed for a variety of indications, including blunt trauma, technical success was achieved in 57.4% of patients when the lesion was within 2 cm of the left subclavian artery in comparison to 100% for lesions situated more distally.[34] In order to gain adequate proximal fixation, some[39] have routinely deployed endografts across the left subclavian artery. Although covering the left subclavian artery poses little risk of limb threatening arm ischemia,[34, 39] an adjuvant carotid-subclavian bypass has been required in up to 13% of cases[39] and type II endoleaks can occur. The angle of the aortic arch must also be considered in treating lesions close to the subclavian artery. An acutely angled arch may cause difficulty tracking the delivery system[42] as well as increasing the risk of proximal endoleak and compromising distal flow due to "telescoping" or stent deformation.[34] With these anatomic considerations in mind, we reviewed the angiograms of 50 patients with a documented aortic injury. The average proximal neck diameter was 19 mm, the mean curvature at the site of injury was 54 degrees and only 14% of patients had a proximal neck ≥2 cm from the left subclavian artery[30] (Figure 40–3).

These reports, though limited in number and demonstrating the logistic difficulties expected with any new technology, suggest that stent graft repair may play an increasing role in the treatment of these injuries. The Talent (Medtronic AVE, Inc., Sunrise, FL) and Gore (W.L. Gore and Associates, Inc., Flagstaff, AZ) devices are currently being evaluated in the United States and their commercial availability will undoubtedly increase the utility of endovascular repair of these injuries. For the present, endovascular repair of blunt thoracic aortic injuries outside of well-constructed trials should be restricted to life-threatening situations where no other alternative is feasible.

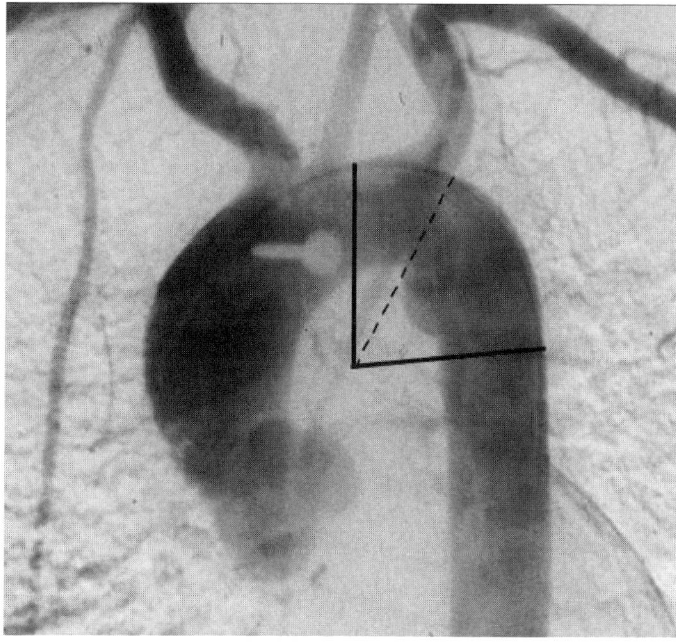

Figure 40–3. Thoracic aortagram demonstrating a typical blunt aortic injury at the isthmus. In considering endovascular treatment of blunt aortic injuries, the distance of the injury from the left subclavian artery and the curvature of the aorta at the site of injury are of primary concern. Although the proximal diameter averages 19 mm, only 14% of such injuries will have a neck ≥2 cm in length. The angle of curvature averaged 54 degrees at the left subclavian artery (dashed line), but will be larger if coverage of the left subclavian artery is required for proximal fixation (solid line).

We currently consider endovascular repair in patients with contraindications to immediate operation and/or injuries such as head trauma that preclude strict blood pressure management.

DELAYED AND NON-OPERATIVE MANAGEMENT

Although immediate operative intervention is warranted in most patients with blunt aortic injuries, there are some patients in whom deferred management may be necessary. In the absence of exsanguinating thoracic hemorrhage, treatment of life threatening abdominal and head injuries before aortic repair is widely accepted. However, longer periods of delayed management may be appropriate in some patients with severe associated injuries or medical comorbidity. Indications for delayed management were initially developed by Akins[43] and subsequently refined by others[8,10] (Table 40–2). Consideration of delayed operative management further requires that the patient have been hemodynamically stable for 4 to 6 hours and show no evidence of an expanding mediastinal hematoma.[2]

There is a continuum of aortic injury extending from subintimal hemorrhage to complete disruption and some injury patterns may also warrant initial non-operative management. Minimal aortic injury has been defined as those with an intimal flap <1 cm and absent or minimal periaortic hematoma.[44] Among 8 patients with minimal aortic injury followed radiographically for 1 to 10 weeks, no aorta related morbidity or

TABLE 40–2. INDICATIONS FOR DELAYED MANAGEMENT OF BLUNT AORTIC INJURY

Advanced Age

Pre-existing Cardiac Disease

Severe Head Injury
    Glasgow Coma Score <6
    Elevated Intracranial Pressure
    Intracranial Hemorrhage

Pulmonary Injury
    PaO_2/FiO_2 Ratio <200
    Positive End Expiratory Pressure (PEEP) ≥ 7.5 cm H_2O
    Intolerant of Single Lung Ventilation

Cardiac Injury
    Wall Motion Abnormalities
    Requirement for Inotropic Support

Refractory Coagulopathy

mortality was noted. Limited data also suggests that small intimal injuries identified by transesophageal echo may also have a benign prognosis.[27] Still other injuries may be associated with risks that exceed the benefits of operative repair. A small defect in an extremely calcified aorta represents a particular hazard.[45] Associated injuries may also preclude repair of injuries involving the aortic arch and requiring hypothermic circulatory arrest. In contrast, patients with a hemothorax larger than 500 cc and no pneumothorax; pseudocoarctation (upper extremity hypertension with diminished femoral pulses—Figure 40–4); a supraclavicular hematoma; or an inability to control blood pressure are at increased risk of early rupture and warrant urgent operation.[10,25]

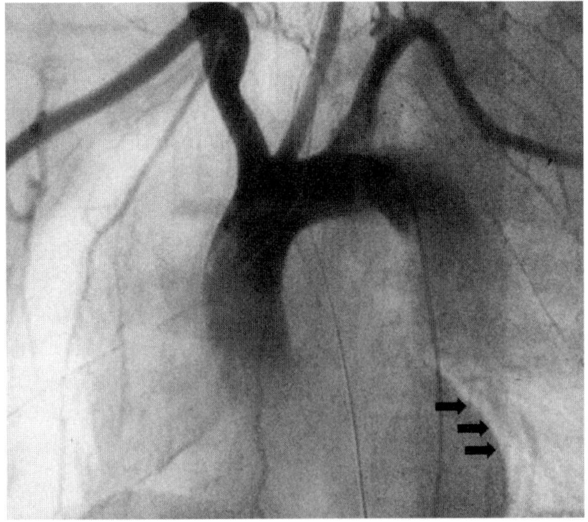

Figure 40–4. Thoracic aortagram showing complete transection of the thoracic aorta with near complete occlusion of the distal lumen by the associated flap (black arrows). Such pseudocoarctation with upper extremity hypertension and diminished femoral pulses is associated with a high risk of rupture and warrants immediate surgical intervention.

Rigorous blood pressure control is critical in the selective management of blunt aortic injury. Manipulation of left ventricular systolic ejection dynamics ($\Delta P/\Delta t$) presumably reduces aortic wall tension and shear stress as reflected by a decrease in the upslope of the arterial pressure tracing.[18] Beta-blockers are therefore recommended as first line agents with vasodilators added if the systolic blood pressure remains elevated despite maximal beta blockade. Although maintaining a systolic blood pressure below 120 mm Hg appears to significantly reduce the incidence of rupture, aiming for a systolic pressure 10 to 20 mm Hg lower than baseline may be more practical.[2,8,18] If significant head injury is present, intra-cranial pressure monitoring should be employed to ensure an adequate cerebral perfusion pressure. Appropriate anti-hypertensive therapy should be continued indefinitely until the injury is either repaired or resolved.

Serial radiographic examination should be performed every 2–3 days for the first week in patients selected for delayed operative management. In the absence of progression, further radiological and clinical surveillance should be performed at least every 6 months. Although spiral CT has proven to be the most useful modality in following these injuries,[8] others[27] have successfully used transesophageal echocardiography for this purpose. Some aortic injuries may resolve under observation, while others will ultimately become chronic pseudoaneurysms. Unfortunately, there is little data regarding those features most likely to predict progression. Injury progression, enlargement of a pseudoaneurysm, or the development of symptoms mandates operative intervention.

The literature includes over 500 patients managed in a delayed fashion, and of these, approximately 10% were managed entirely non-operatively.[2] Three surgical groups have reported in-hospital aortic rupture rates of $\leq 5\%$ with selective delayed repair.[46–48] In our experience, up to 20% of patients are candidates for delayed or non-operative management based on associated injuries or premorbid conditions.[8] Of 145 patients evaluated over 16 years, delayed or non-operative management was undertaken in 30. Fifteen patients underwent delayed aortic repair a median of 3 days following injury, while 15 were never operative candidates and were observed. Three of 15 patients (20%) in the delayed operative group demonstrated progression of the initial injury, with 1 rupturing and 2 demonstrating enlargement of a pseudoaneurysm within 5 days of injury. Five of 15 patients (33%) in the non-operative group died, all due to non-survivable head injuries. No deaths among the unoperated patients were due to aortic complications and at a median follow-up of 2.5 years, 5 of the injuries are stable chronic pseudoaneurysms while 5 have completely resolved. Maggisano[10] similarly reported an aorta-related mortality rate of 4.5% among those selected for delayed operative repair. Thirteen patients were managed entirely non-operatively with small chronic pseudoaneurysms at 1 to 4 years of follow-up. Overall hospital mortality, excluding those patients arriving in extremis, was only 17% using a selective approach in comparison to an average mortality rate of 26% in the literature. Based on our experience we have made the following observations: apparently "small" lesions can rupture; the maximum risk of rupture appears to be within the first 5 days after injury; non-operative therapy is reasonable if blood pressure can be controlled; serial follow up with radiographic studies is critical in the first week following injury; and operative versus non-operative management should be based on injury location and comorbidity rather than size alone.

CONCLUSION

Although the natural history may be different than described in early reports, blunt aortic injury is still associated with high mortality rates. Operative repair remains the standard of care in these patients and experience has validated certain technical principles. Left heart bypass should be used in those cases where it is technically feasible and cannulation should be performed prior to dissection, particularly if control proximal to the subclavian artery is required. Injuries ≤1 cm from the left subclavian should be controlled between the left common carotid and subclavian arteries. The role of endovascular repair is rapidly evolving, although blunt thoracic aortic injuries do have special considerations such as proximity to the left subclavian artery and the curvature of the aortic arch. No commercial thoracic devices are currently available in the United States, although a significant future role for these devices is likely. Finally, although improvements in surgical care have reduced the incidence of complications such as paraplegia, it is clear that immediate operative repair may be risky and technically difficult in at least some of these patients. Deferred operative intervention with aggressive blood pressure control may be appropriate in some especially high-risk patients.

REFERENCES

1. Fabian TC, Richardson JD, Croce MA, et al. Prospective study of blunt aortic injury: Multicenter Trial of the American Association for the Surgery of Trauma. *J Trauma.* 1997;42: 374–380.
2. Mattox KL, Wall MJ, Jr. Historical review of blunt injury to the thoracic aorta. *Chest Surg Clin N Am.* 2000;10:167–182.
3. Nagy K, Fabian T, Rodman G, et al. Guidelines for the diagnosis and managment of blunt aortic injury. An EAST practice management guidelines workgroup. *J Trauma.* 2000;48: 1128–1143.
4. Shkrum MJ, McClafferty KJ, Green RN, et al. Mechanisms of aortic injury in fatalities occurring in motor vehicle collisions. *J Forensic Sci.* 1999;44: 44–56.
5. Brundage SI, Harruff R, Jurkovich GJ, et al. The epidemiology of thoracic aortic injuries in pedestrians. *J Trauma.* 1998;45:1010–1014.
6. Razzouk AJ, Gundry SR, Wang N, et al. Repair of traumatic aortic rupture. *Arch Surg.* 2000; 135:913–918.
7. Parmley LF, Mattingly TW, Manion WC, et al. Non-penetrating traumatic injury of the aorta. *Circulation.* 1958;17:1086–1101.
8. Holmes JH, Bloch RD, Hall RA, et al. Natural history of traumatic rupture of the thoracic aorta managed nonoperatively: A longitudinal analysis. *Ann Thorac Surg.* 2002;73: 1149–1154.
9. von Oppell UO, Dunne TT, DeGroot MK, et al. Traumatic aortic rupture: Twenty-year metaanalysis of mortality and risk of paraplegia. *Ann Thorac Surg.* 1994;58:585–593.
10. Maggisano R, Nathens A, Alexandrova NA, et al. Traumatic rupture of the thoracic aorta: should one always operate immediately? *Ann Vasc Surg.* 1995;9:44–52.
11. Karmy-Jones R, Carter YM, Nathens A, et al. Impact of presenting physiology and associated injuries on outcome following traumatic rupture of the thoracic aorta. *Am Surg.* 2001;67:61–66.
12. Read RA, Moore EE, Moore FA, et al. Partial left heart bypass for thoracic aorta repair. *Arch Surg.* 1993;128:746–752.
13. Sturm JT, Hankins DG, Young G. Thoracic aortography following blunt chest trauma. *Am J Emerg Med.* 1990;8:92–96.
14. Hunink MG, Bos JJ. Triage of patients to angiography for detection of aortic rupture after blunt chest trauma: cost-effectiveness analysis of using CT. *AJR Am J Roentgenol.* 1995;165: 27–36.
15. Mirvis SE, Bidwell JK, Buddemeyer EU, et al. Value of chest radiography in excluding traumatic aortic rupture. *Radiology.* 1987;163:487–493.

16. Kram HB, Wohlmuth DA, Appel PL, et al. Clinical and radiographic indications for aortography in blunt chest trauma. *J Vasc Surg.* 1987;6:168–76.
17. Sturm JT, Luxenberg MG, Moudry BM, et al. Does sternal fracture increase the risk for aortic rupture? *Ann Thorac Surg.* 1989;48:697–698.
18. Mattox KL. Red River anthology. *J Trauma.* 1997;42:353–368.
19. Gammie JS, Shah AS, Hattler BG, et al. Traumatic aortic rupture: Diagnosis and management. *Ann Thorac Surg.* 1998;66:1295–1300.
20. Symbas PJ, Horsley S, Symbas PN. Rupture of the ascending aorta caused by blunt trauma. *Ann Thorac Surg.* 1998;66:113–117.
21. Mirvis SE, Shanmuganathan K, Miller BH, et al. Traumatic aortic injury: diagnosis with contrast-enhanced thoracic CT-five-year experience at a major trauma center. *Radiology.* 1996;200:413–422.
22. Pretre R, Chilcott M. Blunt trauma to the heart and great vessles. *New Engl J Med.* 1997;336:626–632.
23. Mirvis SE, Bidwell JK, Buddemeyer EU, et al. Value of chest radiography in excluding traumatic aortic rupture. *Radiology.* 1987;163:487–493.
24. Mirvis SE, Shanmuganathan K, Buell J, et al. Use of spiral computed tomography for the assessment of blunt trauma patients with potential aortic injury. *J Trauma.* 1998;45:922–930.
25. Clark DE, Zeiger MA, Wallace KL, et al. Blunt aortic trauma: signs of high risk. *J Trauma.* 1990;30:701–705.
26. Blackmore CC, Zweibel A, Mann FA. Determining risk of traumatic aortic injury: How to optimize imaging strategy. *AJR.* 2000;174:343–347.
27. Kepros J, Angood P, Jaffe CC, et al. Aortic intimal injuries from blunt trauma: resolution profile in nonoperative management. *J Trauma.* 2002;52:475–478.
28. Ahrar K, Smith DC, Bansal RC, et al. Angiography in blunt thoracic aortic injury. *J Trauma.* 1997;42:665–669.
29. Feczko JD, Lynch L, Pless JE, et al. An autopsy case review of 142 nonpenetrating (blunt) injuries of the aorta. *J Trauma.* 1992;33:846–849.
30. Carter Y, Meissner M, Bulger E, et al. Anatomical considerations in the surgical management of blunt thoracic aortic injury. *J Vasc Surg.* 2001;34:628–633.
31. Jahromi AS, Kazemi K, Safar HA, et al. Traumatic rupture of the aorta: Cohort study and systematic review. *J Vasc Surg.* 2001;34:1029–1034.
32. Forbes AD, Ashbaugh DG. Mechanical circulatory support during repair of thoracic aortic injuries improves morbidity and prevents spinal cord injury. *Arch Surg.* 1994;129:494–497.
33. Karmy-Jones R, Carter Y, Meissner M, et al. Choice of venous cannulation for bypass during repair of traumatic rupture of the aorta. *Ann Thorac Surg.* 2001;71:39–41.
34. Rodrigues Alves CM, da Fonseca JH, de Souza JA, et al. Endovascular treatment of thoracic disease: patient selection and a proposal of a risk score. *Ann Thorac Surg.* 2002;73:1143–1148.
35. Dake MD, Miller DC, Semba CP, et al. Transluminal placement of endovascular stent-grafts for the treatment of descending thoracic aortic aneurysms. *N Engl J Med.* 1994;331:1729–1734.
36. Fujikawa T, Yukioka T, Ishimaru S, et al. Endovascular stent grafting for the treatment of blunt thoracic aortic injury. *J Trauma.* 2001;50:223–229.
37. Kato N, Dake MD, Miller DC, et al. Traumatic thoracic aortic aneurysm: treatment with endovascular stent-grafts. *Radiology.* 1997;205:657–662.
38. Semba CP, Kato N, Kee ST, et al. Acute rupture of the descending thoracic aorta: repair with use of endovascular stent-grafts. *J Vasc Interv Radiol.* 1997;8:337–342.
39. Orend KH, Kotsis T, Scharrer-Pamler R, et al. Endovascular repair of aortic rupture due to trauma and aneurysm. *Eur J Vasc Endovasc Surg.* 2002;23:61–67.
40. Rousseau H, Soula P, Perreault P, et al. Delayed treatment of traumatic rupture of the thoracic aorta with endoluminal covered stent. *Circulation.* 1999;99:498–504.
41. Ruchat P, Capasso P, Chollet-Rivier M, et al. Endovascular treatment of aortic rupture by blunt chest trauma. *J Cardiovasc Surg (Torino).* 2001;42:77–81.
42. Bruninx G, Wery D, Dubois E, et al. Emergency endovascular treatment of an acute traumatic rupture of the thoracic aorta complicated by a distal low-flow syndrome. *Cardiovasc Intervent Radiol.* 1999;22:515–518.

43. Akins CW, Buckley MJ, Daggett W, et al. Acute traumatic disruption of the thoracic aorta: a ten-year experience. *Ann Thorac Surg.* 1981;31:305–309.
44. Fabian TC, Davis KA, Gavant ML, et al. Prospective study of blunt aortic injury: helical CT is diagnostic and antihypertensive therapy reduces rupture. *Ann Surg.* 1998;227:666–676.
45. Camp PC, Shackford SR. Outcome after blunt traumatic thoracic aortic laceration: identification of a high-risk cohort. Western Trauma Association Multicenter Study Group. *J Trauma.* 1997;43:413–422.
46. Pate JW, Gavant ML, Weiman DS, et al. Traumatic rupture of the aortic isthmus: program of selective management. *World J Surg.* 1999;23:59–63.
47. Warren RL, Akins CW, Conn AK, et al. Acute traumatic disruption of the thoracic aorta: emergency department management. *Ann Emerg Med.* 1992;21:391–396.
48. Pierangeli A, Turinetto B, Galli R, et al. Delayed treatment of isthmic aortic rupture. *Cardiovasc Surg.* 2000;8:280–283.

41

Management of Upper Extremity Vascular Trauma

Richard R. Keen, MD, John D. Keen, MD, and Mitchell J. Cohen, MD

Trauma remains the fourth leading cause of death in the United States. After lethal impact injuries to the central nervous system, exsanguination from intra-thoracic vascular injuries is the next most common cause of death in trauma victims.[1]

The trend that is important to vascular surgeons is that their role in the management of vascular trauma is increasing by default. In the past, general surgeons with training in vascular surgical techniques had performed the majority of the operative treatments for traumatic vascular injuries. As the vascular experience of general surgeons both in training and in practice continues to decrease, fewer general surgeons with training in the management of vascular injuries will be available. The number of general surgeons who are trained in the management of vascular trauma will be compromised even further if endovascular technology, including the use of covered stents, takes on an increasing role in the treatment of vascular trauma.

In the current economic and practice environment, the treatment of vascular problems needs to be efficient, cost-effective, and durable.[2] Of all of the medical and surgical problems that vascular surgeons manage, the operative treatment that perhaps is the most cost-effective is the management of vascular trauma.[3] The cost-effectiveness of an intervention is measured by the incremental societal resource cost in dollars for every quality adjusted life year (QALY) saved, the ratio by which cost-effective decision analysis is performed.[4] The lower the value for the dollars per QALY, the better, as this lower ratio may reflect either a lower cost or a very effective outcome. Usually treatments costing $50,000 per QALY are acceptable.[4]

The outcome for the treatment of vascular trauma is life salvage or functional limb salvage.[5] In calculating the cost per QALY saved, the incremental cost for providing a treatment is divided by the number of years a person will live with the benefit of this treatment after the treatment is completed. The 2 variables that are most important in determining a low ratio of cost per QALY saved for a particular intervention are; 1) a durable, dramatic change in outcome (functional limb salvage vs. amputation) and therefore quality of life, and; 2) treatment at a young age (life vs. death). The successful operative treatment for vascular trauma produces dramatic outcomes reflected in durable life and limb salvage in predominantly young individuals, making the overall treatment of vascular injuries cost-effective.[6]

EVALUATION AND INITIAL TREATMENT OF UPPER EXTREMITY VASCULAR TRAUMA

The vascular system of the upper extremity begins and ends in the chest. Any discussion of upper extremity vascular trauma needs to include the management of injuries to the intrathoracic great vessels at the thoracic inlet.

The innominate artery and the proximal portions of the subclavian arteries lie within the bony thorax and exit through the cervicothoracic inlet (Figure 41–1).[7] The subclavian arteries enter Zone I of the neck as these arteries exit the thoracic inlet. The majority of both the right and left subclavian arteries lie within Zone I of the neck, which extends from the sternal notch to the top of the clavicles (Figure 41–2).[8]

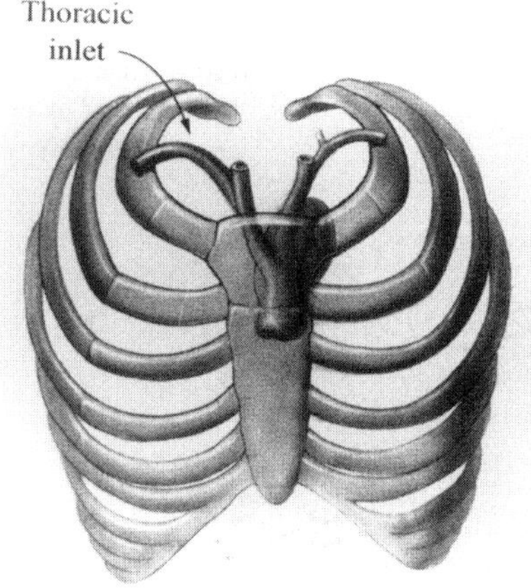

Figure 41–1. The innominate artery and the proximal portions of the subclavian arteries lie within the bony thorax and exit through the cervicothoracic inlet. (Reprinted with permission from Trunkey DD, Meyer DM, Brusel KR. Thoracic inlet and mediastinal injuries. In: Thal ER, Weigelt JA, Carrico CJ, eds. *Operative Trauma Management.* New York: McGraw Hill;2002:110–121.)

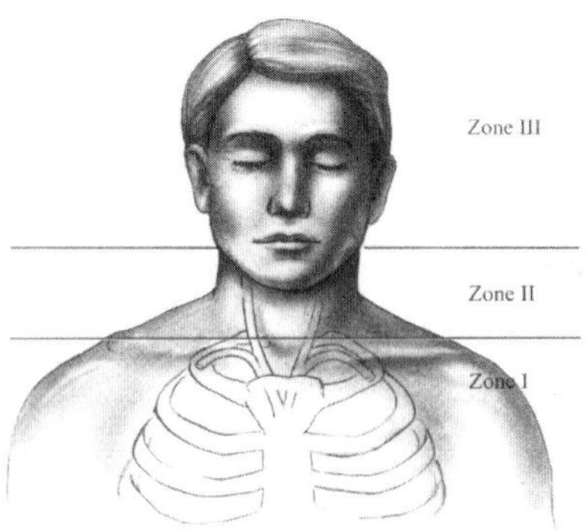

Figure 41–2. The subclavian arteries enter Zone I of the neck as these arteries exit the thoracic inlet. The majority of both the right and left subclavian arteries lie within Zone I of the neck, which extends from the sternal notch to the top of the clavicles. (Reprinted with permission from Trunkey DD, Meyer DM, Brusel KR. Thoracic inlet and mediastinal injuries. In: Thal ER, Weigelt JA, Carrico CJ, eds. *Operative Trauma Management.* New York: McGraw Hill;2002:110–121.)

Injuries to the innominate and subclavian arteries and veins are among the most difficult acute clinical problems faced by vascular surgeons. In patients reaching the hospital, the overall mortality of these injuries approximates 50%. These injuries may present as transections, partial lacerations, intimal defects with small pseudoaneurysms, and as arteriovenous fistulas.[9]

Successful management of upper extremity vascular injuries that occur within the cervicothoracic inlet depends upon surgical expertise in 3 areas: 1) rapid, immediate resuscitation; 2) recognition and delineation of the location, extent, and complexity of the injuries; and 3) prompt operative or endovascular intervention that permits control of the hemorrhage and repair of the injured vessels.[10] Options are dictated by the patient's condition on presentation to the emergency department or trauma unit.

Early Management and Resuscitation

Expeditious treatment needs to be pursued for any patient with suspected upper mediastinal vascular injury. Any evidence of airway compromise or hemodynamic instability is treated with endotracheal intubation. Penetrating injury of the intrathoracic vessels that can cause immediate exsanguination externally or into the chest can just as readily present as a hematoma confined at high pressure within the medistinum. Hemodynamic stability in patients with an intrathoracic great vessel injury is an illusion the would make Houdini proud!

If intravenous resuscitation fails to stop cardiovascular collapse and cardiac arrest ensues, then immediate emergency department anterolateral thoracotomy is the treatment for exsanguinating hemorrhage due to an intrathoracic vascular injury. Left anterior thoracotomy in the fourth interspace is performed with the patient in the supine position. This maneuver permits access to the descending thoracic aorta, which is clamped. Cross-clamping of the descending thoracic aortic increases afterload and therefore myocardial and cerebral perfusion. This procedure can buy time while the source of the hemorrhage is located and controlled and the resuscitation continued. The left thoracotomy can be extended rapidly across the sternum into the right chest which permits opening the chest like a clamshell. This maneuver provides rapid access to the intrathoracic great vessels for direct control of hemorrhage.

The limitation of this approach (tranverse thoractomy) is that direct access is compromised to the vessels at the apex of the chest and the thoracic inlet. Preload may be temporarily improved but valuable time can be lost with this approach in the setting of injuries beyond the most proximal portion of the subclavian arteries or veins, as this approach will not permit direct control of hemorrhage from these vessels. Therefore, we believe that the role of left anterolateral thoractomy in the emergency or trauma unit or even in the operating room is limited to the setting of cardiac arrest or impending arrest.

Patients presenting in severe shock with a systolic blood pressure of less than 50 mm Hg should be transported immediately to the operating room and explored through a transverse thoracotomy or preferably, a median sternotomy (Figure 41–3). In exsanguinating patients with suspected or known subclavian artery or vein injury, immediate vascular control can be obtained by manual pressure through an anterior thoractomy or median sternotomy (Figure 41–4).

Patients with mild to moderate shock with a systolic pressure of between 50 and 90 mm Hg should be rapidly resuscitated while preliminary imaging studies, such as chest x-ray and cervical spine films are obtained. If shock persists or recurs, resuscita-

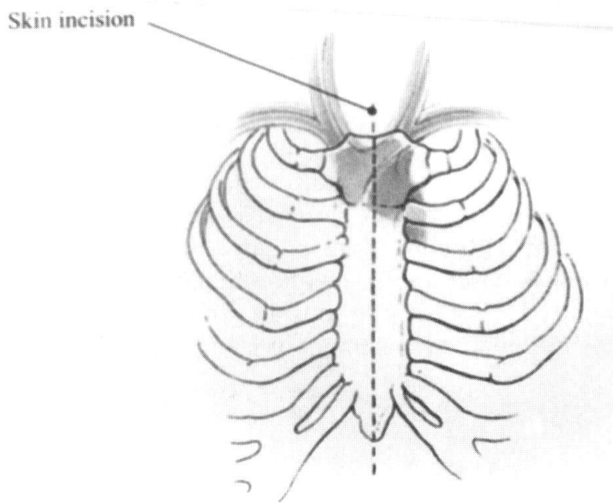

Figure 41–3. Median sternotomy is the preferred initial incision for exposure and control of *all* vascular injuries caused by midline penetrating wounds that involve the thoracic inlet. Injuries to the innominate artery and veins, and the proximal right *and left* subclavian arteries to the level of the origin of the vertebral arteries are readily approached by way of a median sternotomy. (Reprinted with permission from Trunkey DD, Meyer DM, Brusel KR. Thoracic inlet and mediastinal injuries. In: Thal ER, Weigelt JA, Carrico CJ, eds. *Operative Trauma Management.* New York: McGraw Hill;2002:110–121.)

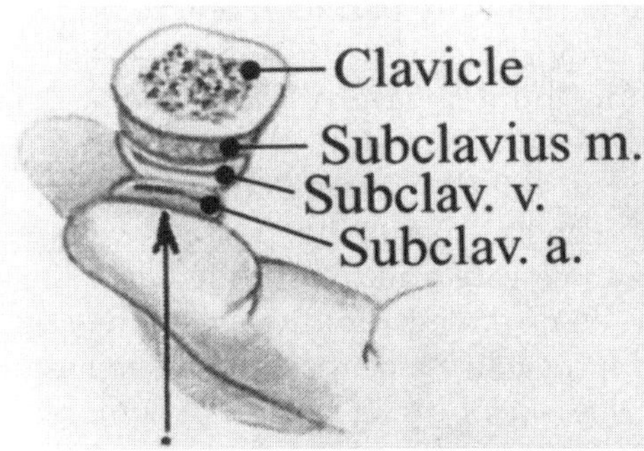

Figure 41–4. In exsanguinating patients with suspected or known subclavian artery or vein injury, immediate control can be obtained by manual pressure through an anterior thoractomy or median sternotomy. (Reprinted with permission from Trunkey DD, Meyer DM, Brusel KR. Thoracic inlet and mediastinal injuries. In: Thal ER, Weigelt JA, Carrico CJ, eds. *Operative Trauma Management.* New York: McGraw Hill;2002:110–121.)

tion should be continued in the operating room. If the patient shows signs of hemodynamic stability, further diagnostic imaging studies can be undertaken.[11]

Imaging to Localize the Injury

There are specific, real benefits to preoperative vascular imaging if time permits. The path of projectiles can provide some clue as to the potential vascular structures that could be injured, but because bullets and shrapnel can ricochet inside the chest like marbles in a box, we have found presumed projectile paths to be misleading.

For a patient with evidence of hemodynamic stability, aortic arch arteriography and selective great vessel proximity arteriography performed in the angiography suite has served as the standard method for evaluating the intrathoracic upper extremity arteries, including the innominate and subclavian arteries in the thoracic inlet. Arteriography is sensitive and specific for diagnosing intrathoracic arterial injuries.[8,9] Delayed venous phases of the angiogram also can be used to diagnose intrathoracic venous injuries.

An additional advantage of arteriography performed in the angiography suite is simultaneous placement of an occluding balloon catheter proximal to the area of arterial injury. This balloon catheter can be inflated at any time and proximal occlusion of the injured vessel can be achieved if the patient's hemodynamic condition rapidly deteriorates.

We anticipate that the role for arteriography in the management of upper extremity vascular trauma will evolve from a primarily diagnostic modality to a technology that will be used predominantly for therapeutic interventions.[12] As endovascular technology continues to improve, arteriography may be undertaken as much for diagnostic purposes as for anticipation of performing a specific endovascular therapy.

The imaging modality that may rapidly replace arteriography in the diagnostic evaluation of vascular trauma is helical CT angiography. Multi-detector helical CT angiography, a fast and non-invasive imaging technique, is sensitive and specific in the diagnosis and localization of upper extremity vascular trauma.[13] Whether CT angiography will be as sensitive as conventional arteriography in diagnosing subtle defects remains to be determined. We anticipate using multi-detector technology CT angiography to evaluate potential intrathoracic vascular injuries in the new Cook County Hospital. We expect that this technology will eliminate the need for arteriography in the majority of patients with possible thoracic vascular injuries who require arteriography at the present time.

OPERATIVE STRATEGY: THE "INCISION DECISION"

Obtaining proximal control before directly tackling the vascular injury is the cardinal rule of vascular trauma management. When in doubt, for presumed intrathoracic upper extremity vascular injuries, perform a median sternotomy.

Median sternotomy is our preferred initial incision for exposure and control of *all* vascular injuries caused by midline penetrating wounds that involve the thoracic inlet, including the left subclavian artery. Injuries to the innominate artery and veins, and the proximal right and left subclavian arteries to the level of the origin of the vertebral arteries are readily approached by way of a median sternotomy.

Midline splitting of the sternum often is required in order to obtain proximal control of the injured vessel prior to exposing the area of injury. In our experience, median sternotomy provides much better exposure to the vessels in the superior mediastinum than any other approach. If proximal control is obtained before encountering exsanguinating hemorrhage, then the likelihood for a successful outcome is high, regardless of the location of the injury. Sternotomy is fast, and most importantly, permits excellent exposure to the heart, aortic arch, innominate artery and veins, and *both* subclavian arteries to the level of the origins of the vertebral arteries.

Past claims that sternotomy can not be used to get proximal control of the left subclavian artery simply are not true. The keys to using a median sternotomy to obtain proximal control of the left subclavian artery are to do a complete sternotomy and to open the sternal retractor as widely as possible. This permits approaching the left subclavian artery from the left lateral aspect of the sternotomy. Both the left subclavian and left common carotid arteries arise beyond the pericardial reflection so clamp placement at the origin of the left subclavian artery will not be blocked if this technique is used. However, because the origins of the left common carotid and left subclavian arteries are in such close proximity, it can be difficult to clamp the origin of the left subclavian artery on the aortic arch with a partial occluding clamp without also clamping the origin of the left common carotid artery. Other authors who perform a large amount of vascular trauma have also recognized the advantages of median sternotomy over the infamous trapdoor incision for left subclavian artery exposure.[7, 14]

The open treatment of subclavian injuries illustrates the step-wise approach that should be followed in addressing upper extremity vascular injuries. The operative treatment of upper extremity vascular injuries often requires two incisions. One incision is used for proximal control of the injured artery that does not decompress any associated hematoma. A second incision directly over the area of the injury only is made after proximal control is achieved. A variation of this theme is illustrated in a step-wise approach to subclavian artery injuries.

Following complete median sternotomy and placement of a sternal retractor, only the left subclavian artery proximal to the origin of the vertebral artery is accessible through this incision. Exposure of the entire left subclavian artery following sternotomy is possible after adding a second supraclavicular incision extension (Figure 41–5).[15] A 5 cm left supraclavicular extension of this incision divides the left neck strap muscles and the sternocleidomastoid, exposing the left innominate vein, the left internal jugular vein, and the medial portion of the left subclavian vein. Dividing the left innominate vein exposes the first portion of the left subclavian artery. Exposure of the proximal right subclavian artery requires division of the right internal jugular vein. Exposure of the second portion of the left subclavian artery posterior to the anterior scalene muscle requires division of this muscle, with care taken to preserve the left phrenic nerve which lies on its dorsal aspect. Exposure of the second portion of the left subclavian artery also may be facilitated by division of the left internal jugular vein, but with attention to preserving the terminal portion of the vein, as this location is where the thoracic duct inserts into the posterior aspect of the left internal jugular vein. The vagus nerves also lie anterior to the subclavian arteries and these also may be encountered in the dissection. Arteriography certainly is helpful in localizing the injury in relation to the vertebral artery and therefore facilitates planning of the operative approach.

Injuries to the middle and lateral portions of the subclavian artery require either a supraclavicular incision or direct incision over the clavicle combined with clavicle resection (Figure 41–6). We prefer clavicle excision in the exposure of mid- and distal subclavian artery injuries and for the exposure and repair of all subclavian vein injuries. Injuries to the mid-subclavian artery that are close to origin of the vertebral artery still should be addressed with a median sternotomy (for proximal control) followed by a supraclavicular incision or clavicle resection. The subclavian artery that vascular surgeons are used to seeing in older adults in the elective setting is truly a "subclavian" or even an "infraclavian" artery in younger trauma victims. This makes supraclavicular exposure difficult in the setting of hemorrhage. Claviculectomy is the fastest way to get exposure of the middle and lateral subclavian artery and especially the subclavian vein. Our experience with clavicle excision in the management of both subclavian trauma and Paget-Schroetter disease has demonstrated to us that the morbidity of clavicle resection is low. Others have reported similar results with clavicle resection.[16]

Injuries to the first portion of the axillary artery (between the clavicle and pectoralis minor) and to the second portion of the axillary artery (posterior to pectoralis

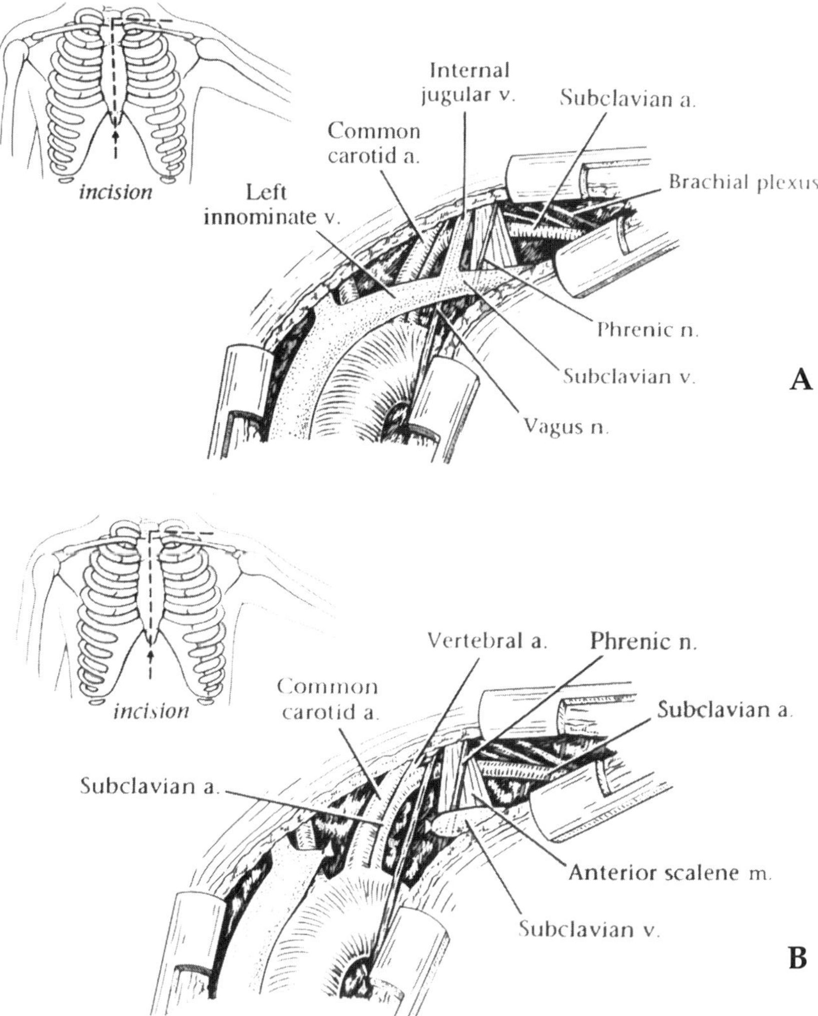

Figure 41–5. Exposure of the entire left subclavian artery by way of median sternotomy. **(A)** Following complete median sternotomy and placement of a sternal retractor, a 5 cm left supraclavicular extension of this incision divides the left neck strap muscles and the sternocleidomastoid, exposing the left innominate vein, the left internal jugular vein, and the medial portion of the left subclavian vein. **(B)** Dividing the left innominate vein exposes the first portion of the left subclavian artery. Exposure of the second portion of the left subclavian artery requires division of the anterior scalene muscle. Care is taken to preserve the vagus and phrenic nerves, which lie anterior to the subclavian artery. (Reprinted with permission from Hajarizadeh H, Rohrer MJ, Cutler BS. Surgical exposure of the left subclavian artery by median sternotomy and left supreclavicular extension. *J Trauma.* 1996;41:136–139.)

minor) can be obtained using the same infraclavicular incision used for axillofemoral bypass. We approach injuries to the third portion of the axillary artery (at the level of the medial and lateral humeral circumflex arteries on arteriography) by first obtaining proximal control of the axillary artery through an infraclavicular, pectoralis major splitting incision. Once proximal control is obtained, we perform a second curvilinear incison along the anterior border of the axillary hair line and the lateral border of pectoralis major, as one would use for an axillary dissection, to obtain direct access to the

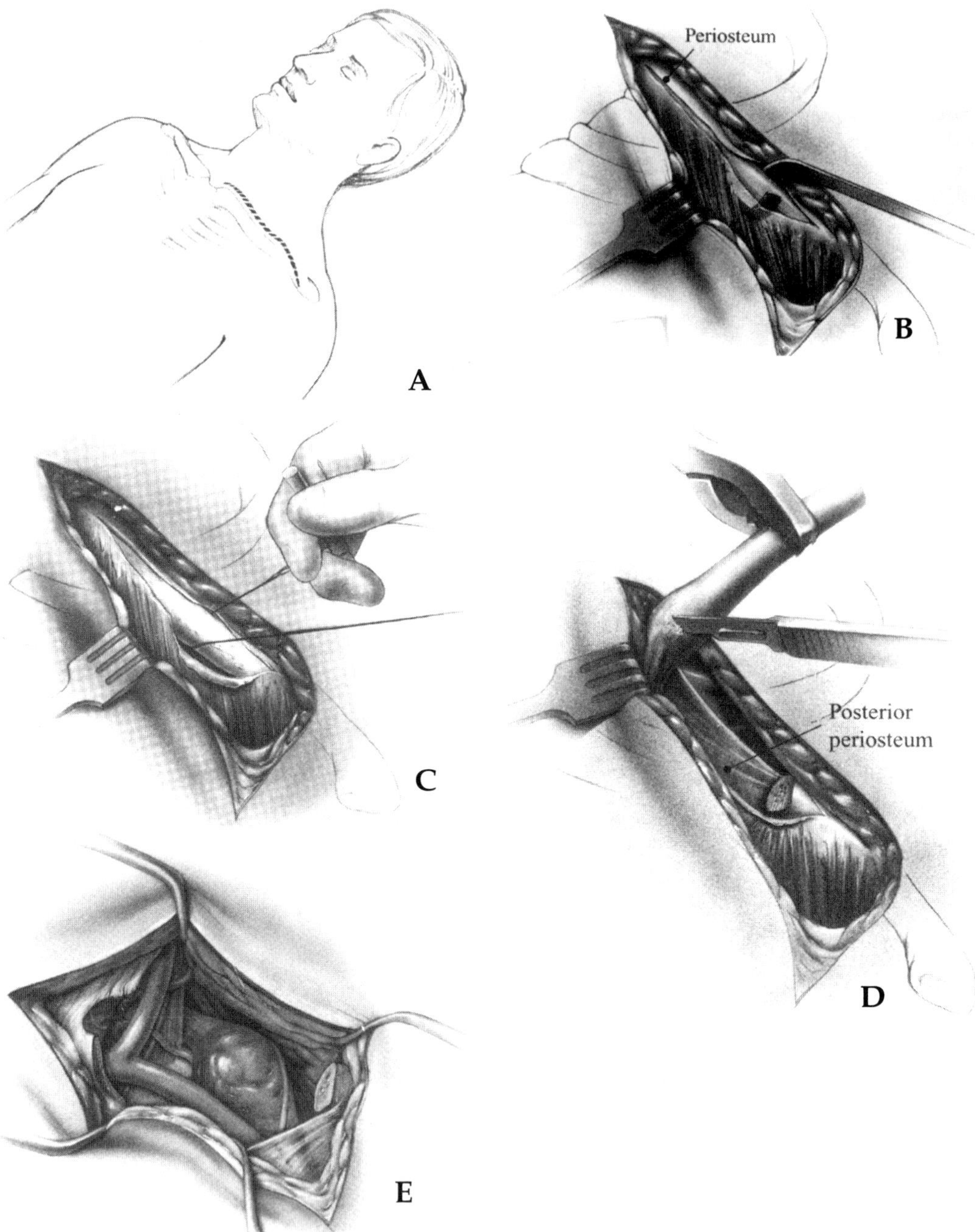

Figure 41–6. The subclavian artery lateral to the origin of the vertebral artery is outside of the thoracic inlet and cannot be approached or repaired by a median sternotomy alone. **(A)** The subclavian artery that lies in the supraclavicular fossa in older adults tends to be more retroclavicular or even infraclavicular in younger trauma patients, making supraclavicular exposure difficult in the setting of hemorrhage. **(B)** The periosteum of the clavicle is incised and the subclavius muscle detached. **(C)** A Gigli saw is used to transect the clavicle at the junction between its middle and distal thirds. **(D)** The sternoclavicular ligaments are incised and the medial clavicle is disarticulated off of the manubrium. The posterior periosteum is preserved. **(E)** Claviculectomy is the fastest way to get exposure of the lateral subclavian artery and especially the subclavian vein. (Reprinted with permission from Trunkey DD, Meyer DM, Brusel KR. Thoracic inlet and mediastinal injuries. In: Thal ER, Weigelt JA, Carrico CJ, eds. *Operative Trauma Management.* New York: McGraw Hill;2002:110–121.)

injury. Injuries to the proximal brachial artery can be approached with an extension of this axillary incision distally along the medial upper arm.

Hematomas within the axillary sheath can cause a compartment syndrome. The axillary sheath is small and non-compliant. Any bleeding within this space can cause a compartment syndrome manifest as compression symptoms to the nerve roots of the brachial plexus, particularly the median nerve. A compartment syndrome with compression of the brachial plexus by a tense hematoma within the axilla explains why some patients with arterial bleeding confined to the axilla present with an anesthetic, paralyzed arm within 30 minutes of the injury. These findings of an insensate, paralyzed arm are not due to arm ischemia but rather to the direct force of the hematoma on the nerve roots contained within the axilla or upper arm. This direct pressure causes ischemia to the nerve and necessitates prompt operative exploration and decompression.

The diagnosis of axillary artery injuries can be missed unless a high index of suspicion is maintained. The axillary artery is relatively inaccessible to direct examination physical and duplex examination, especially in often uncooperative patients who are unenthusiastic about the placement and pressing of an ultrasound transducer over the region of their recent injury. For these reasons, we continue to find arteriography to be very helpful in the diagnosis of axillary artery injuries, and other locations when there is evidence of an arterial injury but the exact level of the injury is not clear. This scenario has come into play with increasing frequency more recently with the larger percentage of trauma victims having sustained multiple gunshot wounds.

The other group of axillary artery injuries where arteriography is helpful is in shotgun wounds. Because of the associated soft tissue injury, these vascular reconstructions are best performed with extra-anatomic tunnels. A special situation occurs with shotgun wounds, which for some unknown reason have a tendency to injure arteries in the axilla and upper arm.[6] Reconstruction of these injuries usually requires treatment with a vein bypass routed in an extra-anatomic location, such as retrohumeral.[17]

Injuries to the brachial, radial, and ulnar arteries are approached through standard incisions that most vascular surgeons are familiar with because of their role in the creation of vascular access for hemodialysis.[18] Injuries at the antecubital fossa are common. An S-shaped incision starting from the medial upper arm and extending across the antecubital crease permits safely obtaining proximal control of the brachial artery and repairing an injury at the level of the antecubital fossa through one incision (Figure 41–7). Tourniquets or Esmark bandages are another technique for achieving proximal control for distal upper extremity arterial injuries.

The ankle-brachial or brachial-brachial index is considered part of the screening physical examination in patients with extremity vascular trauma. The limitation of the pressure index is the lack of sensitivity in detecting arterial pseudoaneursyms. Reports professing the safety and adequacy of the screening physical exam in the detection of occult vascular injuries are handicapped by the peppering of the vascular literature with reports of the late complications of occult vascular injuries that lead to adverse outcomes.[19]

UPPER EXTREMITY TRAUMA: TO REPAIR, OR NOT TO REPAIR

Arterial and venous injuries can be either ligated, repaired primarily, or repaired with interposition grafts composed of either saphenous vein, arm vein, or prosthetic material. Severe injuries to the innominate and subclavian arteries may require repair with

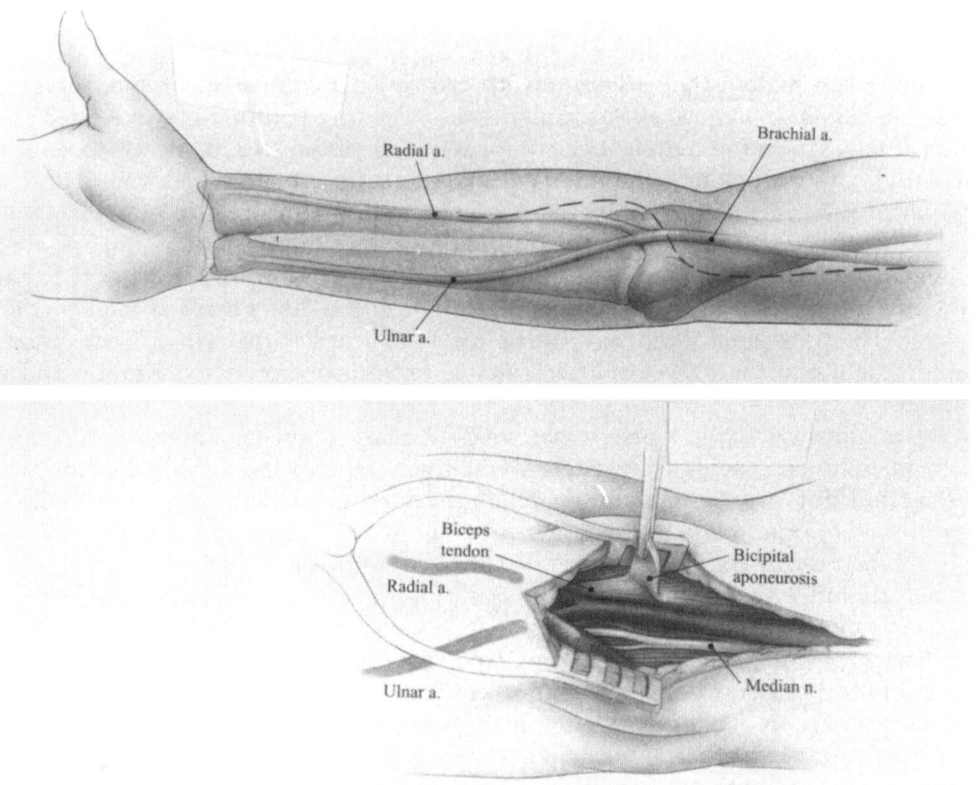

Figure 41–7. An S-shaped incision starting from the medial upper arm and extending across the antecubital crease permits obtaining proximal control of the brachial artery and repairing an injury at the level of the antecubital fossa through one incision. (Reprinted with permission from Owings JT. Upper extremity vascular injuries. In: Thal ER, Weigelt JA, Carrico CJ, eds. *Operative Trauma Management.* New York: McGraw Hill;2002:398–409.

PTFE grafts. Alternative autogenous conduits are panelled vein grafts or spiral grafts, but the frequent urgent nature of the procedure may preclude a complex autogenous reconstruction for these larger vessels. The innominate and subclavian vein injuries can be complex to repair. Vein ligation is a reasonable approach in these cases. In fact, vein ligation can be performed in nearly all venous injuries in the upper extremity so long as the venous collateral network is not compromised by extensive soft tissue damage or other injuries. Once the patient is stabilized and vascular control has been obtained, advantages certainly exist for autogenous reconstructions.[6]

Ligation of the subclavian artery has been reported. We find that repair with prosthetic material can be performed fast enough in these cases that arterial ligation is seldom necessary. The upper extremity arterial injuries that one may elect to ligate are radial artery transections, depending on the arterial supply provided by the ulnar artery. Because the ulnar artery is the predominant supply to the hand, we perform reconstruction of the ulnar artery.

Concomitant neurologic injuries usually are observed and not repaired at the time of the repair of the vascular injury. Elective nerve exploration and repair can be undertaken at a later time, depending on the recovery of neurologic function.

OUTCOMES

Injuries to the axillary artery and brachial artery are not associated with the same high frequency of limb loss as is seen with injuries to the popliteal artery. However, because of the high association of upper extremity vascular injuries with associated neurologic injuries, the long-term disability experienced upper extremity vascular trauma is high.[20] In general, 50% of patients with upper extremity vascular injuries have associated neurologic deficits. Only half of these acute neurologic deficits resolve, leaving approximately 25% to as many as 67% of victims of upper extremity arterial injuries with repaired vascular injuries but severely compromised upper extremity function.[20, 21]

ENDOVASCULAR THERAPY

Endovascular treatments have the potential to dramatically improve the outcomes for the most severe cases of upper extremity vascular trauma, especially for trauma involving the intrathoracic great vessels, the cervicothoracic vessels in Zone I of the thoracic inlet, and the subclavian and axillary vessels. Endovascular therapy has the potential to decrease the incidence of what is the second leading cause of traumatic death (Figure 41–8).[22] The cost-effectiveness ratio would be low (and beneficial) for any significant advance in the treatment of these often lethal injuries that predominantly affect young adults.

In order for endovascular therapy to accomplish this goal, the treatment would have to become much faster, for the patients that potentially could be saved are those succumbing to exsanguination. In the largest series to date that utilized endografts for the treatment of upper extremity vascular arterial injuries in 9 patients from South

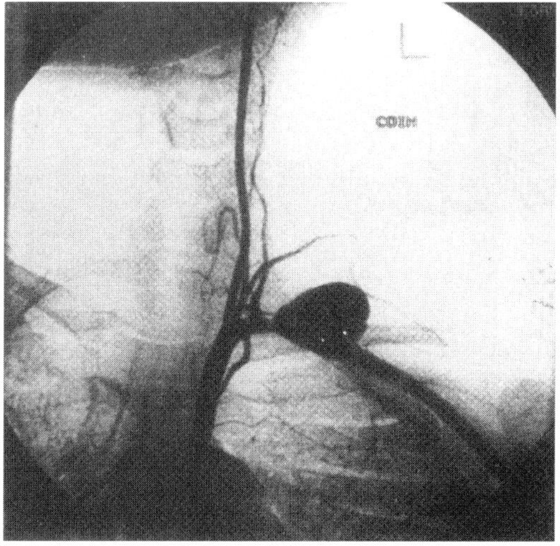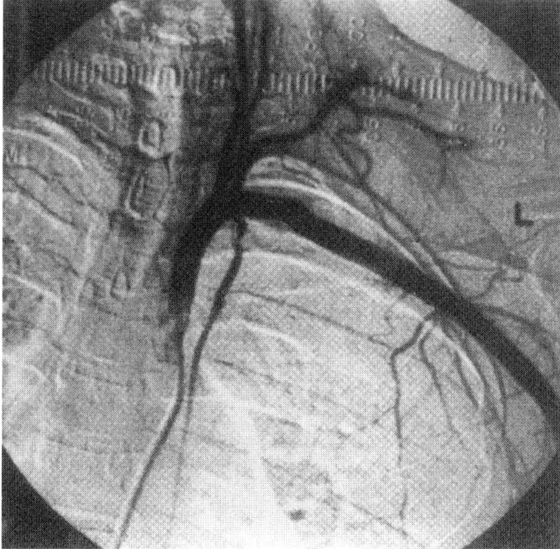

Figure 41–8. Treatment of a pseudoaneurysm of the middle portion of the left subclavian artery with an endograft. **(A)** Selective left subclavian arteriogram demonstrates a pseudoaneurysm; **(B)** Following treatment with an endograft, complete exclusion of the injury is seen. (Reprinted with permission from DuToit DF, Strauss DC, Blaszcyk M, et al. Endovascular treatment of penetrating thoracic outlet injuries. *Eur J Vasc Endovasc Surg.* 2000;19:489–495.)

Africa, the duration of the these 9 endovascular procedure ranged from 77 to 179 minutes, within a mean of approximately 2 hours. The mid-term durability of these endografts placed for trauma has been good, but long-term data are lacking.[12] One limitation in applying endovascular therapy to the management of vascular trauma has been an economic disincentive in using these devices in trauma victims.

The available technology has improved dramatically with the further refinement of covered stents (Figure 41–9). The Viabahn (Gore) endograft consists of thin PTFE inside of a flexible nitinol stent. This self-expanding endograft is inserted through 8 French to 12 French sheaths and deployed by pulling a fiber which opens the grafts from distal to proximal.[23, 24]

Further improvements or more experience or both are needed with this (or another) endograft that could permit the use of this type of endovascular device in patients *in extremis*. The possibility exists that the adverse outcomes seen with the majority of the vascular trauma at the thoracic inlet and the thoracic outlet could be improved. This technology remains more than a siren's song.

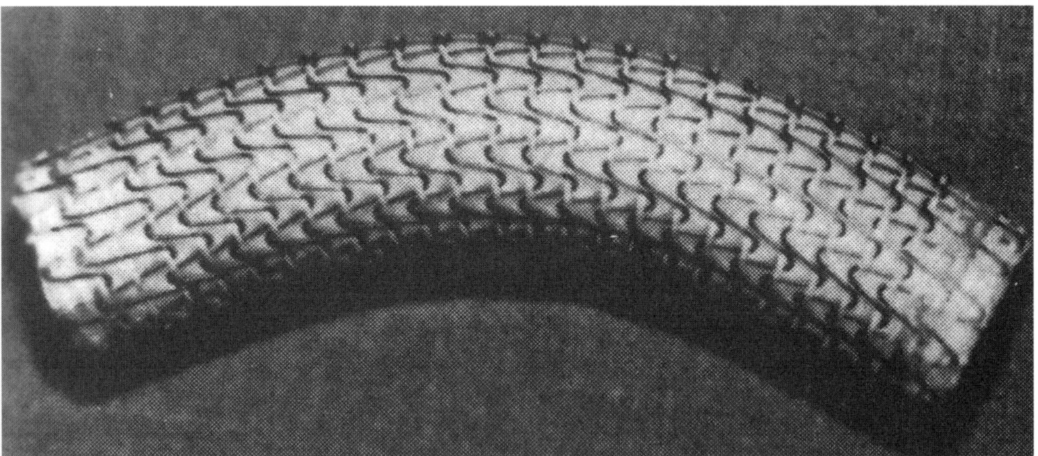

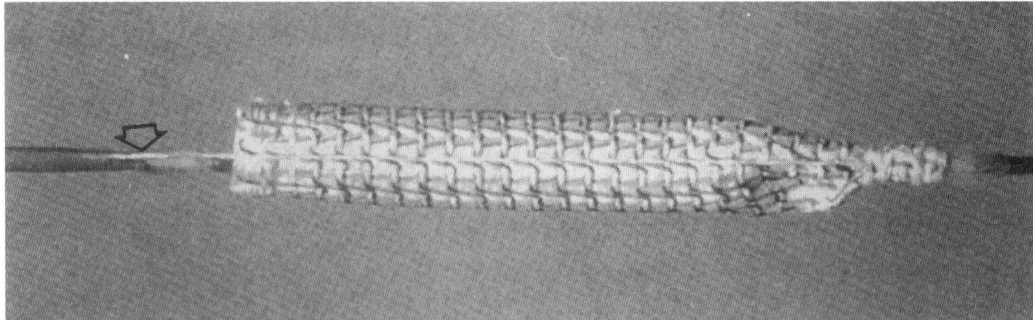

Figure 41–9. The Viabahn (Hemabahn) endograft. **(A)** This stent-graft consists of thin ePTFE inside of a flexible nitinol stent. (Reprinted with permission from a)Burger T, Meyer F, Tautehahn J, et al. Initial experience with percutaneous repair of popliteal artery lesions using a new PTFE stent-graft. *J Endovasc Surg.* 1998;5:365–372.) **(B)** This self-expanding endograft is deployed by pulling a fiber (arrow) and deploys trailing end to leading end. (Reprinted with permission from Bartorelli AL, Trabattoni D, Agrifoglio M, et al. Endovascular repair of iatrogenic subclavian artery perforations using the hemobahn stent-graft. *J Endovasc Ther.* 2001;8:417–421.)

REFERENCES

1. Johnansen K. Diagnostic choices in vascular trauma. In: Pearce WH and Yao, JST, eds. *Advances in Vascular Surgery*. Chicago: Precept Press; 2002:539–550.
2. Yao JST, Pearce WH. Preface. In: Yao, JST and Pearce WH, eds. *Practical Vascular Surgery*. Stamford, CT: Appleton & Lange; 1999:xv.
3. Patel ST, Kent KC. Cost-effectiveness of carotid endarterectomy in the prevention of stroke. In: Yao, JST and Pearce WH, eds. *Practical Vascular Surgery*. Stamford, CT: Appleton & Lange; 1999:171–184.
4. Keen JD, Keen RR. The cost-effectiveness of exclusion arteriography in extremity trauma. *Cardiovasc Surg*. 2001;9:441–447.
5. Keen JD, Dunne PM, Keen RR, et al. Proximity arteriography: cost-effectiveness in asymptomatic penetrating extremity trauma. *J Vasc Interv Radiol*. 2001;12:813–821.
6. Keen RR, Meyer JP, Durham JR, et al. Autogenous vein graft repair of injured extremity arteries: early and late results with 134 consecutive patients. J Vasc Surg. 1991;13:664–668.
7. Trunkey DD, Meyer DM, Brusel KR. Thoracic inlet and mediastinal injuries. In: Thal ER, Weigelt JA, Carrico CJ, eds. *Operative Trauma Management*. New York: McGraw Hill; 2002:110–121.
8. Monson DO, Saletta JD, Freeark RJ. Carotid vertebral trauma. *J Trauma*. 1969;9:987–999.
9. Lim LT, Saletta JD, Flanigan DP. Subclavian and innominate artery trauma. A five year experience with 17 patients. *Surgery*. 979;86:890–897.
10. Marin ML, Veith FJ, Panetta TF, et al. Transluminally placed endovascular stented graft repair for arterial trauma. *J Vasc Surg*. 1994;20:466–473.
11. McIntyre WB, Ballard JL. Cervicothoracic vascular injuries. *Sem Vasc Surg*. 1998;11:232–242.
12. Veith FJ, Ohki T, Cynamon J, et al. Endovascular grafts in the management of vascular injuries. In: Pearce WH and Yao, JST, eds. *Advances in Vascular Surgery*. Chicago: Precept Press; 2002:403–411.
13. Soto JA, Munera F, Cardoso N, et al. Diagnostic performance of helical CT angiography in trauma to large arteries of the extremtities. *J Comput Assist Tomogr*. 1999;23:188–196.
14. Demetriades D, Chahwan S, Gomez H, et al. Penetrating injuries to the subclavian and axillary arteries. *J AM Coll Surg*. 1999;188:290–295.
15. Hajarizadeh H, Rohrer MJ, Cutler BS. Surgical exposure of the left subclavian artery by median sternotomy and left supreclavicular extension. *J Trauma*. 1996;41:136–139.
16. Green RM, Waldman D, Ouriel, et al. Claviculectomy fpr subclavian venous repair: long-term functional results. *J Vasc Surg*. 2000;32:315–321.
17. Marone L, Nigri G, LaMuraglia GM. A novel technique of upper extremity revascularization: the retrohumeral approach. *J Vasc Surg*. 2002;35:1277–1279.
18. Owings JT. Upper extremity vascular injuries. In: Thal ER, Weigelt JA, Carrico CJ, eds. *Operative Trauma Management*. New York: McGraw Hill;2002:398–409.
19. Perry MO.Complications of missed arterial injuries. *J Vasc Surg*. 1993;17:399–407.
20. Brown KR, Jean-Claude J, Seabrook GR, et al. Determinates of functional disability after complex upper extremity trauma. *Ann Vasc Surg*. 2001;15:43–48.
21. Keen RR, Meyer JP, Schuler JJ, et al. Early and late results in the treatment of extremity vascular repair: patency, limb salvage, and function. In: Flanigan DP, ed. *Civilian Vascular Trauma*. Philadelphia: Lea & Febinger; 1992;465–472.
22. DuToit DF, Strauss DC, Blaszcyk M, et al. Endovascular treatment of penetrating thoracic outlet injuries. *Eur J Vasc Endovasc Surg*. 2000;19:489–495.
23. Burger T, Meyer F, Tautehahn J, et al. Initial experience with percutaneous repair of popliteal artery lesions using a new PTFE stent-graft. *J Endovasc Surg*. 1998;5:365–372.
24. Bartorelli AL, Trabattoni D, Agrifoglio M, et al. Endovascular repair of iatrogenic subclavian artery perforations using the hemobahn stent-graft. *J Endovasc Ther*. 2001;8:417–421.

42

Venous Thromboembolism in Vascular Injury

Michael A. West, MD, PhD

INTRODUCTION

Venous thromboembolism continues to be a frequent cause of morbidity and less frequently of mortality after major traumatic injuries.[1–3] Specific information regarding the late incidence of deep vein thrombosis (DVT) or pulmonary embolism (PE) after major vascular injury is not readily available. In many reports it can be difficult to separate thromboembolic complications of acute vascular injuries or their management from late complications. Nonetheless, the basic principles relating to the pathogenesis of thromboembolic complications after traumatic injuries should be familiar to all vascular surgeons. This brief review will focus on the pathophysiology of post-traumatic venous thromboembolism with an additional emphasis on factors that may be associated with treatment of major vascular injuries. In addition, the current recommendations regarding post-traumatic DVT/PE prophylaxis will be discussed.

Deep vein thrombosis is encountered frequently in patients sustaining major traumatic injuries.[1–3] Autopsy series of patients dying after injury suggest that as many 65% have evidence of DVT,[4] with an incidence of PE in the range of 10–15%.[5,6] More recently, surveillance studies using venography or duplex techniques have found an 8–14% incidence of DVT and a 1.5–3% incidence of PE.[2,7–9] In many instances DVT were found despite appropriate prophylactic therapy (see below). Thromboembolic complications are noted even more frequently with severe blunt injuries than after penetrating injuries.

The increased incidence of thromboembolic complications after traumatic injuries is not surprising. Virchow described his triad of factors associated with development of venous thrombi in 1856. Those factors include: 1) Hypercoagulability; 2) Decreased blood flow (stasis); 3) Intimal injury. In most instances of severe trauma all 3 pathophysiologic factors delineated by Virchow are present. Even elective surgery is associated with demonstrable increases in the coagulability of blood.

Hypercoagulability is well documented after experimental traumatic injuries. This enhanced activation of coagulation pathways may be partially due to release of tissue factor (TF) in response to injury.[10] After trauma, coagulation is favored due to both enhanced coagulation (demonstrable as decreased antithrombin III levels and enhanced D-dimer formation) and due to decreased fibrinolysis.[3,11] Enhanced coagulability of blood is seen almost immediately after injury. To a large extent these alterations may be acutely beneficial to patients that have sustained massive traumatic injuries, however these same "adaptive" alterations complicate post-injury management.

Stasis is another major factor favoring the formation of blood clots. Venous stasis is associated with a higher incidence of formation of DVT. Stasis on the arterial side, or following arterial repair, may also occur as a complication of traumatic injuries, however it presents as acute or subacute ischemia. Arterial thrombosis requires prompt operative or lytic interventions to restore blood flow. In the case of peripheral vascular injuries the first priority for minimizing venous stasis is restoration of adequate arterial inflow. The surgical technique chosen for management of venous injuries can dramatically impact the incidence of thromboembolic complications. For example, ligation of venous injuries is associated with a much higher incidence of DVT and post-phlebitic complications than primary repair. Delayed fasciotomy can also increase the incidence of DVT/PE. Aside from the acute injury, many patients are at risk for stasis later in their clinical course due to immobilization or paralysis.

Intimal injury can result from several factors after traumatic injuries. These include, direct injury to the vessel (laceration, intimal tear, contusion) or ischemic injury from shock or delayed restoration of blood flow to an injured extremity. In many cases of blunt injury to the extremity, vascular injury results from "penetrating trauma" from nearby bone fragments. Surgeons need to maintain a high index of suspicion in the face of associated orthopedic or neurologic injuries.

RISK FACTORS

The risk factors for thromboembolic are most clearly delineated for patients undergoing elective surgical procedures. Even so, these risk factors and an understanding of the pathophysiology of DVT permit us to identify trauma patients at enhanced risk for thromboembolic complications. In general, patients are divided into low, moderate, high and very high-risk groups. Table 42–1 summarizes these risk factors. Patients without any specific risk factor would be classified as "low" risk (not shown in Table

TABLE 42–1. RISK FACTORS FOR DVT

Factor	Moderate Risk	High Risk	Very High Risk
Age	>40	>50	>70
Injury	Extensive Soft Tissue Trauma	Pelvic Fracture	Severe Pelvic Fracture
	Lower Extremity Fracture	Tib/Fib Fracture	Multiple (>3) Long Bone Fx
	No venous injury	Venous Injury	Extensive Venous Injury
Other Factors	Immobilization	Spinal Cord Injury	Spinal Cord Injury with paralysis
	Estrogen Therapy	GCS <8	
	Malignancy		
	Blood Transfusion		
ISS	>9	>16	

42–1). This classification scheme is most useful for determination of the type of prophylactic measures that should be employed to minimize thromboembolic complications. In addition, patients with a past history of venous thromboembolism should be considered to be at significantly increased risk.

Iatrogenic interventions often place patients at additional risk for thromboembolic complications. There is excellent data documenting that the presence of femoral vein catheters enhance the risk for lower extremity thrombi.[12,13] Although the exigencies of emergency venous access may necessitate insertion of lower extremity access catheters these should be avoided whenever possible and always removed at the earliest possible time. Catheters in the subclavian and internal jugular veins have also been associated with development of DVT in these vessels.[12]

PROPHYLAXIS

Several measures have been employed prophylactically to decrease the incidence of thromboembolic complications (see Table 42–2). In most cases these measures are designed to counteract one or more of the factors in Virchow's Triad. Decisions regarding the institution of prophylactic measures must be balanced against the risks of these interventions in light of the injuries sustained by the patient. In most cases there are not evidence-based recommendations for these measures specifically in trauma patients. In all cases prophylactic measures will be most effective if instituted early, in as much as almost half of all post-traumatic PE occur within the first week after injury.[14] In many cases early mobilization may be one of the most effective measures that can be employed to decrease the development of DVT. It is important to recognize that decisions regarding ICU sedation, ventilation mode, management of orthopedic injuries and many other "routine" management decisions impact whether patients can be mobilized.

Sequential compression devices (SCD) have been widely employed in trauma patients and in post-operative elective surgical patients.[15–18] These devices probably work by increasing blood flow in the lower extremities and by enhancing fibrinolytic activity.[19] There is no risk of increased bleeding with SCD, making them ideal for use in multiply injured patients or individuals with spinal cord injury or closed head injury. Ironically, the presence of lower extremity fractures may prevent use of SCD in patients who could benefit from them. Another closely related device designed to compress the venous plexus in the foot may be an alternative in patients with leg fractures, however recently the utility of these devices has been questioned. In many in-

TABLE 42–2. MEASURES FOR DVT PROPHYLAXIS

Moderate Risk	High Risk	Very High Risk
Compression Stockings	Compression Stockings	Compression Stockings
SCD	SCD	SCD
± Unfract Heparin*	LMWH*	LMWH*
	Surveillance Duplex	Surveillance Duplex
		IVC Filter
		(Possibly) Warfarin*

*if no contraindication to anticoagulation

stances SCD devices are combined with compression stockings, although good objective evidence to recommend this combination is lacking.[17]

Anticoagulation with various forms of heparin has been documented to decrease thromboembolic complications in elective surgical patients. In most instances anticoagulation is contraindicated in injured patients with closed head injury, major pelvic fractures, evidence of ongoing hemorrhage or spinal cord injury. Prophylaxis with low dose unfractionated heparin (5000 U sq q8–12 hours) may be appropriate in patients identified to be at low-moderate risk for DVT/PE. More recent data suggests that fractionated, low molecular weight heparin (LMWH) is more effective in patients at high risk for post-traumatic DVT.[20] Appropriate prophylactic doses for LMWH are: 30 mg of enoxaparin sq q 12 hours[20] or 120 IU/kg of dalteparin sq q 12 hours.[12] Neither have specific FDA-approved indications for post-traumatic DVT prophylaxis, however both have shown effectiveness after elective surgical procedures. Studies are ongoing to determine if or when LMWH could be safely employed in patients with closed head injury or spinal cord injury, but preliminary results are encouraging.[21–23] There is good evidence that anticoagulation with warfarin can be used in patients with severe pelvic fractures that require prolonged immobilization.

A major ongoing controversy in trauma patients concerns which subgroup would benefit from insertion of a vena caval filter.[14,24–27] Vena caval filters have been shown to significantly decrease the incidence of PE in the face of venous thrombi in the proximal veins. Several studies have been performed documenting that patients at very high risk for venous thromboembolism and PE benefit from prophylactic insertion of vena caval filters. In addition, caval filters should be inserted in patients that develop a PE while on prophylactic or therapeutic anticoagulation. It should be noted that patients with a caval filter are at increased risk for distal clot formation and should be anticoagulated if there are no contraindications (e.g. head injury, etc.).

DIAGNOSIS

The appropriate treatment in the face of a documented DVT is generally much more straightforward. In this setting concerns about the possible risks of anticoagulation must be interpreted in light of the known presence of a DVT or PE. There is now good evidence documenting the sensitivity (>95%) and specificity of relatively simple, non-invasive bedside surveillance techniques to identify DVT in high risk populations.[28–30] Bedside duplex examination of the proximal veins every 5–7 days has been shown to detect asymptomatic proximal clots in a significant number of trauma patients in the high and very high risk groups. Basically, this technique uses both flow and imaging duplex modalities to identify the presence of a flow-limiting, non-compressible luminal defect. When all 3 parameters are present there is a very high degree of correlation of duplex imaging with the results from venography. If proximal clots are identified then anticoagulation, with or without placement of an IVC filter should be done.[31]

Contrast venography remains the "gold standard" for diagnosis of DVT,[20–32] however from a practical standpoint it is seldom employed outside of research studies in trauma patients due to the inconvenience, cost and need to expose patients to contrast agents. An additional "problem" with use of venography is the conundrum of what to do about the frequent detection of distal calf thrombi. Use of duplex methods have largely supplanted venography in ICU patients.

Currently dynamic spiral CT scanning[33–35] has largely replaced pulmonary angiography and/or ventilation perfusion (V/Q) scans for diagnosis of PE.[35] Both spiral CT and pulmonary angiography will demonstrate filling defects in the pulmonary vasculature. V/Q scans are generally reported in terms of low, indeterminate or high probability for a PE. The presence of a PE is unlikely with a low probability V/Q scan, however many critically ill or injured patients will have concomitant pulmonary findings that limit the utility of this diagnostic modality. It should also be noted that in many instances confirmation of a PE may not be necessary in the presence of a documented DVT unless it would alter therapy.

OPERATIVE APPROACH TO VENOUS INJURY

The incidence of late DVT and post-phlebitic syndrome is lowest if lateral venorrhaphy, rather than ligation, can be performed for venous injuries. Isolated distal vein injuries probably have minimal impact on thromboembolic complications, however operative decisions regarding treatment of proximal extremity or truncal venous injuries can have a profound impact on the incidence of these complications.[36–39] Direct compression proximal and distal to the venous injury facilitates visualization of the extent of the injury[40,41] or insertion of a balloon catheter may also be employed.[42] In large proximal vessels or the IVC, direct pressure at the site of injury may permit placement of sutures at either end of the injury. Traction on these sutures may allow the surgeon to position a vascular clamp, thus allowing precise repair of the injury. Contused or non-viable vessel wall should be debrided. Care is take to avoid compromising the luminal diameter by more than 25%. Occasionally an interposition vein graft may be necessary to avoid this, however the clinical stability of the patient and presence of other injuries must be weighed in this choice (see below) because it may significantly prolong the operation. Although frequently mentioned there is probably limited uses for "spiral" interposition grafts.[43] With extensive damage to the vena cava an externally supported PTFE graft may facilitate repair.

Clinical instability of multiply injured patients may dictate a "damage control" approach to venous injuries and in this setting ligation may be the best option.[44,45] It should be recognized that proximal ligation is often accompanied by massive, sometimes uncontrollable, edema of the distal extremity. In the setting of proximal ligation "prophylactic" fasciotomy should be strongly considered and the extremity should be closely monitored for viability, as amputation may be required. Data suggests that late thrombotic sequelae are decreased even if attempted venous repair results in acute thrombosis because the lumen may recanalize.[46]

CONCLUSION

Venous thromboembolism is frequently encountered in patients with traumatic injuries. Injuries to the arteries and veins increase the likelihood for development of these complications. Patients at increased for venous thromboembolism should have appropriate prophylactic measures instituted as soon after injury as possible to minimize the risk for PE or late sequelae from DVT.

REFERENCES

1. Meissner MH. Deep venous thrombosis in the trauma patient. *Semin Vasc Surg.* 1998;11:274–282.
2. Knudson MM, Collins JA, Goodman SB, et al. Thromboembolism following multiple trauma. *J Trauma.* 1992;32:2–11.
3. Rogers FB. Venous thromboembolism in trauma patients: a review. *Surgery.* 2001;130:1–12.
4. Sevitt S, Gallagher N. Venous thrombosis and pulmonary embolism: a clinicopathologic study in the injured and burned patients. *Br J Surg.* 1961;48:475–489.
5. Fitts WT, Lehr H, Bitner RL et al. An analysis of 950 fatal injuries. *Surgery.* 1964;56:663–668.
6. Coon W. Risk factors in pulmonary embolism. *Surg Gynecol Obstet.* 1976;143:385–390.
7. Geerts W, Cook D, Selby R, et al. Venous thromboembolism and its prevention in critical care. *J Crit Care.* 2002;17:95–104.
8. Velmahos GC, Kern J, Chan LS, Oder D, et al. Prevention of venous thromboembolism after injury: an evidence-based report—part I: analysis of risk factors and evaluation of the role of vena caval filters. *J Trauma.* 2000;49:132–138; discussion 139.
9. Shackford SR, Davis JW, Hollingsworth-Fridlund P, et al. Venous thromboembolism in patients with major trauma. *Am J Surg.* 1990;159:365–369.
10. Miller-Graziano CL, Lim RC, Chin M. Generation of tissue factor by patient monocytes: correlation to thromboembolic complications. *Thromb Haemost.* 1981;46:489–495.
11. Line BR. Pathophysiology and diagnosis of deep venous thrombosis. *Semin Nucl Med.* 2001;31:90–101.
12. Davidson BL. Risk assessment and prophylaxis of venous thromboembolism in acutely and/or critically ill patients. *Haemostasis.* 2000;30:77–81; discussion 63.
13. Vavilala MS, Nathens AB, Jurkovich GJ, et al. Risk factors for venous thromboembolism in pediatric trauma. *J Trauma.* 2002;52:922–927.
14. Rogers FB, Shackford SR, Wilson J, et al. Prophylactic vena cava filter insertion in severely injured trauma patients: indications and preliminary results. *J Trauma.* 1993;35:637–641; discussion 641–632.
15. Winemiller MH, Stolp-Smith KA, Silverstein MD, et al. Prevention of venous thromboembolism in patients with spinal cord injury: effects of sequential pneumatic compression and heparin. *J Spinal Cord Med.* 1999;22:182–191.
16. Knudson MM, Lewis FR, Clinton A, et al. Prevention of venous thromboembolism in trauma patients. *J Trauma.* 1994;37:480–487.
17. Otero R, Uresandi F, Cayuela A, et al. Use of venous thromboembolism prophylaxis for surgical patients: a multicentre analysis of practice in Spain. *Eur J Surg.* 2001;167:163–167.
18. Cook D, Laporta D, Skrobik Y, et al. Prevention of venous thromboembolism in critically ill surgery patients: a cross-sectional study. *J Crit Care.* 2001;16:161–166.
19. Knight MT, Dawson R. Effect of intermittent compression of the arms on deep venous thrombosis in the legs. *Lancet.* 1976;2:1265–1268.
20. Geerts WH, Jay RM, Code KI, et al. A comparison of low-dose heparin with low-molecular-weight heparin as prophylaxis against venous thromboembolism after major trauma. *N Engl J Med.* 1996;335:701–707.
21. Norwood SH, McAuley CE, Berne JD, et al. Prospective evaluation of the safety of enoxaparin prophylaxis for venous thromboembolism in patients with intracranial hemorrhagic injuries. *Arch Surg.* 2002;137:696–702.
22. Norwood SH, McAuley CE, Berne JD, et al. A potentially expanded role for enoxaparin in preventing venous thromboembolism in high risk blunt trauma patients. *J Am Coll Surg.* 2001;192:161–167.
23. Deep K, Jigajinni MV, McLean AN, et al. Prophylaxis of thromboembolism in spinal injuries—results of enoxaparin used in 276 patients. *Spinal Cord.* 2001;39:88–91.
24. Hak DJ. Prevention of venous thromboembolism in trauma and long bone fractures. *Curr Opin Pulm Med.* 2001;7:338–343.
25. Montgomery KD, Geerts WH, Potter HG, et al. Practical management of venous thromboembolism following pelvic fractures. *Orthop Clin North Am.* 1997;28:397–404.

26. Zwaan M, Lorch H, Kulke C, et al. Clinical experience with temporary vena caval filters. *J Vasc Interv Radiol.* 1998;9:594–601.
27. Rogers FB, Strindberg G, Shackford SR, et al. Five-year follow-up of prophylactic vena cava filters in high-risk trauma patients. *Arch Surg.* 1998;133:406–411; discussion 412.
28. Cipolle MD, Wojcik R, Seislove E, et al. The role of surveillance duplex scanning in preventing venous thromboembolism in trauma patients. *J Trauma.* 2002;52:453–462.
29. Knudson MM, Morabito D, Paiement GD, et al. Use of low molecular weight heparin in preventing thromboembolism in trauma patients. *J Trauma.* 1996;41:446–459.
30. McCoy KL, Gahtan V, Kerstein MD. Use of venous duplex scans to evaluate symptoms of deep vein thrombosis: an analysis of ultrasound usage by various medical specialties. *Am Surg.* 1999;65:417–420.
31. Bick RL. Proficient and cost-effective approaches for the prevention and treatment of venous thrombosis and thromboembolism. *Drugs.* 2000;60:575–595.
32. Leclerc JR, Geerts WH, Desjardins L, et al. Prevention of venous thromboembolism after knee arthroplasty. A randomized, double-blind trial comparing enoxaparin with warfarin. *Ann Intern Med.* 1996;124:619–626.
33. Raskob GE, Hull RD. Diagnosis of pulmonary embolism. *Curr Opin Hematol.* 1999;6:280–284.
34. Lipchik RJ, Goodman LR. Spiral computed tomography in the evaluation of pulmonary embolism. *Clin Chest Med.* 1999;20:731–738, viii.
35. Cook D, McMullin J, Hodder R, et al. Prevention and diagnosis of venous thromboembolism in critically ill patients: a Canadian survey. *Crit Care.* 2001;5:336–342.
36. Burch JM, Richardson RJ, Martin RR, Mattox KL. Penetrating iliac vascular injuries: recent experience with 233 consecutive patients. *J Trauma.* 1990;30:1450–1459.
37. Barkun JS, Terazza O, Daignault P, et al. The fate of venous repair after shock and trauma. *J Trauma.* 1988;28:1322–1329.
38. Hobson RW, 2nd, Yeager RA, et al. Femoral venous trauma: techniques for surgical management and early results. *Am J Surg.* 1983;146:220–224.
39. Blumoff RL, Powell T, Johnson G, Jr. Femoral venous trauma in a university referral center. *J Trauma.* 1982;22:703–705.
40. Degiannis E, Velmahos GC, Levy RD, et al. Penetrating injuries of the abdominal inferior vena cava. *Ann R Coll Surg Engl.* 1996;78:485–489.
41. Turpin I, State D, Schwartz A. Injuries to the inferior vena cava and their management. *Am J Surg.* 1977;134:25–32.
42. Graham JM, Mattox KL, Beall AC, Jr., et al. Traumatic injuries of the inferior vena cava. *Arch Surg.* 1978;113:413–418.
43. Pappas PJ, Haser PB, Teehan EP, et al. Outcome of complex venous reconstructions in patients with trauma. *J Vasc Surg.* 1997;25:398–404.
44. Moore EE, Burch JM, Franciose RJ, et al. Staged physiologic restoration and damage control surgery. *World J Surg* 1998; 22:1184-1190; discussion 1190–1181.
45. Asensio JA, McDuffie L, Petrone P, et al. Reliable variables in the exsanguinated patient which indicate damage control and predict outcome. *Am J Surg.* 2001; 182:743–751.
46. Blumoff RL, Proctor HJ, Johnson G, Jr. Recanalization of a saphenous vein interposition venous graft. *J Trauma.* 1981;21:407–408.

XIII

Venous and Lymphatic Disorders

43

The Management of Lymphatic Disorders

Peter Gloviczki, MD, Thom W. Rooke, MD,
Gail L. Gamble, MD, Audra A. Noel, MD, and
Karen L. Andrews, MD

Lymphatic disorders such as chronic lymphedema and chylous effusions are difficult and frustrating to treat and frequently impossible to cure. Vascular surgeons, physical therapy physicians, vascular internists, general practitioners, and pediatricians treat patients with chronic lymphedema, which is both a physical disability and a psychological problem for the patient. To focus efforts to treat this difficult disease, in the past decade in the US lymphedema clinics have been established in many institutions. Physical therapy has been the most effective way to manage lymphedema but many places embraced a multidisciplinary approach. Multidisciplinary lymphedema centers, run primarily by physical therapy physicians, like the one at the Mayo Clinic, bring together expertise of both medical and surgical disciplines.

In this chapter we discuss evaluation and treatment of the most frequent lymphatic disorder, chronic lymphedema, and review current attempts at lymphatic reconstructions in patients with primary chylous disorders and abnormalities of the thoracic duct.

CHRONIC LYMPHEDEMA

Chronic lymphedema develops as a result of impaired lymphatic transport, most frequently due to congenital or acquired obstruction of lymph vessels and the lymph-conducting elements of lymph nodes. Protein-rich extracellular fluid accumulates in the subcutaneous tissue when the collateral lymphatic circulation becomes insufficient and when all compensatory mechanisms, including the tissue macrophage activity or drainage through spontaneous lymphovenous anastomoses, have been exhausted. The deficient transport of tissue fluid containing lymphocytes, plasma proteins, immunoglobulins, and cytokines results in a chronic inflammatory process in the skin and subcutaneous tissues.

Classification of Lymphedema

Chronic lymphedema can be primary, idiopathic, or secondary, due to a known underlying cause. Primary lymphedema occurs when there is aplasia, hypoplasia, or primary fibrotic occlusion of the lymph vessels or lymph-conducting element of the lymph nodes, the latter occurring at any age, although most frequently at puberty.[1] Congenital lymphedema is usually observed at birth, but before the age of 1 year. The hereditary form of congenital lymphedemas is called Milroy's disease. Primary lymphedema praecox presents between the ages of 1 and 35 years while lymphedema tarda is defined as primary lymphedema occurring after the mid-30s. Worldwide, filariasis is the most common secondary lymphedema. Additional etiologies include other infections, affecting the lymph vessels and lymph nodes, trauma, insect bite, tumor, surgical excision of nodes for biopsy, or to remove tumor metastases or radiation treatment to lymphatic tissue. In the United States, post-surgical and post-radiation upper limb edema is the most common secondary lymphedema, with incidence rates varying from 2–24% of those treated for breast cancer.[2]

Lymphedema may also be classified based on clinical severity of the disease.[3] Grade I edema is entirely reversible, it is pitting and it can be cured temporarily by limb elevation. Grade II edema is partially pitting, does not completely reduce with elevation and some degree of subcutaneous fibrosis is present. Grade III edema is associated with severe fibrosis and even sclerosis of the skin and subcutaneous tissues is present. Mechanical treatment to reduce swelling in this stage is challenging.

Bilateral lymphedema should be differentiated from edema caused by systemic disease, such as congestive heart failure, liver or renal disease, and fluid retaining medications such as anti-inflammatory drugs or some antihypertensives. In unilateral limb swelling, acute deep venous thrombosis, chronic venous insufficiency such as post-thrombotic syndrome, vascular malformation, limb hypertrophy, reflex sympathetic dystrophy, and lipedema are included in the differential diagnosis.

Evaluation of Lymphedema

Clinical presentation is usually so characteristic, that the diagnosis of lymphedema in most patients can be established based on a detailed history of the disease and physical examination. The patient with lymphedema usually presents with unilateral swelling of the lower limb, where the edema is non-pitting and swelling is usually pain-free. As mentioned before, Grade II chronic lymphedema does not resolve overnight. Unlike venous edema, there is often involvement of the foot and toes, producing the characteristic "buffalo-hump" appearance of the foot and squaring of the toes. Although there is sometimes a pinkish discoloration of the skin, cyanosis and skin ulcerations are rare. Long-standing edema leads to thickening of the skin, hyperkeratosis, with verrucal-like appearance frequently draining lymph and giving the appearance of "elephantiasis" in end-stage disease.

Imaging studies in patients with chronic lymphedema are used selectively, depending on the age of the patient, the presentation of the disease and whether surgical treatment is planned or not. Non-invasive evaluation includes duplex scanning to exclude venous disease and computed tomographic (CT) scan to diagnose underlying benign or malignant tumor or lymphadenopathy. Magnetic resonance imaging is useful to exclude vascular malformation or soft tissue tumors and it is a good test to confirm enlargement of the subcutaneous compartment due to lymphedema. Lymphoscintigraphy will confirm, if needed, that edema is lymphatic in origin.[4–8]

Lymphoscintigraphy is performed with radio labeled antimony trisulfide colloid (technetium 99m-labeled Sb2S3 colloid) or labeled human serum albumin, injected into the interdigital space of the hands or feet. The body is then imaged with a dual-headed gamma counter. At our institution, the sensitivity of the semiquantitative interpretation is excellent (92%) with a specificity of close to 100% for the diagnosis of lymphedema.[5,6] It remains the test of choice to differentiate lymphedema from edemas of other origin.

Contrast lymphangiography is rarely performed today for obstructive lymphedema, and is usually reserved for preoperative evaluation of patients with lymphangiectasia and chylous complications. We have used contrast lymphangiography selectively for preoperative assessment of chronic lymphedema before lymphatic microsurgery.[9,10] It helps define anatomy and the exact site of patent major lymphatic channels. Potential complication of contrast lymphangiography is a progression of lymphedema due to inability of the lymphatic system to clear the lipid soluble contrast material.

Treatment of Lymphedema

The aim of the treatment is to reduce or minimize the swelling, to treat and prevent infectious complications, such as cellulites or lymphangitis, to restore function and cosmetic appearance of the limb and to prevent a fortunately rare late complication, the development of lymphangiosarcoma. A delay in treatment or prolonged non-compliance with conservative measures frequently contributes to the deterioration of the patient's condition.

Non-surgical management

Skin care and treatment of any infection, specialized massage techniques to promote the movement of lymph, compression therapy and elevation and exercises to reduce swelling and supplement the massage are the key components to most comprehensive physical therapy program.[11,12] Contraindications to intensive compression treatment or massage are acute infections, malignancy, congestive heart failure, or acute deep venous thrombosis.

Skin Care

Skin care is essential, and local treatment of any fungal foot infection will decrease the risk of lymphangitis. These patients are prone to develop infection, which is usually caused by group D Streptococcus, susceptible to penicillin. It is likely that factors such as weak antigenic stimulation of regional lymphocytes and reduced extravascular macrophage function contribute to increased risk of infections. The limbs should be washed regularly with soap and water and kept moist with an alcohol-free emollient cream.

Massage

Manual Lymphatic Drainage is just 1 way to describe the specialized massage techniques used today to increase lymphatic transport of the limb.[11,12] The techniques are aimed at dilating the existing collateral lymphatics to carry more lymph and protein to more proximal areas of the body, where lymphatic transport is normal. The more proximal body areas are massaged first, followed by distal massage of the limb. Optimal results from massage therapy can be expected in patients without significant fibrosis of the skin and subcutaneous tissues.

Compression bandages and garments

Graduated compression treatment can be performed with garments and bandages and with intermittent compression pumps. The applied pressure is greater at the distal end of the limb, and is gradually reduced toward the proximal end to create a pressure gradient. The aim of compression treatment is to increase total tissue pressure, which will increase the hydrostatic pressure gradient from the tissues to the initial lymphatics and between the distal and the proximal lymph collectors. The 2 main forms of bandages include elastic (high-stretch compression e.g., Ace Bandage™) bandages, with a high resting pressure but a low working pressure. They are tight after placement but stretch in response to daily exercise. Low-elastic or low-stretch compression bandages have a low resting pressure and a high working pressure. They provide comfortable support after placement and the real advantage is that they promote lymphatic flow better since total tissue pressure is increased with muscle contraction.

Compression bandages are preferred over garments during massage treatments, when the volume of the limbs changes during a short period of time. We usually recommend stockings or garments that cover the affected area completely and exert a pressure of 30 to 40 mmHg or 40 to 50 mmHg at the ankle.

Elevation and exercise

Elevation of a lymphedematous limb is one of the most effective treatment of lymphedema. In hospitalized patients we use a lymphedema sling, for home care we recommend a foam wedge to elevate the leg or lifting the end of the bed to increase the hydrostatic pressure gradient and promote lymph transport of the limb.

Swimming is one of the best exercises to help lymphatic flow, but any muscle exercise, combined with non-stretch external compression, will help lymphatic transport. We should keep in mind, however, that muscle exercise will increase arterial flow to the limb as well, which will increase lymph production.

Intermittent pneumatic compression therapy

Compression pumps, similar to massage, increase total tissue pressure in edematous limbs. While they also promote lymph flow, a portion of the fluid, because of the higher pressures, is pushed into the capillaries, back to the blood. This may result in accumulation of higher concentration of protein in the interstitial tissues. In some patients, therefore, a more rapid recurrence of the edema may be observed. A limitation of compression pumps in the management of lymphedema is that they cannot apply pressure to areas of the trunk adjacent to draining lymph nodes. Since high pressures are generated by the pump, it may promote infection or sudden swelling of the genitalia due to movement of the fluid there through lymphatic collaterals. Patients should undergo pump treatment under regular supervision, usually as a home treatment, between sessions of massage therapy.

Drug treatment

Antibiotics are used to reduce or prevent infection. Since fungal infections increase the chances of lymphangitis, if local treatment is not effective, systemic antifungal treatment is indicated. For acute lymphangitis and cellulitis (erysipelas) intravenous high dose penicillin is usually effective. For prevention in patients with recurrent infections, we recommend a program of 1 week per month prophylaxis of Penn VK 250 or 500 mg. q.i.d. For those with a penicillin allergy, a first generation cephalosporin or erythromycin is given.

Diuretics to decrease interstitial fluid should be used cautiously, and as short- term treatment only. Diuretics do not change interstitial protein content and edema reaccumulates rapidly. Benzopyrones looked promising to enhance fluid return by macrophage stimulation with increased proteolysis in the superficial tissues. They have been reported to reduce edema in both upper and lower extremities.[13] Side effects, including abnormal liver enzymes have also been reported and the claimed benefit was not confirmed by a Mayo Clinic study.[14] Benzopyrons are not approved in the US.

SURGICAL TREATMENT

Excisional Operations

Surgical excision of the excess tissue or operations to increase lymphatic drainage is rarely performed today in most centers. The main indication for excisional operations is impaired function of the limb due to its large size and weight in patients, not responding sufficiently to intensive medical management. Another indication is excision of the excess skin and subcutaneous tissue after successful compression treatment. In the US, Miller reported the best results in larger series of patients, who underwent excisional operation for chronic lymphedema.[15]

Microvascular techniques have allowed surgical attempts at direct lymphatic reconstructions, performance of lymphovenous anastomoses,[9,10,16–28] or lymphatic grafting[29–33] (Figure 43–1A–D). Unfortunately, patients with primary lymphedema usually have diffuse disease and are not considered candidates for reconstruction. Efforts to increase lymph transport by transfer omentum or a segment of ileum (mesenteric bridge operations) to the affected areas to promote neolympho-lymphatic communications have limited applications.

Lymphovenous Anastomoses

Patent lymph vessels distal to an occluded (or excised) lymphatic tissue segment are required for lymphovenous anastomoses. Venous hypertension is a contraindication to this type of reconstruction. An ideal candidate is a patient with a proximal pelvic lymphatic obstruction with dilated infrainguinal lymph vessels. Anastomoses in the leg are performed usually between the superficial medial lymphatic bundle and tributaries of the saphenous or the femoral vein (Figures 43–1A–B, 43–2A–B), using microsurgical tehnique and operating microscope. Anastomoses using normal femoral lymph vessels and a tributary of the femoral vein in experiments yielded a patency rate of 50% at 3 to 8 months after surgery in our experience.[16] In 14 patients who underwent lymphovenous anastomoses at the Mayo Clinic for chronic lymphedema, only 5 limbs, 4 with secondary lymphedema, maintained the initial improvement at an average of 46 months after surgery.[9] Because of equally good or better results obtained with compression treatment, we currently perform this operation at the Mayo Clinic only in patients with large, dilated distal lymph vessels, usually due to lymphangiectasia. However, experience from other centers indicates that clinical improvement can be achieved with lymphovenous anastomoses in obstructive lymphedema (Table 43–1).[16–28] In O'Brien's

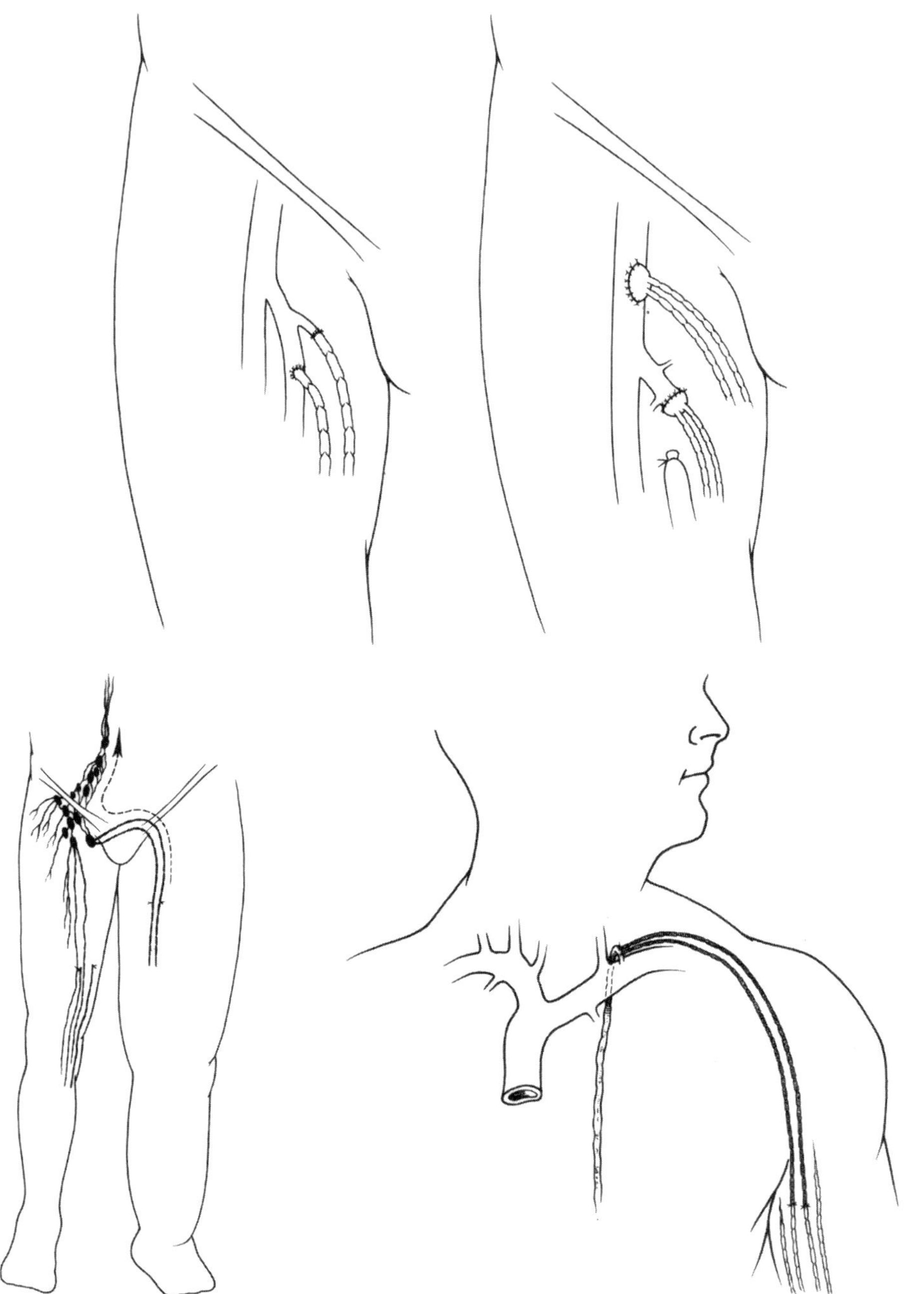

Figure 43–1. Reconstruction for lymphatic obstruction in secondary lymphedema. **(A)** End-to-end and end-to-side lymph node-vein anastomosis. **(B)** End-to-end and end-to-side lymph vessel-vein anastomosis. **(C)** Cross-femoral lymph vessel transposition for secondary lymphedema of the left lower extremity. **(D)** Treatment of postmastectomy lymphedema with transplantation of 2 lymph channels from the lower to the upper extremity. (With permission of Mayo Foundation).

series from Australia, 73% of the patients had subjective improvement and 42% experienced long-term improvement.[18] Campisi and associates have reported on 665 patients with lymphedema, treated with lymphovenous anastomoses, with subjective improve-

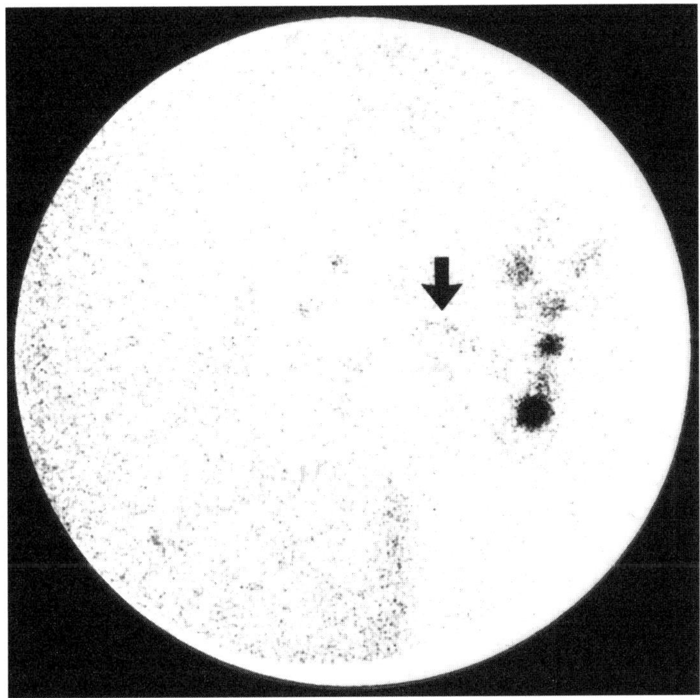

Figure 43–2. Lymphoscintigram 3 months after suprapubic lymphatic grafting for secondary lymphedema of the right lower extremity. Labeled colloid was injected into the right foot only. Arrow indicates suprapubic graft. Note intense filling of the left inguinal nodes. Preoperative lymphoscintigram in this patient showed no activity at the groin. L, lymphatic graft. (With permission from the Mayo Foundation.)

ment in 87% of their patients.[27] Four-hundred-forty-six patients were available for long-term follow-up and the authors observed persistent volume reduction in 69% and discontinuation of conservative measures in 85%. The authors emphasized that microsurgical reconstruction has to be performed early in the course of the disease, when intrinsic contractility of the lymphatics are still maintained and before extensive chronic inflammatory changes in the subcutaneous tissue develop. Lymphoscintigraphy in Campisi's experience showed improved lymph transport and fast disappearance of the tracer at the anastomosis site.

Lymphatic Grafting

The advantage of using lymphatic vessels for bypass of the obstructed lymphatic segment is that lymph coagulates much less than blood, and chances of patency are better than with lymphovenous anastomoses. The technique was pioneered by Baumeister in Germany, who performes this operation in patients with unilateral secondary lymphedema of the lower extremities or in those with postmastectomy lymphedema of the arm (Figure 43–1C–D).[29–33] The lymphatic grafts are harvested from the healthy leg of the patient. It is important to document normal lymphatics in the donor leg with lymphoscintigraphy before considering surgery.

In postmastectomy lymphedema bypass between the arm and the supraclavicular lymphatics is performed using grafts harvested from the superficial medial bundle of the leg. Unilateral lower limb edema is treated by transposition of 2 or 3 normal lymphatic trunks in the thigh to the contralateral groin lymphatics (cross-femoral graft-

TABLE 43–1. CLINICAL RESULTS OF MICROSURGICAL LYMPHATIC RECONSTRUCTIONS

First author, year	No. Patients	Extremity Upper	Lower	Type of Operation	Follow-up (mo)	Excellent or Good Clinical Results %
Krylov, 1982	50	+		LVA	?	30
Nieuborg, 1982	47	+		LVA	6-12	68
Gong-Kang, 1985	91		+	LVA	24*	79
Zhu et al., 1987	48		+	LVA	6–52	33
	185		+	LVA	6–52	73
Gloviczki, 1988	6	+		LVA	36.6*	50
	8		+	LVA		25
O'Brien, 1990	46	+		LVA		54
	30		+	LVA		83
	6†	+		LVA	51*	33
	8†		+	LVA		50
Baumeister, 1990	36	+		LG	>12	33
	12		+	LG	>24	8
Campisi, 2001	231	+		LVA	>7 years* in 446 patients	83%
	446		+	LVA		
Campisi, 2001	133			LVL	"Log-term" in 95 patients,	
			+		max. years	15

*Mean.
†Lymphovenous anastomosis plus excisional procedure.
LVA, Lymphovenous anastomoses; LG, lymphatic grafting; LVL, lymphatic-venous-lymphatic graft with autologous vein
(Adapted and revised from Gloviczki P. The Management of Lymphatic Disorders (Section XVIII). In: Rutherford RB (ed). *Vascular Surgery*, 5th edition. Philadelphia: WB Saunders; 1995:1883–1949.)

ing). In a report of 55 patients undergoing such procedures, 80% of the patients were noted by Baumeister to have improvement after a mean follow-up of 3 years.[32] Lymphoscintigraphy can demonstrate graft patency (Figure 43–2). Baumeister et al. reported later on 127 limbs in 122 patients with microsurgical lymphatic grafting (79 with arm edema, 48 with lower extremity edema).[32,33] Most patients with arm edema experienced a decrease in volume measurements. In our limited experience with this operation, we observed long-term patency of suprapubic lymphatic graft (Figure 43–2), although graft patency was followed by short-term clinical improvement only.

Vein grafting

Campisi reported on using saphenous vein grafts to bypass lymphatic obstruction.[34, 35] In 133 patients autologous vein grafts were implanted, performing the anastomoses between the vein graft and the lymph vessels using microsurgical techniques. Excess volume reduction was higher in patients, who underwent operation in the early stages of lymphedema. Of the entire group, greater than 75% improvement was noted in 47% of the patients and greater than 50% in another 34%. Long-term follow-up was available in 95 patients and improvement was documented in 81% (Table 43–1). The incidence of lymphangitis has also decreased after surgery. Unfortunately, results of late graft patency, studied with lymphoscintigraphy, were not reported.

Autotransplantation of Free Lymphatic Flap

Autotransplantation of normal lymphatic tissue to a site deficient of lymphatic nodes and vessels is an attractive idea to enhance lymph transport. Trevidic and Cormier performed autotransplantation of a contralateral free axillary lymph node flap in the axillary fossa in patients with postmastectomy lymphedema.[36] The flap included the inferior axillary nodes, and a portion of the latissimus dorsi muscle with a segment of skin. The flap was supplied by the subscapular artery and vein, which were anastomosed to the subclavian artery and vein at the recipient side. Only 1 of 19 grafts failed and improvement was documented in 75% of patients. Lymphoscintigraphy showed improved lymphatic transport in 75% of the patients and contrast lymphography demonstrated the development of new lympholymphatic anastomoses in some patients. Further experience and longer follow-up with this operation are needed to assess its efficacy.

PRIMARY CHYLOUS DISORDERS AND THORACIC DUCT OCCLUSIONS

Surgical recontruction of the lymphatic system has been attempted in patients with primary chylous disorders and in those with obstruction of the thoracic duct. Primary developmental abnormalities of the lymph vessels (lymphangiectasia, obstruction) or secondary causes (tumor, trauma) lead to congestion of the mesenteric lymphatic circulation, and chyle, rich in chylomicrons and proteins accumulate in abnormal areas of the body.[37–41] Disruption of the lymphatics causes chylous fistulae to the skin (chylocutaneous fistula) or to the pelvis or urether (chyluria) or effusions such as chylothorax or chylous ascites. Rupture of the distended lymph vessels or lymphatic cysts into the lumen of the bowel may manifest in protein loosing enteropathy. Primary chylous reflux is the term used to describe retrograde flow in the incompetent lymphatic system due to lymphangiectasia and loss of lymphatic valve function.

Most patients are at the early teens at the onset of symptoms, since the disease is congenital. Mean age of 35 patients, 15 males and 20 females, who were treated surgically for primary chylous disorders at the Mayo Clinic was 29 years.[37] The patients presented with lower limb edema (54%) due to reflux of chyle and poor lymphatic transport, dyspnea (49%) due to pulmonary lymphangiectesis or reflux of chyle into the lungs, scrotal or labial edema (43%) and abdominal distention (37%) because of chylous ascites.

Many patients are malnourished since important lipids, protein, calcium, and cholesterol is lost in the chyle. Loss of lymphocytes and immunoglobulins will cause compromise of the immune system and the patients become susceptible to infections.

Evaluation

Just as with primary lymphedema, history and physical examination will frequently reveal the diagnosis. Chest x-ray shows pleural effusion, paracentesis or thoracentesis reveal milky fluid, rich in albumin and lipids. Computed tomography confirms the effusion and may identify an underlying malignancy. The dilated lymphatics (megalymphatics, lymphangioleimyomatosis) are better seen with magnetic resonance imaging. We use both lymphoscintigraphy and, as mentioned before, contrast lymphangiography in surgical candidates to define the anatomy of the lymphatics, diagnose thoracic duct occlusion and localize the site of the lymphatic leak.

Non-surgical Management

Patients with lymphedema due to chylous reflux are managed the same way described previously. Limb elevation is these patients is very effective, but upright position will restore edema almost immediately due to reflux of chyle into the lower limbs. Diet rich in medium chain triglycerides or sometimes parenteral nutrition is given to decrease production of chyle. Diuretics are frequently needed in large doses in advanced cases. We have used furosemide and aldacton in high doses in several patients. Paracentesis or thoracentesis is frequently needed and always should be done before surgical treatment is contemplated.

Surgical treatment

We recently reported results of surgical treatment of lymphedema in 35 patients with primary chylous disorders.[37] In 4 patients with lymphangiectasia and reflux of chyle, we performed lymphovenous anastomoses. In 2 of these patients a saphenous vein interposition graft was used, with good early result (Figure 43–3). The rationale to place an interposition vein graft with competent valves is to avoid reflux of the venous blood into the incompetent lymphatic system. Additional surgical procedures for these patients includes ligation and excision of the refluxing and ruptured lymphatics, and lymphatic cysts, placement of a peritoneo-venous shunt, and sclerotherapy of the dilated lymphatics. In our experience two-thirds of the patients with primary chylous disorders demonstrated durable clinical improvement after surgical treatment.

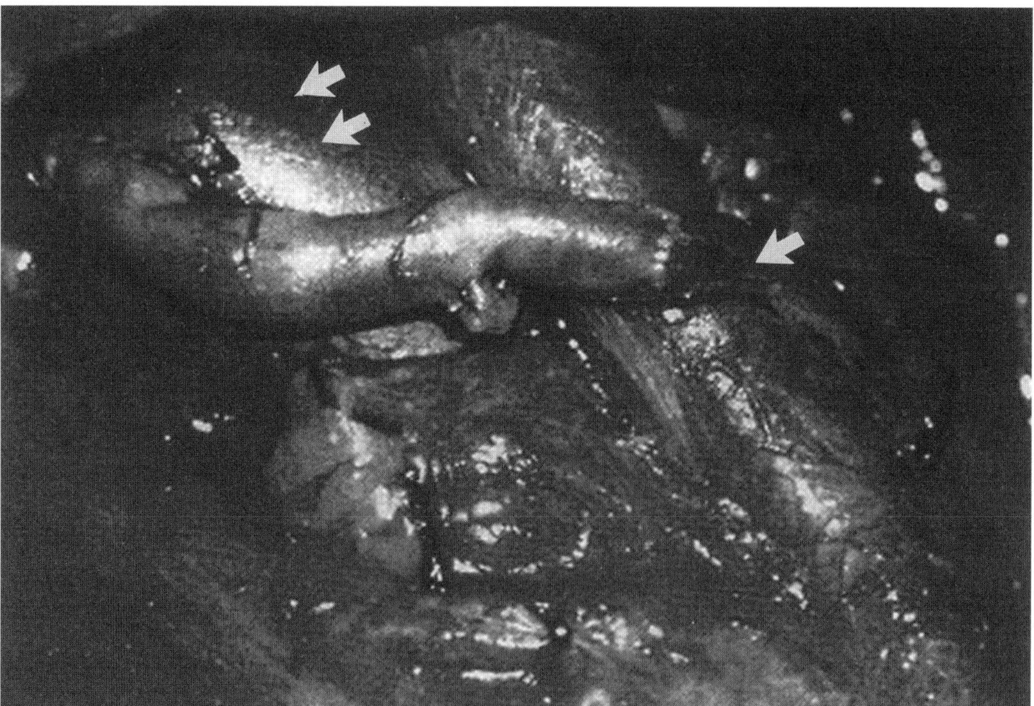

Figure 43–3. Saphenous vein interposition graft from a dilated lymph vessel (single arrow) to the right common iliac vein (double arrows). This patient had lymphangiectasia, chylous reflux and chylocutaneous fistulae (With permission of the Mayo Foundation)

A special type of lymphovenous anastomosis is the thoracic duct–azygos vein anastomosis, that can be attempted to reconstruct the duct and improve lymphatic transport when the upper thoracic duct is occluded. Through a right posterolateral thoracotomy, an anastomosis between the lower thoracic duct and the azygos vein is performed in an end-to-end fashion, with 8–0 or 10–0 non-absorbable interrupted sutures and magnification using loupes or the operating microscope. Only a few patients with this operation have been reported,[40,41] and we have performed successfully this operation in 2 patients.[10] Browse reported 2 successes in 3 patients who underwent thoracic duct reconstruction.[41] Kinmonth suggested that the anastomosis alone is not effective for decompressing the thoracic duct and that ligation of the abnormal mediastinal lymphatics and oversewing of the sites of the lymphatic leak are also necessary.[40] In occasional patients, occlusion of the thoracic duct at the jugulo-subclavian junction can contribute to ascites or chylous effusions. Microsurgical anastomosis between the thoracic duct proximal to the occlusion and the internal jugular vein can be performed, with good technical result (Figures 43–4A–C).

CONCLUSION

Chronic lymphedema and chylous disorders continue to be difficult pathologies but progress in the understanding and management of lymphatic diseases has been significant. Physical therapy is the mainstay of treatment of lymphedema, microsurgical re-

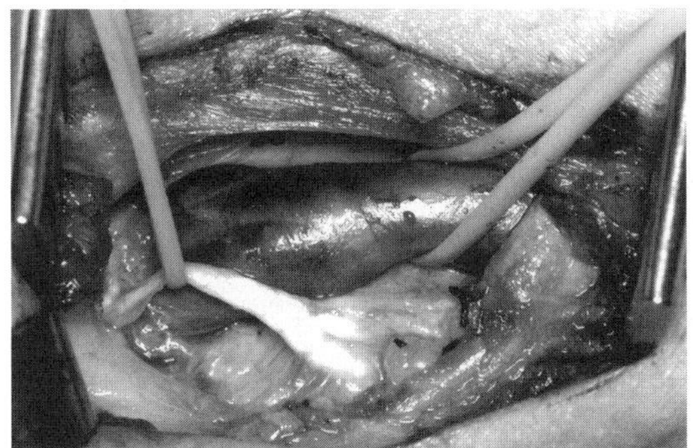
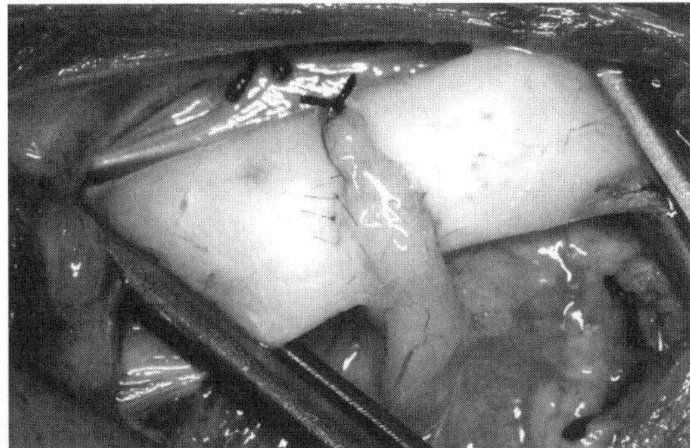
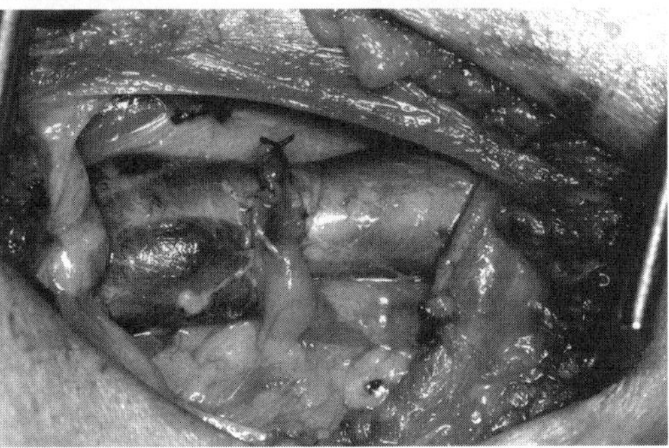

Figure 43–4A–C. Thoracic duct—internal jugular vein anastomosis in a patient with recurrent ascites and occlusion of the thoracic duct at its junction with the jugular vein. **(A)** Chyle filled thoracic duct dissected next to the internal jugular vein. **(B)** Completed anastomosis between the duct and the jugular vein, showing filling of the excluded vein segment with chyle. **(C)** Final picture of completed anastomosis, after removal of clamps.

constructions are rarely performed and only in a few centers worldwide. Patients with primary chylous disorders have more success with surgical treatment which provides durable success in two-thirds of the operated patients. Occasionally, reconstruction of the obstructed thoracic duct can be performed with good result.

REFERENCES

1. Gloviczki P, Wahner H. Clinical diagnosis and evaluation of lymphedema. In: Rutherford RB (ed). *Vascular Surgery (5th edition)*. PhiladelphiaWB Saunders: 2000;2123–2142.
2. Petrek JA, Hulan MC. Incidence of breast carcinoma related lymphedema. *Cancer.* 1998;83:2776–81.
3. Foldi M. Classification of lymphedema and elephantiasis. 12th International WHO/TDR/FIL Conference on Lymphatic Pathology and Immunopathology in Filariasis, Thanjavur, India, 1985. *Lymphology.* 1995;18:159.
4. Stewart, G, Gaunt JI, Croft DN, et al. Isotope lymphography: a new method of investigating the role of the lymphatics in chronic limb oedema. *Br J Surg.* 1985;72:906.
5. Gloviczki P, Calcagno D, Schirger A, et al. Noninvasive evaluation of the swollen extremity: Experiences with 190 lymphoscintigraphic examinations. *J Vasc Surg.* 1989;9:683.
6. Cambria RA, Gloviczki P, Naessens JM, et al. Noninvasive evaluation of the lymphatic system with lymphoscintigraphy: A prospective, semiquantitative analysis in 386 extremities. *J Vasc Surg.* 1993;18:773.
7. Williams WH, Witte CL, Witte MH, et al. Radionuclide lymphangioscintigraphy in the evaluation of peripheral lymphedema. *Clin Nucl Med.* 2000;25:451–464.
8. Witte CL, Witte MH. Diagnostic and interventional imaging of lymphatic disorders. *Int Angiol.* 1999;18:25–30.
9. Gloviczki P, Fisher J, Hollier LH, et al. Microsurgical lymphovenous anastomosis for treatment of lymphedema: A critical review. *J Vasc Surg.* 1988;7:647–652.
10. Gloviczki P, Noel AA. Lymphatic reconstructions. In: Rutherford RB (ed) *Rutherford's Vascular Surgery, 5th edition.* Philadelphia: W.B. Saunders Company; 2000:2159–2174.
11. Gamble GL, Rooke TW, Gloviczki P. Nonoperative management of chronic lymphedema. In: Rutherford RB (ed). *Rutherford'sVascular Surgery (5th edition)*. Philadelphia, WB Saunders, 2000;2142–2153.
12. Foldi E, Foldi M, Weissleder H. Conservative treatment of lymphoedema of the limbs. *Angiology.* 1985;3:171–180.
13. Casley-Smith JR, Morgan RG, Piller NB. Treatment of lymphedema of the arms and legs with 5,6-benzo-[alpha]-pyrone. *N Engl J Med.* 1993;329:1158–1163.
14. Loprinzi CL, Kugler JW, Sloan JA, et al. Lack of effect of coumarin in women with lymphedema after treatment for breast cancer. *N Engl J Med.* 1999;340:346–350.
15. Miller TA, Wyatt LE, Rudkin GH. Staged skin and subcutaneous excision for lymphedema: A favorable report of long-term results. *Plast Reconstr Surg.* 1998;102:1486.
16. Gloviczki P, Hollier LH, Nora FE, et al. The natural history of microsurgical lymphovenous anastomoses: An experimental study. *J Vasc Surg.* 1986;4:148–156.
17. Nielubowicz J. Olszewski W. Surgical lymphaticovenous shunts in patients with secondary lymphoedema. *Br J Surg.* 1968;55:440.
18. O'Brien BMcC, Shafiroff BB. Microlymphaticovenous and resectional surgery in obstructive lymphedema. *World J Surg.* 1979;3:3–15.
19. Puckett CL, Jacobs GR, Hurvitz JS, et al. Evaluation of lymphovenous anastomoses in obstructive lymphedema. *Plast Reconstr Surg.* 1980;66:116.
20. Huang GK, Ru-Qi H, Zong-Zhao L, et al. Microlymphaticovenous anastomosis for treating lymphedema of the extremities and external genitalia. *J Microsurg.* 1981;3:32–39.
21. Jamal S. Lymphovenous anastomosis in filarial lymphedema. *Lymphology.* 1981;14:64.
22. Krylov V, Milanov N, Abalmasov K. Microlymphatic surgery of secondary lymphoedema of the upper limb. *Ann Chir Gynaecol.* 1982;71:77.

23. Nieuborg, L. *The Role of Lymphaticovenous Anastomoses in the Treatment of Postmastectomy. Oedema.* Alblasserdam, The Netherlands: Offsetdrukkerij Kanters BV;1982.
24. Ho LC, Lai MF, Kennedy PJ. Micro-lymphatic bypass in the treatment of obstructive lymphoedema of the arm: case report of a new technique. *Br J Plast Surg.* 1983;36:350–357.
25. Gong-Kang H, Ru-Ai H, Zong-Zhao L, et al. Microlymphaticovenous anastomosis in the treatment of lower limb obstructive lymphedema: analysis of 91 cases. *Plast Reconstr Surg.* 1985;76:671–685.
26. Campisi C, Tosatti E, Casaccia M, et al. Lymphatic microsurgery (in Italian). *Minerva Chir.* 1986;41:469–481.
27. Campisi C, Boccardo F, Zilli A, et al. Long-term results after lymphatic-venous anastomoses for the treatment of obstructive lymphedema. *Microsurgery.* 2001;21:135–139.
28. O'Brien BMcC, Mellow CG, Khazanchi RK, et al. Long-term results after microlymphaticovenous anastomoses for the treatment of obstructive lymphedema. *Plast Reconstr Surg.* 1990;85:562–572.
29. Kleinhaus E, Baumeister RGH, Hahn D, et al. Evaluation of transport kinetics in lymphoscintigraphy: Follow-up study in patients with transplanted lymphatic vessels *Eur J Nucl Med.* 1985;10:349–362.
30. Baumeister RG, Siuda S, Bohmert H, et al. A microsurgical method for reconstruction of interrupted lymphatic pathways: Autologous lymph-vessel transplantation for treatment of lymphedemas. *Scand J Plast Reconstr Surg.* 1986;20:141–146.
31. Baumeister RG, Siuda S. Treatment of lymphedemas by microsurgical lymphatic grafting: what is proved? *Plast Reconstr Surg.* 1990;85:64–74.
32. Baumeister RGH, Frick A, Hofmann T. 10 years experience with autogenous microsurgical lymphvessel-transplantation. *Eur J Lymphology.* 1991;6:62.
33. Baumeister RGH, Fink U, Tatsch K, et al. Microsurgical lymphatic grafting: First demonstration of patent grafts by indirect lymphography and long term follow-up studies. *Progress in Lymphology.* 1994;27:787.
34. Campisi C, Boccardo F, Alitta P, et al. Derivative lymphatic microsurgery: indications, techniques, and results. *Microsurgery.* 1995;16:463–468.
35. Campisi C, Boccardo F, Zilli A, et al. The use of vein grafts in the treatment of peripheral lymphedemas: long-term results. *Microsurgery.* 2001;21:143–147.
36. Trevidic P, Cormier JM. Free axillary lymph node transfer. In Cluzan RV (ed): *Progress in Lymphology.* Amsterdam, Elsevier Science Publishers, 1992;13:415–420.
37. Noel AA, Gloviczki P, Bender CE, et al. Treatment of primary chylous disorders. *J Vasc Surg.* 2001;34:785–791.
38. Browse NL. The diagnosis and management of primary lymphedema. *J Vasc Surg.* 1986;3:181.
39. Rockson SG. Lymphedema. *Amer J Med.* 2001;110(4):288–295.
40. Kinmonth, J. B. Chylous diseases and syndromes, including references to tropical elephantiasis. The Lymphatics: Kinmonth, J. B. *Surgery, Lymphography and Diseases of the Chyle and Lymph Systems, 2nd ed.* London; Edward Arnold: 1982;221–268.
41. Browse NL, Wilson NM, Russo F, et al. Aetiology and treatment of chylous ascites. *Br J Surg.* 1992;79:1145–50.

44

Superficial Venous Thrombosis

Vita Sullivan, MD and Thomas W. Wakefield, MD

Superficial venous thrombosis is also known as superficial thrombophlebitis and formerly phlebothrombosis. These terms refer to thrombosis of part of a superficial vein, more often in the lower extremities and most commonly associated with varicose veins. The incidence of clinically recognized superficial venous thrombosis in the United States is thought to exceed 125,000 cases per year.[1] Superficial venous thrombosis is a deceptively benign disease and for decades received little attention in the medical literature. It is now recognized as an entity that contributes to significant morbidity since it is associated with chronic post-thrombotic syndrome. Superficial venous thrombosis can even lead to death secondary to pulmonary embolism (PE), particularly if located in the above knee segment of greater saphenous vein extending into the deep venous system.

ANATOMY

The superficial veins of the lower extremity include the greater and lesser saphenous veins. Both originate at the dorsal venous arch of the foot. Branching sites and valve number are highly variable. The greater saphenous vein begins as the confluence of veins draining the medial aspect of the foot just anterior to the medial malleolus and travels subcutaneously in a straight line approximately 1 to 2 cm posteromedial to the tibia. It joins the femoral vein 2 to 4 cm lateral to the public tubercle and inferior to the inguinal ligament at the fossa ovalis. In 5–10% of individuals, the greater saphenous vein may exist in duplication as 2 separate trunks that form a single vein at its origin in the ankle and at its termination in the groin. The lesser saphenous vein arises behind the lateral malleolus from a confluence of veins that drain the lateral foot. The lesser saphenous vein is a subcutaneous structure that curves toward the midline of the posterior calf, then ascends vertically to join the popliteal vein behind the knee near the head of the gastrocenemius muscle. The lesser saphenous vein may also send branches into the thigh which anastamose to branches of the greater saphenous vein. In contrast, the deep veins of the lower extremity parallel arteries, bearing the same names. Perforating veins connect the deep and superficial systems by traversing the fascial layer between these anatomically distinct compartments at the level of the ankle and lower calf (Cockett's perforators), usually 10 cm or so below the knee joint (Boyd's perforator), the distal thigh (Dodd's or Huntarian perforator), and the saphenofemoral junction (Figure 44–1). Notably, there is significant anatomic variation in perforating veins. In the upper extremities the superficial veins include the cephalic and basilic veins. In the neck the superficial veins are comprised of the external jugular veins. The majority of superficial venous thrombosis occurs in extremity veins, which shall be the focus of this discussion.

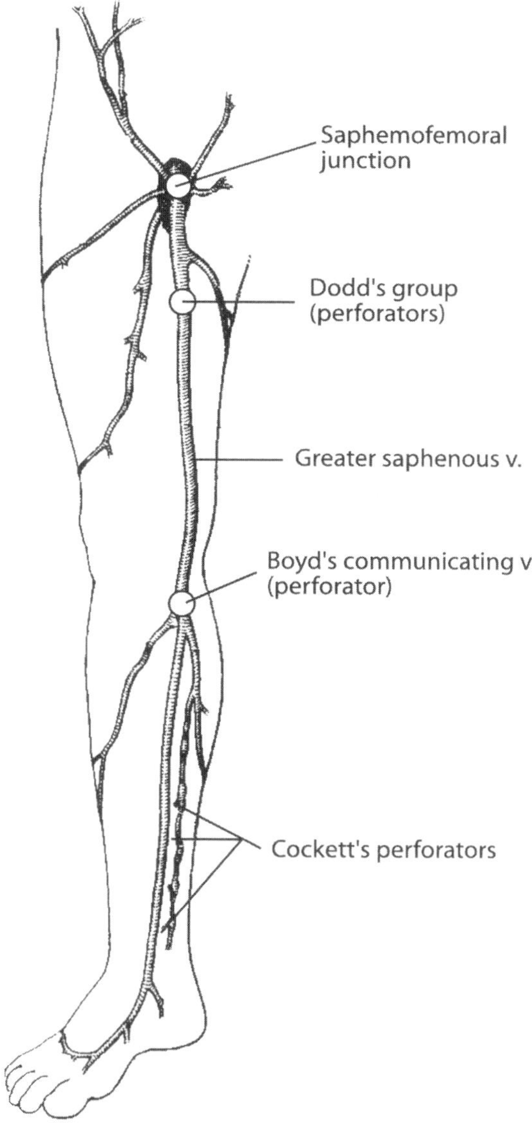

Figure 44–1. Location of major perforators.

Venous valves fragment the column of blood from the foot to the heart, and when unopposed (valvular insufficiency) the column of blood can lead to pressures of 110 to 120 mm Hg at the ankle. One unique feature of veins is their delicate bicuspid valves. The deep veins contain more valves than the superficial veins and the distal lower extremity contains more valves than the proximal lower extremity. The greater saphenous and lesser saphenous systems contain 8 to 10 valves with an anatomically constant valve located just distal to the saphenofemoral venous junction. Valves are present in venules as small as 0.15 mm in diameter. Valves are oriented to direct flow toward the heart and from superficial to deep in order to prevent reflux. Valves in the upper extremity are less important for venous function. The loss of valvular function in a lower extremity secondary to thrombosis confers far greater consequences than loss of upper extremity valvular competence. Perforatoring veins which connect the deep and superficial venous systems also contain valves.

Veins contain muscular fibers as well as collagen but are less elastic in nature than arteries. The smooth muscle is arranged in both circular and longitudinal fashions, and, in general, the amount of circular muscle proportionately reflects the pressure with which a particular vein must contend. Hence, lower extremity veins have more muscle present in their walls as opposed to veins in the thorax, neck, or upper extremities. Venous pathophysiology involves both obstruction and valvular insufficiency.

CLINICAL PRESENTATION

The incidence of clinically recognized superficial venous thrombosis in the United States is thought to exceed 125,000 cases per year.[1] Lutter et al. reviewed 1,412 ultrasound examinations for acute venous thrombosis and noted a 19% incidence of superficial venous thrombosis.[2] There is no gender difference or left versus right predisposition.[3–6] The clinical appearance of superficial venous thrombosis is typically obvious. It involves a painful, firm, palpable cord with an area of inflammation and/or tenderness along the axis of the affected vein, and sometimes localized and/or generalized edema (Figure 44–2). In 1 retrospective review of 43 patients with superfi-

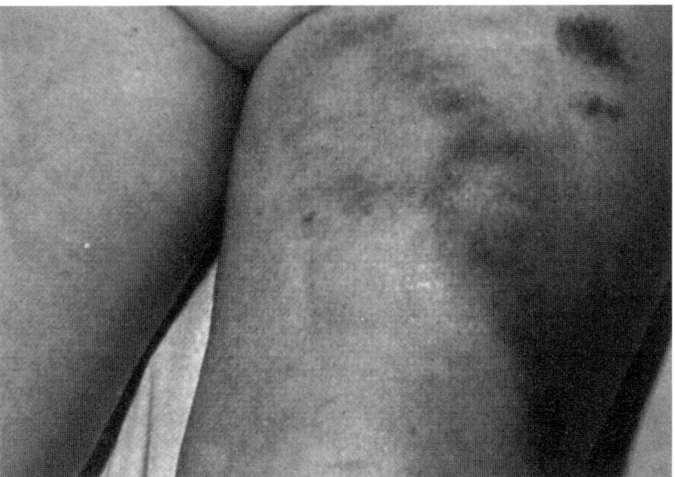

Figure 44–2. Typical example of Superficial Venous Thrombosis (used with permission from from Walker FW. Superficial Thrombophlebitis. In *Color Atlas of Peripheral Vascular Diseases.* Page 91).

cial venous thrombosis, 100% had associated pain, 46% had localized swelling, and only 15% had generalized swelling.[7] There may be a history of venous puncture or intravenous canalization (particularly in upper extremity thrombophlebitis), contrast media or pro-phlebitic medication infusion (peripheral parenteral nutrition, diazepam, pentobarbital, colony stimulating factor), trauma (especially in lower extremity thrombophlebitis associated with varicose veins), physical inactivity, use of oral contraceptives, occult or known malignancy, or infections.

The inflammatory reaction associated with superficial venous thrombosis usually takes weeks to subside. The thrombosed vein may be tender for months. Recurrence rates of superficial venous thrombosis have been estimated at 15–20%.[4,8,9] The introduction of duplex ultrasound imaging in 1982 by Talbott helped further elucidate the complicated nature of superficial venous thrombosis, particularly in relation to its involvement with deep venous thrombosis (DVT). Extension into the deep venous system is not predictable by history or physical findings.[7]

SUPPERATIVE SUPERFICIAL VENOUS THROMBOSIS

Usually supperative venous thrombosis is associated with an intravenous catheter or multiple puncture sites secondary to intravenous drug abuse, most often occurring in an upper extremity. The clinical presentation is similar to that of non-suppurative thrombophlebitis though often there is also pyrexia, leukocytosis, and/or bacteremia. When associated with signs of sepsis, supperative thrombophlebitis becomes known as septic thrombophlebitis. Local intravenous catheter site infections occur up to 8% of the time and bacteremia is detected in approximately 1 of every 400 intravenous catheterizations.[10] Immunocompromised and burn patients are particularly susceptible to septic thrombophlebitis The diagnosis is confirmed with expression of purulent material from the site. The most important factor to decrease the incidence of supperative superficial venous thrombosis is to limit intravenous catheter placement to 48 to 72 hours. The treatment consists of removal of the cannula, warm compresses, elevation, complete excision of the affected venous segment with open packing, and tailoring of intravenous antibiotics.

SUPERFICIAL VENOUS THROMBOSIS
ASSOCIATED WITH VARICOSE VEINS

Varicose veins were first referenced in the Ebers papyrus dated 1550 B.C.E. Hippocrates discussed management of varicose veins in his treatises. Varicose veins affect more than 20 million Americans and constitute the most common vascular disorder of the lower extremities. No other animal except man is afflicted by lower extremity varicosities, likely secondary to the evolution of erect stature and bipedal movement. Varicose veins can be large, tortuous and bulging, or small spider like telangectasias. Varicose veins that arise spontaneously are known as primary varicose veins and are predisposed by obesity, physical inactivity, hypertension, positive family history, pregnancy, female sex, and advanced age. Secondary varicose veins result from chronic venous insufficiency usually from damaged valves from previous thrombosis, tumor, trauma, or congenital versus acquired arteriovenous fistulas.[11] Varicose veins manifest with pain, aching of the lower extremities after prolonged use, vague feelings of fullness, and occasionally edema. Initial treatment of both primary and secondary varicose veins includes elastic compression stockings, elevation, and exercise.

Varicose veins are highly associated (50 to 93%) with superficial venous thrombosis, most commonly below the knee.[9,12] Superficial venous thrombosis of a varicose vein is easily recognizable on physical exam as a hard, tender, erythematous, palpable cord. The area can be indurated and edematous and may be associated with cellulitis. If there is no associated cellulitis, thrombosis of a varicose vein can be treated with non-steroidal anti-inflammatory medications (NSAIDs), elevation, elastic compression stockings, and heat for relief of discomfort. If a superimposed cellulitis develops then antibiotics should be added. Superficial venous thrombosis of a varicose vein may lead to erosion of the overlying skin with bleeding, which then becomes an indication for surgical intervention. Surgical intervention is contraindicated in individuals with arteriovenous fistula, arterial insufficiency, lymphedema, cellulitis, and Klippel-Trenaunay Syndrome in the absence of a deep venous system. In addition, varicose disease is notably a pre-operative risk factor (2–3x increased risk) for development of deep venous thrombosis and warrants venous thrombosis prophylaxis.[13]

Above the Knee Superficial Venous Thrombosis

Above knee superficial venous thrombosis is thought to represent a more serious condition. It has a predilection to evolve into the deep venous system and can lead to pulmonary embolism. Surgical therapy for superficial thrombophlebitis was first recommended at the beginning of the twentieth century.[14] Historically, above the knee superficial venous thrombosis was treated with flush saphenofemoral junction ligation and stripping of the phlebitic segment. More current reviews of the literature suggest that anticoagulation is superior to surgical intervention for minimizing complications and preventing subsequent DVT and PE development, though in cases where anticoagulation is contraindicated or in the presence of unremitting pain, surgical intervention still offers a viable alternative.[15]

Extension of thrombophlebitis within the superficial venous system (proximally or distally but not into the deep venous system) has had little attention in the literature, particularly with respect to different surgical techniques. Only Belcaro et al. addressed this in the current literature by noting a decreased rate of superficial thrombus extension both at 3 months (0% versus 14.1%) and 6 months (1.4% versus 7.7%) in patients who were treated by ligation, stripping of the phlebitic vein, and perforator interruption as opposed to those treated only with flush ligation at the saphenofemoral junction.[16] The rate of superficial extension in the group treated by ligation, stripping, and perforator interruption was also lower than that seen in patients who received only anticoagulant therapy (1.4% versus 7% at 6 months). This suggests that ligation in combination with stripping and interruption of perforators is superior with respect to superficial thrombus extension, thus resulting in symptomatic pain relief more rapidly than conventional medical therapies.[16–18]

Progression of superficial venous thrombosis into the deep venous system is postulated to occur by 3 pathways: via the saphenofemoral junction into the common femoral vein, via the knee perforators into the popliteal vein, and via the ankle perforators into the tibial and peroneal veins. Chengelis noted that 90% of propagation occurred via the saphenofemoral junction or at the popliteal as compared to only 10% occurring at the level of the malleolus.[19] The rate of extension into the deep venous system in a literature review of management of above knee superficial venous thrombosis was 3.4% in a group treated with ligation versus 2.2% in a cohort treated with anticoagulation, with an overall rate of 3.1%.[15]

The incidence of DVT associated with superficial venous thrombosis on presentation is estimated between 0.75% and 40%.[2,4,9,12,16,19–23] Since the advent of duplex ultrasound imaging the estimates of concurrent superficial venous thrombosis with associated DVT are in the middle of this range. A 100% correlation between duplex and venography has been noted by Lohr.[7] The association of a noncontiguous DVT with superficial thrombophlebitis has been estimated to be as high as 25% to 75% in those patients who present with involvement of both the deep and superficial venous systems.[2,12,17] There is no correlation between the initial symptom development of superficial venous thrombosis and the time of diagnosis of concomitant DVT.[13]

SUPERFICIAL VENOUS THROMBOSIS AND PULMONARY EMBOLISM

Superficial venous thrombosis causing PE was first noted by Richter in 1905.[20] In 1952, Herman reported the lethality of PE secondary to superficial venous thrombosis and also recommended surgical treatment. Pulmonary embolism, the most lethal and under recognized complication associated with this entity, has been estimated to occur from 0 to 17%.[2,4,8,14,18–20, 22] Only one series by Lutter et al. noted predisposing risk factors to be significantly associated with a more complicated course. These risk factors were: bilaterality of superficial thrombophlebitis, age greater than 60, male sex, history of DVT, immobility, presence of systemic infection, and location in the greater saphenous vein.[2]

The benefits of anticoagulant therapy include its effective prevention of PE, minimal reported morbidity, and potential preservation of the greater saphenous vein for future use as a bypass conduit, although post-phlebitic vein when used as conduit has been shown to be associated with early failure in distal lower extremity bypass grafting.[24] The preservation of greater saphenous vein and recanalization rates on anticoagulant therapy have not been well studied to date.

HYPERCOAGULABLE STATES AND SUPERFICIAL VENOUS THROMBOSIS

Primary hypercoagulable states are inherited disorders with great unevenness in penetrance. They include disorders such as Antithrombin III deficiency, Factor V Leiden mutation, Prothrombin 20210A gene mutation, Protein C and Protein S deficiencies, disorders of tPA, abnormal plasminogen, dysfibringoenemia, Factor XII deficiency, and lupus anticoagulant and anticardiolipin antibody syndrome. All primary hypercoagulable states can have superficial venous thrombosis as a significant or presenting clinical sign (except purpura fulminans and Coumadin necrosis).[25] Patients with primary hypercoagulable states may not respond to initial therapy of superficial venous thrombosis, therefore a hypercoagulable investigation should be considered in patients with ascending or worsening thrombosis. If the hypercoagulable work-up is positive, the decision for long-term anticoagulation can then be made on an individual basis.

The increased incidence of hypercoagulability associated with superficial venous thrombosis is estimated as high as 35% based on 2 rounds of testing.[6] This increased incidence is likely secondary to increased awareness and better testing for primary hypercoagulable states. The risk of superficial venous thrombosis in the absence of varicose veins, malignancy or autoimmune disorders was 13-fold higher for deficiencies of inhibitors of coagulation (Antithrombin III, Protein C or S), 6-fold higher for the Factor V-Leiden mutation, and 4-fold higher for the prothrombin gene mutation.[26] The incidence of hypercoagulability associated with superficial venous thrombosis approaches that seen in DVT. Thus, the same indications for hypercoagulable work-up in patients with DVT should be applied for patients with superficial venous thrombosis (unexplained venous thrombosis in individuals <45 years of age, recurrence, thrombosis of inferior vena cava, mesenteric, hepatic, renal, portal or cerebral veins, or a positive family history).

Secondary hypercoagulable states can also present with superficial venous thrombosis and include: malignancy, pregnancy, use of oral contraceptives, Behcet's disease, Mondor's disease, Buerger's disease, infectious agents, intravenous catheters, and intravenous drug use.[10] Notably, pregnancy was the most frequent risk factor associated with superficial venous thrombosis at the time of diagnosis in one study.[26] In pregnancy, the rate of superficial venous thrombosis parallels that of DVT and a marked preponderance of thrombotic events is notable in the first postpartum week.[27]

Conditions that may mimic superficial venous thrombosis include sarcoid granulomas, cutaneous polyarteritis nodosa, dermatophyte cellulitis, and Kaposi's sarcoma with hyperalgesic pseudothrombophlebitis in HIV positive patients.

MONDOR'S DISEASE

In 1869, Fagge first described the clinical findings associated with Mondor's disease or superficial venous thrombosis of the breast. In 1939, Henri Mondor first noted the clinical significance of the disease. Mondor's disease (also known as superficial thrombophlebitis of the breast) is an uncommon disorder whose true incidence is unknown. It is characterized by the sudden onset of localized chest pain that is exacerbated by movement and followed by the appearance of palpable, tender, often visible, cord-like structures in the thoracoepigastric or lateral thoracic veins. Young females between the ages of 20–50 are most commonly affected. No correlation to race or family history has been noted.[28] The clinical entity often has an antecedent history of trauma or surgical biopsy though no true etiology is known. A list of postulated etiologies related to Mondor's disease is varied and largely speculative but include: idiopathic, injury (iatrogenic versus traumatic), infection, muscular strain, pendulous breasts, tight undergarments or bandages, carcinoma, adenopathy, radiation, intravenous drug abuse, and/or shaving. Accurate diagnosis is based on history and physical exam and must be distinguished from breast malignancies. There are no consistent mammographic or laboratory findings. Biopsies have been noted to show sclerosis of the involved vein with intimal and adventitial thickening, luminal obstruction and connective tissue proliferation and inflammatory cell infiltration. Typically, when not associated with malignancy, Mondor's disease is a benign, self-limited condition which usually resolves in 2 to 8 weeks.[10,28] Treatment typically consists of warm compresses, NSAIDS and close follow-up. Treatment is largely palliative and does not alter the duration of the disease. There are suggestions that younger age tends toward earlier resolution of symptoms and larger, pendulous breasts are associated with a longer clinical course.[28]

THROMBOANGIITIS OBLITERANS

In 1908, Leo Buerger first described a disorder of presenile spontaneous gangrene secondary to vascular insufficiency and termed it thromboangiitis obliterans (Buerger's disease).[29] It has an estimated prevalence of 13 in 100,000.[30] The disease is a nonatherosclerotic segmental inflammatory disease which commonly affects the small and medium-sized arteries, veins and nerves of the arms and legs.[30] More prevalent in the Middle East and Far East, clinical criteria for diagnosis of thromboangiitis obliterans include: onset before 50 years of age, distal extremity arterial disease, exclusion of hypercoagulable states, exclusion of diabetes mellitus and autoimmune disorders, and for purposes of the current discussion, the frequent occurrence of superficial migratory venous thrombosis. Additional criteria include tobacco use, and possible Raynaud's phenomenon. Diagnosis is based on clinical evaluation, laboratory evaluation to exclude hypercoagulable states along with autoimmune disorders and diabetes, arteriography of all extremities, and rarely biopsy. The course is progressive requiring amputation in persistent tobacco users. Patients typically present with distal extremity claudication and progress to rest pain and ulceration. Superficial venous thrombosis occurs in approximately 40% of patients with thromboangiitis obliterans.[30] The thrombosis may be migratory and can parallel disease activity. Women with tromboangiitis obliterans have a higher association with migratory superficial venous thrombosis likely confounded by pregnancy their higher incidence of varicose disease, and use of oral contraceptives. Histologic examination demonstrates inflammatory occlusive thrombi with micorabscesses and giant cells. Angiographic studies of the arteries of all 4 extremities can differentiate Buerger's disease from atherosclerosis. It is not uncommon to see angiographic abnormalities in limbs that are not clinically involved. Notably, these angiographic findings are suggestive for the disease but may also be seen in scleroderma, rheumatoid vasculitis, connective tissue diseases and antiphospholipid antibody syndrome. The main form of treatment is cessation of all nicotine containing products. Anticoagulation frequently fails to control the disease. The role of surgical revascularization is usually not possible secondary to the distal nature of the disease, although it may be attempted if a target vessel exists. The role of sympathectomy in treating pain and preventing amputation remains unclear.

SUMMARY AND SUGGESTIONS FOR CLINICAL MANAGEMENT GUIDELINES

- *Suppurative Superficial Venous Thrombosis*
  - usually secondary to intravenous catheter placement
  - the best therapy is prevention—removing intravenous catheters within 48 to 72 hours of placement
  - treatment consists of cannula removal, warm compresses and elevation; if cellulitis is noted add antibiotics; if purulent discharge is noted with bacteremia or sepsis then excise the entire involved segment, pack open, allow to heal by secondary intention, and tailor antibiotics according to cultures
- *Superficial Venous Thrombosis Associated with Varicose Veins*
  - treat with NSAIDs, elevation and elastic compression stockings
  - if a superimposed cellulitis develops then antibiotics should be added
  - if bleeding occurs secondary to erosion through the skin direct pressure will most often arrest bleeding and surgical excision can occur at a later time.
- *Above Knee Superficial Venous Thrombosis Associated with or without Varicose Veins*
  - obtain bilateral duplex examination to assess for associated DVT,
  - if the superficial venous thrombosis is located above the knee but is not approaching the saphenofemoral junction then medical therapy with heat, ele-

vation, elastic compression stockings and NSAIDs can be employed, though
close follow-up and repeat duplex scanning within 1 week is recommended
- if the superficial venous thrombosis is approaching the saphenofemoral junction then anticoagulant therapy should be considered for 6 weeks to 3 months
- if the saphenofemoral junction is involved or there evidence of DVT then anticoagulation for 3–6 months is recommended
- if there is a contraindication to anticoagulation then flush ligation at the saphenofemoral junction and stripping of the phlebitic vein should be considered
- if PE is documented then anticoagulation for 6 months is recommended
- *Unexpected SVT*
  - complete duplex scanning of the deep and superficial venous systems of both limbs to rule out concomitant DVT should be obtained
  - hypercoagulable work-up should be considered in patients without a history of: associated trauma or inactivity, veinipuncture site or canalization, malignancy, varicose veins; and in those individuals with: severe thrombophlebitis, recurrence, family history of thrombosis, early age at presentation, resistance to therapy[10,25]
  - treatment should include heat, elevation, elastic compression stockings, and NSAIDs; should ascending progression be noted a repeat duplex should be obtained; if associated DVT is diagnosed then therapy should include anticoagulation for 3–6 months.

REFERENCES

1. Vitti MJ, Barnes RW. Nonoperative treatment of acute superficial thrombophlebitis and deep femoral venous thrombosis. In: Ernst CB SJ, ed. *Current Therapy in Vascular Surgery*. St. Louis: Mosby, 1995:888–889.
2. Lutter KS, Kerr TM, Roedersheimer LR, et al. Superficial thrombophlebitis diagnosed by duplex scanning. *Surgery*. 1991;110:42–46.
3. Lofgren EP, Lofgren KA. The surgical treatment of superficial thrombophlebitis. *Surgery*. 1981;90:49–54.
4. Hafner CD, Craneg JJ, Krause RJ, et al. A method of managing superficial thrombophlebitis. *Surgery*. 1964;55:201–206.
5. Kerr TM, Cranley JJ, Johnson JR, et al. Analysis of 1084 consecutive lower extremities involved with acute venous thrombosis diagnosed by duplex scanning. *Surgery*. 1990;108:520–527.
6. Hanson JN, Ascher E, DePippo P, et al. Saphenous vein thrombophlebitis (SVT): a deceptively benign disease. *J Vasc Surg*. 1998;27:677–680.
7. Lohr JM, McDevitt DT, Lutter KS, et al. Operative management of greater saphenous thrombophlebitis involving the saphenofemoral junction. *Am J Surg*. 1992;164:269–275.
8. Husni EA, Williams WA. Superficial thrombophlebitis of lower limbs. *Surgery*. 1982;91:70–74.
9. Ascer E, Lorensen E, Pollina RM, et al. Preliminary results of a nonoperative approach to saphenofemoral junction thrombophlebitis. *J Vasc Surg*. 1995;22:616–621.
10. Samlaska CP, James WD. Superficial thrombophlebitis. II. Secondary hypercoagulable states. *J Am Acad Dermatol*. 1990;23:1–18.
11. Gloviczki P, Merrell SW. Surgical treatment of venous disease. *Cardiovasc Clin*. 1992;22:81–100.

12. Jorgensen JO, Hanel KC, Morgan AM, et al. The incidence of deep venous thrombosis in patients with superficial thrombophlebitis of the lower limbs. *J Vasc Surg.* 1993;18:70–73.
13. Guex SE. Thrombotic complications of varicose veins. A literature review of the role of superficial venous thrombosis. *Dermatol Surg.* 1996;22:378–382.
14. Gjores J. Surgical therapy of ascending thrombophlebitis in the saphenous system. *Angiology.* 1962;13:241–243.
15. Sullivan V, Denk PM, Sonnad SS, et al. Ligation versus anticoagulation: treatment of above-knee superficial thrombophlebitis not involving the deep venous system. *J Am Coll Surg.* 2001;193:556–562.
16. Belcaro G, Nicolaides AN, Errichi BM, et al. Superficial thrombophlebitis of the legs: a randomized, controlled, follow-up study. *Angiology.* 1999; 50:523–529.
17. Plate G, Eklof B, Jensen R, et al. Deep venous thrombosis, pulmonary embolism and acute surgery in thrombophlebitis of the long saphenous vein. *Acta Chir Scand.* 1985;151:241–244.
18. Williams RD Zollinger RW. Surgical treatment of superficial thrombophlebitis. *Surg Gynecol Obstet.* 1964;118:745.
19. Chengelis DL, Bendick PJ, Glover JL, et al. Progression of superficial venous thrombosis to deep vein thrombosis. *J Vasc Surg.* 1996;24:745–749.
20. Krause U, Kock HJ, Kroger K, et al. Prevention of deep venous thrombosis associated with superficial thrombophlebitis of the leg by early saphenous vein ligation. *Vasa.* 1998;27:34–38.
21. Blumenberg RM, Barton E, Gelfand ML, et al. Occult deep venous thrombosis complicating superficial thrombophlebitis. *J Vasc Surg.* 1998;27:338–43.
22. Sover ER, Brammer HM, Rowedder AM. Thrombosis of the proximal greater saphenous vein: ultrasonographic diagnosis and clinical significance. *J Ultrasound Med.* 1997;16: 113–116.
23. Prountjos P, Bastounis E, Hadjinikolaou L, et al. Superficial venous thrombosis of the lower extremities co-existing with deep venous thrombosis. A phlebographic study on 57 cases. *Int Angiol.* 1991;10:63–65.
24. Filippone ND, Shah DM, Welch HF, et al. Chronic venosus obstruction as a factor in the early failure of bypass grafts in the leg. *Am J Surg.* 1980;140:671–674.
25. Samlaska CP, James WD. Superficial thrombophlebitis. I. Primary hypercoagulable states. *J Am Acad Dermatol.* 1990;22:975–89.
26. Martinelli I, Cattaneo M, Taioli E, et al. Genetic risk factors for superficial vein thrombosis. *Thromb Haemost.* 1999;82:1215–7.
27. McColl MD, Ramsay JE, Tait RC, et al. Superficial vein thrombosis: incidence in association with pregnancy and prevalence of thrombophilic defects. *Thromb Haemost.* 1998;79:741–742.
28. Pugh CM, DeWitty RL. Mondor's disease. *J Natl Med Assoc.* 1996;88:359–63.
29. Buerger L. Thrombo-angiitis obliterans: a study of the vascular lesion leading to presenile spontaneous gangrene. *Am J Med Sci.* 1908;136:567–80.
30. Olin JW. Thromboangiitis obliterans (Buerger's disease). *N Engl J Med.* 2000;343:864–869.

45

Mesenteric Venous Thrombosis: Current Concepts in Diagnosis and Treatment

Mark D. Morasch, MD

Mesenteric venous thrombosis (MVT) is largely considered to be the least common cause of acute mesenteric ischemia. This entity is responsible for less than 10% of clinically significant cases of mesenteric ischemia and is found in fewer than 1 in 1,000 laparotomies.[1,2] Earlier reports suggested that mortality rates for MVT could be as high as 50% but more recent reports have found this disease process to be much less likely to be fatal than other forms of mesenteric ischemia (Table 45–1).[2–6] In addition, the widespread use of CT scanning has led to more frequent diagnosis of benign subclinical acute or chronic forms of MVT. Because MVT may not be suspected and, therefore, not diagnosed in many patients, its true incidence remains unknown but the incidence

TABLE 45–1. LITERATURE REVIEW OF ACUTE MVT, MANAGEMENT, MORTALITY

Author (year)	No. of Patients	Bowel Resection	Nonoperative	Anti-coagulation	30 Day Mortality (%)
Sack (1982)[11]	9	9	0	6	2 (22%)
Wilson (1987)[4]	16	10	3	6	8 (50%)
Montany (1988)[5]	6	5	1	6	3 (50%)
Clavien (1988)[12]	12	12	0	12	5 (42%)
Kaleya (1989)[7]	22	22	0	22	7 (32%)
Harward (1989)[13]	16	5	11	7	3 (19%)
Levy (1990)[14]	21	19	2	17	8 (38%)
Grieshop (1991)[15]	15	5	10	9	2 (13%)
Rhee (1994)[2]	53	30	19	33	14 (27%)
Morasch (2001)[6]	23	8	14	19	7 (30%)

of symptomatic MVT over a 20-year period was reported to be 2 in 100,000 admissions in one report.[7] MVT can occur at any age but it seems to be more common in the sixth and seventh decades and there appears to be a slight male preponderance.[8]

Commonly, patients with MVT present with abdominal pain. This can be sudden in onset but frequently begins insidiously and worsens progressively. Approximately one-half of patients with clinically significant MVT have abdominal pain that lasts anywhere from 1 week to 1 month before they seek medical attention and another one-quarter report abdominal pain that has lasted for more than a month. In our 2001 review, only 16% of our patients developed peritonitis from intestinal necrosis and just 2 patients died from massive bowel infarction.[6] Declining mortality rates may be the result of more aggressive treatment and earlier diagnosis; it is also quite possible, however, that we now more readily diagnose a more benign form of the disease because of widespread use of CT scanning. Improved image resolution of high-speed CT and MRI has likely added to their sensitivity, making diagnosis of MVT more common. An apparent increase in the incidence of MVT along with declining mortality may be due to improved diagnostic capabilities rather than an actual increase in disease frequency.

Traditionally, an objective diagnosis of MVT has been difficult to establish. A mild leukocytosis with a left shift and a slightly elevated lactic dehydrogenase level are usually the only abnormalities present. Other laboratory values such as serum amylase are usually unremarkable. Plain films of the abdomen will usually show a nondescript ileus pattern with dilated fluid-filled bowel loops. The diagnosis of MVT usually requires a high clinical index of suspicion and should be followed by some form of non-invasive abdominal imaging. Newer generation contrast-enhanced abdominal CT scanning can accurately detect portal and mesenteric vein thrombosis. CT scanning established a diagnosis in over 90% of the patients in our series who underwent the test.[6] Acute thrombus in the superior mesenteric vein (SMV) is evident on CT as a central lucency devoid of contrast and surrounded by an inflamed and thickened vein wall (Figure 45–1). Other CT findings include SMV dilatation, persistent enhancement of thickened bowel wall, and a well developed collateral venous circulation in more chronic cases. Because of the accuracy and simplicity of CT scanning, we no longer recommend venous-phase angiography as a primary diagnostic modality. MR venography (Figure 45–2) and duplex ultrasound have also been used successfully at our institution to diagnose or confirm the diagnosis of MVT.

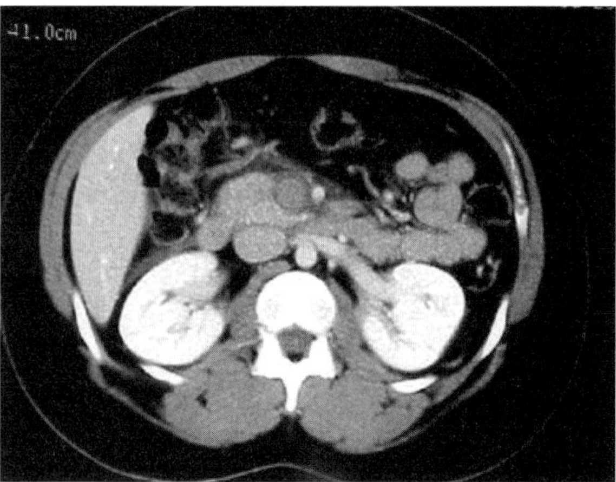

Figure 45–1. CT scan showing typical MVT.

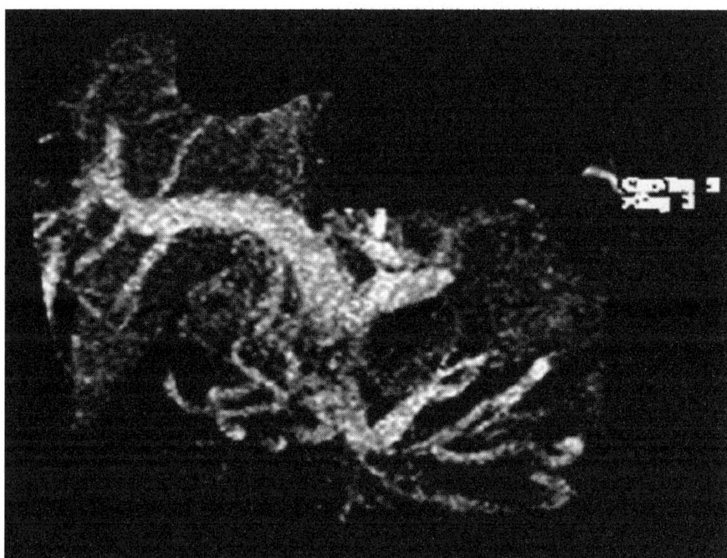

Figure 45–2. MR venogram showing occlusion.

A variety of hypercoagulable states are known to be associated with MVT. The most common associated hypercoagulable states include prior abdominal surgery, the presence of a neoplasm, or deficiencies of the vitamin K-dependent coagulation inhibitors (proteins S and C). Antithrombin III deficiency and Leiden factor V gene mutation are genetic risk factors that have commonly been found in patients diagnosed with MVT. The use of oral contraceptive agents is responsible for approximately 5% of MVT cases (9% to 18% of cases in women).[9] Additional hypercoagulable states that have been associated with MVT are listed in Table 45–2. Past medical history or a fam-

TABLE 45–2. CONDITIONS ASSOCIATED WITH MVT

Direct injury
    Abdominal trauma (blunt and penetrating)
    Postsurgical (particularly postsplenectomy)
    Intra-abdominal inflammatory states (pancreatitis, inflammatory bowel)
    Peritonitis and abdominal abscess

Local venous congestion or stasis
    Portal hypertension/cirrhosis of the liver
    Congestive heart failure
    Hypersplenism

Hypercoagulable states
    Protein C and protein S deficiency
    Antithrombin III deficiency
    Activated protein C resistance (factor V Leiden gene mutation)
    Presence of the 20210 A allele of the prothrombin gene
    Methylenetetrahydrofolate reductase mutations
    Neoplasms (particularly pancreatic and colonic)
    Oral contraceptive use
    Polycythemia vera
    Heparin-induced thrombocytopenia
    Lupus anticoagulant/antiphospholipid syndrome

ily history of pathologic thromboses in combination with abdominal complaints should increase the index of suspicion for MVT. In fact, a hypercoagulable state at diagnosis is much more common in patients with MVT than in patients with deep venous thrombosis (DVT). In a recent update of our 2001 review, 37 of 41 patients (90%) had an identifiable hypercoagulable state and 54% of the patients in this series had some form of factor deficiency associated with hypercoagulability.

Although the natural history of MVT is unknown, it does not appear to have the same ominous prognosis associated with arterial occlusion. In our updated review, the early mortality rate was only 17% and only 2 patients died of massive bowel infarction. At surgery or autopsy the affected segments of bowel appear markedly edematous and darkly reddened (Figure 45–3). The mesentery is thick and rubbery and the thrombotic process is segmental. Sequestered third-space fluid is more extensive than with arterial mesenteric disease. This often-massive sequestration accounts for the significant volume requirements noted in patients who present with an aggressive form of MVT. Fortunately, colonic involvement is rare because of the extensive collateral venous drainage from the large bowel.[10]

In our review, treatment ranged from observation and bowel rest with or without anticoagulation to extensive bowel resection with venous thrombectomy. Our updated review also included 3 patients who underwent attempted treatment with thrombolytic agents. Thrombolytic therapy carries risk for hemorrhage and has been reported to have a low rate of success unless initiated soon after the thrombotic process begins. At present, we agree with the majority of authors who recommend conservative management for most MVT patients that includes bowel rest and aggressive anticoagulation with heparin and Coumadin (Figure 45–4). Venous thrombectomy and intra-arterial or transhepatic thrombolysis should be reserved for only the most dire circumstances and only when the perceived benefits outweigh the potential risks involved since the vast majority of patients will improve with observation and anticoagulation alone.

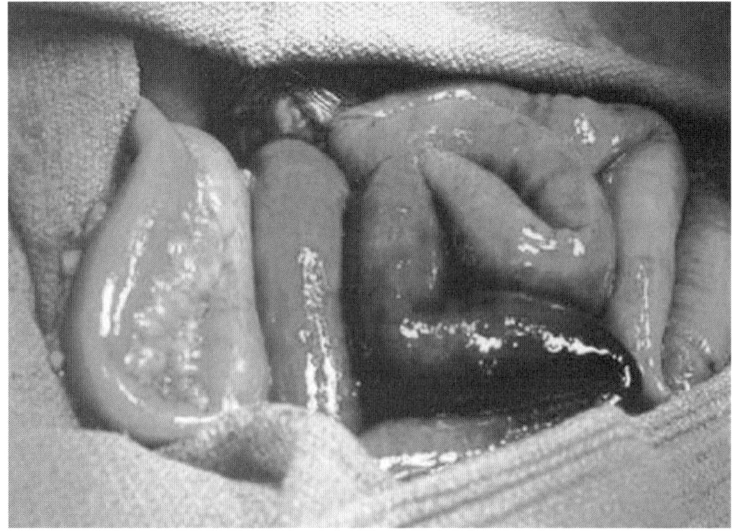

Figure 45–3. Bowel ischemia secondary to MVT.

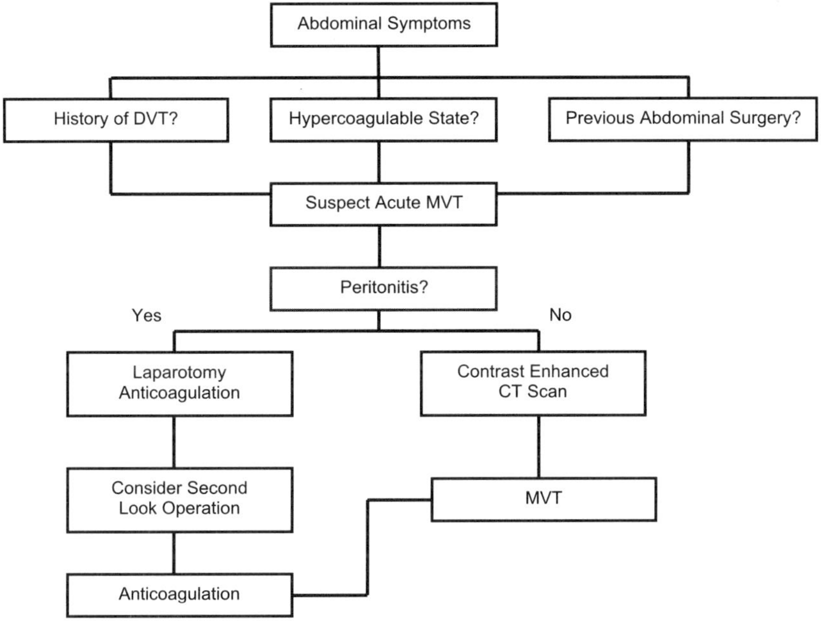

Figure 45–4. Management of acute mesenteric ischemia.

MVT should be suspected in patients presenting with abdominal pain, especially those with known hypercoagulable disorders, history of DVT, or prior splenectomy and these patients should undergo fine-columniation contrast-enhanced CT scanning with close attention to the mesenteric venous phase. Early anticoagulation with heparin followed by Coumadin, usually for life, is recommended to limit thrombosis and reduce the likelihood of recurrent symptoms. Patients found to have asymptomatic or chronic MVT serendipitously on imaging performed for other indications should certainly be evaluated for hypercoagulable disorders and should also be considered for anticoagulation therapy. Indeed, full hypercoagulability screening should be performed in all patients diagnosed with MVT and, properly treated; most of these patients should have a good long-term prognosis.

REFERENCES

1. Kazmers A. Intestinal ischemia caused by venous thrombosis. In: Rutherford RB, editor. *Vascular Surgery.* Philadelphia, PA: WB Saunders; 1995:1288-1300.
2. Rhee RY, Gloviczki P, Mendonca CT, Petterson TM, Serry RD, Sarr MG, et al. Mesenteric venous thrombosis: still a lethal disease in the 1990s. *J Vasc Surg.* 1994;20(5):688–697.
3. Warren S, Eberhard TP. Mesenteric venous thrombosis. *Surg Gynecol Obstet.* 1935;61:102–121.
4. Wilson C, Walker ID, Davidson JF, Imrie CW. Mesenteric venous thrombosis and antithrombin III deficiency. *J Clin Pathol.* 1987;40:906–908.
5. Montany PF, Finley RK. Mesenteric venous thrombosis. *Am Surg.* 1988;54:161–166.
6. Morasch MD, Ebaugh JL, Chiou AC, Matsumura JS, Pearce WH, Yao JS. Mesenteric venous thrombosis: a changing clinical entity. *J Vasc Surg.* 2001;34(4):680–684.
7. Kaleya RN, Boley SJ. Mesenteric venous thrombosis. In: Najarian JS, Delaney JP, editors. *Progress in Gastrointestinal Surgery.* Chicago: Year-Book Medical Publisher; 1989:417–25.
8. Hassan HA. Mesenteric venous thrombosis. South Med J.1999;92(6):558–562.
9. Kumar S, Sarr MG, Kamath PS. Mesenteric venous thrombosis. *N Eng J Med.* 2001;345:1683–1688.

10. Bramwit DN, Hummel WC. The superior venous and inferior mesenteric veins as collateral channels in inferior vena cava obstruction. *Radiology.* 1968;92:90–91.
11. Sack J, Aldrete JS. Primary mesenteric venous thrombosis. *Surg Gynecol Obstet.* 1982;154:205–208.
12. Clavien PA, Harder F. Mesenteric venous thrombis. *Helv Chir Acta.* 1988;55:29–34.
13. Harward TRS, Green D, Bergan JJ et al. Mesenteric venous thrombosis. *J Vasc Surg.* 1989;9:328–333.
14. Levy PJ, Krausz MM, Manny J. The role of second-look procedure in improving survival time for patients with mesenteric venous thrombosis. *Surg Gynecol Obstet.* 1990;170:287–291.
15. Grieshop RJ, Dalsing MC, Ckirit DF, et al. Acute mesenteric venous thrombosis: Revisited in a time of diagnostic clarity. *Am J Surg.* 1991;57:573–578.

46

Evaluation and Management of Recurrent Varicose Veins

B. Mahendran, FRCS (Edin), M. Grouden, MSc,
M.P. Colgan, MD, P. Madhavan, FRCS (Edin),
D.J. Moore, MD, FRCSI, and G. Shanik, MD, FACS

> *"More is missed by not looking than by not knowing"*
> Thomas Mc Grae (1870–1935)

Varicose vein surgery is one of the commonest procedures performed under general surgical and specialist vascular surgical services. Despite advances in diagnosis and surgical technique, significant recurrence rates of 20–40%[1-6] are reported. The variation in the reported incidences of recurrence may vary due to differences in definition of recurrence or due to completeness of patient follow-up, e.g., patients who are pleased with their result may not attend for follow-up and patients with recurrence may go elsewhere for a second opinion.

The causes of recurrence are numerous and include incorrect pre-operative diagnosis, inadequate surgery and inappropriate supervision of junior staff. Continuation of the disease process leading to true recurrence is unpreventable. One paper reports performance by junior surgeons as being responsible for "persistent incompetence rate of 41%."[2] Surgery for varicose veins is the most litigious of surgeries performed by general and vascular surgeons and recurrent veins account for a large percentage of claims. Reasons include unrealistic expectations by patients and inadequate explanation by the surgeon of realistic results and associated complications. Adequate pre-operative evaluation and appropriate surgery by trained personnel is an ideal that can be achieved. This chapter discusses the evaluation and management of recurrent varicose veins.

EVALUATION

Recurrent Varices After Surgery (REVAS) is a consensus document,[3] which defines recurrent veins as "the presence of varicose veins in a lower limb previously operated

"""

on for varices (with or without adjuvant therapies)." REVAS recommends 3 levels of diagnosis to clearly define and characterize the recurrent veins. **Level I** is a thorough history, clinical examination and continuous-wave Doppler examination; **Level II** involves non-invasive investigations such as Duplex imaging and **Level III** invasive investigations such as phlebography and ambulatory venous pressure measurements. It also recommended expansion of the CEAP classification to define sites, nature and sources of recurrence, in addition to magnitude of reflux and other possible contributory factors. Clinical diagnosis remains essential but the use of imaging techniques is paramount.

Colour-coded Doppler imaging is a safe and accurate method of assessing both the superficial and deep venous systems. It provides both anatomical and hemodynamic information with precise identification and localization of sites of reflux. In our practice Doppler imaging is mandatory for patients with recurrent varicose veins.

Accurate evaluation of patterns of recurrence is important, as the surgical intervention is different for each pattern. Vessels are assessed for patency and the patient is asked to perform a Vasalva maneuver to check for the presence of reflux. There are several different ways of performing these maneuvers and the reliability of the results is operator-dependent. Our patients undergo assessment of their deep veins, with emphasis on patency, compressibility, and incompetence. We then image the SFJ to determine if it has been adequately ligated, followed by the thigh saphenous vein, to determine patency and incompetence and the presence of residual main branches. Particular attention is paid to the presence of an incompetent mid-thigh perforator. Careful assessment of the popliteal fossa is important when examining patients with primary or recurrent varicose veins since it is notorious for its anatomical variation. Where possible patients are scanned standing with their knee slightly flexed. In addition to the anatomical variations that are encountered in the popliteal fossa, the termination level of the short saphenous vein can vary considerably from patient to patient.

Two studies of the non-invasive findings in recurrent varicose veins were carried out in our unit, one in 1993–94 and the second in 2001–02 as part of an ongoing varicose vein waiting list initiative. Five types of recurrences related to the sapheno-femoral junction and LSV were noted where there had been previous reported ligation of the SFJ.[1]

- The sapheno-femoral junction was widely patent and incompetent
- There was evidence of neovascularization at the groin and this fed into a patent incompetent thigh saphenous or a residual branch
- A residual "stump" was imaged at the previously ligated SFJ
- The thigh saphenous vein was patent and connected by small branches in the groin to the common femoral vein
- The sapheno-femoral junction was adequately ligated, however, the thigh saphenous or a branch was patent and fed by an incompetent mid-thigh perforator

The distribution of findings in each study is illustrated in Table 46–1. The most frequent finding was that of an intact, incompetent sapheno-femoral junction or long saphenous vein, highlighting the importance of good surgical technique. These findings are very similar to those of others.[4,5,6] Darke[4] studied the morphology of recurrent varices using Doppler and venography and found SFJ incompetence in 48%, while the long saphenous vein was involved in 80% of cases. Two limbs had recurrence from

Table 46-1. Sites of recurrences in cases of previously ligated sapheno-femoral junctions

Site	1993/1994		2001/2002	
	No.	%	No	%
SFJ	40	56	45	48
LSV	20	28	28	30
SPJ only	8	11	12	13
Concomitant SPJ	22	31	14	15
Total studied	72		94	

pelvic incompetence. Bradbury[5] and co-workers examined 148 limbs with recurrent veins and found an intact SFJ in 72% of the 71 limbs that underwent repeat groin dissection and a patent LSV in 43% of the 120 limbs, which had undergone previous SFJ ligation.

Plethysmography

Plethysmography provides a quantitative measure of venous function. Photoplethysmography measures venous refilling time and may be useful in separating superficial and deep venous incompetence, however correlation with other non-invasive tests is poor. Air plethysmography provides hemodynamic information from the whole leg. It will separate the contribution made by reflux, obstruction, and the calf muscle pump. Its main use is in assessing chronic venous insufficiency.

Phlebography

Where Duplex alone is inconclusive, varicography is performed, by injecting contrast directly into the varicose veins to provide additional information. This is very useful in difficult cases such as, where the termination of, below knee varicosities is in question, due to unrecognised anatomical variations. It is also a standard investigation where peri-vulval veins are found suggesting an intra-abdominal origin of incompetence.

Ascending and descending venography is performed in centers with a vested interest in recurrent varicose veins surgery, to define recurrence and delineate valvular incompetence in both superficial and deep veins. This provides a map of the lower limb and pelvic venous system to plan appropriate and staged procedures for each level.

Lymphoscintography is very useful in defining possible delayed lymphatic drainage as further surgery may tip the balance and result in permanent postoperative swelling.

MANAGEMENT

Management may be conservative or operative. Support stockings are beneficial in alleviating the symptoms of venous hypertension. Where recurrences are minor with no junction incompetence sclerotherapy may provide excellent results. In many cases the patient is unwilling to accept the cosmetic appearance and is anxious for surgical re-intervention.

Sapheno Femoral Junction / Neovascularisation

If there is evidence of an intact sapheno-femoral junction, incompetent branches or in some instances of neovascularisation, it is necessary to re-explore the groin. If however an incompetent thigh perforator alone is found to be filling a patent incompetent thigh long saphenous vein, and the SFJ is adequately ligated then exploration of the groin is not necessary.

When re-exploring the groin, the incision is placed above the original scar and dissection is carried down to the femoral vein. Further dissection proceeds along the medial and lateral border of the femoral vein to identify all the tributaries and avoid potential complications by entering the previous operative field without control. The dissection is carried downwards until the long saphenous vein or a patent branch is identified. The SFJ or stump is carefully dissected, the branches or LSV are ligated and the junction flush ligated with non-absorbable sutures. The LSV if present is then stripped retrogradely. These procedures are not without complications, which include. major nerve and vessel injury, occasionally uncontrolled bleeding and infrequently deep vein thrombosis and secondary lymphoedema.

Neovascularisation or formation of thin walled immature veins (cavernoma), in the scar tissue of groin dissection has been enthusiastically described.[7] This led to the proposal of forming a partition covering the saphenofemoral junction. Cribriform fascia has been used historically. Use of pectineus fascial flap, has been described by Sheppard[8] and Gibbs.[9] Glass[10] initially proposed using artificial material as a barrier. Various materials including Dacron, PTFE and Silicone rubber have been used to form a partition. However, these barrier methods have not been proven to be effective in containing groin recurrence.[11]

Long Saphenous Vein

If the groin is adequately ligated but the LSV not removed then the patent long saphenous with or without its perforator is identified and marked on the skin pre-operatively. Through a small transverse incision in the thigh the site of the perforator is explored and it is ligated subfascially. The lower end of the long saphenous vein is dissected out and a stripper passed through in a retrograde fashion as far as the upper end. The long saphenous vein is then stripped retrogradely. This procedure can be repeated for other prominent branches or for a duplicated long saphenous vein system.

Perforators and Below-Knee Varices

Perforator surgery is performed only when there is a significant perforator present as demonstrated by duplex and in the presence of significant skin changes and/or ulceration. Linton's procedure involves placing a liberal vertical incision along perforators and the varicosity fed by the perforators. The dissection continues down to the deep fascia, which is then incised to demonstrate the perforators and their junctions. The ligation is carried out in the sub-fascial plane and the varicosity along with part of the perforator is excised. Modification to Linton's incision, like DePalma's or Cockett's has reduced wound complications such as flap necrosis and wound infection. However with the advent of Sub-fascial Endoscopic Perforator Surgery (SEPS)[12] this procedure is only done selectively.

SEPS was introduced by Fischer[13] and Hauer[14] and is a minimally invasive procedure where perforators are ligated with significantly reduced morbidity. A small 2 cm incision is made in the fascia under vision and video-controlled scope with fibre optic lighting is inserted subfascially, to demonstrate the perforators, which are then interrupted by endoscopic technique with small ports placed remotely. Advantages are clearly, reduced morbidity over the open procedure. Complications include wound infection and nerve injuries and occasionally deep vein thrombosis. Duplex guided sclerotherapy has been used with some success.[15]

Graduated compression stockings are adequate in the presence of below knee varices where patient compliance is good. Local avulsions as day case surgery or sclerotherapy can be performed as an outpatient procedure where varices are small.

Deep Vein Incompetence

In chronic venous disease deep venous pressure is high either due to post-thrombotic syndrome or primary deep venous reflux, leading to the formation of varicose veins and/or ulceration. In some cases valvuloplasty may be considered. This involves the surgical plication of the commissural attachment of the incompetent valves, with resultant valvular competence. Kistner pioneered venous valve reconstructive surgery in the presence of deep venous insufficiency.[16,17] The original technique has been evolved by, Raju[18] and Sottiurai[19] but controversy still surrounds both its indications and also its durability.

Venous valve reconstruction is usually performed in the presence of intractable leg ulcers and in recurrent varicose veins where deep venous insufficiency is the major aetiological factor. Raju et al. report similar results for these various procedures.[18]
- Internal valvuplasty—venotomy and valve commissural repair
- Prosthetic sleeve—external wall support of the valve bearing segment
- External valvuplasty—adventitial dissection and valve commissural repair
- Axillary vein transfer—interposition of a competent axillary vein segment
- Angioscopic repair—angioscopy assisted trans-commissural repair

Pelvic Venous Incompetence

The role of pelvic venous channels has been described, which can cause persistent recurrence if not recognised. Surgical procedures either open or laparoscopic, are effective. However, coil embolisation of these veins should be treatment of choice.

NEW TRENDS IN VENOUS SURGERY

Innovation in the technique of varicose vein surgery is mostly industry driven. There is no single novel approach that can tackle all aspects of the disease process. Each new invention or "gadget" targets a particular issue, which may not be adequately addressed by conventional surgical techniques. Three new technological advances are worth mentioning here, though studies are currently underway to evaluate their efficacy

Laser Ablation / Radio Frequency Ablation

Endo-luminal thermal ablation of the long saphenous vein is the end point of these techniques where the probe, employing either laser or high frequency radio waves, is placed in the long saphenous vein retrogradely and withdrawn while producing intense local heat. Advantages include a reduced operative morbidity and its performance under local anaesthetic. Its main drawback is the fact that the SFJ and branches are left intact.

Foam Sclerotherapy

"A cure for varicose veins with a single injection" is the novel concept of injecting sclerosing foam into the long saphenous vein, pioneered by Tessari.[20] This is achieved by mixing air and sodium tetradecylsulfate in syringes to form foam with microbubbles. This is then injected under local anaesthetic, into the long saphenous vein from the lower end under duplex guidance at the groin. The spillage of sclerosant into the femoral vein is avoided by continuous monitoring. Small spillages are reported not to be harmful. The foam was found also to enter and fill incompetent branches and incompetent perforator veins, thus providing a complete obliteration of the incompetent superficial venous system.

Advantages include the absence of haematoma formation due to LSV stripping with its concomitant morbidity, and avoiding nerve injuries. This procedure carries inherent risk of venous thrombosis, pulmonary emboli, skin necrosis, occular scotomas, and varicophlebitis. Recanalisations of the veins may occur leading to recurrence, however the procedure can be repeated if necessary.

TriVex System (Smith & Nephew Inc., MA, USA)

While the other 2 methods deal with the incompetent long saphenous vein, the TriVex system targets one of the widely loathed procedures among surgeons and patients alike, the stab avulsions of below knee varicosities. The patients are usually warned to their dismay during conventional procedures, that they would swap their varicosities for scars. Multiple incisions and avulsions lead to pain, haematoma formation and scarring. An associated complication is the incidence of nerve injury even in the hands of adept surgeons. Missed varicosities result in unsatisfactory residual veins and cause recurrence.

The Trivex system is based on the promise of reducing these complications, leading to fewer incisions and complete excision of varicosities thereby reducing the associated morbidity and recurrence. Trans-illuminated Powered Phlebectomy (TIPP),[21] is performed by a device containing, a rotating tubular blade in a protective sheath, facing a lateral window. The procedure involves insertion of the transillumiator, which has a fibreoptic light channel set at a 45 degrees angle and another channel through which saline and local anaesthetic mixture can be infused under pressure to produce tumescence in the subcutaneous space. The instrument transilluminates the skin to show silhouette of the veins. The powered tissue dissector is then inserted through another incision and triangulated to excise of varicosities within the arc of both these instruments. The dissector cuts and digests the varicosities under vision, with immediate aspiration by suction. A randomized controlled trial is currently underway in our institute comparing conventional surgery with TriVex.

Early results are encouraging. Tumescent anaesthesia is very effective in reducing the incidence of haematoma formation and post-operative pain and total surgery time is reduced.

CONCLUSION

Varicose veins are the price paid by humans to walk erect. Recurrent varicose veins are a cross, borne by any surgeon performing varicose vein surgery. Much research has been done on venous hemodynamics and operative technique, however the rate of recurrence has not significantly altered over the decades. Thorough history, physical examination, and appropriate investigations are essential if results of repeat surgery are to be optimized. Complications, though relatively infrequent, do occur and new techniques may help reduce these in the future. Realistic expectations must be emphasized as recurrence though multi-factorial is inherent and not correctable and freedom from ongoing varices is unfortunately only obtainable by ongoing maintenance.

REFERENCES

1. Grouden MC, Colgan MP, Moore DJ, Shanik GD. The Value of Duplex Scanning in Patients with Recurrent Varicose Veins. *J Vasc Tech.* 1996;20:137–139
2. Lees T, Singh S, Beard J, et al. Prospective audit of surgery for varicose veins. *Br J Surg.* 1997;84:44–46.
3. Perrin MR, Guex J, Ruckley CV, et al. Recurrent varices after surgery (REVAS), a concensus document. *Cardiovasc Surg.* 2000;8:233–245.
4. Darke SG. The Morphology of Recurrent Varicose Veins. *Eur J Vasc Surg.* 1992;6:512–517.
5. Bradbury AW, Stonebridge PA, Ruckley CV, et al. Recurrent varicose veins: correlation between preoperative clinical and hand-held Doppler ultrasonographic examination, and anatomical findings at surgery. *Br J Surg.* 1993;80:849–851.
6. Labropoulos N, Toulouakis E, Giannoukas AD, et al. Recurrent varicose veins: Investigation of the pattern and extent of reflux with colour flow duplex scanning. *Surgery.* 1996;119: 406–409.
7. Nyamekye I, Shephard NA, Davies B, Heather BP, Earnshaw JJ, et al. Clinicopathological evidence that neovascularisation is a cause of recurrent varicose veins. *Eur J Vas Endovasc Surg.* 1998;15:412–415.
8. Sheppard M. A procedure for the prevention of recurrent saphenofemoral incompetence. *Aust N Z J Surg.* 1978;48:322–326.
9. Gibbs PJ, Foy DMA, Darke SG. Reoperation for recurrent saphenofemoral incompetence: a prospective randomised trial using a reflected flap of pectineus fascia. *Eur J Vasc Endovasc Surg.* 1999;18:494–498.
10. Glass GM. Prevention of saphenofemoral and saphenopopliteal recurrence of varicose veins by forming a partition to contain neovascularisation. *Phlebology.* 1998;18:494–498.
11. Bhatti TS, Whitman B, Harradine BK, et al. Causes of re-recurrence after polytetrafluoroethylene patch saphenoplasty for recurrent varicose veins. *Br J Surg.* 2000;87:1356–1360.
12. Kalra M, Gloviczki P. Subfascial endoscopic perforator vein surgery: who benefits? *Semin Vasc Surg.* 2002;15:39–49.
13. Fisher R. Prognosis in endoscopic perforans vein excision in postphlebitic syndrome. *Wien Med Wochenschr.* 1994;144:258–260.
14. Hauer G, et al. Endoscopic subfascial dissection of a perforating vein. *Surg Endosc.* 1998;2:5–12.
15. Guex JJ. Ultrasound guided sclerotherapy for perforating veins. *Hawaii Med J.* 2000;59:261–262.
16. Kistner R. Surgical repair of a venous valve. *Straub Clin Proc.* 1968;24:41
17. Kistner RL. Surgical repair of the incompetent femoral vein valve. *Arch Surg.* 1975;110:1336.
18. Raju S, Fredricks RK, Neglen PN, et al. Durability of venous valve reconstruction techniques for primary and postthrombotic reflux. *J Vasc Surg.* 1996;23:357–367.
19. Sottiurai VS. Surgical correction of recurrent venous ulcer. *J Cardiovasc Surg.* 1991;32:104–109.
20. Tessari L, Cavezzi A, Frullini A. Preliminary experience with a new sclerosing foam in the treatment of varicose veins. *Dermatol Surg.* 2001;27:58–60
21. Arumugasamy M, McGreal G, O'Connor A, et al. Technique of transilluminated powered phlebectomy-a novel, minimally invasive system for varicose vein surgery. *Eur J Vasc Endovasc Surg.* 2002;23:180–182.

47

Techniques of Bedside Vena Caval Filter Placement

Albert D. Sam II, MD, Thomas C. Naslund, MD, and Jon S. Matsumura, MD

Vena cava filters (VCFs) have been used for nearly 30 years for the prevention and treatment of venous thromboembolism. With a pulmonary embolism (PE)–free event rate of 96%,[1] VCF placement has been shown to be an effective means of reducing PE in high-risk individuals whom anticoagulation therapy is contraindicated. Formerly placed in the operating room through surgical cutdowns, most filters are now placed in the operating room or angiography suite percutaneously with fluoroscopic guidance. As technology has advanced, a growing number of institutions now insert VCFs at the patient's bedside, providing convenience and potentially increased safety and reduced cost.[2–4]

Techniques used at the bedside to guide VCF placement include portable fluoroscopy, intravascular ultrasound (IVUS) and surface duplex scanning. All allow for detailed evaluation of the inferior vena cava (IVC) with the latter 2 avoiding the use of a radiocontrast agent. Carbon dioxide has been used at the bedside with fluoroscopy to avoid nephrotoxicity in those at risk.[4] More importantly, bedside VCF placement avoids the need to transport critically ill patients to the angiography or operating suite. In this chapter we describe advantages and disadvantages of methods of bedside placement and review our experience with IVUS-directed placement.

RATIONALE FOR BEDSIDE FILTER PLACEMENT

Bedside VCF placement has several potential safety factors similar to advantages that have led to widespread practices of bedside tracheostomy, gastrostomy, and right heart catheterization. In the critically ill intensive care unit (ICU) patient cohort, most have multiple invasive monitors and indwelling catheters that need frequent observation, which is more difficult during transport (Figure 47–1). Some also may have endotracheal intubation, spinal or intracranial drains, feeding tubes or other lines that may become dislodged during transportation. Transport-associated neurologic injury may occur in those with intracranial hypertension or unstable spinal segments, and patients with non-fixated pelvic or long bone fractures may experience bleeding. Transfer out of the ICU hinders treatment of hypothermia, aggressive resuscitation, alternative modes of ventilation and delicate management of hemodynamic drips.

Factors leading to an apprehension in accepting bedside techniques of VCF placement include perceived increased infectious risk, inability to adequately image or access the vena cava, and fear of filter misplacement. To date none of these risks has been shown to be a significant problem in a large published series. One real limitation practitioners may face is availability of portable equipment and/or technical staff.

FLUOROSCOPIC-GUIDED PLACEMENT

One solution to transporting a patient to an angiography suite or to an operating room is to perform bedside procedures using portable fluoroscopy. The technique requires a portable C-arm and is more convenient if ICU beds are specifically designed with a fluoroscopic window.[2] Lead aprons and radiology technicians are necessary with this technique. Unfortunately, many hospitals are not equipped or staffed for this type of support. Limited image quality due to metal frames in intensive care beds, radiation scatter, transfer to a fluoroscopy table, potential radiocontrast nephrotoxicity, and insufficient bedside space are additional difficulties with this method. At some centers, however, this is a viable alternative. A prospective trial at one such center reported their experience in 25 consecutive trauma patients. No intra- or postoperative complications were reported. Compared to placement within the operating room or radiology suite, cost analysis revealed savings of $1844 and $2245 respectively.[2]

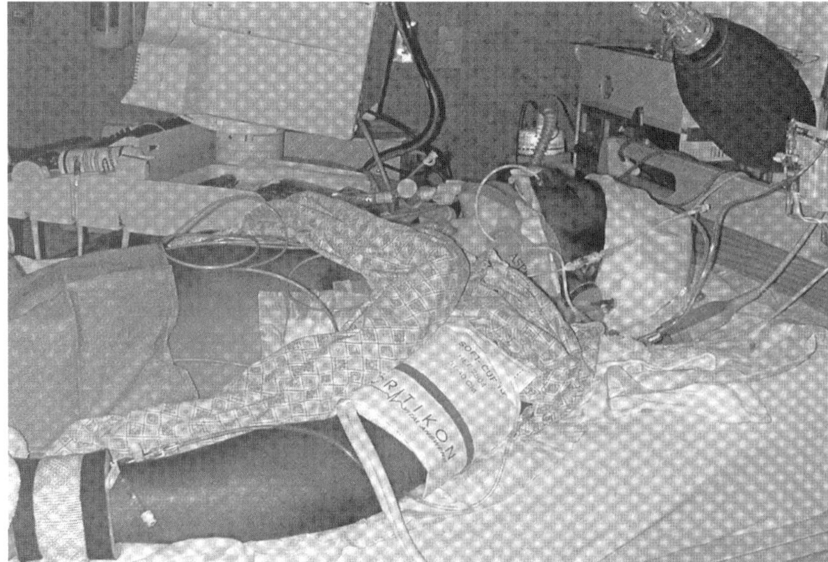

Figure 47–1. A multitrauma patient in the intensive care unit whose transport to the operating room or interventional suite would be potentially hazardous.

Carbon dioxide (CO_2) may also be used as a contrast agent for bedside fluoroscopic-guided VCF placement as it has been demonstrated to be a safe contrast medium and has no associated nephrotoxicity. Sing et al. has reported excellent efficacy and safety results using carbon dioxide in a prospective trial involving critically ill trauma patients.[5] In their series of bedside VCF placement, a subset of patients (those with renal insufficiency or diabetics receiving contrast load in the preceding 24 hours) receiving CO_2 as a contrast agent proved successful in 26 of 27 patients. The sole failure was in an obese patient where cavography was obscured by excessive bowel gas.

When these techniques can be used at the patient's bedside, practitioners retain the benefits of familiarity with fluoroscopic visualization.

Jugular access is also an option with this technique as the transition through the mediastinum can be readily visualized. The primary drawbacks are the requirements for fluoroscopy-ready beds, portable C-arm machines, and technicians at a practitioner's particular institution.

DUPLEX-GUIDED PLACEMENT

Technique

The patient is properly placed in the comfortable supine position used for an ultrasound examination of the abdomen. It is helpful if the patient has had meals or tube feedings discontinued for 6 to 8 hours to minimize bowel distension that limit caval visualization. Venous access can be obtained using either a femoral or a jugular approach. The patient is prepped and draped in sterile fashion and the operator positions him/herself properly for gaining venous access. A vascular ultrasound technologist images the vena cava and identified, its diameter is noted and the renal veins are located. The right renal artery can be a key structure to identify as it passes posterior to the IVC near the level of the right renal vein. A long guidewire can be visualized as it is passed into the infra-renal vena cava. The filter and delivery system are then carefully passed over the guidewire. It is helpful to simultaneously image the right renal vein-infra-renal cava junction as the apparatus is positioned (Figure 47–2).

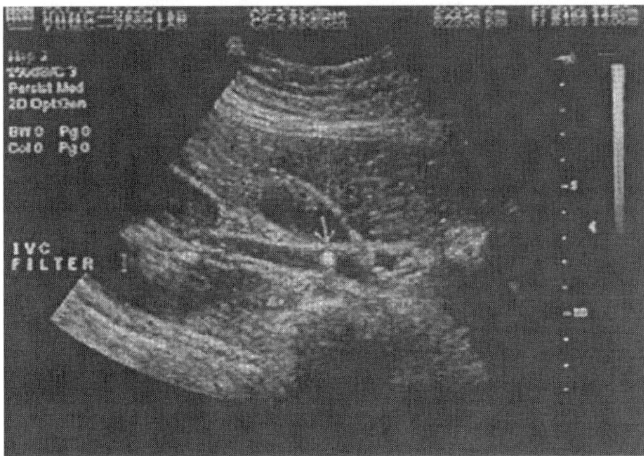

Figure 47–2. Greenfield filter tip (arrow) at right renal vein-inferior vena cava junction. With permission: *J Vasc Surg.* 2002;35:286–291.

Once the delivery system is positioned properly, the filter can be deployed under direct visualization (Figure 47–3). The delivery system is removed in the usual fashion and a portable plain x-ray of the abdomen may be obtained to confirm proper filter placement. Some centers forego the x-ray, having become confident in the reliability of the duplex technique.

Discussion

The use of transcutaneous duplex ultrasonography to visualize the IVC during placement of caval filters is the most popular method to be adopted by many centers.[6–8] Duplex ultrasonography is readily available in most hospitals and vascular surgeons often have a familiar working relationship with duplex technicians. Filter placement can be performed in the vascular laboratory or, if preferred, the apparatus can easily be transported to remote areas of the hospital. In addition, radiocontrast nephrotoxicity and ionizing radiation are not a concern when ultrasound is used. Newer generation ultrasound machines easily image the iliac veins and the IVC can usually be adequately visualized for delivery and placement of a caval filter. Furthermore, the duplex scanner is more convenient for surgeon and staff compared to bulky portable C-arms. Vanderbilt University's vascular surgery service recently reported their preferred bedside method using duplex-guided IVC filter placement.[9] Of the 325 consecutive patients assessed, 12% were found to be unsuitable for duplex-guided placement due primarily to visualization difficulties. Of the 284 patients undergoing filter placement, only 4% experienced complications related to either filter misplacement (n=6), clinically significant access site thrombosis (n=1), filter migration (n=1), bleeding (n=1), or IVC occlusion (n=3). In this series, follow-up data revealed only 1 patient who developed a pulmonary embolic event that occurred in a patient with a misplaced filter. Calculated average cost savings was estimated to be $2,388 per procedure ($4,558 vs. $2,170—angiography suite vs. bedside respectively). These impressive results with duplex ultrasound establish this modality as useful for the placement of VCFs.

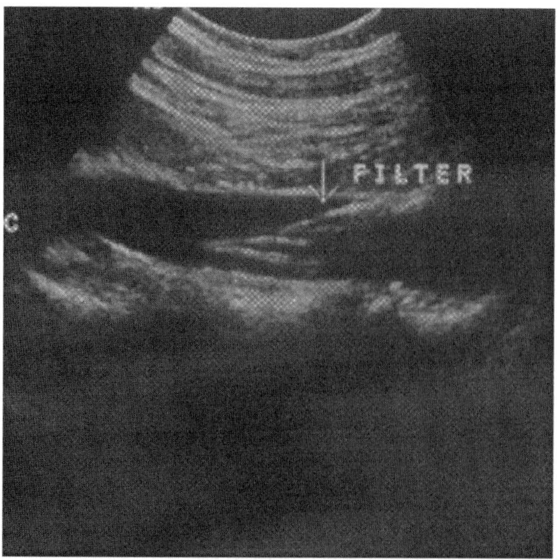

Figure 47–3. Filter deployed in inferior vena cava. With permission: *J Vasc Surg.* 2002;35:286–291.

IVUS-GUIDED PLACEMENT

Technique

After draping, IVUS catheter premeasurement is performed to the precise length of the over-the-wire percutaneous femoral Greenfield filter deployment system (Figure 47–4).[10,11] Premeasurement permits placement of external markers during IVUS pull-back assessment, which will directly correlate with the subsequent deployment device length and position. A single groin puncture method is used in all patients. After femoral vein cannulation, a J-tipped guidewire is passed into the central venous circulation and then exchanged for a floppy-tipped super stiff wire (through a 5F-angled guidecatheter). The monorail IVUS catheter is then passed over the super stiff wire to the level of the right atrium. Venous anatomy is examined by pullback technique, and the landing zone (Figure 47–5) between the renal veins and iliac vein confluence is marked on the immobilized drape, a long mark for the renal veins and a short mark for the iliac confluence.

This is confirmed with a second pullback run with particular attention to guidewire position appearing directly adjacent to the IVUS catheter. This maneuver verifies a pathway length similar to the deployment sheath. The 8F sheath is removed, the tract serially dilated, and the deployment sheath inserted. The VCF is then deployed in the cephalad end of the landing zone after removal of the guidewire. The guidewire is removed immediately before deployment to avoid entrapment of the wire. Gentle pressure is applied for less than a minute until the foot of the bed is raised to obtain hemostasis. By minimizing external compression, we believe this may reduce the frequency of insertion site thrombosis. We have not performed jugular access by IVUS imaging alone.

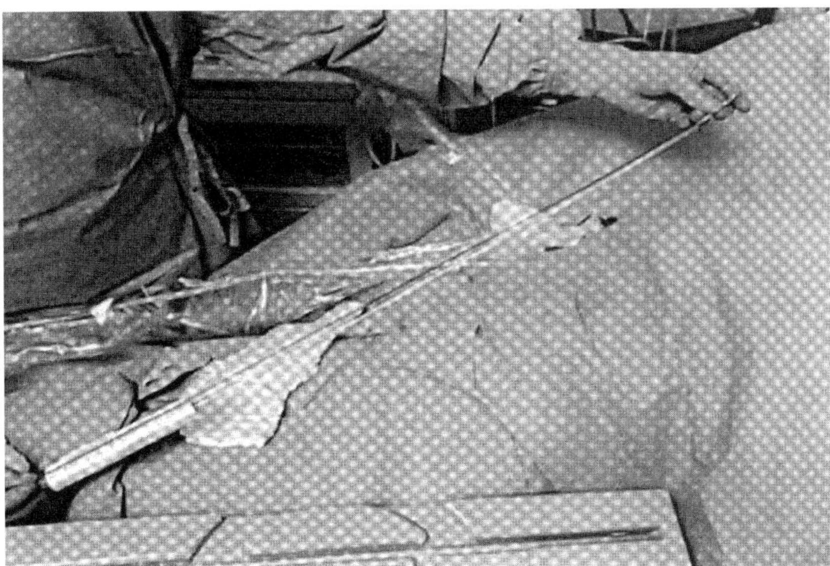

Figure 47–4. Premeasurement. IVUS catheter is placed alongside VCF deployment device, and a Steri-Strip is placed on IVUS catheter the precise length of the device away from tip of IVUS probe. With permission: *J Vasc Surg.* 2001;34:21–26.

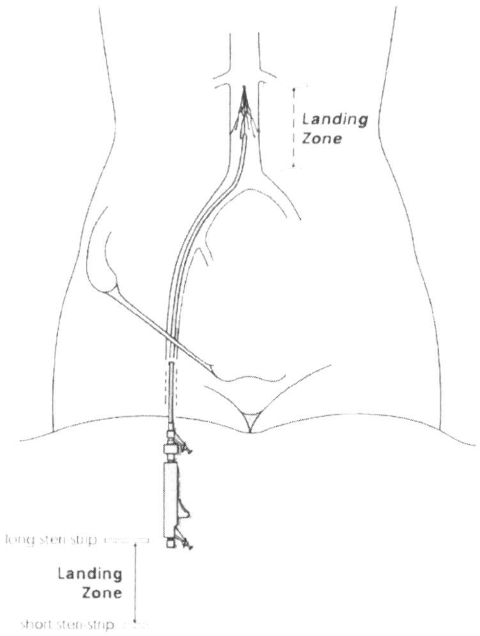

Figure 47–5. Schematic depiction of "landing zone" between long and short Steri-Strip, corresponding to length of IVC between renal vein confluence (craniad) and iliac bifurcation (caudad), respectively. Steri-Strips are used as markers on the immobilized drapes within which VCF will be placed. To ensure accurate placement, take care to aim past the renal vein marker. With permission: *J Vasc Surg.* 2001;34:21–26.

DISCUSSION—THE NORTHWESTERN EXPERIENCE

In the last 5 years we have placed 32 VCFs by an IVUS-directed technique. Compared to duplex ultrasound, IVUS requires only a single operator and caval visualization is not effected by obesity, overlying abdominal wounds, bowel distention and abdominal packing. In our original report 24 of 26 patients (92%) underwent successful placement of the VCF in the infrarenal IVC in accordance with Northwestern University's institutional review board guidelines.[3] With experience, the procedure takes 10 to 20 minutes after obtaining venous access—totaling 40 to 50 minutes including draping, prepping, and documentation. Immediate confirmation of VCF placement with a portable abdominal radiograph showed only 1 patient to have had filter tilt greater than 13 degrees. There was no limb asymmetry.

In one instance a filter was erroneously deployed into the iliac vein. One patient experienced an acute insertion site DVT within the first week that completely resolved by 29 days after VCF placement. Another patient presented with bilateral lower extremity edema and cyanosis 56 days after the procedure. A duplex scan showed an acute IVC occlusion, which appeared to be caused by trapped thrombus. This patient was treated with warfarin sodium (Coumadin) for 6 months, with the filter recanalizing 5 months after initial diagnosis. No other major adverse events related to VCF insertion occurred within 30 days. No clinical pulmonary emboli have occurred. One death due to respiratory failure occurred on postprocedure day 9 in a patient with a history of a right pneumonectomy who underwent a left thoracotomy for spinal fusion.

The primary disadvantage of IVUS is the lack of widespread experience with IVUS technology and thus the lack of familiarity with image interpretation required for filter placement. The technique requires extensive experience with guidewire manipulation and also the deployment system. Another disadvantage of IVUS compared to duplex ultrasound relates to its increased cost due to the catheter (roughly $600/catheter). Compared to conventional placement in the OR /angiography suite, IVUS still provides an average savings of $880 per procedure in our series.[3]

SUMMARY

Bedside VCF placement is feasible and safe regardless of the method chosen to visualize the IVC. Fluoroscopy, duplex ultrasound and IVUS-directed methods have all been shown to have certain advantages and disadvantages Portable fluoroscopy allows a traditional method of bedside IVCF placement but requires a large portable machine. Duplex is both simple and inexpensive but body habitus, external wounds, and bowel gas can limit visualization. Only IVUS placement used allows convenient portable equipment, requires no technician support, and permits visualization of the IVC with VCF placement regardless of surface or bowel gas issues.

CONCLUSION

Vena caval filter placement may be performed at the bedside in critically ill patients. Of the various means of placement, physicians should select that method most suitable to their particular hospital resources and their base of experience.

REFERENCES

1. Greenfield LJ, Proctor MC. Twenty-year clinical experience with the Greenfield filter. *Cardiovasc Surg.* 1995;3:199–205.
2. Tola JC, Holtzman R, Lottenberg L. Bedside placement of inferior vena cava filters in the intensive care unit. *Am Surg.* 1999;65:833–838.
3. Ebaugh JL, Chiou AC, Morasch MD, et al. Bedside vena cava filter placement guided with intravascular ultrasound. *J Vasc Surg.* 2001;34:21–26.
4. Sing RF, Cicci CK, LeQuire MH, Stackhouse DJ. Bedside carbon dioxide cavagrams for inferior vena cava filters: preliminary results. *J Vasc Surg.* 2000;32:147.
5. Sing RF, Jacobs DG, Heniford BT. Bedside insertion of IVC filters in the intensive care unit. *J Am Coll Surg.* 2001; 192:570–576.
6. Sato DT, Robinson KD, Gregory RT, et al. Duplex directed caval filter insertion in multitrauma and critically ill patients. *Ann Vasc Surg.* 1999;13:365–371.
7. Nunn CR, Neuzil D, Naslund TC, et al. Cost-effective method for bedside insertion of vena caval filters in trauma patients. *J Trauma.* 1997;43:752–758.
8. Cheanvechai V, Marshall BE, Flinn WR. Bedside insertion of the IVC filter. In Peter Gloviczski (ed). *Perspectives in Vascular Surgery and Endovascular Therapy.* New York: Thieme; 2002:21–35.
9. Michael S.Conners III, Stacey Becker, Raul J.Guzman, et al. Duplex scan-directed placement of inferior vena cava filters: A five-year institutional experience. *J Vasc Surg.* 2002;35:286–291.
10. Oppat WF, Chiou AC, Matsumura JS. Intravascular ultrasound-guided vena cava filter placement. *J Endovasc Surg.* 1996;6:285–287.

11. Oppat WF, Morasch MD, Matsumura JS. Vena caval filter placement in critically ill patients using intravascular ultrasound. In Yao JST, Pearce WH (eds). *Modern Vascular Surgery*. New York: McGraw-Hill; 2000.

48

Retrievable Vena Caval Filters for Venous Thromboembolism

Lazar J. Greenfield and Mary C. Proctor

The saying that everything old becomes new again is being demonstrated with vena caval filters. More than 30 years ago, it became possible to place devices in the inferior vena cava (IVC) that would prevent thrombus from embolizing from the lower extremities to the lungs. Among the earliest devices, all but the Greenfield Stainless-steel Filter (GSF) were associated with a high rate of adverse events and were withdrawn from the market. While the majority of these devices were intended to be permanent, a few like the Eichelter Sieve were tethered and intended to be removed once the risk of pulmonary embolism (PE) had abated (Figure 48–1). Over the next 20 years, vena caval filters were considered to be permanent implants. Outcomes for patients with a Greenfield filter demonstrated a consistent, low rate of caval occlusion from 2% to 5%, while preventing recurrent PE in 96% to 99% of patients.[1,2]

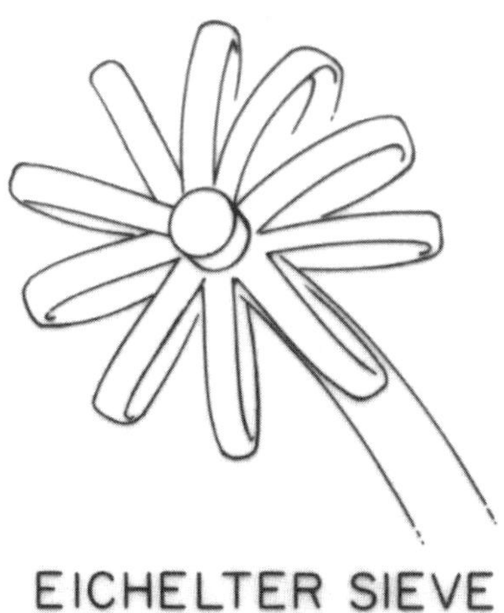

Figure 48–1. The Eichelter sieve was one of the first tethered vena caval filters designed for temporary use.

Two factors were largely responsible for the expansion of indications for filter placement. First, the excellent outcomes experienced by patients who received the filter and secondly, the development of smaller insertion systems that simplified placement. The latter was made possible with the use of the Seldinger technique enabling percutaneous placement of dilators and sheaths. These factors led to a significant increase in the variety and number of filters placed for expanded, softer indications.

As the market expanded 3 additional devices received FDA approval. The Vena Tech and Simon Nitinol filters retained the conical design while the Bird's Nest filter provided a screen of wires to capture emboli (Figure 48–2). Hemodynamic testing of various filter designs has shown an association between the number of trapping levels and the rate of IVC occlusion.[3] The complications and poor outcomes reported with some devices were apparently related to their design and outweighed the potential benefits. As a result, some physicians began to recalculate the risk/benefit calculus of filter placement. This led to reconsideration of a potentially retrievable device. This was especially attractive when the indication for filter placement was purely prophylactic, when the perceived the period at risk was thought to be very short or for very young patients.

To support this logic, several assumptions must be made. First, that it is possible to identify the duration of risk for thromboembolism. Second, that the risk from the long-term placement of the filter exceeds the risk of subsequent PE. Third, that the function of the retrievable filter is equivalent to that of a permanent device. Finally, that the risks associated with retrieval do not exceed the risk of permanent placement and that the additional cost is justified. As yet, the literature provides little in the way of evidence to support these assumptions or to establish a clear advantage for temporary devices.

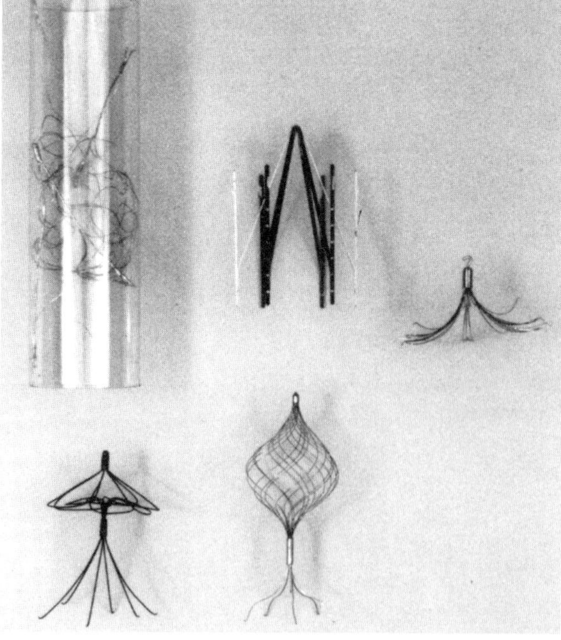

Figure 48–2. Collection of vena caval filters including the Bird's Nest (upper left), VenaTech (upper center), and Simon Nitinol (lower left) currently approved by the FDA. The Amplatz (upper right) and Gunther basket (lower right) were withdrawn from the U.S. market.

NEW RETRIEVABLE FILTERS

Retrievable devices fall into 2 groups; *temporary* filters that must be removed after several days or *optional* devices which may be left permanently or retrieved as determined by the physician. Temporary devices have their greatest appeal when used during a procedure that leaves the patient at high risk for thromboembolism such as during thrombolytic therapy or mechanical thrombectomy. Optional devices are frequently used with young trauma patients, during pregnancy or during treatment for malignancy.

Early devices such as the Amplatz filter and the Gunther basket are shown in Figure 48–2. These devices were tested with disappointing results in small clinical studies and withdrawn from further evaluation. Devices of current interest include the Gunther Tulip filter (Cook, Indianapolis, IN), and a new device designed by Nitinol Technologies and being developed by CR Bard called the Recovery filter. These devices represent the second generation of removable filters.

No published data are available for the new Nitinol filter from Bard. It has a 2 stage trapping system comprised of a lower cone and an upper level of wire struts that may also facilitate centering of the device within the IVC (Figure 48–3). It is superior to the current Simon Nitinol filter in that is does not have the central spoke that added considerable interference to blood flow and was a nidus for fibrin deposition. The filter is held in place by the radial force of the upper struts. Because the device is currently undergoing clinical evaluation prior to FDA submission, limited data are available regarding its performance making it difficult to evaluate. It is characterized as an optional filter allowing removal for a period of 4 weeks or longer. Based on its design, it should function well to trap both small and potentially lethal emboli. However, it does have a double trapping level that has been shown to increase turbulence and stagnation within the filter, slow thrombus resolution and contribute to caval or filter occlusion.[3] As with other filters with dual trapping surfaces, the clinical sequelae do not always become evident during the 30 day evaluation studies, often taking 6 to 12 months for caval occlusion to be diagnosed.

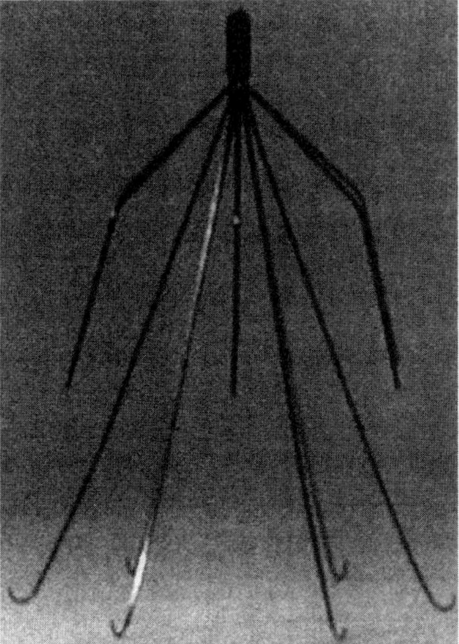

Figure 48–3. The new Nitinol Recovery filter has a 2-stage trapping system. No published data are available for this device.

The retrieval system has 9 wire limbs covered by a thin polymer covering. It is made in 2 sizes and inserted through the jugular vein via a 10 or 20F sheath. The device is advanced over the upper tier of the filter to separate it from the IVC and then advanced to cover the lower cone. With the filter encased, the entire system is removed.

The Gunther Tulip filter referred to as the MReye filter has been evaluated and approved for use in both Europe and Canada (Figure 48–4). Although the filter was approved for use in the US, the retrieval system has not been made available. The filter has 4 legs with short hooks that fix it to the IVC. The upper level is comprised of elongated wire loops extending along 3/4s of the strut length. It has twice the number of filter wires as the conical filters. While the manufacturer suggests that this is an advantage, hemodynamic modeling shows that this design may be associated with increased flow disturbance and the potential for a higher rate of caval occlusion. In vitro studies with this device showed a significantly greater clot-capture rate compared to competitive filters suggesting the potential for filter obstruction. The 6% incidence of caval occlusion in clinical studies appears to support this hypothesis.[4]

The filter is removed with a 13 French system designed specifically for this device. A hook at the top of the filter allows it to be snared by the hook from the retrieval system, a platinum loop collapses the struts, and a sheath is then extended over the filter. The short strut-hooks are freed from the vena caval wall and the device is retracted into the recovery system and withdrawn from the jugular access site. Animal studies demonstrate retrieval to be a simple and safe procedure.

Millward[5] reported a preliminary study of this device in 15 patients, all but 1 with DVT or PE. Nine patients underwent retrieval from the jugular approach after a mean time of placement of 8 days. The retrieval procedure required between 2 and 13 minutes of fluoroscopy time and there were no complications. One filter had a small thrombus proximal to the hook and the remainder were clear. Post-retrieval histologic examination revealed resolving thrombus adherent to the filter legs, which was up to

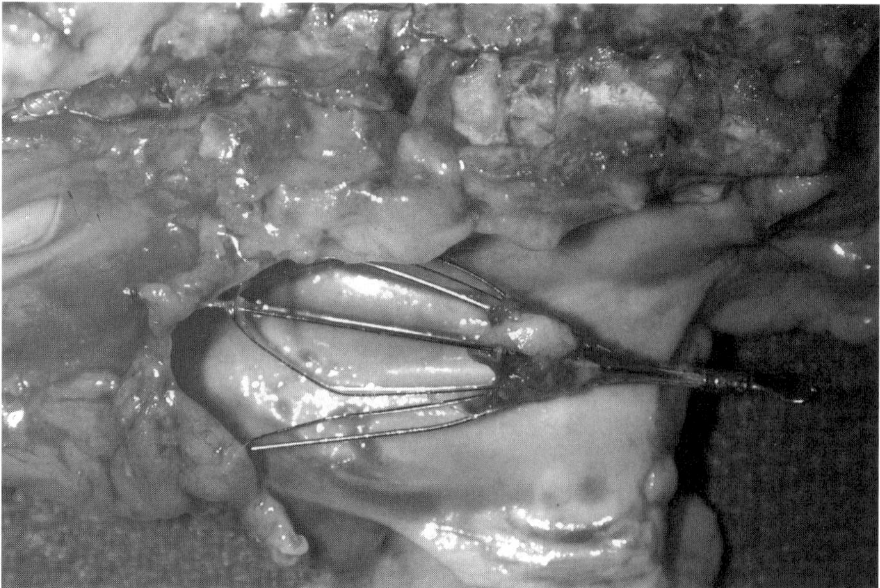

Figure 48–4. The Gunther Tulip filter is designed to be retrievable but the retrieval system has not been approved in the U.S. The filter shown is an autopsy specimen (Courtesy of Dr. Oja, University of Toronto).

30 mm in length and 2–3 mm in width. Eight months following removal, 1 patient developed recurrent DVT. Five patients with a continued contraindication to anticoagulation did not undergo retrieval and underwent follow up at a mean of 1 month. One had an IVC occlusion with thrombus to the level of the filter and the rest were patent.

Neuerburg et al.[4] conducted a larger study in 83 patients with a higher rate of prophylactic indications. Thirty-three patients had 30-day follow-up and the remainder were studied between 30 days and 3 years after placement. Event rates for migration and tilt were low. Caval perforation was documented in 3 patients, 1 of which was related to a 90 degree rotation of the filter within the IVC. Caval occlusion was documented in 8 of the 75 patients with follow up (11%), all occurring within 2 weeks of placement. One was associated with a massive fatal PE 2 days following insertion and there were 2 non-fatal PE. Only 5 of the filters were retrieved; 3 due to misplacement at insertion and 2 that were planned for removal at 6 and 11 days.

Millward reported on the 90 patient Canadian Registry of the Gunther Tulip. The demographics and indications for placement were typical of the filter population. Retrieval was successful in 51 patients after a mean implantation time of 9 days and outcomes were available for 37 patients. Eight percent of patients required placement of a permanent filter over the next 17 to 167 days. Additional follow up was available for 25 of the patients in whom the filter was left in place. The only adverse event was a 5% filter occlusion rate.

A more recent report by Ponchon[6] reviewed the prophylactic use of the Tulip filter in 10 patients without thromboembolism. Mean time to explant was 8 days. Two filters could not be retrieved due to caval thrombosis and a continued contraindication to anticoagulation while a third filter became acutely angled within the IVC preventing removal.

It appears that the Tulip filter can be retrieved safely without damage to the IVC. However, it demonstrates little benefit over standard devices with respect to adverse events including perforation, 10% caval occlusion and a 4% incidence of recurrent PE that developed within 2 weeks of placement. Additionally, 8% of patients required placement of a second, permanent filter.

The Tempo filter was a temporary device that underwent initial studies in the US (Figure 48–7). Bovyn[7] reported early results in 66 patients with a mean implant time of 30 days. There were no PE but IVC thrombosis developed in 15% and migration in 7.5%. Rossi[8] reported 3 migrations of this device to the right atrium which were fatal for 2 patients. A fourth patient had a 50 mm cephalad migration. A death during the clinical evaluation of the filter in the US led to early termination of the study with no subsequent evaluations.

Several European centers have reported experience with other types of retrievable filters. In most cases, the studies included several available devices but the outcomes were reported for the group as a whole. Linsenmaier[9] reported on a group of 50 temporary filters including the Gunther, Tulip and Antheor devices which were removed between 1 and 12 days following placement. Thrombus was present in 18% with 2 PE, 2 migrations, and 1 IVC thrombosis.

A series of 188 patients were followed by Lorch et al.[10] The majority were placed prior to thrombolytic therapy with a mean insertion time of 5 days. The devices included the Guenther, Antheor, and Prolyser filters. The incidence of adverse events was high including 4 fatal PE. There was a 16% rate of filter thrombosis and migration in 5%. Additional procedures were performed to clear the filters prior to removal including thrombolysis and aspiration. Overall, 5% of patients required placement of a permanent filter.

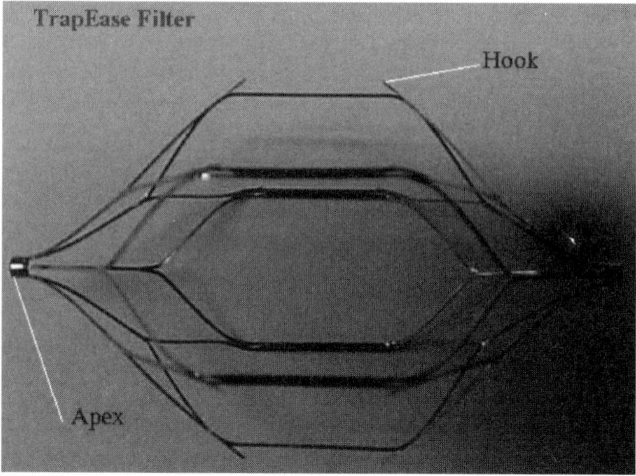

Figure 48–5. The recently approved TrapEase filter which is designed to trap emboli against the wall of the vena cava.

FILTER DESIGN AND TESTING

Few series report the bench and animal testing methods used during filter development. Exceptions include Lorch[11] who did comparative in vitro studies, Pavcnik[12] who performed in vitro and in vivo tests and Stecker,[13] Kuszyk,[14] and Hosaka[15] who reported in vivo evaluations. While none of these devices is available in the US, the studies identified areas for improvement that may lead to future approval.

Evaluation of the design and function of vena caval filters varies from one manufacturer to another. The current FDA approval requirements leave room for significant differences in the sophistication of the testing methodology. At the end of the day, regardless of whether a device is intended as a permanent, optional or temporary vena caval filter, it must trap significant emboli without becoming occluded, allow for clot resolution, and remain fixed within the IVC. In addition, optional and temporary devices must meet the additional burden of safe retrieval over an appropriate period of time. Since this is a new area, appropriate performance standards remain to be established.

DISCUSSION

Economic considerations have largely been ignored, but are important and remain to be evaluated. Retrievable devices are priced within the range of permanent filters and the costs associated with placement are similar. Measuring the IVC, identifying caval anomalies and determining the appropriate site for placement must be carried out. Patients with temporary filters attached by a tether may require 1 or more additional devices if they continue to require prolonged protection. These devices have a high risk of infection at the tether site and should the patient become septic, they have to be removed or replaced. This doubles or triples the cost. In other cases, the period at risk may exceed the limit for use and another device must be placed. Finally, an interventional procedure is required at the time of removal. Should a thrombus be found in the filter, it may be necessary to lyse the clot or subject the patient to a surgical procedure to remove it. Therefore, there is no economic advantage for using these retrievable devices.

The concept of a retrievable filter was developed in an effort to reduce adverse events associated with the permanent devices such as IVC thrombosis, metal fatigue, insertion site thrombosis, or migration. Careful review of the available literature suggests that these new devices have comparable or higher adverse event rates relative to the Greenfield filters (GF). Data from the Michigan Filter Registry demonstrate that problems with the GF develop soon after placement. The longer a filter is in place, the lower the incidence of recurrent thrombosis or caval occlusion. The rate of GF limb fracture is less than .01% and in our experience has not been associated with clinical sequelae.

The indications for use of a retrievable filter remain unclear. Various authors suggest use with thrombolytic infusion or during mechanical thrombectomy to prevent PE. This may be the most appropriate assuming that patients remain candidates for anticoagulation treatment of the DVT. Other indications include a temporary contraindication to anticoagulation, young trauma patients with limited risk of PE who never develop DVT, patients who develop DVT in the late stages of pregnancy, as prophylaxis for patients with malignancy undergoing chemotherapy or radiation therapy or in any situation in which the period of risk is short. There has not been sufficient time to evaluate each of these indications and the lack of FDA approval for any of the retrieval systems means that experience will remain limited in the near future.

Recently the TrapEase filter was granted 510K approval based on claims of comparability to a marketed device (Figure 48–5). However, within a year, one-quarter of the adverse event reports received by the FDA regarding filters were of occlusion of the vena cava with this device, and in 4 cases, this resulted in death. This situation emphasizes the need for comprehensive evaluation of new IVC filters. Just because a device is not necessarily intended for permanent placement, it must still meet all of the standards for permanent implantation in addition to proving that it can be removed successfully. The burden of proof should include the short and long-term consequences of removal to demonstrate that retrieval has no long-term complications of its own. To demonstrate that a device can be removed implies that removal is the best management of the problem, that the period of DVT/PE risk has been appropriately calculated and that patients are no longer at risk.

CONCLUSIONS

The fate of retrievable filters will not be decided rapidly. Although the original concept of temporary filter placement was to minimize complications and risk, reported clinical experience indicates that the short-term complications are actually greater and the long-term consequences unknown. Many theoretical and practical issues must be resolved including indications, materials, cost/benefit, and utility. Just as permanent filters gained support as evidence of efficacy and safety accumulated over time, experience with these new devices needs to be gathered and evaluated, allowing evidence-based decisions to guide this new practice.

REFERENCES

1. Greenfield LJ, Proctor MC, Cho KJ, et al. Extended evaluation of the titanium Greenfield vena caval filter. *J Vasc Surg.* 1994;20:458–465.

2. Greenfield LJ, Proctor MC. Twenty-year clinical experience with the Greenfield filter. *Cardiovasc Surg.* 1995; 3(2):199–205.

3. Couch GG, Johnston KW, Ojha M. An in vitro comparison of the hemodynamics of two inferior vena cava filters. *J Vasc Surg.* 2000;31(3):539–549.

4. Neuerburg JM, Gunther RW, Vorwerk D, et al. Results of a multicenter study of the retrievable tulip vena cava filter: early clinical experience. *Cardiovasc Intervent Radiol.* 1997;20:10–16.

5. Millward SF, Bhargava A, Aquino J, et al. Gunther tulip filter: preliminary clinical experience with retrieval. *JVIR.* 2000;11(1):75–82.

6. Ponchon M, Goffette P, Hainaut P. Temporary vena caval filtration preliminary clinical experience with removable vena caval filters. *Acta Clin Belgica.* 1999;54(4):223–228.

7. Bovyn G, Gory P, Reynaud P, et al. The Tempofilter: a multicenter study of a new temporary caval filter implantable for up to six weeks. *Ann Vasc Surg.* 1997;11(5):520–528.

8. Rossi P, Arata FM, Bonaiuti P, et al. Fatal outcomes in atrial migration of the Tempofilter. *Cardiovasc Intervent Radiol.* 1999;22:227–231.

9. Linsenmaier U, Rieger J, Schenk F, et al. Indications, management and complications of temporary inferior vena cava filters. *Cardiovasc Intervent Radiol.* 1998;21(6):464–469.

10. Lorch H, Welger D, Wagner V, et al. Current practice of temporary vena cava filter insertion: a multicenter registry. *JVIR.* 2000; 11(1):83–88.

11. Lorch H, Zwaan M, Kulke C, et al. In vitro studies of temporary vena cava filters. *Cardiovasc Intervent Radiol.* 1998;21:146–150.

12. Pavcnik D, Uchida BT, Keller FS, et al. Retrievable IVC square stent filter: experimental study. *Cardiovasc Intervent Radiol.* 1999;22(3):239–245.

13. Stecker MS, Barnhart WH, Lang EV. Evaluation of a spiral nitinol temporary inferior vena caval filter. *Acad Radiol.* 2001;8(6):484–493.

14. Kuszyk BS, Venbrux AC, Samphilipo MA, et al. Subcutaneously tethered temporary filter: pathologic effects in swine. *JVIR.* 1995;6:895–902.

15. Hosaka J, Roy S, Kvernebo K, Enge I, et al. In vivo evaluation of the adjustable temporary venous Spring filter and the RF02 temporary filter. *Acad Radiol.* 1999;6:343–351.

Index